NUMBER 350

THE ENGLISH EXPERIENCE

ITS RECORD IN EARLY PRINTED BOOKS
PUBLISHED IN FACSIMILE

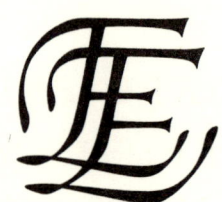

WILLYAM BULLEYN

BULLEINS BULWARKE
OF DEFECE AGAINSTE ALL SICKNES
SORNES AND WOUNDES

LONDON 1562

DA CAPO PRESS
THEATRVM ORBIS TERRARVM LTD.
AMSTERDAM 1971 NEW YORK

The publishers acknowledge their gratitude
to the Trustees of the British Museum
for their permission to reproduce
the Library's copy

(Shelfmark: 432.1.10)

S.T.C. No. 4033
Collation: ¶4, a-q6, r4, Aa-Hh6, Ii4; A-G6, H5.H6, I6, I-O6

Published in 1971 by
Theatrum Orbis Terrarum Ltd.,
O.Z. Voorburgwal 85, Amsterdam
&
Da Capo Press
- a division of Plenum Publishing Corporation -
227 West 17th Street, New York, 10011
Printed in the Netherlands
ISBN 90 221 0350 1

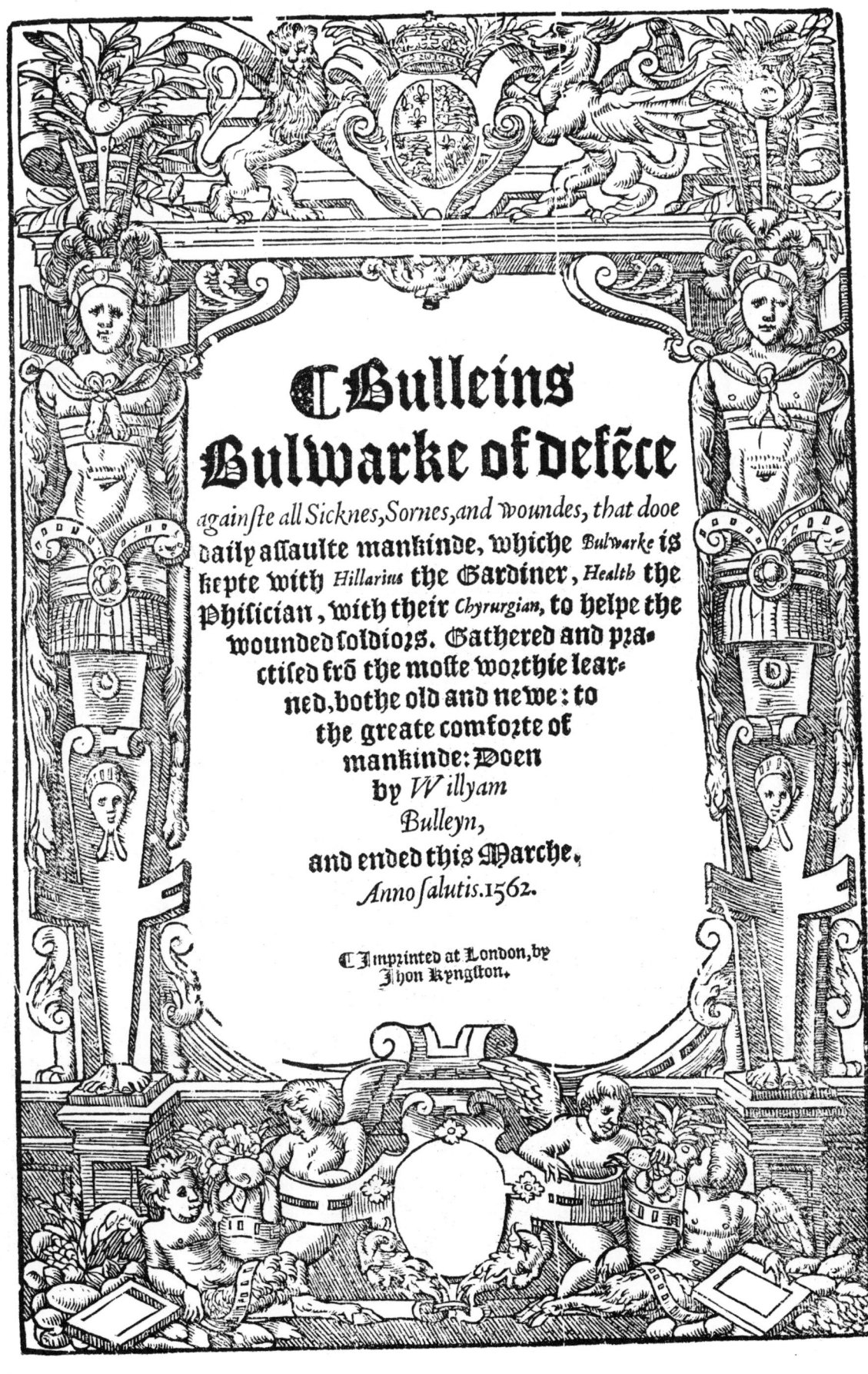

Bulleins
Bulwarke of defēce

againste all Sicknes, Sornes, and woundes, that dooe daily assaulte mankinde, whiche Bulwarke is kepte with Hillarius the Gardiner, Health the Phisician, with their Chyrurgian, to helpe the wounded soldiors. Gathered and practised frō the moste worthie learned, bothe old and newe: to the greate comforte of mankinde: Doen by *Willyam Bulleyn*, and ended this Marche. *Anno salutis*. 1562.

Imprinted at London, by Jhon Kyngston.

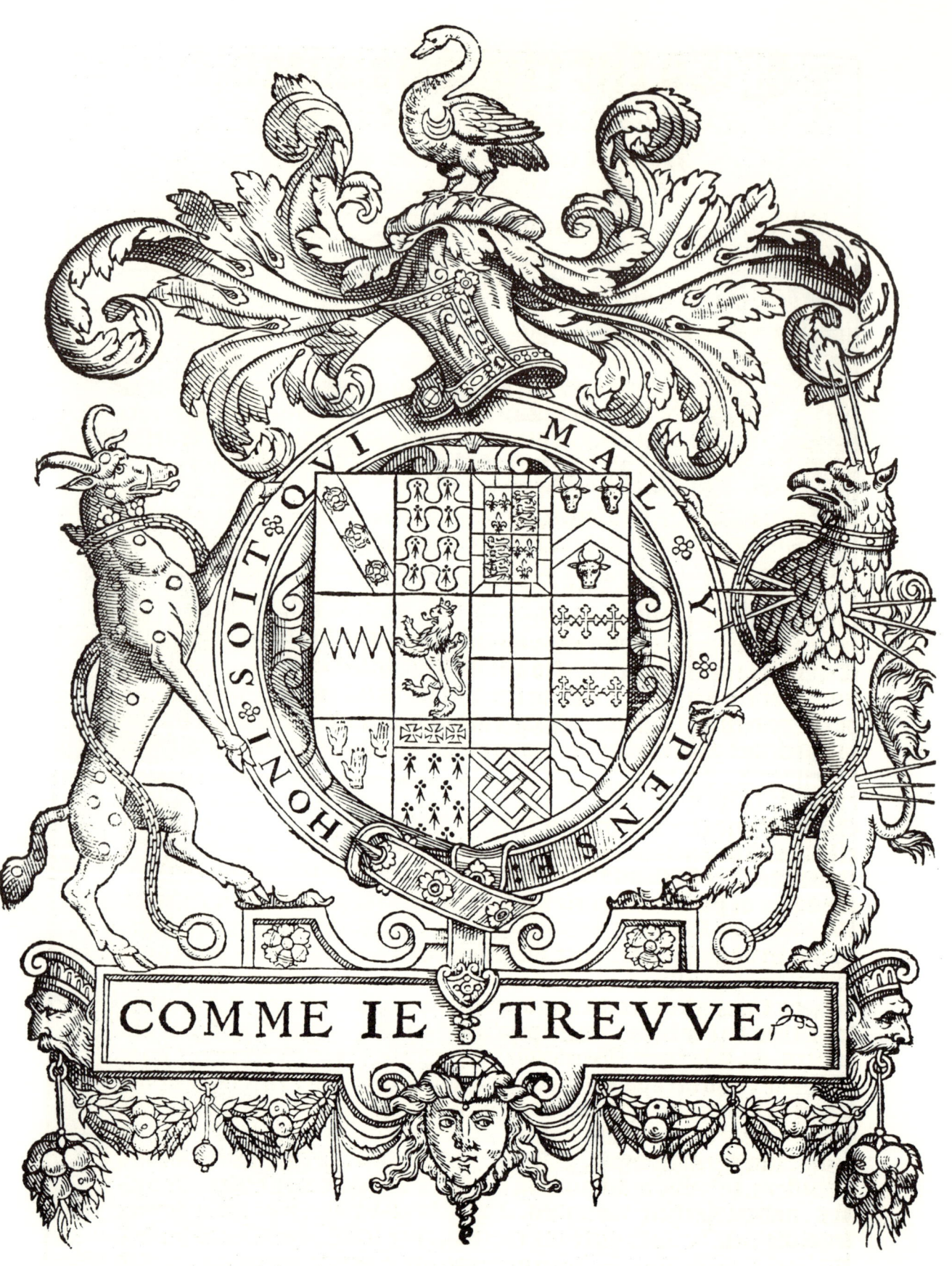

¶ To the right honorable

Lorde Henry Cary, Baron of Hunsdon, Knight of
the moste noble order of the Garter.
VVillyam Bulleyne witheth all
healthe, and perfect
felicitie in
Christe.

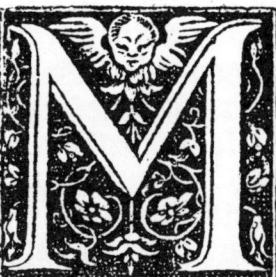Ankinde, whiche is called of the Philosopher, *Microcosmos, orbiculum,* or a little worlde, hauyng in it self, either miserie, felicitie, or a meane: although it be of the moste beautifull forme, and fairest in shape, excelling al other liuyng creatures vpon the yearth. And also is rightly indued with goodlie giftes of Nature, in whose braine is fixed, the iewell called Reason: the mother of Art and Science: by whom be wrought and inuented maruellous thinges, whereby our eternall God is perceiued, in vs his creatures. More aboundantly then in the high lightes moueable, and fixed in the firmament of heauen: whose naturall influences be knowen vnto mankinde. Euen so bee the vertues of euery creature here in yearth: as Beast, Foule, Fishe, Serpent Trees, Plantes, Fruictes, Flower, Herbe, Grasse, Gumme, Stone, and Metall. There is nothyng so secrete hidden, within the minerals of the yearth, or lurkyng so lowe vnder the floodes of the Sea: but by meanes and policie, thei are brought to vse. Their names, qualities, and natures, are knowen, vnto the wittie hedde of mankinde, to this ende, to helpe mankinde, in the tyme of his bodily infirmitie. These God hath ordained by his diuine prouidence, that euery creature sencible, and incensible, should serue his beste creature, mankinde. To this ende, that he should serue hym, in rightousnesse and holinesse, all *Luke.i,* the daies of his life, for these his giftes. And the Philosopher saieth, *in libro de cælo & mundo. Deus & Natura nihil frustra agunt.* GOD and Nature doeth nothyng in vaine, but are euer woorkyng and dooyng: he the principall cause, and thei his effecte. Yet for all these singuler vertues, giuen to manne, through the continuaunce of time, calamities of this worlde, woundes in the bodie, corrupcion of the Aire, aboundaunce of humours. &c. Thesame Mankinde dooe decaie, dye, and retourne vnto the duste, and become as though he had neuer been: although he bee neuer so honorable, yea or poore, death doeth make equalitie betwen them. Euery mannes course is appoincted, thei can not prolong their *Job. xiiii.* tyme: notwithstandyng, God hath ordained sonderie meanes, by his ministers, to helpe mankinde in the tyme of sicknes, to ease their paines, and heale their woundes. And I beyng a childe of the common wealthe, am bounde vnto my mother, that is, the lande, in whom I am borne: to pleasure it, with any good gift, that it hath pleased God

C.ii. to

The Epistle dedicatorie.

to bestowe vpon me, not to this ende, to instructe the learned, but to helpe the ignoraunt, that thei maie resort to this little *Bulwarke*, whiche I doe dedicate vnto your honourable Lordshippe. Where as thei shall not be onely defended in the same, from sicknes and woundes: but also beyng wounded, through cruell assaulters of this *Bulwarke*, or sicke, eftsones, here thei shall haue at hande, all maner of *Cordials*, and wholesome salues. Whereby thei shalbe the abler, to kepe this holde, against all bodily euils: whiche I dooe call Sorenes, and Sicknes, for whose sakes, I haue builded this little Fort, callyng it my *Bulwarke*. Not beyng able to builde any bigger woorke of defence, against sickenes, or euill diate: as that manne of worthie memorie, Sir Thomas Eliot knight did, when he builded his *Castle of Health*, a booke verie profitable. Would God, that all menne of worshippe in their calling, were the like disposed to their countrey, as he was: and many moe, whose names I dooe commende vnto the reader, within this little *Bulwarke*. And although there will be many parauenture, bothe malicious, spitefull, and cankered of mynde: that bothe with slaunder and disdaine, will laie their Batrie, against this Forte, I shall be able euer to repulse thē, through your good Lordshippes good aide. For I haue builded it verie lowe, wantyng neither the strength of ordinaunce, prouision of victualles, and the pollicie of the moste worthie Capitaines, and good Souldidiours: as *Hyppocrates, Galen, Dioscorides &c.* Now finally, I shall moste humbly desire your good lordship, to take this simple boke, in an argumēt of my good zeale and loue, that I bare vnto you, for your goodnes toward me. For if I were otherwise able, to gratifie your honor, accordyng to my bound duetie: I would not leaue it vndoen, as knoweth God, who euer giue your Lordship, continuaunce of honour, and prosperous healthe. From London. Marche, 1562.

Your Lordshippes euer to commaunde.

Willyam Bulleyn.

To the good reader
VVillyam Bulleyn sendeth
Salutacion.

For as moche good reader, as fower yeres last past, I promised (in a boke of myne, called the *Gouernment of Health*, whiche I dedicated to a knight of great worshippe in the North, called sir Thomas, the Baron of Hilton) to sette forthe an other booke of healthfull medicenes. Euen so, by the space of one yere nexte after thesame, I trauailed to performe my promes made, and so finished my copie: which copie did perishe in Shipwracke, and so my labour was loste. And not onely my labour, but also my life, by sondrie malicious and deuilishe inuencions, by, and through one William Hilton: in nature, brother to the forsaied Baron of Hilton, but in condicions, nothyng at all, for he wanted his gentlenes, and good nature. Now, after God had deliuered me, from the great perill of this manne, that is to saie: conspiryng of my giltles death, and hurtles life, towardes him and his. Eftsones this man attempted an other newe despleasure, against me for debte: colouring his malice, by a pretence of lawe. By whiche accion, finally I was imprisoned, my thought a longe tyme (for there are but fewe gestes, that haue pleasure in soche Innes.) And beyng in this prison, me thought I had not onely conuenient tyme, but also a quiete conscience: to trauell, in renuyng my late booke, or loste copie, whiche in deede, I am not able to finishe. Beyng preuented with so many troubles, and lettes of my saied enemie, whose doynges at large, I commit to silence. Least I should seme to write, a storie or Tradige, or els a discripcion of his folie, in the place of Phisicke: no lesse also can I, but declare some cause of my lette, and why my booke came not foorthe or this tyme, where as I promised. But blame me not, good reader, although I put hym in my booke, which would haue put me from this life. And this booke, whiche I haue doen, gentle reader, take it in good parte, I praie you, for that is my desire.

First, I haue made you a booke of Simples, as herbes, fruites. &c. For I had no small pleasure, in the natures of theim, beyng moued of the Heathen men, so to doe: whose names doe, and euer shall remain: emong soche as reade of Simples. *Galen* commedeth vnto vs, the loue and cunnyng that *Orphius Museus, Hesiodus Homerus*, and *Rufus Ephesus*, had in herbes. Who can forget *Lysimacus*, a worthie noble capitaine to Alexander, whiche, when he was wounded verie deepe, founde an herbe, whiche healed hym & called thesame herbe, by his owne name: *Atemisea* a noble Quene called Mugworte, after her owne name. *Helena* founde first the bertue of *Enulacampana*. Gentian, was named by kyng *Gentian of Ilyrica*, with many mo noble men and women, whiche delited in the flowers, and frutes

To the Reader.

tes of the grounde, many of them you shall finde in the Simples. I cā not forget Attalus, the king of the lesse Asia. And Euax a king of Arabi, which writte good bookes, to Nero the Emperour: with many good workes of Compoundes. Emong all, Dioscorides a noble knight of Egipte, whiche serued Anthonius and Cleopatra, like a worthie Souldiour in the fielde: and excelled all other, in the noble knowlege of herbes. &c. Let vs not forget, the passyng wisedome of Salomon, whiche had knowlege moste excellent, in naturall Philosophie, aswell as Morall: and taught the Quene of Saba all the vertues of herbes. How worthie were Archalaus, Capadocia, and Agamemnon Argiuorum, whiche were noble kinges, yet wer thei Heathen, sauyng Salomon. Whose chief delites, wer not in Bacchus banketes, or Venus game: but spent their time pleasauntly, in the swete fieldes emong fruites, flowers, and Spices of delite. Would God in soche vertues, the Christians, wer their equalles. When you haue redde the Simples folowyng, then approcheth the Chirurgyan, Plaster, and Salue prepared readie, to make whole the wounded man. Hyppocrates, Galen, and Auicen to finishe his cunnyng cure. Then cometh the Apothicarie, Nicholaus, with riche Cordialles, Pilles, Electuarys, and Purgacions of eche kinde, with his maister the Phisician. Whiche doe dispense euery medicen in tyme place, quantitie, and good order, to his paciente with good diate, trauell, slepe: and finally, the perturbacions of the minde. At which place good reader, I should haue declared of other Judgementes, as Pulse, Urine. And the proper cures of euery Feuer, afflictyng of the bodie: whiche hereafter, by Goddes grace, I shall bryng to passe, if tyme will suffre me to liue. And vntill soche tyme, moste gentle reader, take this in good parte, from the handes of hym, whiche thinke it well bestowed vpon you, if curteslie you doe receiue the same againe. Thus fare ye well. Yours euer to his power.

Willyam Bulleyn.

⁋ Soche faultes as be committed, shall shortly be reformed in this booke.

¶ The Aucthours,
Capitaines, and Souldiours of this
Bulwarke.

Moyses.
Dauid.
Salomon.
Esdras.
IESVS Chrystus.
Lucas Euangel.
Paulus Apost.
Hyppocrates.
Galenus.
Lycimacus rex Macedo.
Auicen.
Dioscorides.
Auaroyes.
Rasis.
Ruellus.
Isaac.
Theophrastus.
Fulgentius.
Mesuæ.
Paulus Aegineta.
Arnoldus de noua Comen.
Pandect.
Leonardus Futchius.

Conradus Gesnerus.
Petrus Andrias Matthiolus.
Leonellus Fauentinus.
Iulianus Moristica.
Nicolaus Prep.
Nicolaus Myrepsi.
Ioh. Placatomus.
Ioh. Tagaultius.
Iacobus Hollerus.
Marianus.
Plato de Legibus.
Exenophon.
Pompeus Mela.
A. Gellius.
Strabo.
C. Plinius Secundus.
Persius.
Textor. offic.
Ouid.
Virgil.

xliij. in nomber.

THE BOOKE OF SIMPLES.

Fol.j.

Marcellus.

Frste of all,my frende *Hillarius*, bicause I haue no small grief in my breast:I shall desire you,to shew me the nature of an herbe called *Asaron*,which I trust will help me by the waie of vomitte.

Azarabaccha or wild Nardus.

Hillarius.

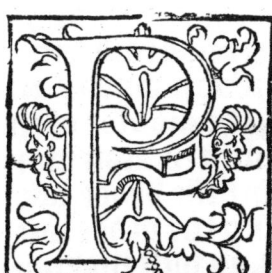

Linius remembring this herbe *lib.xj.cap.xiij.* and *lib.21.cap.6.* emõg al other flowers or herbes saith he:it is vtterly refused,& not worthy to be preferred,emong pleasaunt garlandes,or swete nosegaies,bicause of the basenesse, and bitternesse of his nature. In forme saith he,it is not vnlike vnto Iuie leaues:notwithstanding it is rounder,softer,and broder,it is moch like vnto *Vngula*,called foles foote. *Dioscarides* with whõ none haue euer been comperable hetherunto, for the excellent inuencion,and knowlege of herbes,*lib.i.cap.ix.* saieth the leaues be of the foresaid forme. And is so hote,that it doeth behemently bite the tong,but in vertue it prouoketh brine, helpeth the dropsie, and painfull ache of the huckle bone, called *Sciatica*. Vi. dragmes of the rotes of *Asaron*, sodde in swete water, drinke thesame water, and then it will drawe forthe the termes in women.*Galen lib.vi.simpli.medi.* speaking of the rootes of *Asari* saith thei bee like to *Acorus*, but that is maruellous,it should so bee:for *Acorus* will not prouoke strong vomites, as *Asaron* wil. Therefore *Dioscorides* haue saied the truthe, and *Mesue* saith,that *Asaron* haue the vertue of *Elleborus*,to purge bothe vp and doune, Choller and fleume, whiche *Acorus* can not doe so:it is hot and drie in the third degree. In Latin it is called *Vulgago*, prouoke brin,clense the matrix,helpeth the liuer from al grief, raines stomack,belly & splen.&c.in the laude therof,hauyng these vertues as I haue said frõ *Dioscorides* & *Mesue*,*Marcus Æmileus* affirmeth thesame,saiyng:

Azarabaccha is broader in Italie,then here in Englande.

Azaron prouoketh termes,and helpeth Sciatica

Azaron doe help the liuer and stomacke

Est Asaron Græcè vulgago dicta Latinè,
Hæc calidæ & siccæ virtutis dicitur esse
Tertius est illi gradus,vt dicunt in vtroq̨,
Prouocat vrinam potaq̨, menstrua purgat
Hocq̨ modo iecoris medicatur sumpta dolorj:

Here haue three notable learned men,declared the vertue of *Asaron*. Furdermore, if the iuce of sixe leaues, bee strained with a pinte of whaie, specially of Goates milke, and drinke it in the mornyng. This drinke in Sommer,will caste forthe yellowe choller,and vnnaturall fleume. For in Sõmer vomentes ought to be taken,to clense the vpper parts, as the lower members be purged,by electuary in winter. Furdermore xxx.grene leaues steped in newe wine al the night,and strained in the mornyng:drinke this against all the aboundaunce of humours in the breaste, or precordiall partes,in this maner. Powre this wine into a close potte,with a pece of fatte Porke,and seeth thesame:then let the

Asaron in Grece, Vulgago in Latine, hote and drie in the.iii. degree, prouoke brine, and purge termes mestrual and taketh awaie the paines of y̨ liuer.

xxx.leaues do serue in infusion but other waies three, fower,or fiue doe suffice.

a.i. wine

paciente eate of the Porke, and then drinke the wine, or els the wine maie be drunke after the Porke, simplie deluted or steped all the night with the leaues, and neuer to bee sodden with the Porke. This will helpe the Jaudes, & if it be drunke of any bodie, which haue a tercian being first digested: and specially not on the sicke daie, it will clene deliuer frō the said tercian, in the beginninges of *Hydrops*, timpanies, quotidiās, grene sicknes, and quartens, wormes, swelling in the stomack there is no better remedie, then to drinke this, as in the maner aforesaid: For a weake frantike brain, commyng of an extreme cold, when melancholie is placed in the mancion of reason, through whiche, the principall sences be obscured and darkened. Shaue the moulde of the hedde, and wache the same with wine, wherin Calamintes, Rosemary *Lignum Aloes*, and *Asaron* haue been sodden, and then anoint the hedde with the oiles of Males, Mintes, and *Asaron* warme, purging the hedde with pilles of *Hiara simplex*, and to abstain from soche meates, as will ingender melancholie, or make exalacion, or smoke vp into the braine. The iuce of *Asaron* tempered with *Nil.* called Misseltow, and strained with a little Rosewater, will clense the darke sight of the iyen, and make thē clere. And thus I doe ende of herbe *Asaron*, whiche haue vertue against choller: would God it had the like effect, to clense disdaine, rankor and malice, so that grace, that most precious herbe, might be replanted again in eche mans breast, which the deuill haue supplanted through pride.

Asaron good againste Dropsie, Feuers, & frāsy.

The Arabians calle that Nill, whiche wee name Viscum or Missltowe, Lib. primo Paradox. Cap. xxvi.

Marcellus.

What is *Asplenon*, called *Scolopendrion*, or *Citrache*, and *Hemyonitis* leaued like Dragon and *Phyllitis*, called Hartes tongue good for?

Hillarius.

This herbe *Asplenon*, no herbe maie be compared therewith, for his singuler vertue, to helpe the sicknes, or grief of the Splene, the place of melancholie. It is called *Scolopendrion*, of a speckled worme with many fete. This herbe is a small Ferne, growing emong stones, neither hauing stalke, flower, or sede: the leaues be yellowe by neath, and greene aboue. There is an other herbe of the same vertue, for the splen called *Hemionitis*, whose leaues be moche like Dragong, with many small rotes: these said herbes dieth not, and be hot in the first, and drie in the second degree. Goodly sirups are made of thē for the splene, thet be very good in decoccion for the same: if one doce drinke of this herbe sodden in Wineger, by the space of. 40. daies, then it haue vertue to cōsume ỹ splen: this herbe haue vertue to help the Jaundes, stone, strangurie, hicket, or winde, & *Capper* barkes, *Tamarice* rotes, *Scolopendrion*, & *Scilla* sodē by art together, wil help the splen. Ther is an herbe called *Phyllitis*, or Hartes tong, growing in darke places, whiche is partly of ỹ nature of ỹ said herbes, which haue singuler vertu, bothe for man & beast, to be drunke against poison: and bloodie flixes, or flowing of termes immoderat in womē. But many now adaies, haue soche passiōs of the splen Cancred with melancholie, corrupted with disdain, & with goldē wordes, louing onely from the splen, and not frō the hart, and giueth eche

Asplenon good for the Splene.

Hemyonitis leaued like Dragon.

Diosco. lib. 3. Copi. 134.

Galen lib. 5. Sim. medica. Capi. xii.

The splenaticke loue.

other

The boke of Simples. Fol. ij.

other the curtisie of the tongue, without the consent of the hart, and thus I cōclude of Hartles tongue, & Harts tongue, the one of comfort the other of decay. *Lingua fallax non amat veritatem, & os lubricum operatur ruinas.* — *Prouer. 27. d.*

Marcellus.

What is the vertue of wormewodde? that bitter herbe called *Absinthium*.

Hilarius.

Absinthium is a comen herbe, it is of diuers kindes, as *Ponticum*, and *Romanum*. &c. it is hotte in the first, and drie in the seconde, and it is very bitter, and beyng dried, kepeth clothes from wormes and mothes, and the Sirups therof eaten before wine, preserueth men frō dronkenesse, if it be sodden in vyneger, it wil helpe the sores ȳ bredes in ȳ eares, being layd warme vpon it, it is to be dronke against swelling of ȳ stomacke. And *Ophthalmia* which is a sicknes of the eye, is greatly helped with wormewod, if it be stamped & made luke warme with Rose water, and put into a cleane walnut shel, the sirup healeth the bluddy fluxe bounde to the belly, it doth helpe a colde stomacke, if it be dronke. v. daies, euery morning twoo sponefull of the sirup, it is also good against the dropsie. And thus saith *Auicen*, Figges Cockle, Wormwod, and Niter stamped together, and made in a plaster, is good against the disease of the Splene, and also killeth wormes in the belly, vsed in the foresaid maner, one dram of the pouder may be dronke at once in wine, it hath many goodly vertue, as the wine therof beynge dronke agaynst dropsies, coldnes of the stomacke, winde, swellinges, as if a handefull be sodden in. viii. pounde of cleane water or wine, in a vessel of siluer, glasse or stone, putting in swete Calamus, Cinamom the flowers of Cassia, Suinance, Spikenarde & Dates of eche. ʒ. iiii. beaten all together and sodden, as is aforesaied, or els these thinges put in a vessell of new wine with a linnen bagge, and so kepte close ii. monthes, and afterwarde dronke of them that haue either the yelow Jaunders, paynes in the raines, lothesomnes of the stomacke, stoppyng of termes, swellyng after meate, continuance of vomites, colde passions of the hart. &c. this vertue hath wormewod wine saith *Dioscorides, libro quin. Cap. 40.* Furthermore gather a. li. of wormwod leaues, & stampe it in a morter of stone, and then put vnto the same. li. iiii. of the best white sugar, and so beate them together vntil they be come to one substaunce, kepe this in a close potte or glasse. And this is the vertue therof, saieth that well learned mā *Mathiolus*, it helpeth the dropsie, if ȳ pacient eate euery day of this half an ounce. iii. houres before meate, and this I haue knowen many helpte saith he, and as for the vertu of the syrup of wormewod, it shal come in his place accordingly

Marcellus.

What is the vertue of Anisseede?

Hilarius.

It is muche lyke vnto Fenell seede, and is called Roman Fenell, it is warme and sweete, and hotte in the seconde, and drie in the thirde degree, the new seedes be best, it engendreth vital seede, it

Marginalia: Wormewod. — Sore eares. — For the eyes — Bluddi flux. — Colde stomackes. — Dropsies. — *Auicen, lib. 2.* — *Simp. 2.* — For the splē. — Wormewode hath many vertues. — A goodli medicen for Hydro. — *Galen de sim.* — Openeth the raines.

a.ii. openeth

The booke of Simples.

openeth the stoppyng of the raynes and Matrix, beynge dronke with Ptisantes or cleane temperate wine, this herbe or seede is comfortable in sweet compounded medicines or pouder for shortnesse of breth, and sorenesse of the lunges, and also is good to be sodden in Ptisātes, made of Barlie, to be dronke in the feuer Quotidian bredde of fleume, it ingendereth Milke in the breastes dronke with sweet wine or milke prouoketh vrine, maketh sweete breath, and is good against the Collike or winde of the great guttes, being dronke with good white wine and Sugar, and also stoppeth the whites which runneth oftentimes from the bodies of women, the pouder thereof, with the pouders of Fenell, Gallinga, Spicknarde, Thamoris, Nutmegges, and graines of Parradice, called Cardamon, tempered with wheate flower, water and red wine, and so baken in manchedes or cakes, bee moste holsome to be eaten of them which haue the runyng of the raynes, wastyng of nature, moyst dropsies, or in them in whome the humour of fleume dothe greatly abounde, through homidite, winde or colde, & this was proued to helpe a Lady whiche was sicke of a Tinpanie, and was syr Thomas the Barrone Hiltons wife, within the Bisshopbrike of Durisme, whiche vsed this breade duryng one halfe yere, and also ones a moneth was purged with holsome Electuariis accordyng, and bloud letting, and thus I conclude of Anisede, the beast cometh from Egipt.

A good remedie for the runyng of the raines.

Marcellus.

What is the vertue of Mouse eare, which is lyke the eare of a Mouse and full of heere, in forme muche like the eare of a Mouse.

Hilarius.

AN herbe commonly knowen, colde and moyst in the first degree, as *Galen* saith, a decoction of this herbe sodden in water with sugar, is good against the fallynge sicknes, beynge oftentimes dronke and put a leafe therof into the nose, it will prouoke sternutacion or neesyng, whiche wonderfully doeth clense the baines, and sodden in white Wine, Pthisane or Burrage water, with Sugar candy, this is good against paines in the throate, *Angina*, as, *Dioscorides* writeth but littell of this herbe. And *Galen* saith, in the .vii. lib. of Simples, þ it is drie in the seconde degree, and it groweth in Maye vpon Hilles, Medowes, and way sides, saith *Mathiolus* vpon *Dioscorides*. Futhermore if it be stamped with Madder and the great Plantin rootes, & an herbe called the Sheperdes purse, and so sodden in redde wine and strayned out, and so puttyng a littell drinke warme, this is also good against the blouddy fluxe, or a broken vayne within the body of one, whiche haue fallen into some depe place, and this was proued of a yong man dwellyng in new Castell, whiche fell into a deepe coale pit, whose vtward woundes were healed by an auncient practisour called Mighel a Frencheman, whiche also is cunnynge to helpe his owne countrey disease, that now is to commonly knowen here in Englande, the more to be lamented: But yet dayly increased, whereof I entende to speake

Falling sicknesse.

Nesyng.

Mousheere helpeth the throte.

Against the bloudie flixe.

Michell the Chyrurgian of Newcastle

The booke of Simples. Fol.iij.

speake in the place of the Pore.
Marcellus.
What is the vertue of Garlyke?
Hilarius.

GArlyke is very hot and drie in the fourthe degree, it troubles the stomacke of Cholorike men, it is hurtfull to the eyes and head, it increaseth drines, but it will prouoke vrine, and is good to be layd vpon the bityng of a Snake, or Adder, it is good for the Emeroides, applied to the sore place beyng first stampte, if it be sodden, the stinke therof is taken from it, but the vertue remaineth to be eaten againſt the coughes and paine in the lunges, it cutteth and consumeth corrupt flume, and bringeth sleape, it is not good for hotte men, and women with children, or nurses geuyng mylke to children: but *Galen* calleth it the common peoples Treakell. If Sanguine men do eate much of it, it will make them to haue redde faces, but it is a speciall remedy agaynſt Poyson, and a hot plaster applied to the bityng of a madde Dogge, made of Garlyke helpeth it: if it be dronke killeth wormes in the belly. And Garlike stamped with Mastike, and put into the mouth dothe aſwage dolour of the teeth. Garlike dried or burnt into pouder, and tempered with Hony and Beares greace, is good to anoynt a baulde head to recouer heere: and all this and more reporteth *Dioscorides*, which excelled in herbes. *Plinius* reporteth if it be stamped and made in a Gargarismi, it healeth *Angine*, it helpeth the throate, with Oyle of Quinces and so warme applied to the belly is good againſt the Collicke and the bluddy fluxe. New Ale and Garlyke, killeth wormes to be dronke: it is good to be eaten agaynſt the fallyng euell. And Garlyke healeth Fistulaes tempered with Pitche Brimstone and Rosen, made hotte in a tente. With such like vertue as *Plinius, Ætius, Galen. &c.* reporteth: but it is a groase kinde of medicine, verie vnpleasant for fayre Ladies, & tender Lylly Rose colloured damsels, which often time profereth sweet breathes before gentle wordes but both would do very well.

Garlike.

Prouoketh vrine.
Bityng of a Snake.
Hemerodes.

Coughes.

Corrupte flume.

Againſt poysone.

For tothache

To increase heare.

A medicene for the Scull

Marcellus.
What is the vertue of Hony? the fruites of Bees labour and their Sommers trauell.
Hilarius.

AVEROYS saith, Hony is hotte and drie in the seconde degree, and doth clense very much, and is a medicinable meate, most chiefly for olde men and women, for it doth warme them and conuerte in them good bloud. It is not good for Chollerike persons, because of the heate and drines: they do greatly erre that say Hony is hot and moyſt, but if it be clarified from his waxe and drosse, and kepte in a close vessel, theris nothyng likquid vpon the earth that
a.iij. remayneth

Auerois in.5.
Simeon Sethi
It for chollerike persones
Honie is an heauely dew.
Auicen in.ii. can.cap.504.

The booke of Simples.

remaineth lenger. And this precious iewel Hony hath euer ben more praised, for it will conserue and kepe any fruite, herbe or roote, or any other thyng that is put into it, an exceading longe time. *Plinius* writeth of a Monster which was long kept in Hony in *Clauious* daies. Meruelous is the worke of God, Hony beyng an heauenly dewe that falleth vpon flowers and leaues as *Auicen* saieth, and is neither iuce of leaues nor fruites, but only the heauenly dewe, wherunto the Bees in sommer in dew time gather the saied Hony, and lay it vp in store, in theyr curious houses builded, wheras they dwell together in most goodly order. O Bees, Bees, how happier are you then many wretched men, which dwell neuer together in vnitie and peace, but in continuall discorde and quietnes, as Virgell saith: *En quo disiosdia ciues produxerit miseros.* Beholde whither discorde hath brought wretched Citizens. But now to speake of the most excellent vertues of Hony, it is good in the meates of them whiche be flugmatike. Hony newly taken out of the Comes is partly laxatiue, & clarified Hony doth binde and drie vp flume, and kepe the bodies of flugmatike and old persons from corruption. The best Hony is gathered in the spryng time, the second in Sommer but that which is gathered in winter is ill and hurtefull. One parte of Hony, and some parte of water sodden together vntill the frothe be all scommed of, and when it is colde, kepe it in a cloase stone pot, this drinke (saieth *Galen*) is holsome for Sommer, it clenseth the Lunges, & preserueth the body in health, *Oximel simplex,* and *Compositum*, be made with Hony: and so be many mo thynges, whiche be made of great bertue. Also the aucthour of the *Pandect*, saith Hony poured into a new wounde eftesones is clensed and made whole. Hony mingled with a littell Salte, and warme poured into the eare, killeth wormes that bredeth there: the same also killeth Lice, if childrens heads be anoynted therwith. Rub younge childernes gommes with cleane Hony euery daye and it will easely cause their teeth to growe. Hony mingled with oyle of Roses, and so dronke incontinently, will cause one to bomit whan they haue eaten any benom thinge, as rotten Mouthrimpes, called Fungas. &c. Also *Gargarismus* and *Suppositus* be made of Hony, the one doeth clense the throate, and the other doth relaxe the belly. There is an infection in the skinne, through the corrupcion of the lyuer, whiche is called *Serpigo*, oftentimes in the paulme of the hand, chiefly in the right hande specially in Cholerike persons, whiche is helped with Hony mingled with Coste, and anointed warme euery day twoo times. Also the distelled water of Hony hath vertue to make cleane the skinne of them whose faces be vncleane: but moste chiefly if it be stilled with stronge Vineger, Mylke, and the Vrine of a boye, & so with a spunge washe the face to bedwarde, and let it drie in of it selfe. The goodly oyntment called the *Vnguentum Egiptiacum*, whiche clenseth all corrupt humores, and woundes beyng rotten within, the chief thing in this oyntment is Hony, it is meruelous that they which vse to eat Hony daily, & daily anoint their stomackes with oyle of wormewod, should either dis

The booke of Simples. Fol. iiij.

die sodenly, or liue paynefully, or be euell colloured in their faces. The people of Walles doe vse to drinke Mede and Metheglyne, and vnder heauen there is no fayrer people of complexion, nor cleaner of nature. Anointe the head beyng new shauen with Beares greace and Honie mingled together, preserueth the heere from fallyng. Hony of Roses is a goodly Medicine, outwardly in woundes, and inwardly clenseth flume, mundifieth the stomacke, and openeth the mouthe of the vaynes, and also is good to put in the eies to clense them.

welchemens drinke.

To encrease Heare.

Marcellus.

I Did neuer here any thing so greatly commended as thou hasse commended Hony: if it be true that thou hast spoken, there be but fewe thinges maye be compared to it, for the excellent vertue of it.

Hilarius.

BE not in doubt of the truth therof, for the best Aucthours haue taught me, and dayly experience moueth me, thus muche to reporte of Hony, I ought to thinke no shame therof. In asmuche as the God of heauen and earth, maker of all creatures, did geue his people of Israel no greater blessyng then a lande which did flow with Milke and Hony. And often times amongest the blessinges of God, sweet Hony is rehersed. The Prophet Dauid in the Psalmes, do ofte name Hony, and the Hony combe, making a comparison betwene it and the worde of God. In some of the holy Sacrifices, Hony was brought in for an offerynge, before the Lorde God into his holy Temple, the strong Nazareth of God Judge of Israell: that mightie prince Samson, loued wel Hony as appeareth after he had slaine the Lyon, he did eate the Hony which he founde in his carcase, so did his father and his mother of the same Hony, it was a deuine omen of the wisedome and learnyng that afterwarde came vnto Plato, when in his Cradell, Bees brought Hony vnto his mouthe. who was greater amonge men then S. Iohn Baptist, what was his most foode: it was wilde Hony. How many plesant verses hath Virgill written vpon Bees and Hony, who euer did excel *Plinius secundus,* in the nature of Creatures, and as it playnly appereth in his. xi. booke, declaryng of a worthy man called *Aristomachum,* which so wonderfully loued Bees, that he did nothynge, but onely by the space of. lxiii. yeares obserue the natures and properties of Bees, and in the same booke saith he, the bees haue many Kinges with smal Coronets on their heads about whom the great agmen or swarme do cluster and fleeth into the fieldes, and cometh home in order, bringinge their treasure with them: the elder Bees do builde with in ye Hiues, hauyng therin a Mistres or Queene to set them to worke, which neuer go fro home, but place euery thyng in order, the younger do bring their stuffe to Hiue, non of them be idel euery one of them haue a house to dwell. vi. cornered in fashion, they will suffer no filthinesse to be amongest them, nor straungers to dwell

Exodus.

Psalmes.

Iudic. 14.

Plini. lib. 11. cap. 9.

Xenophon, in his booke of Houshold.

The propertee of a good huswyfe.

I. iiii. with

The booke of Simples.

Bees maintain no strangers, for they bee not profitable.

within their Citie or common wealth. They also punish them with stinging, that hurt their Princes, and thei haue prouidence of wether when it is faire and foule. Also they haue seces of smellyng, for if any of them be loste in the fielde, they folow their felowes by the sweete ayre, they be scant perfit of hearyng, but yet as appereth they heare, when thei doo muster at the soundes of Basens: their greatest delight is in Tyme and Balme, and therfore about Athens is the best Hony

Plinii.lib.xi. Capi.xii.

in the worlde, as *Plini* saith, and in the Islande called *Calydne*, and also in *Meleta*, would God saith he that we had ye Honi in the same nature that it falleth from the heauens. Yea rather would to God that idle people would take Bees for an example to labour, and subiectes to obay. &c. What shall I speake more of the properties of Bees, and of their good natures, prouidence and cunning, nothing els *Marcellus*? but these simple verses folowyng.

The kyng of Bees and his armie.

A Noble Prince there is, vvhose vvelth and vvorke excell,
More then all other earthly vvightes, that in the vvorld do dvvell,
Saturne blacke and colde, hath taught him for to flie
The hory Frostes and snovves vvhite, and darknes of the skie.
Sagittarius and Pisses lorde, Iouis called by name,
Doth cunnyng geue vnto this prince, hovv he his house should frame.
The red flamyng bloudy Marce, the Lorde of vvarre and strife,
Doth teache this kyng his host to traine, vvith sharpe dartes all their life,
O happie Sol vvith golden beames, vvhose glorie doth excell,
Thou arte the candell of this vvorlde, and darknes doth expell.
Thou makest glad this littell kyng, in fielde vvhen he doth ride,
No horse he hath but vvynges to flie, thou only art his guide.
VVhen he doth sounde his vvarlike tune, in Hiue vvhere he doth dvvell,
His souldiers muster all of heapes, the starres they do excell.
In numbre infinite most faire, the cleare aier do them infuse,
Dame Flora svvete do them reioyse, but Boreas them misuse.
VVith grisly stormes and Hayle harde, he breakes their tender bones,
No helmets haue, nor shieldes they beare, to kepe them from harde stones,
vvhan stormes be past and Venus come, the banisher of colde shovvers,
vvith pretie hornes, and tender vvinges, thei playe among the flovvers.
The Beane flovvers make them glad, the Lilly make them gaye,
Their chief delight is Time and Balme, most glad they are of May.
For Marcurie do geue them mirthe, vvhen Gemeny doth embrace,
From risyng sunne to Titans fall, labour is all their grace.
In flovvred Fieldes and Motley meades, vvhere vvhit doe grovve in grene,
The heauenly devves, that in night dovvne fall, is gathered vp of Beene.
Ioue doth reyne from virgelij this precious heauenly gyfte,
vvhom Bees doe knovv, and to Hiue doe beare, vvith vvinges fliyng svvift.
And then they make this goodly meate, Manna fallen from heuen.
The singes, xii. vvith Bees do vvorke, so do the Planets seuen.

Marcellus.

The boke of Simples.

Now you haue well declared what Hony is, is ther any vertue in the Combes or Ware.

Hillarius.

GALEN saieth, in the .vi. booke of Simples, Ware is good for plasters, not only in drying, but also peraccidense, it moisteth, and is vsed for outwarde Medicines, but not for inwarde medicines: but *Dioscorides* reporteth that Ware doeth mollifie and warme the body, and .x. graines waight droken with the syrup of Planten is good for the blouddy fluxe, it also drieth the Mylke in womens breastes, and to conclude there be but few Emplasters that can be without the helpe of Wax. It hath also been abused in churches, chaples and temples offered by the ignorant, before the blinde.

Dioscorides libr secundo. capi.lxxvii.

Mercellus.

I do know Sage by name, because it doth grow in my garden and is vsed in my kitchin, but Christ doth know, the vertu therof is hidden fro me.

Hillarius.

This noble herbe called *Eleliss bacon*, *Saltuia*, or Sage, as it shoulde appeare by *Theophrastus* there bee twoo kindes of Sage, the one of the garden whiche is roughe, longe and broade leaues, whiche sayth *Mathiolus*, I suppose to be the female herbe, the other Sage which is shorter, narower, with twoo small eares in the beginnyng of their leaues, whiche the sayd *Theophrastus* cal *Sphacelo*, whom *Mathiolus* clepeth the male herbe, and of this groweth greate plenty in Italy, in the toppes of Mountaines, in the noble countries bothe of *Apulie*, and *Calabrie*, so dooe there almoste in euerye Garden in Englande. This herbe is hot and drie saieth *Aetius*, so saieth *Galen*, and some notable practisioners do say, that perfume of Sage doeth stop the inmoderate flux menstrual *Agrippa* did call this the holy herbe, because it was so good to women, not only inexpulsynge euell matter from the Matrix: but also in reteinyng the vitall seede of generation whereby consepcion is made perfect. If a woman drinke the iuce therof with a littell Salte and Suger sodden together, foure daies before, and after, the vse with her husbande, geuyng the man the like quantite, before the time of procreation, without doubt consepcion foloweth. It is saied, sometime there was so great a pestilence in a Citie of Egypt, that through the poyson therof few were lefte a liue, but when the Plage was seased, the younge women were compelled to drynke the wine, or iuce of Sage, through whose vertue they were conceaued with children, hauyng the helpe of man, that in the ende, the Citee was replenished againe, and filled with people of their owne generacion. Sage saieth *Orpheus* .z.iiii. mingled with cleane clarified Hony, & eaten of an emptie stomacke, dothe incontinently stop the bloud that cometh from the breast, stomacke, or lunges, breaking out of the mouth

Sage. Libr.vi.cap. ii.de Plan. Liber.iii. Dioscorides.

Libr.6.simp.

The iuce of Sage helpeth consepcion.

To stoppe bloud runnyng at the mouthe.

with

The booke of Simples.

with cruent vomites. There is a sicknes with in the body, called Tabes, which is a great corruption of humours, through foule matter & bloud mingled together, whose beginnyng comes from the headde through a continuall rume, and doth Apostumate and wounde the Lunges, through whose putrifaction by littell, and by littell, all the membres of the body consumeth, through drinesse, leanesse, and continuall coughe, with paines in the breast, and shortnesse of the wynde, the remedie therof some time hath bin with Sage in this maner.

An excelent Pill agaynst Apostumacio of the Lunges, Rume, or consumption, whiche helped Bulle the aucthour of this booke

Take Spicknard, Ginger, of eche .ʒ.ii. seede of Sage .ʒ.viii. dried, beaten fine in pouder, with the foresaied spices, and .ʒ.xii. of long Peper in like maner, and .ʒ.i. of old Asser, and the iuce of Sage, and so make your Pille in a cleane morter, and take euery mornyng fastyng .ʒ.i. of this, and as much at night, drinking after it pure cleane Sage water, and this is the best Pille that euer I did knowe, and helped me in a great sicknesse in Suffolke, where some time I dwelled. This herbe also prouoketh vrine, clenseth flume, expulseth winde, drieth vp dropsie, helpeth the Paulsie, strengthen the sinewes, and purgeth bloud, if it be sodden in runnyng water. Roche Alam, and Woodbinde lea-

To kil Canker and queceth Robin goodfelowes Feuer.

ues, it killeth the Canker in the mouthe, and also quecheth the great heate and burning, stinke, filthe, and matter, that oftentimes cometh through corruption of nature, or meritrix maner, doth chaunce into the secrete places of men or women, is helped this way, puttinge in a littell of the pouder of Astrologia rotunda: for asmuch as it drieth, it is put into Pigges, which be most moyst of nature to drie vp their humidite or moyster withall, which els be euell for Flugmatike parsons.

Auicen.3. trac cap. i.

The incomparable vertue is so excellent of this herbe, that the great learned fathers of Salarn, did write these wordes to ye late famous Prince kyng Henry the eight, in the laude therof saiyng. *Cur moritur homo, cui saluia Crescit in horto?* Inquerynge why mortall men should die, whiche haue Sage in their Gardens, but because no herbe hath power to make me immortal: they say furthermore. *Contra vim mortis non Crescit medicina in hortis.* And thus I doe conclude of this vertuous herbe Sage. Whose wine beynge dayly dronke, is good against the faulyng sicknesse. And the comon Sage Ale, rightly brewde with Sage, Squinans, Spicknarde, Calamus, Fenell seedes, and Bettony, is very hollsome for the Flugmatike, Dropsie, winde Collike, rawnesse of the stomacke with indigestion.

Marcellus.

What be the vertue of Onions in their kindes?

Hillarius.

Onions prouoketh slepe. Longe. Onions.

They do make thin the bloud, and bringe sleape, they be not good for Cholerike men. The longe Onion is more vehementer then the rounde, and the Redde more then the white the Graye more then the Greene, and the rawe more then the sodden, or preserued in salt, although they cause sleape very painfull

The booke of Simples. Fol.vj

full and troubelous, hot in the thirde degree, but they warme & clenſe the ſtomacke, bringeth good collour to the face, and then it muſte bee good for the new Greene ſicknes, and doth very well prouoke vrine, & being roſted, and warme aplied to the painfull harde Emerodes, efteſones it doth open them, if vineger warme be put to them, and cleane pilled or taken from the ouer rinde and ſkinne, and cutte of bothe the endes, and caſt into water, remainyng in it one houer, and ſo ſliſe it: this doth take away the behement ſharpneſſe, that els would hurt the eies and head, and beyng applied with Hony, Rue, and Salt, al incorporated together to the wounde bitten of a Dogge, it healeth it ſoone. Leekes purge the bloud in Marche, and paineth the head, and be not greatly praiſed, for their iuce is euill ſaieth *Dioſcorides*. The head beyng anointed with the iuce of them, keepeth heare from faulynge, there is muche varietee of this Onion amonge writers, ſaith *Plinius*, but this ſhall ſuffice, for vs Engliſhmen. There be great plentie of good Onions that be brought from Flaunders, called ſainct Homars Onions. So there be very many growyng in Holland in Lincolne ſhere, and in the towne of Duriſme in the North countrey.

To clenſe the ſtomacke.

Grene ſickenesse. Onions doe heale the Emeroides.

For bityng of a Dogge. Leekes.

Heere from failyng.

Where plentie of Onions doe growe.

Marcellus.

What is the vertue of Fenell?

Hillarius.

IT hath powre to warme in the third degree, & drie in ye firſt, & maketh ſweet ye breath: the ſeede eaten oftentimes vpon an emptie ſtomacke, dothe helpe the eye ſight. The rootes cleaue waſhed be very holſome in Potage, & is good in Tiſants. The greene or red tufts, growyng vpon the ſtalkes, ſodden in Wine, Potage or Ale, helpeth the bladder, raignes, and breaketh the ſtone: encreaſeth Mylke in womens breaſtes, and ſeede of generacion. It is good to vſe Endiue or ſuche like with it, becauſe it is very hotte, and it is very good to waſhe ones feete to bedwarde. It is good in Barbars bathes, and waſhing water, with Balme and Baies The ſyrup is very good and holſom, it helpeth a Flegmatike ſtomacke. And Fenell, Parſely, and Watercreſſes, of eche like quantitie ſtamped together, pouringe white wine to them, & the crums of Barly breade, ſtading al one night in a ſtone morter, the next day being ſtrained, clarified and drunke, this will clenſe the raignes from grauel, ſtone, and choler, & cauſe one to make much water that hath the ſtrangurie. It is good for fat men to open the beſſels, as Vaynes, and Guttes. There be two kindes of Fenell, one *Marathrum*, which is beſt: the other *Hippomarathrum* which is wilde, the ſeede hath greater vertue then the roote.

Fœniculum. Swete breathes. For the eye ſight.

To breake the ſtone. Encreaſeth Mylke. To waſhe feete.

An excellente medicene of Fenel, for the raines and bladder.

For fat folks

Two kindes of Fenel.

Marcellus.

What is the vertue of Purſlin?

Hillarius.

Colde

The booke of Simples.

Purslen is an herbe of a singuler vertue to coole, or quenche Choller.

Cold in the third, and moiste in the second degree. If it be stamped with steped Barly, it maketh a good plaster to coole the hed, iyes, and liuer, in Agues, and hot inflamaciō. To eate of it, it stoppeth fluxes, and quencheth burnyng Choller, extinguishe venerus luste, and greatly helpeth the raines, and bladder, and will kille round wormes in the bellie: and comforteth the matrixe, againste hotte choller, and termes aboundyng. And the iuice is good to drinke in hot Feuers it may be preserued with Salte, and then it is very good with roosted meates. *Plini* saieth, it is supposed to make the sight blunt and weake:

An example of Purslen.

Further he saieth that in Spaine, a greate noble man, whom he did knowe, did hang this Pursline roote on a Threade, commonly about his necke, whiche was troubled of a *Vuela*, and was healed therewith.

Marcellus.
What is the vertue of Dragons?

Hillarius.

Of Dragōs, whiche helpeth againste the pestilēce.

The iuce of Dragōs saith *Dioscorides*, dropped into the iyes, doeth clense them, and causeth moche brightnesse, vnto the iyes of them, whiche haue darke sightes. The water of this herbe, hath vertue against the pestilēce, if it be dronke blood warm with Venice Triacle, or *Mithridatum*. The sauour of this herbe is hurtefull, to women newly conceiued with childe. *Plini* saieth, that who so beareth this herbe vpon them, no venemous Serpent will doe them any harme. This herbe is hotte and drie, and heyng sodden in wine, it healeth a kibed heele, called *Pernio*. And this herbe being brused, and applied with Planten, healeth a newe wounde.

Marcellus.
What is the vertue of *Filipendula*?

Hillarius.

Filipendula haue rounde rootes hangyng vpon smal fine thredes in the yearth.

It is called *Filipendula*, bicause it haue small round rootes, hanging vpon it with thredes in the ground, it is an herbe hote and drie, in the third degree: if it bee sodden in white wine, & dronke, it drieth vp windy places in the guttes, and clenseth the raines of the backe and bladder. And the pouder dronke in wine, is good against the falling euill, and helpeth the yellow Iaundes: the leaues and stalkes sodden in wine and drunke, clenseth the secondes.

Marcellus.
What is the vertue of Violettes?

Hillarius.

Violettes be great coolers and to cold for the harte.

SIMEON SETHI reporteth, that thei doe helpe againste hotte inflamacions of the guttes, hedde, and stomacke, if the cause be of burning Choler: either the water, sirup, or conserue of the said violettes, being eaten or drunke, after the digestion of any hot passion: but vndoubtedly it offēdeth the hart, bicause of the great coldnes. The sauor of the flowers be pleasaunt. The oile that is made

The booke of Simples.   Fol. vj.

made of this herbe, haue vertue to reconsile quiete slepe to thē, whiche haue greuous hote paine in the hedde, Uiolet water, and cleane Sallette oile, of eche one vnce together dronke, clense rotten matter in the stomacke: and coughes, or paine in the lunges. *Good for coughes and short winde.*

Marcellus.

What is the vertue of white Lilles? and water Lilles called *Nimphea.*

Hillarius.

Dioscorides saieth, that the Oile of Lilles doeth mollefie the Sinewes, and the mouthe of the matrix, the iuce of Lilles, Uineger and Honie, sodden in a brasen vessell, doeth make an ointment, to heale bothe newe and old woundes: if the rootes bee rosted, and stamped with Roses, it maketh an heasyng plaster against burnyng of fire, the same roote rosted, hath vertue to breake a pestilence sore, applied hote vnto the sore place, and is drie in the firste degree. The oile of water Lilles bee moiste, sufferente against all hote diseases to anointe the ardente and hote places, and dooeth reconsile quiete slepe, if the forehedde bee anointed therewith: it is holsome for madde men. The seede and roote sodden in wine, stoppeth the immomoderate fluxe menstruall, and for the bloody flixe, as *Dioscorides* and *Galen* saieth. *Libro. viii. Simplicium Medicamentorum.*

Marcellus.

What is the vertue of Chickwede?

Hillarius.

Almoste euery ignoraunte woman doeth knowe this herbe, but there be of diuers kindes, thei be very good to kepe woundes frō apostumacions, stamped, and applied vnto theim, and draweth corrupcion out of woundes, and sodden with vineger, doeth drawe fleume out of the hedde, if it bee often warme put it into the mouthe, and spit it out againe: in the same maner it helpeth the teeth, and sodden in wine and so dronke, it will clense the raines of the backe. *Anagallis or morsus Galline, called Chicke wede*

Marcellus.

What is the vertue of Sorrell? whiche in the North is called sower Dockens.

Hillarius.

Euery one dooeth right well knowe it, and all thei that make grenesause, but the discripcion, I leaue to *Dioscorides*, and *Leonardus Fuchius*, not onely in this herbe, but in all other, and to tell the vertue I wil, it is colde and drie, in the seconde degree, it also stoppeth: it is like Endiue in propertie, because it ouercometh Choller, and is moche commended: It helpeth the yellowe Iaunders, if it bee dronke with small wine or ale, and also quencheth burnyng feuers, to eate of the leaues euery Mornyng in a Pestilence tyme, is moste holsome, if *Rumex lapathus, or acedula, is Sorrell, and Sorrell de bois.*

b.i.   thei

The booke of Simples.

they be eaten fastyng. This herbe doeth *Dioscorides, Galen* and *Auicen* greatly commende, besides the great learned men of this time.

Marcellus.

What is the vertue of Planten or Waybrede.

Hilarius.

Plantago, called arnoglossa

THe greater Planten is the better, it hath seuen great vaines, it is colde and drie, the seedes dronke with red wine, or the rootes sodden therin, stoppeth the blouddy flur, likewise the rootes & leaues being sodden with fayre water, or with Burrage water and Suger, and geue it to him that hath an Ague, either Tercian or quarten, twoo howers afore his fit helpeth it. Proue this, for thus haue I helped many, it is very comfortable for childre that haue great fluxes and Agues, and is a frende vnto the liuer. This herbe is greatly praised of the learned writers. Water Planten rootes, leaues and buddes be holsome for to be dronke against the falyng sicknes.

Marcellus.

What is the vertue of Camamill?

Hilarius.

THis herbe is very hotte, it is dronke agaynst colde windes, and matter being in the guttes, the Egiptians did suppose it wold helpe al colde Agues, and did consecrate the same, as *Galen* saith: also if it be tempered and strained into white wine, and dronke of women, hauyng the childe dead within the body, it will cause present deliueraunce, it doth mightly clense the bladder, and is excellent to bee sodden in water to washe the feete, the oyle is precious, as is declared hereafter.

Marcellus.

What is the vertue of Hoppes.

Hilarius.

Lupus Salictarius bee Hoppes.

THere be Hoppes which doe coole, that be called Lupuli, those that we haue be hot and drie, bitter, sower, hot, saith olde Herballes, and *Fuchius* saieth, thei clense fleume, and cholere, and the water betwene the skinne and fleshe. The sirup will clense grose, raw fleume from the guttes, and is good against obstructions. If the iuce be dropped in the eare, it taketh awaie the stincke of rotten sores, the rootes wil helpe the Liuer, and Splene, being sodden and dronke, the Beere is very good for flegmatike men.

Marcellus.

What is the vertue of Horehounde?

Hillarius.

The boke of Simples. Fol. viij.

IT is an herbe hotte and drie, if it be sodden with fayre water, Suger or Hony, and straine it, this drinke dothe clense the stomack from stinkyng flegme. It is an excellente herbe for women, to clense their monthly termes. The water of this, is good to helpe them which haue a moiste Reume falling from the head vpon the Lunges, beyng often dronke, but it is hurtefull to the bladder and raynes, the sirup therof doth clense the Kinges euill. And also put into the eares doeth greatly comfort the hearing: if the eares be troubled with deafnes, stamped with Hony, and applied to the iyes, it clenseth the sight. *Stinkyng fleume.* / *To helpe a moiste reume* / *Kynges euill* / *To helpe the sight.*

Marcellus.

What is the vertue of Veruen. *Veruen.*

Hillarius.

IT is called the Holy herbe, it drieth and bindeth: if it be sodden with Vineger, it helpeth a disease called S. Anthonies fier, oftentimes washing the pained place. The leaues of Veruen, and Roses, and fresh swines greace stamped together will seace paine and grief in euery wounde, and will kepe woundes from corrupting. It is good for people that haue the Tercian, and Quarten Agues, and thus saith *Dioscorides*. Moreouer he saith the waight of a.z. of this herbe with three halfepeny wayghtes of Olibanum, and put in.z.ix. of old wine tempered together, & dronke fortie daies of this quatite fastyng, it will helpe diseases called the kinges euill or payne in the throate. *Wilde fire.* / *To kepe woundes fro corruption.* / *Against Agues.* / *To helpe the kynges euill.*

Mercellus.

What is the vertue of Rice? *Rice.*

Hillarius.

THere be many opinions concernyng Rice, but I shall stay my selfe with the Iudgement of *Auicen*, Rice saieth he is hotte and drie, and hath vertue to stoppe the belly, it doth norish much if it be sodden with Milke, but it ought to bee steped in water an hole night before. If blanched Almondes be stamped with Rose water streined into theim, and sodden with Cowes Milke, it is very muche norishing: the flower or mele of Irza or Rise, stoppe the bloudy flixe, in drinke or glister. *Auicen, in. ii. can. cap. 78.*

Marcellus.

What is the vertue of Pease, and Beanes? *Beanes.*

Hillarius.

BEanes bee more groser, and fuller of winde, then Pease bee, and maketh euill matter, except thei be well sodden and buttered, and so eaten with the whitest Oniens that maie bee gotten, because thei be harde of digestion, how be it, thei doe make fatte, and partly clenseth, yet thei are not compared with ten- *To make fat*

b.ii. der

The booke of Simples.

der white Peason, well sodden and buttered, or els made in potage, with garden Mintes, and grose Peper, whiche haue vertue to clense the raines of the backe and blader: There is a place in Suffolke called Orfort, where Pease growe on the stones, neuer sowen. Lintelles bee of the same vertue, Barley being cleane hulled, and sodden with milke cleane water, and Sugar, maketh a verie holsome and comfortable potage, for whole chollerike persones, or young people, and of this is moche vsed in the North partes of Englãde, and is called bigge Keale and of cleane Barly and puer water, is made that excellente water called Ptisant.

Ptisant.

Marcellus.

Beates.

What is the vertue of Beates?

Hillarius.

white beates

There be of twoo kindes, and be bothe praise worthie, *Simeon Sethi*, writeth that thei be hote and drie in the third degree, the white be the beste, thei haue vertue to clense, as Niter hath, but euill iuce: the iuce of this herbe with Honie, applied into the nose, do purge the hedde, so doe the lefe, it is an holsome herbe in potage, if it be well sodden, or els it is noisome to the stomacke. if it be parboiled and eaten with Uinegare, it is good against the stopping of the liuer, notwithstanding, the iuce of this herbe doe stoppe the bellie, beyng simplie taken. It is called Bete of Beta, or Ueta, the Greke. B. because of the forme or shape.

Purgynge the head.

Stoppng of the Lyuer.

Mercellus.

Betony.

What is the vertue of Bettony.

Hillarius.

They be of diuers kindes, *Leonardus Fucchius*, doth cal the swete Giloflowers by the names of Bittony, but the one semeth to talke of that whiche is commonly knowen of the people, called the lande Betony, which hath vertue to kill wormes within the belly, & helpeth the quarten, clenseth the Matrix, and hath vertue to heale the body within, if it be brused, it is of so greate effecte, if it be sodden with wormewod in white wine to purge Fleume, it is hot, in the first degree, and drie in the seconde.

To kill wormes.

For bruses.

Mercellus.

Sauerie.

What is the vertue of Sauerie.

Hillarius.

It is hot and drie in the thirde degree, if the grene herbe be sodden in water, or white wine, and dronke, these be his vertues to make Lyuer softe: to clense Dropsies, colde Coughes, clenseth womens diseases, and seperateth the dead child from the mother, *Dioscorides* and *Galen* saith, also Germander is not much vnlike the vertue of this herbe.

Lyuer softe.
Cold coughs
Dead childre

Marcel-

The booke of Simples. Fol.ix.

Marcellus.
What is the vertue of Muſtarde or Sinapium?

Hilarius.

PLINIVS dothe greatly alow it ſaying, that ther is nothing doth perce more ſwifter in to the braine then it doth. Honye Vineger, and Muſtarde tempered together, is an excelente Gagariſme to purge the head, tethe, and throte. Muſtarde is good agaynſt al the diſeaſes of the ſtomacke, or lunges, winde, fleame and rawneſſe of the guttes, and conduceth foode into the body prouoketh vrine, helpeth the Palſie, waſteth the quarten, drieth vp moyſte rumes, applied plaſterwiſe vnto the head. Honye and Muſtarde helpeth the coughe, and is good for them that haue the fallyng ſicknes: And tentes of Vineger and Muſtarde put into the noſe helpeth the Palſie. Notwithſtanding the common vſe of Muſtarde is a cruell enemie vnto the eye, many moe vertues haue I red of Muſtarde, but the occaſion of time hath vnhappely preuented, not only my large diſcription in this, but alſo in many other ſimples.

Muſtarde.

To purgoſe the head.

Falling ſicknes.
Palſie.
Euell for the eyes.

Marcellus.
What is the vertue of Sention, or Groundeſill?

Hillarius.

IT is of a mixte temperature, it cooleth and partely clenſeth. If it be ſtamped and ſodden in water, and drinke it with your potage, it will purge hot choller: this done with Saffron & colde water, ſtamped and put into the eies, it will drie the runnynge drops of them: and prepared plaſterwiſe, it helpeth many greuous woundes. *Dioſcorides* ſaith, that the heads of Sention with the flowers, and a littel wine and Manna, tempered together, healeth the woudes that be in the ſinewes. The flower of this herbe, hath white heere, & when the winde bloweth it away, then it appereth like a balde headded mã therfore it is called Senecio.

Sention.

Hot choler in the ſtomacke
To helpe the eyes.

Dioſcorides lib.iiii.capit. x.Cii.xcii.
For woudes

Marcellus.
What is the vertue of Cucummers?

Hilarius.

THey be (truly) in the ſeconde degree very moyſt, and colde, the ſeedes be very good to be geuen in hot ſickneſſes. The pouder of ẏ ſame ſeedes dronke in cleane wine, is good againſt diuers hot paſſions of the harte. This fruite will cauſe one to make water well. The roote dried, and the pouder therof dronke in water & Honie prouoketh vomit. If thei be moderately eaten, thei bring good bloud. Tempered with Hony, and anoynte the eyes, that helpeth a diſeaſe called Epinictidas, which troubleth men, with ſtrange ſightes in the night: the beſt of this fruite is that which beareth the beſt ſeede, the ſauour

Cucumers.

To prouoke vrine.
Vomit.
Good bloud.

Epinictidas.
Mellons.

b.iii.

The booke of Simples.

Raw herbes

sauour of them is holsome. Mellons, Citruls, Pompens, and this kinde of Pepins, or great apples, be much vsed in Englād, and is more common, then profitable, because they vse to eate them raw. Englishmen beyng borne in a temperate region, enclininge to colde, may not without hurte eate rawe herbes, rootes, and fruites so plentifull, as many men which be borne farre in the Southe partes of the worlde, which be most hot of stomacke: therfore eate these fruites boyled, or els baken with Hony, Peper, and Fenell seedes, or suche like: there be an other hot kinde of bitter Cucumbers which do purge, called Colocynthis. The Aple beyng steeped in Ptisant water, durynge twelue howers, and so strained, and dronke in the mornyng halfe a pint, doo purge Melancholy, and Choler, adust and vitriall fleume, but it is a very groase purgation, but the Trochis of Coloquintida is better to purge with. But. ʒ.i. of the pouder of Coloquintida sodden wt Mirrhe and Ote water, and Hony to a thicknes: maketh a goodly Pill to purge fleume and Choler, it is good in Glisters for the same purpose, sodden with Vineger, this kept in the mouthe, killeth wormes in the teeth. The Oyle of this is good to anoynte the paines in the Huckel bone called *Eschiatica*. It also killeth wormes in the eare, this is moste bitter to the mouth and stomacke it killeth wormes in the belly, both in Emplasters and drinke. The Arabians cal this herbe Chandel, but in latten *Cucurbita siluestris*.

Coloquitida.

Dioscorides lib.iiii.capit. Clxx.

Mathiolus super Dioscoridem.

Marcellus.

Cabage.

What is the vertue of Cabage, or *Brassica?*

Hillarius.

Ius Brassica soluit cuius substantia stringi.
To binde.
Laxatiue.
To clense Leprosie.

Cabage is of twoo properties, of bindyng the bellie, and makyng laxatiue, the iuce of Cabages lightly boiled in freshe Beefe brothe is laxatiue, but the substaunce of this herbe is harde of digestion, but if it bee sodden twise, the brothe of it will binde the bellie, if it be tempered with Allume: This herbe hath vertue to clense a newe redde Leprosie, laid vpon the sore place, in the maner of a plaster, but to conclude of this herbe, the brothe of it hath vertue, to kepe a man from dronkennes, as *Aristotell, Rasis*, and *Auicen*, doth reporte, eaten before meat or drinke. And this is good to make potage withall, and is a profitable herbe in a common wealthe, whiche the Fleminges sell dere, but we haue it growe in our owne gardens, if we would preferre our owne commoditie before idelnesse, and not suffer weedes to grow where herbes should be plāted. If Fenegrice and this be sodden plaster waies it helpeth the Goute. The leaues sodden with Hony, healeth Vlcers and Cankers, and killeth wormes in the belly. Therbe sonndry kindes of wortes, bothe Garden, Fielde & See, much like to eche other in vertue. There be great plentie growing betwene Albrought and Horthford in Suffolke vppon the Sea shore.

Aristote. iii. probl.
Auicen, ii. cā.
rasis. iii. al.

Dioscor. li. 4.

Marcellus.

what

The booke of Simples.   Fol.x.

What is the vertue of Rue, or herbe Grace?
    Hillarius.   *Rewe called herbe grace.*

I tell thee this herbe is very hot and bitter, and doth burne, because of his hotnesse in the thirde degree. If a littell of this Rue be stamped and sodden in wine and dronke, it is an excellent medecine against Poyson and Pestilence. With Roses and Wineger, and Rue stamped together, & put into a forhead clothe or Biggen, & applied unto the Temples of the head or forhead doth seace greuous payne in the head. And in like maner it helpeth the bityng of Serpentes, and of Dogges, stamped with Wineger, manie nice people can not abide it, crying fie it stinkes. The seede of this herbe beten in pouder, and put in fresshe clarified Butter, and Pitche melted together, is good for them to drinke that are brused. The seed of this Rue beyng dried, and beaten into pouder, with the pouders of sweet Callamus and longe Pepper, sodden in white Wine, this being dronke warme, helpeth the winde in the small guttes.

Poyson. Payne in the hedde. Against biting of Dogges, and serpentes. Bulleins experience many tymes.

    Marcellus.
What is the vertue of Lettice?   *Lettice.*
    Hillarius.

It doeth mightly encrease Mylke in womans brestes, and therfore it is called Lettice, as *Marciall* saith, first shalbe geuen to the vertue and power, To encrease milke in womens breastes euerie hower. Lettice is an herbe, colde and moyst, and very comfortable for a hotte stomacke, bringeth sleape, molifieth the belly, the drier it be eaten, the better it is. I meane if it be not muche washed in water, adding cleane salet Oyle, Suger, and Wineger to it, it abateth carnal luste: and muche use of it, dulleth the sight. The seede is precious against hot diseases, dronke with Ptisantes. There is an herbe called Rocket gentill, that partely smelleth like a Foxe, whiche is very hot, an encreaser of seede, this herbe must alwaies be eaten with Lettice. The roote therof sodden in watter will draw foorth broken bones, & will helpe the coughe in yonge children. The seede vehemently doeth expell urine dronke in white wine, and killeth wormes, and tempered with an Oxe gaule, to clense blacke spottes in the face or skinne after stripes.

To encrease Milke. Comforte against hote choller in the stomacke. Ill for sight. To abate the luste. An encrease of seede. Broken bones. Cough. Diosco. lib. ii. Cap. cxxxiiii.

    Marcellus.
What is the vertue of Mintes?   *Mintes.*
    Hillarius.

Mintes be of two kindes, garden, and wilde Myntes, they be hotte unto the thirde degree, and drie in the seconde degree. Garden Mintes be best: the pouder of this with the iuce of Pomgranets, stoppeth vomittes, helpeth sighyng, clenseth hotte choller. Three braunches of this sodden with wine, doth healpe repletion dronke fastyng. This iuce tempered with good Triakel, and

Stoppyng of vomites. Repletion. To kill wormes. Bityng of a Dogge. To helpe the Collike.

    b.iiii.   eaten

The booke of Simples.

eaten of children in mornynges, will kill wormes, and stamped with salte, and applie it to the bityng of a Dogge, it will heale it. It is holsome sodden with windie meates & Peason. &c. and soddē in posset ale with Fenell, it encreaseth vitall seede. It is not beste for Chollerike complexion, but good for fleugmatike, & indifferent for Melancholie, and it will stoppe bloud, stamped and aplied to the place: the iuce of Mintes be beste to mingle in a medicen against poison, the pouder of Mintes are good in potage to helpe digestion, & to make swete breath.

To make swete breth.

Marcellus.

Dandelyon. What is the vertue of Dandelion, or House teeth?

Hilarius.

The heao. *Sowthistell* IT is temperate, colde, and drie, with Roses and Vinegar tempered together, it helpeth the hedde in hote diseases, the Sowethistell called *Soncus*, hath the same vertue, and so hath Cicorie, if thei bee sodden, thei lose the bellie, and quencheth heate, whiche burneth in the stomacke, and defendeth the hedde from hote smokyng vapours, and purgeth yellowe choller, and rebateth venerus and fleshely heate, and is good to be sodden, and dronke in hote burning Agues, though this herbe bee commonly knowen, and counted of many as a vile wede, yet it is reported of *Dioscorides*, to bee an excellent herbe, and is called Lions teeth.

To loose the belly.

Yellowe choler. *Burnynge Agues.*

Marcellus.

Hysop. What is the vertue of Hysope?

Hilarius.

Dioscor. lib. 3.

Siknes in the lunges, *Old coughes* *Rotten humours.* *To helpe the Splene.*

AN herbe commonly knowen, growyng in gardens, and hote in the third degree, it hath vertue to make humours thinne and warme: sodden with Figges, Rewe, and Honie, in clene water, and dronke, it greatly helpeth the sicknes in the lunges, olde coughes, rotten humours, drippynges vpon the lunges, sodden with Erius, and graines of Paradice, called the Cardamon, it mightelie purgeth, and bryngeth good colour, Figges, Salt, Nitrum, and Hysoppe stamped together, and applied to the Splene, helpeth it moche, and taketh awaie the water, that runneth betwene the skin, and the fleshe: sodden with Oximel, it clenseth fleume. How be it, *Galen* writeth but little of this herbe in his eight booke of simples, but saith that it is drie, and hote in the thirde degree. But this herbe was vsed in the olde Testamente, in the tyme of the bloudie Sacrifice. And the holy Prophet in his .li. Psalme, saieth vnto almightie God: Sprinkle me oh Lorde, with Hysop. &c. God graunte vs all to haue soche blessed plantes, of that Hysop in our gardens, whiche haue vertue to heale al sicknesses of the soule, defiled with sinne.

Fleume.

Marcellus.

Wyne. What is the vertue of Wine?

Hilarius.

The boke of Simp'es. Fol. xj.

Hillarius.

HIPOCRATES saith, of a customable thing cometh lesser hurt then thinges not vsed, wherof I gather that they whiche drinke wine moderately with measure doeth profit them muche, and maketh good disgestion, but those people that vse to drinke wine seldome times, be distempered. White wine if it be cleare is holsome to be dronke before meate, for it preserueth the body and perseth quickely to the bladder, but if it be dronke vpon a full stomacke, it will rather make oppilacion, or stoppyng of the meseraites, because it doth swiftly driue foode downe, before nature hath of him selfe disgested it: and the nature of white wine is of lesse warmenesse. The seconde wine is pure Claret, of a cleare Jacent, or yelow choler, this wine doth greatly norish and warme the body, and it is an holsome wine with meate, & is good for flegmatike folke, but very vnholsome for younge children: for *Galen* saieth *Vinum pueris inimicum*, because it heateth aboue nature, and hurteth the head. Nor for them whiche haue hot Liuers, or paines in the head, occasioned of hot vapours, or smokes, for it is like vnto fier, and flare. The thirde is blacke or depe Redde wine which is thicke, a stopper of the belly, a corrupter of the bloud, a breder of the stone, hurtefull to olde men, and profitable to few men, except they haue the blouddy flur. And for the election of wine *Auicen* saieth, that Wine is best, that is betwene new and olde, cleare, declinyng somewhat to Redde or Amber, of good Odoure, neither sharpe nor sweete, but equall betweene twoo, for it hath vertue not only to make humours temperate, warme and moist, but also to expell euell matter, whiche corrupteth the stomacke and bloud. In Somer it ought to be delaied with pure cleane water, as *Aristotle* saith in his Problemes, and not this, that in drie yeres, wines be best and most holsome: but in watry yeares, the Grapes be corrupted, whiche wine doth bring to the body many euill diseases, as Dropsies, Timpanies, Fluxes, Rumes, windes and such like, as *Galen* saith: And thus to conclude of wine, almightie God did ordaine it for the greate comfort of mankinde, to be taken moderately, but to bee dronke with excesse, it is vnholsome, and is a Poyson most benemous, it relaxeth the sinewes, bringeth Palsie, Fallyng sicknesse, in olde persons, hot Feuers, Franfies, Fightyng, Lechery, & a consumyng of the Liuer to the Cholerike: and generally there is no credence to be geuen to dronkardes, although they be mighty men. It maketh me like vnto monsters with countenaunce like to burning cooles. It dishonoreth noble men, and beggereth poore men, and nearehand killeth as many as be slain in cruell battailes, the more it is to be lamented. *Plato in secundo de legibus* commaunded that non vnder .xxii. yeres olde should drinke wine. And this wise man doth shew a reason saiyng: *Non oportet ignem igni adiicere.* One fier ought not to be put to an other or cupled together, for they will deuoure eche other, because there is no meane betwene them, but extreme in one degree. And the wordes of king Lamuel be these against dronken

Hip. in.il. lib. nphari.

Disgestion.
white wine.
Auerois in.6 colig.
rasis in lib. 26.con.ca 1.

Claret wine warmeth the body.
Galen lib. de tue sani.ca,9
Wyne is an enemie to children.
Red wine corrupteth bloud.

Auicen in.3. prim 2.doc. cap.8.
To know good wine.

When wine is best.
Gen in rrg. acu.

Wyne moderatly comforteth.
A glasse for all excesse wine bibbers to looke in.

Plato ix. 2. legibus.

Prouerb.20.

The booke of Simples.

Prouer. xxxi dronken princes or Judges. *Noli regibus ô Lamuel, noli regibus dare vinum quia nullum secretū, vbi regnat ebrietas ne forte bibant & obliuiscantur iudiciorum & mutent causam filiorum pauperis.&c.* Oh Lamuel it is not fit for kinges, it is not for kinges to drinke wine. For there is no secret where dronkenes raineth, least thei beyng dronke forget the law: and paruart or change the iudgement of poore mennes children. Giue wine to suche as be condempned to death, and wine to suche as mourne, that thei maie drinke it and forget their misery and aduersitie. I conclude that wine is holsome for colde complecctions and cruddie stomackes, euell for cholerike, immoderatly taken: a prince to princes, and a confounder of Judges, and finally the floud of Letha to the afflicted, to make them forget their miseries.

Letha a flud whose water did cause men to forget the thues whan thei drik of it

Marcellus.

waters. What is the vertue of the common water of Ryuers, springes and fountaynes. &c.

Hillarius.

Gal.3. de vic. acu.libr.ii. sen.ii. Water is one of the foure elementes, more lighter then earth, heuier then fier and ayre. But this water which is here amonges vs in Riuers, Pondes, Springes, Fluddes and Seas, be no pure waters, for they be mingled with sundrie ayres, corruptions, grosenes, and softnes. Notwithstandyng in all our meates and drinkes, water is vsed, and amongest all liuyng ceatures cannot be forborne, both Man, Beast, Fishe, Fowle, Herbe. &c. haue neede of water. And *Auicen* saith, the clay water is pure, for the clay clenseth the water: that water is better then the water that runneth ouer grauell or stones, so that it be pure Clay and voide of corruption. Also waters running towarde the East be pure, comyng out of hard stony Rockes, and a pinte of that water is lighter then a pinte of the standyng water of Welles or Pooles, the lighter the water, the better it is. Also waters that is put in wine. &c. ought first to be sodden, or it be occupied, and so the fier doeth clense it from corruption. Standyng waters, and waters runnyng neare vnto Cities and Townes, or Martish groundes, woddes, and fennes, be euer full of corruption, because there is so muche filthe in them of Carrions, and rotten dunge. &c. The hier the water doth fall, the better it is, Ise, and Snowe water be very groase, and be hurtefull to the bodies of men and beastes. To drinke colde water is euell, for it will stoppe the bodie, and engender Malancholie. Salt water clenseth a man from Scabs, Iche, and moyste humours, it killeth Lice, and wasteth bloud betwene the skinne and the flesh, but it is most hurtfull to the stomacke: but the vapour and smoke of it is good for them that hath the dropsie. If one that is bitten with a mad Dogge, bee sodenly caste into a swifte runnyng Riuer, and so plunged vp and downe, three or foure times, hangynge by the waste in a stronge Linnen cloth, it wil helpe him by the reason of the great sudden feare, in that Melancholy passion, saith *Dioscorides.* And *Auicen* saieth

what kinde of water is best.

Auicen,lib.ii fen.iii.de dispossicionibus.

Salt water healeth scabs

water

The booke of Simples. Fol.xij.

water wherin steele is quenched, is good to bee geuen to him that is bitten with a mad Dogge. Also *Auicen* sayth, who so euer is bitten of a mad Dogge, and is behemently afraide when he seeth his face in a vessell of water, and knoweth him self, it is a sygne that he shall not die. Also bathes for the clensyng of the corrupt bodies of men, be made of cleane water, without water, men were more defiled then beastes, for it is a nutriment of euery liuyng creature, sensible, and insensible. There is a riuer runnyng at Rome called Tiber, whose water is of suche vertue, that it will remayne in a vessell of stone, by the space of an hundred yeares vncorrupted, as saieth *Petrus, Andreus, Mathiolus*, vpon *Dioscorides*. There was sometime neare vnto that auncient and old Citie called Agrigentum, sacred welles, whiche were of suche vertue, that the water brought foorth suche precious Oile, that the bodies which were anoynted therwith, were clensed of sundrie and diuers diseases. Let vs not be forgetfull of that noble riuer Tagus in Spain, in who swimeth diuers kindes of fishes, vnder whose stremes, lieth plentie of golden sandes, what shall we say, vnto the capital Riuer of al this worlde called *Nilus*, runneth all *Ethiopia* and Egipt, in which Egipt ther is no Rayne, but only the swellyng and ouerflowyng of that fludde, which being falne downe within his bankes, eftesones great plentie of spices, Herbes, Plantes, and fruites do grow, in so muche that the people of the lande doo liue with out any greate trauell, payne, or labour, the cause of the aboundaunce, and swelling of this famous riuer saith *Galen*, is when the Snowes be melted, through the greate heate of the sonne in the Mountaines of *Ethiopia*, the *Ocian* mightie sea of all the worlde, the mother of fishes, strauge monsters, stones of diuers natures, seperature of landes, enuironer of Ilandes, the water therof through a long continuall boyling ouer the fier, is couerted into salt. Also in the Northe partes of Scotland nere and vpon the said *Ocian* sea stickes, braunches, and bordes of broken shippes, falling into the same Sea, vpon these thinges be engendered foules or birdes, whiche wee commonly call Brantes, or Barnakles, a kinde of small Geese, whiche we do se commonly in this Realme all of one coulere and bignes, their Egges were neuer seen amongest vs, thei haue none other generation then I haue saied: although to the incredible and ignorant, it semeth vntrue, whose fantesies I force not of, but of the truth. There be also waters in the North partes of the *Ocian* sea, which doth frese for euer more, whose Ice is nothing els but Christall, for Christall is of no other generation. There be waters of an other nature here in England called *Aquæ Calidæ*, or the hotte Bathes, at a place so named called Bathe, whose water doth neuer freese through extreme coldnesse, but is euer warme, which hath vertue to helpe sore, scabed, mangie, if I may so terme them: many haue come thither lame, and haue gone away without corruption of the flesh, contraxion of sinewes, lamenes of limmes, or weakenesse of nature, and this is a blessyng of God amongest vs, to haue so precious a iewell. There is a well neare hande

The goodlie vertues of cōmon water.

Of Nilus that noble flood.

The cause why Nilus doc flowe.

The cause of Barnacles.

The cause of Cristall.

The effectes of the bathes at the toune of Bathe.

of

The booke of Simples.

of the like effecte at Buckestone, whose water hath doozn many and sundry good cuers, bothe to the sore, and lame: yet these waters are reported to be so gentill ẏ they will not vsurpe or steale from Guiaacū his vertue and good seruice, whiche it daily doeth to his Neapolitan, French, or English fredes, you knowe what I meane. What shal I say more of water of deepe welles, which be warme in winter, by the reason that heate is in the bowels of thearth, ẏ colde in Sōmer, because heate is aboue the yearth. There is a noble well called *Alyssus* in *Accadia*, and who so drinketh of this water, shalbe deliuered of the venome or bityng of madde Dogges. There be diuers welles at Nantwiche. ꝛc. wherof is made great plentie of good white Salt, very riche and profitable to our common wealth. I will not forget the well of Silo and the sacred floud of Jordaine, whiche was the first water of Baptisme where as Jesus Christ our Sauiour was Baptised himself, whose beginning is from the heades of Jor, and Dan, or from a fountaine called *Paneade* so named of *Cæsaree*, in this Riuer is plenty of good fishes, it is a swete noble floud where Christe Jesus our sauiour, did shewe miracles. But *Asphaltites* saieth *Plini*, will suffer nothing to sincke into it, Bull nor Cammell, ꝛc. in this floud is plenty of Bytumen where was Sodome and Gomor, somtime the deade Sea. And thus I make an ende of water on the yearth: Raine water is bindyng and stoppyng of nature, water is a very good seruaunt, but it is a cruell maister.

Marcellus.

What is the vertue of Beere and Ale?

Hilarius.

Ale doeth engender groase humoures in the body, but if it be made of good Barley malte, ẏ of holsome water, ẏ very well sodden, and stande. v. or. vi. daies, vntill it be cleare, is holsome, especially for hotte Cholorike persones hauyng burning Feuers. But if Ale bee very swete and not wel sodden in the bruing, it bringeth inflamacion of winde, and fleum into the belly. If it be very sower, it nippeth and freateth the guttes, and is euill for thei yes, to them that be very flegmatike, Ale is very groase, but to temperate bodies, it encreaseth bloud, it is partly laratiue and prouoketh brine. Cleane brued Beere, if it be not very strong, brued with good Hoppes doeth clense the body from corruption, and is very holsome for the Liuer, it is an vsuall or common drinke in moste places of England, which in deede is hurte, and made worse, with many rotten Hoppes, or Hoppes dried like dust, which cometh from beyonde sea: but although there come many good Hoppes from thence: yet it is knowen that the goodly fieldes, ẏ fruitfull groundes of Englande doe bryng foorthe to mannes vse, as good Hoppes as groweth in any place of the worlde, as by proofe I knowe in many places of the Countrey of Suffolke, where they brewe their Beere with the Hoppes that growe vpon their owne groundes, as in

a place

Side notes:

Guiacū is of greater vertue thā Bath or Burstons wels, against the nosegate of Naples.

The ded sea.

Although Beere ẏ Ale be cōpoundes yet I haue here placed thē after water, whereof thei receiue their greatest substaunce.

The boke of Simples. Fol. xiij.

a place called Brisiard, nere to an old famus castle, called Framyngham and in many other places of the countrie. Thus to cōclude of Ale and Bere, thei haue none soche vertue, nor goodnes, as wine hath: and the surfettes whiche be taken of them, through dronkenes, be worse then the surfetes of Wine. Knowe this, that to drinke Ale or Bere, of any emptie stomacke moderatly, hurteth not, but doeth good. But if one be fastyng hungrie, or emptie, and drinke moche Wine, it will hurt the sinewes, and bryngeth Crampe, sharpe Agues, and Palleis, as *Auicen, Auerois & Rasis* saith. The rinsepichers had a good medicen prepared for thē: for the Maior of London, vpon a politike cōsideracion, Anno. 1560. made an order against mightie Bere and Ale: aswell for the health of the cōmons of London, as for their profite. Where at the Ale knightes, wer not little offended, and doe continue still as true soldiours, to the strōg Bere & Ale, which is their capitain, notwithstādyng my lorde maiors decree, as it plainly appereth, in their flushyng, red, coppred noses. For strong Ale haue soche vertue and worthines, that he can not be so persecuted, afflicted, yea, and banished, but his disciples moste constantly wil folowe him, to thende of their liues. Therfore thei shal haue *Bachus* blessing for their labours. But yet thende of Drunkardes and Gluttons bee miserable: therefore my *Marcellus* heare that moste prudent and wisest prince kyng Salomon, saiyng: *Noli esse in conuiuiis potatorum, nec in comessationibus eorum, qui carnes ad vescendum conferunt: quia vacantes potibus, & dantes symbola, consumentur & vestietur pannis dormitatio. &c.* Kepe no companie with Wine bibbers, and riotous eaters of fleshe. For soche as be drunkardes and rioters, shall come to pouertie. And he that is giuē to moche slepe, with ragged clothes. &c. Lo, these be the rewardes of soche cōpanions and vnthriftes.

A lathrhouse of Nunnes.

Surfettes of Ale, & Beare
Auicē.ii. tertra. capi. viii.
Auero. in cō.
Rasis in. iiii.
almen. cap. v.

Marcellus.

Thanke you for your good counsaile, good Hillarius, you haue spoken indifferently: and you haue alledged good writers, but specially Salomon, whose wordes be well placed, againste riotours and drunkardes, with their rewardes, as pouertie, shame, and ragges. &c. For abusyng the good creatures, and blessynges of God, but to vse them in good order, thei be our seruauntes, and we maie take them for our nede. I praie you saie some thyng of bread, whiche is the chief foode, to all liuyng men in this lande.

Hilarius.

The beste bread is made of cleane Whete, whiche groweth in claie ground: lightly Leuened, meanly Salted, and the bread to be baken in the ouen, not extremely hote, lest it be burned. Nor also lesse then meanly hote, leste the bread be heauie and rawe: the lighter the bread is, and the more fuller of the holes, the holsomer it is, *Auerois*, and *Rasis* saie. And also Bread muste neither bee eaten newe baked, nor very stale, or olde, for the one causeth drinesse, thurst, and smokyng in the hedde, troublyng the braines and iyes, through the heate thereof. The other drieth the bodie,

The meane baked bredo, the beste.

Aue. in. v. col.
Rasis in. xxx.
in almū. cap. 3
What bread is beste.

c.i. and

The booke of Simples.

Bread of a daie olde. and bringeth melancholy humours, hurting memorie. The best bread is that, that is of a daie old: and the loues or manchedes, maie neither be great nor little, but meane, for the fire in small loues, drieth vp the moistnes or vertue of the bread, and in greate loues, it leueth rawnes and grosenes. Rede *Galen*, in the properties of bread, sodden bread, whiche is called Simnelles, or Cracknelles, bee very vnholsome, and hurteth many one. Rye bread is windie, and hurtfull to many, therefore it must be well salted, and baken with Anisedes. And cōmonly crustes of bread, be drie and burned: thei doe engender choler aduste and melācholie humours. Therfore in greate mennes houses, the bread is chipped, and so largely pared, that moche of it abused, and shamfully made into sosse for Dogges: whiche would feede a greate nomber of poore people, but many men bee more affectionate to Dogges, then to men. Barly bread doeth clense, and make the bodie leane.

Galen.ii. aliment.capi.ii.
Sodden bread not holsome.

Barly bread.

Yet thus moche more of bread. If a Manchette stande all night in Borage water, and in the mornyng giuen to a man, that is newe fallen madde, it will helpe hym, vsyng it .xiiii. daies: beyng letten blood in Cephalica, a vaine in the forehed. Also a cake or Manchet, made in this maner, and daily eaten. z. viii. halfe in the mornyng, & as moche at night, helpeth *Gomorra passio*, or runnyng of the raines. A pound of fine flower, and the fine dried pouders of Walnuttes, Chestnuttes, Hasill nuttes, Filberdes, Nutmegges, Almondes, and *Pistacia* these .vii. kindes of Nuttes. z. iii. tempered with this meale, and red wine, and so make your bread. There is also a kinde of Bisquit, made with Anisedes holsome for the lunges, or the reumatike persones. Calamus, long Peper Ginger, Spicknard, and Galinga, bee good to put into the breades of them, whiche haue Dropsie, or Tympanie.

Maister Roger Strages Medicene, brought from Uenis, written by a learned Italian Doctour.

Marcellus.

What is the vertue of Peares?

Hillarius.

Peares.

There be of diuers kinds of Peres, heauier then Aples, not good vntill thei be very ripe, vnlesse thei be tenderly rosted, or baken, and eatē after meales. There is a kind of Peares, groing in the Citee of Norwiche, called the Blacke Freres Peare, very dilicious and pleasaunt, and no lesse profitable vnto a hote stomacke, as I hard it reported, by a right worshipfull Phisicion of the same Citee, called Doctour Mansfeilde, whiche saied, he thought those Peares, without all comparison, were the beste that grewe in any place of Englande. *Dioscorides* saieth *Libr.i.Capi.cxxxii*. That all Peares doe stoppe and binde, so doe the leaues, and therefore saieth he, plasters be wholsome made of thē, to stoppe vomites and laxis. There maie Lye bee made of Peare tree braunches, or barkes: whiche is holsom to seeth wilde Peares in, that be called strāgling, or choke Peares. For so sodden, thei do take awaie benome or hurte: the sam_e Asshes dooe helpe men, beyng drunken in white wine, that be almoste strangled with Mousrums, or soche like. Peares haue many names, as Peare Robert, Peare Jhon, Bushops blessynges,

The operacion of Peares

Blacke Freres Peares of Norwiche

Asshes made of wild peretree, the vertue thereof.

The booke of Simples.   Fol.xiiij.

blessynges, with other pretie names. The redde Warden is of greate vertue, conserued, rosted, or baken, to quenche choller.

Marcellus.

What is the vertue of Aples?   Aples.

Hilarius.

Aples be very cold and windie, hard to digeste, engenderers of ill blood, hurtfull to the flegmatike persones, good to cholerike stomackes, if thei be through ripe, but beste if thei be rosted, or bakē and eaten with grose Peper to bedward. Thei bee of many kindes, as Costardes, the grene Cotes, the Pippen, the quene Aple, and so forthe, the distilled water of Aples, Camphere, Vinegar and Milke, is a good medicen, to anoint the faces of children, that haue the small Pockes, when the saied Pockes be ripe, to kepe them from pittes or erres, prouided, that thei haue giuen them in their Milke Saffron, or Mithridatum, so expell the venome, and kepe them from the aire, duryng the saied sicknesse. The pappe of an Aple with Rose water, applied to the iyes, dooe quenche the burnyng, and take awaie the rednes of theim. Aples bee good in Winter, and prouoke brine: eate theim with a little Salte. Tartes of Aples with Anisedes, make swete breath: there is a windy drinke made of it. Cider: Vergis is not greatly to be lauded, albeit, custome doe permit it.

The operacion of Aples.
Dioscorides Lib.i.cap.131.
For cholerik stomacke.
Costarde, grene cote, Pepins.
A medicen for the small Pockes.

Marcellus.

What is the vertue of Peches?   Peaches.

Hilarius.

The leaues be hote, for if thei be stamped in plaster wise, and applied vnto the bellie, thei kill wormes, the fruite is colde, and very good for the stomacke, thei bee good to bee eaten of theim, that haue stinkyng breathes, of hote causes, eaten of any emptie stomacke, as the counsaill of *Galen*, whiche saieth, if thei be eaten after meate, thei doe corrupt, bothe in them selues, and the meates lately eaten, & thei be binders of the bellie: but Quinces bee moste comfortable after meate, and thei doe enclose the stomack, and letteth vapours to ascende into the brain, and stoppeth vomites. Folkes that be swolne in their bodies, & vse to eate quinces with the grose pouder of Gallinga, Spiknard, Callamus, and Ginger, shall receiue comfort, thei maie be eaten before meate, of the said sicke pacientes, as well as after, but moche vse of them, bee not so profitable, as delectable to the eaters of them.

The operacion of Peches
Hot stomack
Againste stinkyng brethes
Quinces wholsome.
Swellinges

Marcellus.

What be the vertue of Quinces? Iny more then thus?   Quinces.

Hillarius.

If thy stomack be very hote, or moiste, or thy bellie laxatiue, then Quinces be good to be eaten before meate, beyng rosted, or eatē colde, and in this case, the tarter be the better, and Pomgarnet-   Pōgranettes.

The operacion of quinces

c.ii.   tes

The booke of Simples

Isaack in per-
ti. die.

tes be of thesame vertue, as Isaac saieth: but eaten after meate, thei doe enclose the stomacke, and moiste the bellie, thei ought not to be vsed in common meates: the custome of thē hurteth the sinewes, but in the waie of medicen thei bee excellent, and the cores beyng taken out, and preserued in Honie, or kept in their musselege, then thei maie long continue, to the vse of rostyng, or bakyng, for thei bee perillous to the stomack eaten rawe, but preserued, thei doe mightely preuaile against dronkenes, thei be colde in the first degree, and drie in the beginnyng of the seconde

Quinces
rawe hurteth

Against dron-
kenesse.

Marcellus.

Cheries.

What is the vertue of Cheries?

Hillarius.

The operaci-
on of Cheries

THE tarte Cheries vndoubtedly, bee more wholsomer then the swete, and eaten before meate, dooe mollifie the bellie, prepare digestion, and thei bee moste excellent againste hotte burnyng choler, thei be good also after meate, and be of many kindes, as blacke red, and pale, the red Cherie partely tarte is beste, *Galen* and *Rasis*, greatly commende this frute. This frute is cold and moiste in the first degree. And the gumme of a Cherie tree, sodden in wine and drunke, haue all these properties saieth *Dioscorides*: helpeth old coughes, giue good colour to the face, sharpe the sight, maketh perfite digestiō, and maketh clene the raines from grauell. *Plinii* saieth, *Libr.xv.Capi.xxv.* it was a straunge thing to se Cheris at Rome, vntill soche tyme, as *Lucullus* the noble Romain banquished *Mithridates*, the kyng of Pontus. And from thens cam Cheris at that time to Rome, whiche was aboute the incarnacion of our Lorde Christ. lxxiii. yeres. And then within fewe yeres after, all Italie was full, & then moste part of Fraunce: and so to this our great Britain chiefly in Kent, whereas greate plentie doe growe yerely.

Against hote
Choller.
Galen de ali-
men.
Ra.lib.xxiii.
Capit.
Diosc. in libr.
i. capi. cxxix.

Marcellus.

What is the vertue of Grapes, Rasines, Prunes, Barberies, Oringes, and Medlers?

Hillarius.

Grapes.

Hippocrates saieth: that the white Grapes, bee better then the blacke, and wholsomer when thei are twoo or three daies gathered from the Vine, then presently pulled from it, and if thei be swete, thei be partly nutratiue, and warme the bodie, and vnto this agreeth *Galen*, and *Rasis*, whiche semeth to commende swete Grapes, aboue Dates, saiyng: although thei bee not so warme, yet thei doe not stop the bodie, or make opelacion as Dates dooe. Thei be wholsome to be eaten before meate, euen as Nuttes bee good after fishe: towardes the Southe, and Southe Easte partes of the worlde, there bee many growyng in diuers Regions, whereof the Wines bee made, the farthest from vs, the hotter Wine, there be very good grapes growyng

Galen de
alimen ii.
Rasis in. iiii.
alman. xx.

The booke of Simples. Fol.xv.

growyng here in Englande, in many places, as partly I haue seen. Raisons of the Sonne, be very wholsome, and comfort digestion, but the stones and rindes, would be refused: and then thei be good for the splen and liuer, so be Aligante. *Rasis* doeth moche commende them, but vndoubtedly, the small Raisons be hurtfull to the splen. Prunes, and Damaseins haue vertue to relaxe the bellie, if thei be swete and ripe, thei doe nourishe very little, but quenche choller. Grapes, Raisones, Prunes, Plumes, and Slowes, if thei be sower, bee all binders of the bellie. And so is the Barbery, called *Oxiacantha*, and Oringes, excepte the saied Oringes be condited with Sugar, and then thei be good coolers, againste hotte choller, whose rindes be hotte, and drie of nature. The fruite called the Medler, is vsed for a medicen, and not for meate, prouoketh vrine, and of nature is stipticke.

Raisones.

To comfort digestion. Splene and Liuer. Swete prunes bee laxatiue, but tarte be bindyng. Oxiacantha, callee the Barbarie. Mespila called the Medler.

Marcellus.
What is the vertue of Capers and Oliues?
Hillarius.

Freshe Capers be hotte, and drie in the seconde degree, and eaten before meates, doe greatly comfort digestion: and bee the beste thynges for the Splene, or to clense melanchollie, so is the oile of Capers to anoint the Splene, or left side, that can be taken. Preserued Oliues in Salte, eaten at the beginnyng of meales, doe greatly fortefie the stomacke, and relaxeth the bellie, clenseth the liuer, and is hote and drie, in the seconde degree. The decoction of Caper barkes, helpe the Splene, beyng dronke.

Capers and Oliues.

Good for the Splene.

Marcellus.
What is the vertue of Aloes?
Hillarius.

There bee twoo kindes of Aloes, one is named *Succatrina*, whiche is like a liuer, clere, brittle, bitter, coloured betwene redde and yellowe: this is beste for medicenes, a little of this tempered with Rose water, and beyng put into the iyes, helpeth the droppyng, and wattrie iyes. Also it is put into many excellent medicenes, laxatiue, as Safron, Mirrhe, Aloes, mingled together, in the forme of pilles, is the moste excellente medicen against the Pestilence, as it is written in this booke folowyng. Honie and Aloes mingled together, doe take awaie the markes of stripes, and also doe mundifie sores, and vlcers, it doeth clense the aboundaunce of choller and fleume from the stomack, it is not good to be taken in Winter. For *Auicen* doeth forbidde it, but in the Spring tyme, or Haruest, the pouder therof, the waight of a Frēch croune, mingeled with the water of Honie, or Mede, and so dronke in the mornyng, it doeth clense bothe Choller and fleume. There is another grosse Aloes, which is good for horse, tempered with Ale, and ministered, aswell to other greate beastes, as horses, the waight of halfe

Aloes.

Two kindes of Aloes.

To help watrie iyes.

Against the Pestilence, called pillule Ruffi. Markes of stripes, in the skinne.

To clense choler and fleme.

c.iii. an

The booke of Simples.

<small>A cause of the Emeroides.</small> an vnce, and thus moche haue I saied of Aloes: but if Aloes be cleane washed, thei be the holsomer, many vnwashed Aloes, will cause Emeroides.

Marcellus.
What is the vertue of Dictamnum?
Hillarius.

It is of a singuler vertue, leaued like vnto Penerial, but greater, and somwhat rough, and tasteth like Ginger, whē it is bitten on: this herbe is incomperable, for his singuler goodnes, in spedy deliueraunce of ded children from their mothers, beyng drunke in syruppe. There be twoo kindes of theim, the one called *Dictamnum*, and the other *Pseudodictamnum*, one of the garden, thother of the field: and haue many rootes, the leaues be onely occupied, and not the staukes, being sodden in wine, it draweth corruption, out of depe woundes, if any man be wounded with Iron: as Dager, spere, naile, piece of harneis, haileshotte, or maile, droppe in the iuce of this herbe, in the saied wounde, and eftsones it will drawe forthe the Iron, therin fixed, so that the paciente drinke of thesame herbe in wine. *Dioscorides* reporteth, that wilde beastes, and Goates emong the Grekes, whē thei were wounded with arrowes, did feede on this herbe, whose vertue caste out the arrowes, and healed the wounde. It will doe the like also to mankinde, if he be not smitten with a mortall wound. The smoke of this Dittan, called *Dictamnum*, do driue awaie any liuyng thing from manne, that are benemous, as Tode, Neute, Skorpion. &c. And the noble Poete Virgil doe greatly cōmende thesame precious herbe, with these pleasaunt swete verses, saiyng:

<small>Dictamnum is a good sodain salue for a souldiour in the fielde.

Dioscorides Lib iii. capit. xxxi.
A maruelus worke of Dictamnum.

Libr. xii. Ænedos.</small>

Hic venus indigno nati concussa dolore
Dictamnum genitrix Cretæ carpit ab Ida,
Puberibus claudem foliis, & flora commentem
Purpurio: non illa feris incognita capris
Gramina, cum tergo volucres hæsere sagittæ.

Mercellus.

I praie you, what is the nature of Helenium, called Enula campana, whiche we common plain people call Alacampano.
Hillarius.

This herbe of worthie memorie, haue thus been called, as some doe saie, from the battaill of Troie: which was before the incarnacion of Gods onely soonne, our God and sauiour Iesus Christ. 1189. And then was named Elenium, of the lamentable pitifull teares of Helena, wife to Menelaus, when she was violētly taken awaie by Paris into Phrigia, hauyng this herbe in her handes. Or as other

<small>Enula cāpana
A fable perhappes.</small>

doe

The booke of Simples. Fol.xvj.

do saie, this noble Helena made a gooly medicen of this herbe, against the dedly venime, or poisone of Serpentes. And Plini reporteth, that Julius Augustus the Emperour, did eate of this daily with his meat. It preuaileth against poison, it dooe comfort the harte, as it is saied: *Enula campana reddit præcordia sana. Auen.* The wine of this herbe, dooe clense the lightes, breast, and lunges: and swallowed with cleane Honie, it causeth to spit, and breaketh winde. Balme and this herbe be great frendes to the harte: and if it be sodden with Rue, it preuaileth against colike, and ruptures, whiche cometh of winde: it is not exactly hote and drie. It is very comfortable in bathes, to wasshe and clense the bodie from filth, itche, skabbes, and kepe the partes of the body warme, and make them redde, that were pale: and is good for *ischiadas* called Siatica, or paines in ye huccle bones, applied plaster waies warme. The roote is of greate vertue, saieth *Galen Libr.vi.Simplic.Medic.* If it bee champed, saieth Plini, fasting in the morning, it will confirme and stablisshe the teeth: and the oile is good against the tourmentes of the guttes, whiche be vexed with winde, and helpeth the sinewes. If any wilde beast fall in any net, died with thesame Enula, thei shalbe poisoned therewith: as *Galen* saieth in his booke *de Theriaca ad pisonem*, but some wisemen doe thinke rather it bee a fable, then a true historie. And thus I dooe ende of this good herbe, whose chief vertue is in the rootes.

A bitter dissinicion.

Auicen.scë. Can.cap.Enulacampana.

Mercellus.

What is a Tassill good for, besides the Clothe workers businesse, within his shoppe.

Hillarius.

A Tasell is called *Dipsacus* in Greke, by a contrary name, for it receiueth in concauite and holonesse, dewe and raine, to releue the drinesse. It is also called *virga pastoris*, Sheperdes rodde, and Fullers Thistell. There bee twoo kindes, one wilde and vnprofitable: the other is a good seruant in the common wealth, for trimming of clothe and cappes, and it is a stiffe Tasell. The rootes and leaues with the prickes, be drie in the seconde egree: if this herbe be sodden in water to a thicknesse, and drawen through a strainer, and sodden againe vnto a more thicknes, this laied vpon chappes, or places opened with winde, as in Marche, it healeth theim. Thesame put into a Fistula, doeth heale it, and taketh awaie Wartes, so saieth *Dioscorides* and *Plini.*

Tassell.

Marcellus.

What doe you saie of an herbe, called *Hypericon?*

Hillarius.

Dioscorides calleth this herbe *Libr. tertio Capitulum. Cliiii. Hypericum, Chamæpityn, Androsæmon, Or Corion,* with soche coppie of names: The seede dooe partely smell like Rosen. If this herbe bee chafed and broken in ones hande, it sendeth forthe a bloodie iuce, saieth he, the seedes be blacke, and the flower yellowe, it groweth in the mo-

Hypericon, S. Jhons herbe, weede grasse, or worte.

c.iiii. neth

The booke of Simples.

neth of July, and August, and is commonly knowen in euery place: and of temperament or nature, is hotte and drie. *Galen* saieth, it prouoketh vrine: all the herbe must be put to the medicen, as to salues, then it healeth moiste and stinkyng putrified sores. And beyng dronke, either the water, the Syruppe, the iuce, or pouder, healeth *Ischiadis*, or the Siatica, of the same minde is *Dioscorides*. But thei must drinke of the sede saieth he, by the space of xl. daies. And this Saincte Jhons worte or herbe, helpeth tartians or quartaines, dronke with wine: the iuce yealeth any burnte place, and is good for the stone. *Asirum, Androsæmum* and *Coris*, be kinsfolke. But the seedes of *Asirum* will purge, thei differ in forme. But for tyme, sauour, place, and nature, thei bee moche like one vnto the other: And are all named emong vs, sainct Jhons worte or herbe.

Galen Libr viii. Simplex. medicamentorum.

Marcellus.

Ur fieldes doe growe full of Scabios, euery mere and balke is full of it in June: Some dooe vse this herbe for the Pestilens, commonly called the plague. Wherefore doe the learned men, as *Dioscorides* and *Galen* saie it is good.

Hillarius.

Scabius for scabbes, it taketh ye name of the propertie, the righte name is Stoebe or Spora there be two kindes of thē.

Scabiosa so named of old tyme, because it is giuen in drinke inwardly, or ointmentes outwardly, to heale scabbes, sores, corrupcion in the stomacke, yea, and is most frend emong all other herbes, in the tyme of the Pestilence, to drinke the water with Mithridatum a mornynges. It stoppeth the bloodie flixe, and Hemeroides, and an ointment made thereof, healeth *Antrax*, called the Carbuncle, or hotte burnyng Pestilence, boche, or fearfull sore. *Galen* saith *Lib. vii. Simplicium medicam.* that it is hot, drie, and bitter. And haue vertue to binde, drie, and stop, it will ioine a freshe wounde together. The iuce dropped into the iye, healeth it, if it be pricked or bleede. It is good to be dropped into foule runnyng moiste eares: it should seme, beyng bothe hotte and drie. If it be sodden in wine, and drunke, it drieth superfluous humors. *Dioscorides* calleth it *Stoebe*, the flowers is like a Blewe or white thrummed hatte, the stalk rough, the vpper leaues ragged, and the leaues next the grose rootes be plainer. Under whom often tymes, Frogges will shadowe theim selues, from the heate of the daie: hoppyng and plaiyng vnder these leaues, whiche to them is a pleasaunt Tente or pauillion, saieth *Aristophanes*, whiche maie a plade, wherein Frogges made pastime.

Marcellus.

Buglose. What is the vertue of Buglosse?

Hillarius.

To comforte the harte. Fransie.

It is an herbe moste temperate, betwene hotte and colde, of an excellent vertue, a comforter of the hart, a purger of melancholie, a quieter of the Fransie, a purger of the vrine, holsome to be dronke in wine, but moste effectually in syruppe, *Dioscorides*, and *Galen* doth greatly commende this herbe, and that doeth daily experience proue.

Marcellus.

Marcellus.

What is the vertue of Basill? — Basill.

Hillarius.

This herbe is warme in the seconde degree, hauyng the vertue of moistnes, and if it be sodden in wine, with Spicknarde, and dronke, it is good against dropsies, windes, fleumes, coldnes of the harte, hardnes of the stomacke. The sauour of Basill doeth comfort the brain and harte, the vse of this herbe in meates, doeth decaie the sight.

— Ozinum or swet oder, or redolent.
Dropsie.
For the brain and harte.

Mercellus.

What is the vertue of Polipodie? — Polipodie.

Hillarius.

If this herbe be soddē with Beates, and Mallowes, in the broth of a Henne, and dronke, it will lose the bellie, and clense fleume, the roote of this herbe, beyng drie, and beaten in fine pouder, and drawen into the nosethrilles, helpeth a disease called *Polipus.* *Galen,* and *Actuarius,* affirmeth that .ʒ.i. of the rootes of Sene, soddē with Polipodie in Mede, or Honie, and so strained, doth purge choller and melancollie, without paine. It is of the like vertue and effecte, sodden in the broth of a Henne, or Ptisane, and is of order temperate, relaxyng.

— Fleume.
Actua in li. de cōpo.med.

Marcellus.

What is the vertue of Burnete? Whiche in Sommer tyme is vsed to bee put in bowles, & glasses of wine, serued at the table.

Hillarius.

It is very pleasaunt to be putte in cleane cuppes, goblettes, or peces, wherein is cleane Frenche wine, it maketh it pleasaunte with the iuce of Lemondes, and good white sugar, it hath golden flowers, grene leaues, purple rootes of the out side, & white within: and doeth drie and binde, and stoppeth the bloody flixe very well.

— Potentylla.

Marcellus.

What is the vertue of Spinage? — Spinage.

Hillarius.

It is an herbe moche vsed in meate, colde and moiste in the first degree: it mollifieth, and maketh softe the bellie, it is good for them that be hotte and drie, and ill for flegmatike men.

— Mollesyng.

Marcellus.

What is the vertue of Vinegar? — Vinegar.

Hillarius.

Vinegar is colde and drie, and is hurtfull for them that bee melancollie, but when it is drunke, or powred vpon an outwarde wounde, it stoppeth the blood, it also killeth hotte apostumacions

— The propertie of vinegar

The booke of Simples.

To helpe goute. cions of *Erisippilas*: it is an enemie to the Sinewes, Vinegar and Brimstone sodden together, is good for the goute, to washe it with all. Vinegar tempered with wolle, helpeth a disease called *soda*, in the hedde, applied warme vnto the place. It is good in Sauce, for warme and moiste men: Vinegar with cleane clarified Honie, *Penidies*, and faire water sodden together, doeth greatly helpe the paines of the throte, lunges, and stoppyng the winde, and quencheth hotte diseases. And sharp Vinegar mingeled with Salte, and put vpon the bityng of a Dogge, doeth heale it: and against poison it is excellent, chiefly to drinke a little thereof against the Pestilence, in a mornyng.

Paines in the throte.

Bityng of a Dogge.

Against the Pestilence.

Mercellus.

Setwall. What is the vertue of Setwall?

Hillarius.

Theophrastus of Setwall.

Vomites strained.

IT is hotte and drie in the seconde degree, and is good, the pouder thereof to be drunke, is moste of effect against the pestilence, except Mithridatum. It is good against poison, winde, chollerike, and colde passions of the harte: and doeth restraine vomites, the waight of .viii.℥. doeth suffice to bee drunke in Ale or Wine, vpon an emptie stomacke.

Marcellus.

Mellilote. Sertula, or kinges croun What is the vertue of Mellilote?

Hillarius.

IT hath vertue to ripe, and is more hotter then colde, Mellilote Flaxesede, Rose leaues, Camphere, and womannes Milke, tempered together, doeth make a goodly medicen, against the hotte inflamacion of the iyes. If this herbe be drunke in wine, it doeth mollifie the hardnes of the stomacke and liuer: the moste excellent plaster against the paines of the Splene, doeth *Mesue* describe, whiche is made of Mellilote. Vinegar, Roses, and Mellilote together, helpeth headache, applied it to the forehedde in a clothe.

For the iyes, stomack, and liuer.
To helpe the Splene.

Marcellus.

Tyme. What is the vertue of Tyme?

Hillarius.

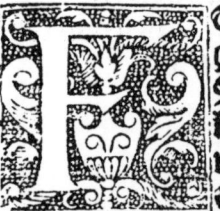T is vehemente of heate, with drinesse in the thirde degree, *Dioscorides* saieth, if it bee drunke with Vinegar and Salt, it purgeth fleume: sodden with Honie or Mede, it hath vertue to clense the lunges, and the breast, matrix raines, and blader, and killeth wormes. The pouder of Tyme eaten in Potage, is holsome for the iye sight: Theophrastus saith, there be twoo kindes of Tyme, thone white, thother blackeshe. There be no flowers growing in feldes or gardens, better beloued of Bene, then the flowers of Time: and that yere wherin the greatest plentie of these flowers be seen, that same yere Honie doth abound,

Theop. lib.ii. Capi. vi.

and

The booke of Simples. Fol.xviij.

and when thei bee scase, and not fertill, then there is little, or no good honie ẏ yere, *Dioscorides* saieth in his .iiii. boke, that *Epithymum* is the flower of the harder Tyme. ʒ.i. of Tyme dried, and beate in pouder, mingeled with .ʒ.iiii. of Orimell, and drunke of an emptie stomach, before diner and supper, helpeth the stomacke, guttes, matrire, and blader: and is good for them that haue redde blered iyes, and for those that bee tourmented of the goute. *Galen* commẽdeth Tyme in his .vi. booke of Simples, so doeth *Aetius* with these commendacions aforesaid. The whiter the Tyme is, with white and purple flowers, the better it is, the blacker the worse. And thus I doe cõclude of Tyme, desirẏng God that we maie spende the tyme well to his glory, and profite of our neighbour, for tyme cannot be called again, but by little and little slippes awaie, thei whiche Godly obserue the tyme, in tyme to come, shall receiue the frutes of their owne labours, with happie liues, quiete myndes, and blessed endes: wheras the shamefull abusers of tyme, and misusers of themselues. Although euill spent time, seme well vnto them, yet their liues be wicked, their labor fruitlesse, and their ende horrible: as ones shall appere whẽ death doeth come, whiche is thende of euery tyme.

¶ Time cannot bee called againe.

Mercellus.

What is the vertue of swete Calamus odoratus, called Calamus Aromaticus?

¶ Swete Calamus odoratus.

Hillarius.

T is an excellent swete roote, and profitable for men, if the Poticares kepe it not, vntill it bee rotten: it is hotte and drie in the beginning, & to the middes of the second degree. It hath power to clense, to drie, and to waste, all windes within the bodie, without hurt. *Galen* doth greatly commende the sauour of it: Thei that drinke of this roote sodden in wine, shall haue remedy of the white Morphewe, and recouer good colours in their faces, and this haue I often proued. It helpeth to clense, purge, and drie, the water that is betwene the skin, and the fleshe: beyng drunke with the sedes of Smalage, Parsely, and Fenell, sodden well together and strained, it helpeth crampes, and sicknenes in the sinewes, being dronke with wine, sodden with Sage and freshe Cappers: it helpeth the coldnes of the splene, liuer, and raines. Also it augmenteth seede of generacion, and purge termes menstrual if the pouder be dronke. What is better in Wormewood, or Sage Ale, then Calamus to be dronke: for them whiche haue the dropsie, as Asclides. &c. It wil expulse and put out sores in the blader, and make the stinkyng brine to be swete: truely it is a noble herbe, but the vertue is in the roote.

¶ To waste winde in the bodie.

¶ A remedy for the white Morphewe.

¶ Seede augmented.

Marcellus.
What is the vertue of Ginger?
Hillarius.

¶ Ginger.

It

The booke of Simples.

Auerois in.v. in coll.
Mesuæ in.iiii distint.

It is hote in the thirde degree, and moiste in the ende of the first, if it be vncolloured, white, and not roten, it is very good, moste chiefly if it bee conserued and grene, as *Mesua* saieth, it maketh warme a cold stomacke, and consumeth windes, helpeth euill digestiō and maketh meate go easely downe into the stomacke.

Marcellus.

Oile Oliues beste.
What is the vertue of oile made of Oliues?

Hillarius.

To digeste colde herbes.
Auerois comēded oile in quito de onis.
Oile of roses.
Againste Fransies.

Grene oile of Oliues, is the mother of all Oiles, whiche doeth drawe into her owne nature, the vertues of herbes, leaues, flowers, fruites, and rootes, sweete Sallet oile is wholsome, to digest colde herbes, and Sallettes, tempered with sharpe Vinegar and Sugar: newe Oile doeth moiste, and warme the stomacke, but olde oile corrupteth the stomacke, and cleaueth to the Lunges, and maketh one hoarse. Oile of Roses, and sharpe Vinegar tempered together, is good to anoint the foreheds of them, that be troubled with extreme heate, or fransie: so that Buglosse be sodden in their Possetale, or els drynke the syruppes of Endiue, or Buglosse. There bee many goodly vertues in compounded oiles, bothe to make hote, and to coole the bodie, whē it is extreme hotte, as the greate learned man *Mesue*, hath described in his *Antidotarii*. Of oiles, you shall haue plentie followyng.

Marcellus.

Rosemarie.
What is the vertue of Rosemarie?

Hillarius.

Kinges euill
The braine comforted.

Rosemarie is an herbe of greate vertue, hotte and drie, sodden in Wine, and dronke before meate: it doeth heale the Kynges euill, or paines in the throte, as *Dioscorides*, and *Galen* saieth. The sauour of it doeth comfort the braine and harte, the flowers of Rosemarie is an excellent Cordiall, called *di Anthos*, and be good after feuers, or for Melancholie men. And the seedes drunke in wine, helpeth the fallyng sicknes, and paines of the breast.

Marcellus.

Agremonie.
What is the vertue of Agrimonie?

Hillarius.

Olde sore.
Bityng of Serpentes.

Dioscorides saieth, that if this herbe with Swines grease, be stamped together, and laied vpon an olde rotten sore beyng hote, it hath vertue to heale it. The seede of this herbe drunke with wine, it is good against the bityng of Serpentes, stoppyng of the Liuer, and bloodie flixe. The syrup of it is good to open the liuer.

Marcellus.

Mugworte.
What is the vertue of Mugworte?

Hillarius.

Mugworte,

Mugworte, Fetherfewe, and Tansie, be very hote and drie, in the seconde degree: Mugworte, Spurge, and Oile of Almondes, tempered plasterwise, and applied colde to the sicke pained stomacke, will bryng health. It is good in bathes saieth *Galen*, it is wholsome for women: it clenseth, warmeth, comforteth the matrixe, and breaketh the stone. *Plini* saieth, it is good againſt bityng of Serpentes, and holsome for trauailyng men, if thei cary it, it lighten them from werines Tansie doeth kill and caste wormes from children, dronke with wine, a colde plaster stamped, and laied vpon the bellie of a woman, whose childe is dedde within her: it will seperate the dedde childe, from the liuyng mother. *Galen* saieth in his sixt booke of Simples, there bee twoo kindes of Mugworte. The one is commonly knowen to vs, the other groweth nere the sea side: thei be bothe of singuler vertues, their waters beyng stilled, their syruppes prepared, bee very wholsome for the corrupted, or stopped matrixe: and also the herbe is good for bathes, in soche purposes for women. And was firste founde of a noble Quene, named *Artimisia*, wife to *Mausolus*, kyng of *Caria*, whiche was bothe learned in herbes and plantes, chaste of life, comely of person: and so loued her husbande, that when he was dedde, she made a sepulcher, whiche was so excellent, costly, and riche, that it was compted to be one of the wonders, and greatest maruailes of the worlde, she called this herbe *Latifolia*, and *Tenufolia*, after her owne name, *Artemisia*.

A paines stomacke.

Breakyng the stone.

Killing wormes in childre

A preset help of a ded child.

To nese.

Marcellus.

What is the vertue of Parseley, and Saxifrage?

Hillarius.

Thei haue vertue to breake the stone: Parseley is hote in the second degree, and drie in the middest of the third. The sede dronk with white wine: prouoketh the menstruall tearmes, as *Dioscorides* saieth, also Smallage hath the like vertue, as furder appereth.

Mercellus.

Now saie on, and shewe to me, my good maister, I praie you, of *Elleborus* the white, and of *Elleborus* the blacke.

Hillarius.

Elleborus *Candidus*, whiche causeth vomites, very stronge and daungerous for conuulcion, and is called *Albus*: because the roote is whitishe, long stalkes, reddishe leaues, with ribbes in them, in the forme of Planten leaues. Many yellowe flowers, growing vpon stalkes, by them selues and growyng in colde groundes. The rootes muste bee gathered in Harueſt: and this herbe is hote and drie, in the thirde degree. And is perilous to bee giuen, to women with childe, olde folkes and children: or to tender people, or in Winter, but in Sommer onely, and

The booke of Simples.

How to correct Elleborus albus.

and before supper. But one dragme, put in Milke or Furmentie: but firste doe thus. Cutte a Radishe roote in the greate ende, cliue it ouerthwarte: then put in your *Elleborus Albus* into it, one night, or twelue howers, then presse it harde, whiche will not onely take the venim, from this *Elleborus*. But also giue it vertue, that it shall not hurte nature, or put the bodie into daunger, whē vomites approcheth. This wil helpe falling sicknes, *vertigo*, Melancholly, madnesse, white Leprosie, windes in the guttes, Dropsie, Timpanie, Goutes, Quartens, Coughes, and many soche like, and maketh neselyng. &c.

Of Elleborus niger.

Elleborus nigar, is called *Melanpodion*, not onely for the blacknes: but the inuenter was called *Melampus*, a keper of goates. It is hote and drie in the third degree, and is planted in the Garden, and is Beares foote: black rough, hearie rootes, like the bushe vpon the breast of a foule, whiche we call the Cocke of Turkaie. It haue all the vertues, that the white haue, and more, three penie waight in pouder dronke, cast forthe wormes, clense fleume, melanchollie, and dropsie. And will clense the matrice, and expulse, or caste forthe the dedde childe. It is good for *Pessares* for women: the iuce is good, for to be put into the eare againste defnes. In plasters, it killeth wormes: the iuce thereof helpeth horse, for the bottes, and Swine that be infected. Or els if it be putte into their eares, it will helpe theim, when thei be pained in their heddes. No beastes dare eate thereof, it is so bitter, nor foules, but onely Quailes: As *Aristotle*, *Auicen*, *Galen*, and *Lucretius* affirmeth. These herbes bee wholsome in outward plasters, to clense melanchollie, and to drie fleume.

Marcellus.
What is the vertue of Centaurie? Or *fell terræ*?
Hillarius.

PLINI saieth, that the syrupe of this herbe, dronke with a little Vinegar and Salt, doeth clense the bodie: the leaues and flowers be of greate vertue, to be sodden, and dronke against all rawe humours of grosse fleumes, waterie, or windie. It doeth clense cruent or bloody matter, within the bodies of men or women: the pouder of this herbe, is good in pessaries for women, causing the dedde childe, to depart from the mother. And is wholsome against the Pestilence, in the tyme of Winter: and is hote and drie, and of two kindes, and healeth bothe olde and newe woundes, as *Galen* writeth to *Papiam*, of the vertue of little Centaurie. This herbe was founde with his vertue, by that olde noble clarke *Chyron Centaurus*, the inuerter of Herbes, Astronomie, and Musike.

Marcellus.
What is the vertue of Penerialle?
Hillarius.

IT is an herbe of moche vertue and profite, hotte and drie in the third degree, *Dioscorides* saieth: if this herbe be sodden with Honie, and Aloes, and dronke. It will clense the Liuer, and purge the blood

The booke of Simples.   Fol.xx.

blood moste chiefly: it helpeth the lunges. *Simeon Sethi* saieth, if a woman drinke it with white Wine: it will also prouoke, and clense the termes menstruall. And is also a very wholsome potherbe, and moche vsed emong Puddyng makers: whiche was inuented of some Phisician, because of the warmnes and goodnes againste melancholie. The iuce with Vinegar, put into the nose, is good againste the Fransie, or Lunatike sicknes.

Marcellus.

What is *Lichen* called Liuerworte, that growe in Welles, darke colde places, and rockes?

Hillarius.

Without all doubte *Lichen* dooe so growe in darcke places, and is called Liuerwort: for it is good against the sicknesse of the Liuer, it is colde and drie. Yet it hath a watrie humour, it is vnpleasaunte in sauour: it stoppeth the bloodie flixe, it healeth a ryng worme, saith *Dioscorides*: stamped with Honie, it helpeth the yellowe Janders, if the mouth and tongue be anointed therwith. The iuce stoppeth woundes from bledyng, *Galen* and *Plini* agreeth to the same.

hepatica lichē called Liuer worte.

Diosco. li. iiii. Capi. xlviii.

Marcellus.

What saie you then of the herbe, belong to the Lunges, called Lungworte?

Hillarius.

Leonardus Fuchius saieth, *Pulminaria* doe growe out of the Oke tree, or stonie places, hauyng softe leaues, the vpper side grene, and the nether whitishe, with little small bladers, vpon the crumpled leaues, and the whole lumpe of this herbe, saieth he, is like the Lunges of mankinde. It is dryyng and bindyng, and not cold and moiste, as some doe affirme: and the reason is, because it growe from the Oke, whiche is of the same nature, and temperamente. And this herbe dooe close newe woundes togither: moste chiefly it helpeth the Lunges, or spittyng of blood, and stoppeth termes immoderate, and the bloodie flure. Mary *Mathiolus* doe saie, that Lungwort haue leaues like to Buglosse: sharp, rough, white spottes, purple flowers, very like to the greate Dogges tongue. It hath the same vertue, that the other haue, and woorketh one effecte: therefore it is no errour, to call theim bothe a like, Lungworte, or *Pulminaria*. Specially, because twoo greate learned men, so call them of their elders and vertues. The last Lungworte, did *Iulianus Marostica*, a noble Phisicion did vse to seeth in water, to the one halfe, puttyng in Sugar, and made a simple syrup, to giue his pacientes, to stoppe spittyng of blood, and to heale sores of the lunges.

Lungworte because it is like the lunges of man.

Super Diosco. lib. 4. cap. 48

Iulianus Marostica his syrupe for the lunges.

D.ii.   Marcellus.

The booke of Simples.

Mercellus.
What saie you then to Mercurie, what is the vertue, and why is it so named?

Hillarius.

Mercurie.

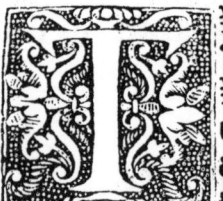

Mercurie helpeth concepcion.

His aunciente inuented herbe, was founde of *Mercurius*, whiche florished about 164. yeres, before Christes birth. He was the sonne of Maia, this man was afterwarde called one of the Goddes, for his wonderous wisedome, and inuencion of Musike, and other Artes. He emong all other herbes, so loued this, that he for the singular goodnes therof, he called it after his owne name, Mercurie. Whereof there bee twoo kindes, male and female: the firste haue blackishe leaues, the second whitishe, thei be hote and drie in the first degree. *Dioscorides* saieth, this doe moue the benefite of the bellie: thei be very good for women, after their naturall termes be past, to drinke either in syrup, or decoction, to helpe concepcion. The male Mercurie for men, the female for women. This Mercurie is very good in glisters laratiue: we call Rumex Mercurie, whiche haue golden Sandes vpon the backeside of the leaues, whiche be also solutiue, and beneficiall for the bellie. Sodden with Mallowes, doe purge the bellie, and expulse fleume, but it anoieth the stomacke, saieth *Plini*.

Marcellus.

Mallowes.

Mallowes so called, *ab emollienda aluo nomen traxit*, it taketh his name of molifiyng the bellie: and thei bee good with Lettis, parboiled and eaten in fine Sallet oile, to molifie the bellie.

Mallowes for nature be very good
To relaxe the bellie, and purge the blood.

Hillarius.

Galen. li. vii. simplic.

Dioscorides and Galen saieth, there bee twoo kindes of theim, one of the garden, whiche is greate with flowers like Roses, called *Bismalue*, and the lesser kinde of the fielde and wood: this herbe is commonly knowen. The more that Mallowes be watrie the lesser thei be of vertue, and the drier the seedes are, the more thei be of stregth. And Mallowes be moiste and slimie of nature, relaxing the bellie, but hurtfull for the stomacke, saieth *Dioscorides*, the leaues with Salt and honie eaten, healeth the paines of the throte, and *Anginæ*. But vsed in woundes or sores, put in no Salte, thei heale the stingyng of Bees: thei bee excellent good in glisters, to purge for the bellie, raines, and stone. The roote sodden and dronke, and eftsones vomited, doe preuaile againste poisone: the leaues stamped, and tempered in oile, dooe

A medicene for womens breastes.

take runnyng vlcers from the hedde. And sodden in brin or pisse, it taketh awaie skurfe, skabbes. &c. from the face. The roote sodden softe, and laied warme vpon a womans breast, with blacke wolle, doe heale the same, whē it aketh, burneth, swelleth, or is harde. So will the leaues

The booke of Simples.   Fol.xxj.

ues, one handfull sodden in Oile and Wine, purge women, saith *Plini*. The leaues sodden in Wine, warme applied to the mouthe of the matrice, after deliueraunce of the childe, doe staie the fallyng doune, and maketh softe. It is good against the feuer, called *Sacra ignis*, the holy fire: whiche we call sainct Anthonies fire. Sodden in Oile and Uinegar: and applied to the member, where as it burneth. The seedes dronke in Wine, doe clense the stomacke from noisomnes, and rotten stinking fleume and melancholie. The iuce often tymes drunke of Mallowes, helpeth from the fallyng euill: and also clense the Lunges, and cause one to speake cleare, saieth *Simeon Sethi*.

    There is also another Mallowe, called *Athæa, Althos* dooe signifie medicene, or remedie: this Mallowe so named, is excellente in vertue. I thinke it to be that, whiche we call the Frenche Mallowe: the leaues and the flowers be hotte and drie, in the first degree, and so be the rootes in the beginnyng of the second degree. Sodden with Swines grece Goose grece, and Terebintin applied to the bellie, to aswage the greuous swellyng, burnyng, or inflation. The same medicene dooe open thynges venemous within the members, that be stopped, saith *Dioscorides*. Seeth the roote in wine, and drinke this wine, it openeth vrine, clense the raines, ease the stone: and is good for *Ischiades*, called Siatica, ruptures, and the bloodie flixe. *Galen* saieth *Lib.vi.Simpli.medicamen.* the seedes be good for the stone and raines: the roote sodden, doe stoppe the bloodie flixe. *Theophrastus* saith, to be drunke in swete wine, helpeth ruptures, and the cough, and with oile, it healeth vlcers. And sodden with fleshe it doeth conglutinate, or ioyne together, thynges seperate within the bodie: and yet it digesteth, looseth, and concocteth crude matter, saieth *Galen*. The leaues sodden in white wine, quencheth the heate, and abateth the swellyng of a womans breast. Who is able to giue more commendacion or praise to any herbe, then to this herbe, for the singular medicen called *Dialthæa*, whiche is in the booke of Compoundes. Mallowes bee commended of all good writers. *Plinius* saieth, that the Mallowes in Arabia, within seuen monethes bee so fertill, and lustie in growyng, that thei be as bigge as staues forthwith, he call the trees. Furder he writeth a marueilous historie of a Mallowe, whiche was monstruous to beholde. There was saie he, in Mauritania, somtyme a garden, where *Hysperides* (whiche were the .iii. doughters of *Atlas*, which kept the garden) wherein grewe Oringes, called the golden Iples, taken awaie by Hercules, in this Garden grewe a Mallowe, twentie foote long: and no man was able to fadom the same. Soche like Mallowes groweth in Inde, & thus I end of Mallowes, good frend *Marcellus*

Althos doe signifie medicene.

Dioscori.lib. iii.capit.146.

Plini.Libr. xix.Capi.iiii.

Marcellus.

Curste fellowes, and tauntyng marchauntes, will saie in dirision skorne, and mockage, when thei bee angrie with others. I care not for theim, no, not a Rushe: is a Rushe of so small an estimacion, and nothyng worth: As it is counted.

                           D.iii.   Hillarius.

The booke of Simples.

Hillarius.

Sir Thomas Rushe.

Rushes doe growe in Fennes, and drie groundes, and bee commonly knowen. And I my self did knowe a Rushe, growyng in a Fenne side, by Orforde in Suffolke, that might haue spente three hundred Markes by yere. &c. Was not this Rushe of good estimacion? A fewe soche Rushes be better, then many greate Trees and Bushes. But *Marcellus* thou dooest not knowe that countrey, where sometyme I did dwell, at a place called Blarall, nere to that Rushe Bushe: I would all the Rushes within this Realme, were as riche in value: it would make a florishing common wealth, and moche plentie, no beggers, but riches, and a golden worlde.

Mercellus.

Pouertie is better emong the common people, then aboundaunce of riches.

THE olde prouerbe is, wishers and woulders, be no good householders: And if there were soche plentie, fare well labour, arte, learnyng, and obedience: But neede is the pricke and whippe, that cause the Plowman to trauell, the Mariner to saile, the Scholemaister to teache. And to conclude, euery manne to labour in his callyng, through whiche labour and industrie, the teachyng of youth, the gouernemente of age, the buildyng of Citees, the mainteinaunce of good lawes: the rewardyng of vertues: the punishement of vices: the defendyng of enemies, and rewardyng of frendes. And obedience to princes be mainteined. Whereas through soche aboundaunce, al wer cast awaie: and euery man would be a maister. Euery one would disdaine seruice: and so at length, all should be tourned into slauery, and the harmonie of the common wealth, should be chaunged into horror,

If harpstrynges were of one degree, vnpleasaunte were that hermonie.

wheras no order is. Example, if all the pipes in the Orgaines, wer of one tune, or one degree vnpleasaunt wer that Musike. But here will I stoppe, and laie a strawe, and fall into my bias againe. I praie thee answere me, what a very Rushe is, whiche groweth in the felde.

Hillarius.

Commonly knowen, and of sonderie kindes, as Rushes growyng in Riuers, and runnyng streames: as there be greate plentie rounde about the Isle of Ely, my natiue countrey, whereof the plain people make Mattes, and horse collers, of the greater Rushes. And of the smaller thei make lightes or Candelles for the Winter. Rushes that growe vpon drie groundes, bee good to strewe in Halles, Chambers, and Galleries to walke vpon, defendyng apparell, as traines of gounes, and Kertles from duste. Rushes be olde Courtiers, and when thei be nothyng worthe: then thei be caste out of the doores, so be many that dooe tread vpon theim. A Rushe is called *Iuncus*, that is a Bulle Rushe, the Rushe bearyng blacke seedes, is called *Atrifer*, whose seedes drunke in Medicen, dooe stoppe flire, and termes immoderate: and the same seedes be good for to cause slepe. *Galen* speakyng of *Iuncus*, he saieth

Old Rushes and old courtiers, be paste pleasure.

Lib.viii. simplic.medica.

the

The booke of Simples. Fol.xxij.

some bare seede, whiche is good in medicen, that is to bring slepe. The other that haue no seedes, be vnprofitable. *Dioscorides* saieth, the seedes of the Rushe of Inde doe bryng slepe, vsed in pocion.

There is also *Iuncus odoratus*, of twoo sortes, *Plini* doe call the first *Triangularis*, it smelleth as swete as the Rose, when it is broken. An other *Rotundus*, the Apothecaries doe call it *Squinantum*, and groweth in *Africa*, but yet *Dioscorides* is of that minde. The beste growe nere to Babilon: because this *Squinantum* is no Englishe herbe, vsed onely of the Apothicaries, we haue it like Ote strawe, and is called *Iuncus*. The flower is *Anthos*, as all flowers be so named in Grece: this herbe, flower, or roote, dronke with Peper, doe helpe the Dropsie, beyng vsed: and is good for the lunges, splene, and raines. The roote of *Squinans* herbe, is hote and drie, and is against winde, collike, dropsie, fleume or crude rawe matter in the bodie, or any member of thesame beaten into pouder, and dronke in wine.

Diosc.li.pri. Capi.xvi.

Marcellus.

O how swete and pleasaunte is Woodbinde, in Woodes or Arbours, after a tender soft rain: and how frendly doe this herbe if I maie so name it, imbrace the bodies, armes and braunches of trees, with his long windyng stalkes, and tender leaues, openyng or spreding forthe his swete Lillis, like ladies fingers, emõg the thornes or bushes. Is this Woodbinde so profitable, as pleasaunt. I praie you tell me.

Woodbinde.

Hillarius.

Woodbinde called *Silua mater, Caprifolium, Lilium inter spinas Periclymenũ*. This herbe is so commonly knowen, that I neede not discribe the forme thereof: for thou hast doen well therof thy self. But to the vertue of this Woodbinde, in temperamente or nature, it is behemently cuttyng and dryyng, as *Galen* saieth, *Libri.viii. Simplic. medicamentorum*, the leaues bee sower. The oile of this is good, to anointe any parte of the bodie, that is nõme or very colde: and the water is good to be drunke against pissyng of blood. And also the Syruppe is good for the Lunges, or one dragme drunke in wine, is very good for the splene, that is stopped, or corrupt lunges. And there is nothyng (in ointmentes for woundes of the hedde) better then this Woodbinde: and Woodbinde water is holsome for sores in the throte and mouthe. And it is saied, that women, whiche vse to drinke plentifull, or moche of this water, it will make them barren.

Sondrie names of wood binde, as Periclymenon, because it winde aboute the next trees and Bushes, that it growes vnto.

Marcellus.

There is a long windyng weede, hauyng the propertie of Woodbinde, in spredyng, windyng, and inbrasyng, or lasyng bushes, braunches and hedges: the leaues somewhat like Iue, and flowers like to white cuppes or belles, what call you it?

Hillarius.

d.iiii.   This

The booke of Simples.

The Belle woodbinde Smylax. Diosco.li.iiii. Capit.xxxv.

THis is called *Heliximus, Smilax*, or *Campanelle*, or the belle woodbinde, *Antonius Muse* saieth, the leaues in likenes, colour and forme, be betwene Mercurie and Planten. But *Dioscorides* saieth, thei be like Iue, and the iuce of the leaues so drunke, or sodden in wine, doe make the bellie laxatiue, and nothing els can I report, but that it is noisom emong herbes and flaxe.

Marcellus.

WHat is the vertue of Senturion, whiche growe almosse in euery Medowe, in Maie and June. Thei haue swete pleasante purple flowers, and of diuers colours, and thei bee sone gone after June come in.

Hillarius.

testiculi canis Dogs stones

THis herbe haue sondrie names, as *testiculus Canis*, or *Orchis*, or in the Grece *Cynosorchim*, *Serapias*, or Dogges stones. In the bishoprike of Durisme, in a place called Warrell there, the people doe call it Crowfoote, although Crowfoote is an other herbe. This *testiculus*, or sauyng your reuerence Ballocke flower, haue twoo stones, and is named *Orchis*, and other three stones, whiche is called *Triorchis*, with many spotted leaues, like a Snake. These be of kindes, male and female, greate and little, of bothe sortes. Some will haue *Satyrion*, whiche you call Senturiō and Dogges tongue, bothe one: but thei do erre, and mistake the matter, that make no distinction betwene them. For there is distaunce betwene them, by the iudgement of the iye: although that in vertue, thei

Libro.iii. in Cap.124.125. 126.127.

be not moche vnlike, and thus saieth *Petrus Andreus Mathiolus*, vpon *Dioscorides* and he doe proue it by this reason: the rootes of Dogges stones, be like other beastes stones, thei be long, twoo hangyng, one higher then the other, that whiche hangeth beneath is full, and will sinke in water, the other stone is hollowe, and will swim). And this conclusion did one maister Jhon Sharman, an auncient good practisioner of Norfolke, shewe me long sins, but the stones of the Satyre be round, without grene, within very white, when the rinde is of, and swelled great, leaued like to the gardē Lilly, but smaller, bedyng to the ground: sone broken, and thre leaues in nomber. Then there is an other of the kind of *testiculi* called *Palma Christi*, whose rootes bee like handes, with fingers.

Satyrus is a beast, hauyng a hedde like a mā, and body like a Goate, and named Godes of the woodes, and thei first foūd this herbe of Venus, to stirre vp carnall luste.

Auicen call theim golden fingers, and be of nature of the greater *testicles*. The greater *testicles* be hote & moiste, and eaten, either in Goates milke, Dia, or Syruppe: thei will prouoke abundantly to *Venus*. But the little kinde, eaten either whole or in pouder, doe quenche, coole, and withstande thesaid *Venus*: and bringeth to dame nature, cold, tremblyng Saturne, whiche is colde and drie. But *Galen* saieth, *Satyrium* or Satires stones, be hote and moiste, swete to tast vpon, and doe as the great *testicles*, and more aboundauntly, and be good against runnyng of the raines, and cōsumption. &c. Giuen to the frātike bodie, or one whose sinewes be weake in hande, in palsie it helpeth theim: The seede. ℈.i. fine in pouder,

pouder drunke in wine, mornyng and euenyng: or diner and supper, vsed a long time, healeth the fallyng euill. *Nicolaus Florentinus* saieth, it helpeth the quartaine, and it stoppeth the bloodie flixe, sodden in redde wine, and healeth stinkyng vlcers, made in plaster. *Diasatiron* is made of this, whiche is of vertue moste excellēt, as appereth in the cōpoundes.

Mercellus.

What is the vertue of *Ligusticum*, called Louage, with the long blacke seedes, and long white rootes?

Hillarius.

THE herbe is great, with large braunches, stalke and leaues smellyng moche like to Smalage, but moche sweter: it is called *Ligusticum*, bicause it was first found in Liguria, and we cal it Louage here in England, the Italian cal it *Ligustico*, the roote, herbe, and seede, brosed and sodden in wine, or the decoction of Ptisane, or Barley water, will clense the lunges, open the vesselles of the vrine: prouoketh termes, or secrete infirmities, healeth woundes thereby, beyng sodden and applied to Phlegmon, or hardnesse in any outward member, is made softe. And warme applied in the maner of a plaster, to the bellie of a woman, whose childe is dedde, eftsones is sent forthe from natures moste secrete Chamber. And the seede finely beaten in pouder, put into some wholsome thinne broth, or wine of a persyng nature, doe skower the raines, clense the splene, and amende the liuer: expulseth the secondes, after the birthe of children, and drieth forthe the winde. *Plini* saith, that the seedes will stoppe the bellie, and is good against the bityng of serpentes. &c. But the seede eaten alone, prouoke vomites, and sometyme therefore saieth he, it muste be giuen with Rewe: and so the seede is good for the dropsie. The rootes sodden and the decoction dronke, is very wholsome for the femenine kinde, for the matrixe, bellie, precordiall, and breaste: It warmeth and make good concoction. Thus I conclude of this *Ligusticum*. But *Galen* saieth, there be twoo kindes of them, the one he calleth *Smirmum*: the other doe grow in the mount of *Amano*, called *Hipposelinum*, which is called Smalage

Fuchius.

Liguria is a part of Italy from the hille Apeninus, vnto the Tuscum Sea. *dios. li. 3. ca. li*

Eritius Cord cal this cōmō Angelica, but *Manardus Epist. lib. xii. Epist. iiii.* doe cal it Alexander, *Ruellus* cal it Louage *Galen. lib. vii simplici.*

Mercellus.

What saie you to *Apium*, whiche is called Smalage?

Hillarius.

THis herbe is named *Hipposelinum*, the greate Persile of Macedon, whiche we name Smalage: other saie, it is *Olus atrum*, whiche is Alexander. Some call it *Smyrnion*, *Marcellus* and *Brasauolus*, doe seme either to mistake, or els vntruely do reporte of this *Hipposelinum*. For thei saie the leaues be rough, and the roote blacke: But *Dioscorides Lib. iii. Capi. lxiiii* doe saie, the roote is white and swete, the leaues be not rough. But *Galen* made very little distinction, betwene *Hipposelinū* and *Smyrnum*: but this is one kind of Persile, the horse

The vertue of Smalage, Louage, Alexander, Persile is to open places, whiche stoppeth vrine & wind

Persile,

The booke of Simples.

Persile, or the Mountain Persile. *Seseli, Smyrnium, Imperatoria, Elaphoboscum*, and Alexander, all these seme to bee Persiles. Some greater, and of more puissancie then other: some cal it wild, some tame. As garden Persile, mountain, water, wood, or hedge Persile, &c. and al these haue power bothe in roote, stalke, leafe, and sede, to open the raines, blader, and to put in euery *Antidotarii*, that moueth vrin, breaketh stone, or clenseth grauell. Or against collike, or stoppyng of the splene, with aboundaunce of melancholie. Sodden in oile any of these rootes, or seedes dronke, it casteth out strong benime or poisone: but the seede is the strongeste part of the herbe. Thei be good to be put into glisters, for the stone, or turmente of the guttes: and in pultases, for swellyng of the legges or armes. And all these be good againste the stingyng of Serpentes, and feuers: swellyng in the stomacke, or dropsie, bothe in plaster, glister, or dronke with cleane white wine, or Ptisan.

<small>The vertues of Persiles.</small>

Marcellus.

There is a stinkyng wede called Dogges tongue, wherefore is the same wede good?

Hillarius.

It is no weede, but a very good herbe, and is called *Lingua Canis*: *Ruellus* and *Futtichius* doe erre, saieth that famous man *Mathiolus* vpon *Dioscorides*, in callyng Dogstongue *Lycopsin*, for it is not so named, but Dogestongue. And there be two of them, as *Mathiolus in Dioscoridem libr.iiii.Cap.Cxxiii.* aboute Adrians daies the Emperour, was found in the sandes, nere vnto Rome. This kinde of Dogestongue, whiche haue neither stalke, flower, nor seede: but out of one roote, there springeth leaues, lowe by the ground, in the compasse of a little weele, like Beane leaues, somewhat white, and with tender soft wolle. This herbe saieth *Petrus Andreas Mathiolus*, is like a widdowe, hauyng no children. But there is another Dogestongue, whiche haue rough seedes, with prickes in the middes like vnto Targettes: whiche seede sodden and dronke, healeth tertian and quartens, and these smell like eche other, and bee colde and drie in the seconde degree. And stamped with olde Swines grease, to make a plaster for a Dogges bityng: It healeth olde and newe cruent bloodie woundes. And mingled with Honie, it preserueth the heere from fallyng: and will quenche burnyng, tempered with vinegar, and sodden in redde wine, either dronke, or make a plaster. It stoppeth the bloodie flixe, and restraineth *Gomorrhæ*, or distillacion of the seede, called nature, vlcers, skabbes, poxe, or soche like. But the firste Dogestongue is the beste, to make pilles withall, for the reume and Catarre. *Galen* make of mencion of this, but *Dioscorides* and others doe.

<small>*Cynoglossum*, Dogestong. But Lycopsin is a kinde of Doggestong, & ca'l:d *Anchusa*. Dioscorides. lib. iiii. Ca.xxiiii</small>

<small>*Fuchius.*</small>

Marcellus.

What is the vertue of *Hippoglossum*, whiche is called *Laurus*, or horse tong, as I haue hard saie, by one that red me a pece of *Dioscorides*.

<small>*diosco.lib.iiii cap. Cxxviii.*</small>

Hillarius.

The booke of Simples. Fol.xxiiij.

Hillarius.

This herbe, or small stirpe, is called *Laurus Alexandrina*, or *Daphne*, the Englishe people call it, the laxatiue *Lauriola*. It dieth not in Winter, it shineth like Iue, or Baies, but is whitish. It beareth the berrie within the leaues, redde: it is hote and drie of nature. It. ʒ. iiii. or. vi. be sodden with *Simphitum*, called Cumphorie, in wine, and so strained and dronke, it will purge the bellie. A little pouder of this, is giuen to childrē in potage, to take awaie the aboundance of humidite, and kill wormes. It make quicke or spedie deliueraunce, in childbirth secondes, and termes, drinke three penie waight, twoo or three tymes saieth *Plini*: *Galen* affirmeth, it forseth vrine. The leaues stamped, and bounde to the hedde, taketh awaie the pain, saieth *Dioscorides*. With this herbe, did that moste noble victorious Alexander, sometyme triumph withall, and his capitaines, be wearyng the diademe. And somtyme the beste herbe of this kinde, did growe vpon the mountain *Idia*, nere to the dolorous citee of Troie in Phrigia.

Lib.iiii.capi. Cxxvij.

Marcellus.

What saie you to *Sanicula*, called *Diapensia*, or the greate fiue leaued leaues, and other fiue leaued herbes?

Sanicula and quinquifoliū.

Hillarius.

Among the herbes for woundes, this is moche praised, and do heale woundes equally, with any other healing flower, roote, or leafe. The toppes of this herbe, is not moche vnlike Straburies, somwhat whitishe, and called *Saniculam a sanandis vulneribus*, of healyng woundes. It groweth in darke places in Maie, and is bitter, hotte, and drie in the seconde degree: The syrup or iuce of this herbe, is very good to be giuen to wounded men, women, and childrē, in small wine, or their other drinke. For it taketh effect both to heale, bothe within and without the bodie: if it be applied hote, vpon a swellyng part or member, it will asswage the same spedely. The iuce thereof is good also for Oxen, milche Keen, and horse that bee broosed, or wounded: either in their drinkes, or applied to the hurte member, or place. There is no spedier remedy to helpe the lunges, then this herbe sodden, and the decoction dronke vpon an emptie stomacke. And what so euer Copharie, called *Symphiton*, can doe in woundes: the same can *Sanicle* called *Sanicula*. It stoppeth the bloody flixe, or helpeth him that haue taken to strōg purgacion: and stoppeth the immoderate runnyng of the raines, now besides this *Diapensia*, wherof we haue spokē. There be her kinsfolkes, called *pentaphilon*, or *Quinquefolium*, haue fiue leaues in nōber. There be three sortes of thē, the great, the meane, and the little: these be commonly knowen, rather by the formes, emong the cōmon people then by their singuler goodnesse, whiche in dede thei haue. As *Dioscorides* saith *lib.iiii.Capi.38.* the rootes well sodden, and drinke the same decoction, helpeth the tartian,

Sanicle healeth woūdes.

Sanicle is good for horse and keen.

The booke of Simples.

tian, and washe the mouthe warme with thesame, and so kept in the mouthe. This taketh the paines from the teeth and stinke, filthe, and vlcers from thesame: and is wholsome in a gargarisme, or for paines in the throte. And if the leaues be well sodde, or the iuce, with Endiue or Planten water, to drinke thesame eight daies, helpeth the yellowe Ianders, in quotidians & quartens, this herbe helpeth, sodden in posset ale. Also for the fallyng sicknes, bicause it is hote and drie, in the third degree: sodden in vinegar, it killeth a tetter or ring worme, it healeth the fistula, tempered with Salte and Honie. Tempered and stamped together, and put into the place or hole: The syrup of this, dronke .xii. tymes, healeth *Angine*, or swellyng in the throte, and stoppe the immoderate fluxe of the bellie, and termes.

A good gargarisme, to washe the throte.

Maister Androwe *Mathioli*, in his cōmentarie vpon *Dioscorides*: coupleth *Fragaria*, called Strauberies, with these fiue leaued herbes. Although thesaid Strauberie haue but three leaues, cold in the first degree, and drie in the seconde. The leaues and rootes, will heale woundes and vlcers: and fluxe of blood, and termes, prouoke vrine, and helpeth the liuer. If thei be sodden in cleane white wine, doe clense the raines and blader: and will clense the mouthe, and strength the teeth, when thei be lose. The distilled water of Strauberies, will clense the darke mistes of the iyen: and also quencheth heat in the face, and taketh awaie redde spottes. And thesame water is wholsome to delaie wine, at dinner and supper: specially for cholorike persones in Sommer. The berie it self beyng ripe, is partly hote and drie, so some learned do affirme but beyng not ripe, thei be cold and drie. These ripe beries strawed into cleane clarified Honie, and put in the pouder of white Peper: dooe helpe them, whiche haue short winde, and pain or straightnes in their breast, or doe vse moche sighyng, saith *Paulus Ægenita*. There be twoo kindes of Strauberies, the greater, and the lesser. Also *Rubus idems*, allowe Brable, called *Ribes*, or *Raspes*, a berie like to the Strauberie: these beries stoppe a fluxe, sodden in redde wine, and dronke often tymes. Nothyng maie be compared to thē, in that case, and quencheth sainct Antonies fire. The leaues stamped, saieth *Dioscorides Lib.iiii. Cap.xxxiiii*, doe heale the Hemeroides, to anoint the place therewith: and also the vertue is to clense and drie. And this frute or leafe, do heale the sores in the mouth and doe close woundes, newe made with any weapon: and this frute stamped, and applied plaster waies to the stomacke, helpeth presently *Cardiaca passio*, and hote paines in the stomack, and the burning paines of the iyes, when thesaid iyes be almoste starte forthe, as thei terme thē. Through greate vomites, fall, footbaule, leape, &c. And thei also kille these foule vlcers, that that crepe through the skinne, growyng vpon the hedde. The flowers of them, with fine clarified Honie, put into the iye, doe cleare the sight, and quencheth heate: drieth vp water, contained in them. And of these *Ribes* called *Raspis*, be twoo kindes, the one with sharpe prickes, whiche is not so effectuall and good, as the other with tender prickes. And thus I ende of these beries, whiche haue the vertue

Fragaria Comaron or the Strauberie, of the swete odour, so named.

To clense the face.

For a shorte winde.

For to heale the Hemeroides.

For Cardiaca passio.

For red iyen

tue of the Mulbery. And thus doth that olde famous Egiptiã knight and most learned man in herbes, that euer was, without all comparison, called *Phacas* or *Dioscorides*, he was subiecte to *Cleopatras* the queene of Egipt, and to *Antonius*, and learned to know herbes in their kindes most truely and commended these herbes and berries aforesaid, whose workes be greatly aduaunsed, and most cunnyngly handled now, by that famous learned Phisicion *Petrus Andreas Mathiolus Senensis. Anno salutis*, 1558.

Dioscorides being an Heathen man, serueth his prince in battell, and yet learned ye knowlege of herbes: But many professing the name of Christ, wil neither serue ye one, or lerne the other, seruauntes to idlenesse, & abusers of tyme.

Marcellus.

What is the vertue of *Arum*, whiche we in Englishe cal Cockowe pintell? And some call it the burning herbe, or dragons mace?

Hillarius.

This herbe is commonly knowen, it groweth in the Sprynge time: leaued like Dragons, in moiste and drie places, and of nature is hotte and drie in the firste degree, and so it is without doubte in the thirde degree. The vertue of this leafe, seede, or roote, tempered with Cowes dunge: it is good to make a plaster againste the goute, saith *Dioscorides*. *Plini* saith the sedes therof finely beatē in pouder & tempred with clene oile, helpeth the sorenes of the eare dropped in, the iuce healeth *polipus* in the nose: and mingled with cleane Honie: It clenseth the darknes of the iyes, and sodden hote with oile, healeth Emeroides, as *Plini* saith, as I haue proued the vertue thereof often tymes.

Aron called Cucko pick.

Marcellus.

What is the vertue of Maidenhere? Called *Tricomanes*.

Hillarius.

IT is an herbe betwene hotte and drie, if it be sodden in Wine, it breaketh the stone: it cleanseth the matrice, bringeth doune the secondes, as *Dioscorides* and *Galen* saith, the syrup of this helpeth the splen and lunges, the beste doeth growe vpon hard rockes. Great plētie growe aboute Chiueat hilles in the North, called *Ordo lucis*: so dooe *Adiantum*, whiche is of thesame vertue.

Maidē heere

Marcellus.

THat herbe whiche you doe call *Symphitum* or Cumphorie, you saied before, *Sanaculum* is equall with it. By this I do gather that this Cumphorie is then equall with Sanaculum. Wherin is their equaltie, in sauour, taste, or other vertues, I praie you tell me?

Hillarius.

NEither like in forme nor tast. Firste in forme the leaues be like Buglosse, yea, or rather to *Solanum*, called the greate night shade leaues, the rootes great and blacke without, and white within flowers yelow. Secondly, the sauour and taste not pleasant, but the vertues agreeth in this point, to heale woundes, yea broken bones because they haue power to draw foorth, and also to glew the seperated flesh together, it groweth in Rockes, euen so in Gardens, it is of twoo kindes. &c. and is hot and drie in the seconde degree. This herbe will draw

Symphitum. Soli lago. Comphory. Consolida. of the healing comfortable herbe so named.

draw foorth filth from the Lunges, if it be sodden in sweet water, & so dronke. And will effectually stoppe the blouddy flixe in menne, and menstrall termes, when thei do abounde in women imoderatly. This herbe assuredly do heale men, when they be faulen from some highe place, if the faule be not deadly. The like it doth to al maner of beasts. Chirurgens can not misse it. Consider also, that there is a lesser kinde of *Symphitum*, of the thirde sorte. *Consolida minor*, which is of the vertue of healing, both within and without the body, and for al broken bones, and doe heale foule sores in the pudent, or secrete places of menne and women. These bee sufferante medicines in meates for the wounded men. These be herbes of great bertues, and excellent in gooduesse for mankinde: and may well procede of the verbe Consolido, of healyng that which was broken, or ioyne together thinges seperated, to comforte or make safe, either in Oyle, Salue, Plaster &c. And thus I do ende of this Symphitum.

To heale a brose, or a faule.

Consildo to heale.

Marcellus.

What is the nature of an herbe, called *Scilla* or *Squilla*? or the sea Onion.

Hillarius.

Here be twoo kindes, whiche of nature be hote and drie, in the seconde degree: and yet of a meruetlous nature. For the outward rinde is berie hote and bitter, and the core is berie colde: therefore thei muste bee caste bothe awaie, after the saied *Scilla* is either rosted, baken, or soddē. For els it is euill, and hurtfull to nature: and thus it must be prepared. Cut of the leaues, whiche be like vnto the leaues of Aloes, but not so groose. The fruit is as great as a boyes head, of *Scilla* which is the greatest kinde. The seconde kinde is lesser, in the bignes of a great Onion or a Peare, and is called *Pancratis*, these bothe springeth or bringeth foorth their yellow flowers three times in the yeare: and in the *Caniculer* daies, roste it vnder the coales in paper, vntill it bee softe, or els bake it in Clay, or els seeth it in shifte of waters, vntill the water leaue bitternesse, then take it foorthe and let it drie in a shadow or darke place, couered with a cleane Linnen clothe, then you maye put to it Orimell, that is cleane Honie clarified, and sharpe Wineger sodden together, whiche is called *Oximel simplex*: and when the *Scilla* and this stande together in a close double glasse in the Sunne, all the *Canisculer* daies, or els to make more spede, to seeth all that is conteined within this glasse, set it in a vessell with hot boiling water, then it is called *Oximel Scillitici*, whiche is of great vertue. This *Oximel* is good to eate of thē whiche haue paines in the head, commyng of cold, or for them whiche be smitten with the fearfull sicknesse, called the Faulyng euill, called *Morbus comitialis*, with opilacion in the head. It also is good for colde, rotten Coughes, and stinking breathes, and chiefly for shorte windes in the spirable partes. It helpeth to aswage the swellyng of the Splen, or the dolour therin: and casteth out filthe from the guttes, that causeth

Goodlie medicenes bee made bothe of Squilla, and of Pancras, whiche is the great and lesser sea oniōs.

The booke of Simples. Fol.xxvj.

seth pain and torment winde in them. But beware of any Bile, or festred sore be not in the guttes, then vse it not to muche. And it killeth smalle wormes in the breast, and also clenseth the raines and bladder mouyng vrine, and healeth the yellow Janders. The wine therof if it be sodden in wine, after it is prepared, it prouoketh vrin, and clenseth the raines, and is good against Dropsies. The oile is good against the Palsey, and coldnesse of the ioyntes, or trembling, for the Splene, and coldnesse of the brain or fete. The vineger clenseth the inward partes, and also killeth Tetters, Ring wormes, and itche in the skinne. The seede beaten into pouder, and eaten with Honie, doth clense the belly. Truly this is an herbe of greate vertue, as saith *Hippocrates. li. ij cap. 167.* and *Galen. li. viij. Simplicium medicamentorum*, and is called the Onion of the Sea. And his roote maketh a molifiyng emplastrum, to make warme and softe, a harde colde sore, commyng of Melancholie, or cold and drie matter.

To heale ringwormes and tetters.

Marcellus.

What is the Marigold, with golden yellowe flowers?

Hillarius.

The Marigold, named *Caltha*, or *Calendula*, because it florisheth al the Kalendes of the yere: and is also named *Sol sequium*, because it openeth his flower, and turneth rounde all the daie after the Son and closeth in his golden beames at night. This herbe nedeth no furder descripcion, it is so commonly knowen: and is hote and drie, the flowers will chaunge the heere, and make it yellowe. And this herbe sodden in wine, drunke warme, moueth sweate, and prouoketh termes menstruall, specially the flowers of this herbe, or the Syrupe. Perfumes of thesame, will doe the like: the smoke of theim to bee made in a close subfumigacion, will dooe thesame. The iuce warme put into the mouthe, helpeth the teeth: if the akyng cometh of colde.

Marigoldes

To moue Sweate.

Marcellus.

What saie you of *Nigilla Romana*?

Hillarius.

This is called *Melanthium*, whiche you dooe name *Nigilla*: for *Dioscorides* doe remember this herbe, in *Libro tertio Cap lxxviij.* callyng it *Githe*, like Poppie. It hath blacke seedes, the leaues moche like Coriander: the knoppes wherin the sede dooe growe, in the toppe haue little hornes, and is hote and drie, in the third degree. Brose it, & smel thereupon, put it in a linen clothe, and holde it to the nose in the mornyng, and it will stop a cold reume: temper it with vineger, and it will take awaie hedache applied thereunto. Euen so it killeth wormes in the bellie, applied therunto plaster waies, mingled with an oxe gaule: and the iuce dropped into the iye, healeth a disease called *Epiphoras*, which is dropping of theim. It is good for to drinke, to clense the lunges, purge termes,

Nygilla.

putteth

The booke of Simples.

putteth awaie winde and collike, and kill wormes, &c. Dronke in wine by the reason of the bitternesse, it maketh waie and quicke passage for the vrine: and skower cleane the bladder, excepte the stone be cōfirmed in it. It taketh paines in the mouthe and teeth awaie. Put in warme *Against poisone.* with Vineger, and preuaileth againste poison, as eatyng of a Spider, or any benim: and dronke in wine or whaie certain daies, it wil drawe milke into breastes of women, clense, and increase the same, with manie singuler vertues: as *Dioscorides, Galen, Plini,* and *Simon Sethi* affirmeth. And *Of Opium made of black Poppie.* wilde Cocle that groweth in corne, is of the same kinde: and the iuce maie be pressed for the, as *Opium*, and preserued to medicen to cause slepe.

Marcellus.

What vertue haue Poppie, I praie you?

Hillarius.

Of Poppie wilde & tame There is wilde Poppie, leaued like Rocked, and flowred like a Rose: it groweth in corne, the seede redde, and is cold nere hand in the fourth degree. *Dioscorides* affirmeth, if this be sodden in water, and applied to the head, or drinke it, reconcileth slepe. It also quencheth S. Anthonies fire, called *Sacer ignis*, or shingles, made in a plaster, w oile of Roses and Vineger, *Acacia* and this sodden together in red wine, doe stoppe the bloodie flixe and termes, whiche be harde to be stopped. But this herbe maketh the memorie verie dulle, to vse it moche: but Saffron, Mirrhe, and the oile of bitter Almondes, tempered with the iuce thereof, warme put into the deafe eare, bryngeth hearyng, if it be *A medicene for sore eyes very excellēt.* not incurable. Rose water, womans milke, and the white of an Egge beaten together put into the eye, doth take awaie dimnesse, burninge rednesse, and swellyng from them, and cleareth the sight. Now the great Poppie, called Papauer of the garden, whiche in Grece is named *Mecon*: there be of theim twoo kindes, white and blacke in theyr *white Poppie is the best.* seedes and flowers, the white is beste, it hath all the vertues and manie more then I haue written of the wilde Poppie. And the seede is good to be tempered with meate, to make bread, to giue to theim that can not sleape, to be put into Milke, and so eaten at night, it stoppeth the belly. *Opium* is made of blacke Poppy, whiche is colde, and is vsed in sleaping medicines: but it causeth deepe deadly sleapes. And thus I doe ende of Poppy, wilde and tame.

Marcellus.

What is Coriander of Nature?

Hillarius.

Coriander. CORION called in Grece, *Coriandrum* in Latten, and beareth a rounde seede, like informe to a worme called *Corus* or *Crinex*, this herbe is commonly knowen, and is colde saith *Dioscorides lib. 3. cap. 62.* It healeth S. Anthonis fier, Carbuncles, and suche lyke burnyng thinges: but *Galen* obseruyng more diligently the nature of this

The booke of Simples. Fol.xxvij

this herbe, whose iudgement the greatest number of the wisest and beste learned do folow vntill this day, do affirme in *lib.8.cap.iiij.de compositione medicame.* that it is al together hote, and saith he: *Si Coriandrum strumas dissoluit quo nam igitur pacto frigidum erit?* that is saith *Galen*, if Coriander doe dissoue or wast the kurnels in the throate called the kynges Euell. By what meanes then shall it be hot: for it is not possible that suche grose hard thinges should be wasted of colde thinges. But this doeth bothe wast, and as *Simion Sethy* affirmeth, the seedes eaten with, or after meate, do so warm the stomacke, and retaineth the meate vntill it be almost concocted. Therfore the conclusion must be nedes true that it is hotte and drie. *Plini* writeth to *Marcus Varro*, Coriander beaten in pouder, and mingled with viner, doeth preserue fleshe from corruption in Summer. But the vertue is in the seedes steeped in vineger and dried. But to drinke muche of the iuce of the herbe, doth take awaye the speche, or causeth madnesse: thus I ende of this Coriander.

<small>Galen do dissente in this place, frō Dioscorides, in ye nature of Coriander.</small>

<small>Plini lib. natu.hist.li.xx. Capi.xx.</small>

Marcellus.

What is *Foenygrece*, called commonly Fenicricke?

Hillarius.

This herbe is like. iij. leaued grasse, and the seede groweth in a longe Codde. The meale or pouder, of the seede of Foenigrece called Fenycrike, hath vertue to molifie. Sodden in sweete water, it quencheth bothe within & without any inflamacion of the body. The same being sodden in sharpe vyneger, and Nitor, applied warme to the left side, asswageth the dolour and paine of the Splene. Euen so it doth the like to the Liuer, hauing Oile of Roses mingled therwith: this seede is vsed in many molifiyng plasters. The decoction dronke, and the seede applied to the belly, doth helpe *Tenasmus*, whiche is a desier to go to the stoole, and can not, or a stinkyng flix. And the Oyle dothe clense spottes and skars in the fleshe or skin, where as woundes haue been, and helpeth Flegmon, whiche is an impostimacion of bloud cōminge of heate, aboue nature, gathered into some place of the body: and is hot in the seconde degree, and drie in the first, saith *Galen : libro.vij.Simpl. medicament*. Of Foenigrece is an excellent *Fomentum* made for the iyen, that be sore or dimme: whiche I haue seen maister Luke make. which is an excellent man, in the cure or regiment for the iyes.

<small>Dioscori. lib.ij.cap.xcv</small>

<small>Tenasmus:</small>

<small>Flegmon.</small>

<small>Maister Luke of London.</small>

Marcellus.

What then of Flax?

Hillarius.

Knowen of euery body, but there be twoo kindes of Flax. the wilde Flax is not good : the common sowne Flax, is good & profitable for linen cloth, without which we shalbe like bestes, bothe at borde & bedde. Linen is comely, bothe for men and specially for women, & more cōmendable in the temple then holly

<small>Flaxe.</small>

e.iij. and

The booke of Simples.

and is called in Greeke Lynon, and our English worde is Linen, the Latten *Linum*, muche like to eche other in name. *Galen* saith, *lib.7.simplic. medica.* The seede of Flax is hotte and moiste in the first degree, yet some what drying in the midst, it hath vertue to molifie, ripe, and breake Apostumes, if it be made in meale, tempered with swines greace and Mallowe rootes, warme applied, in the maner of a plaster. It is vsed in many medicens and glisters, with Oyle of Roses, to clense sharpe costife humours: but it wil make the belly to swell, if it be vsed in the maner of meate, yet it will styrre vp Venus, if it be eaten with Peper and Hony. The decoction therof is holsom to cleanse, molify, and ripe the apostimacion the secret places of women so diseased or pained. The Oyle that cometh therof, hath many vertues: as for Painters, to temper their Coullers with, and for varnishyng of boordes: for the Armorer in makynge cleane Harnisse, and Weapons, and Lampes. Flax Oyle, washed in. iiii. or. vi. shiftes of cleane colde water, beaten with a sticke vntil it turne white, then with a spone take it foorth, for it will swime euer a lofte, and this will heale burninges, scaldinges and hot inflamacions. This Oyle molifieth harde sores, and is good for bone setters for to stregth the sinewes, iointes, and bones, for conuulcion, Hemerodes &c. And if it be dronke after poison, it will caste it foorth by vomittes, and clenseth the stomacke. Flax beinge fine is vsed with Repercussiues, as with Bolearmonie, and whites of Egges. Without Flax, Chirurgians can not worke, nor helpe the eyes, except fine Flax be in it.

The vertue of linte Oile.

Marcellus.

Neckewede.

There is an herbe, whiche light fellowes, merily will call Gallowgrasse, Neckeweede, or the Tristrams knot, or Saynt Iudres lace, or a bastarde brothers badge, with a difference on the left side &c. you know my meanyng.

Hillarius.

Hempe.

What you speake of Hempe? mary you terme it with manie pretie names, I neuer heard the like termes giuen to any simple, as you giue to this, you cal it neckwede. A well I pray you, woulde you know the propertie of this Neckeweede in this kinde, beinge chaunged into such a lace, this is his vertue. Syr if there be any yonkers troubled with idelnesse and loytryng, hauyng neither learnyng, nor willyng handes to labour: or that haue studied Phisicke so longe that he or they, can giue his Masters purse a Purgacion, or his Chist shoppe, and Countinghouse, a strong vomit, yea, if he bee a very cunning practicioner in false accomptes, he may so suddenly, and rashely minister, that he may smite his Father his Maister or his friende &c. into a sudden incurable consumption, that he or they shall neuer recouer it againe, but be vtterly vndone, and cast either into miserable pouertie, prisonment, bankeroute &c. If this come to passe, then the

Many good medicines made of hepe

Perilious practicioners be heredescribed.

best

The booke of Simples. Fol.xxviii

best rewarde for this practicioner, is this Neckeweede: if there be any swashbuckler, common theefe, ruffen, or murtherer past grace, ye nexte remedie is this Lace or Corde. For them which neuer loued concorde, peace nor honestie, this wil ende all the mischief, this is a purger, not of Melancholy, but a finall banisher of al them that be not fit to liue in a common wealth, no more then Foxes amonge sheepe, or Thistels amonge good Corne, hurters of trew people. This Hempe I say, passeth the new Diat, bothe in force and antiquitee. If yonge wantons, whose parentes haue left them fayre houses, goodes, and landes, whiche be visciously, idle, vnlearnedly, yea or rather beastly brought vp: after the death of their saied parentes, their fruites wil spryng foorth which they haue learned in their wicked youthe: then bankets and brothels will approche, the Harlots will be at hande, with dilightes and intisementes, the Baude will doe hir diligence, robbyng not onlie the purses, but also the hartes of suche yongemen, whiche when they be trapped, can neuer skape, one amonge an hundreth, vntill Hempe breaketh the bande amonge these loytring louers. The Dice whiche be bothe smalle and light, in respecte vnto the Coluerying, or double Cannon shotte or Bollet, yet with small force and noyse can mine, breake downe, and destroy, and caste away their one Maisters houses, faire feldes, plesaunt woddes, and al their money, yea frendes and al together this can the Dice do. And moreouer, can make of worshipfullborne Gentilmen, miserable beggers, or theefes, yet for the time a loft syrs, hoyghe childe and tourne thee, what should youth do els? I wille, not liue like slaues or pesantes, but all golden, glorious, may with dame Venus, my hartes delight say they. What a sweete heauen is this? Haue at all, kockes woundes, bloud and nayles, caste the house out at the window, and let the Diuell pay the Malte man, a Dogge hath but a day, a good mariage will recouer all together: or els with a Barnards blowe, lurkyng in some lane, wodde, or hill top, to get that with falshead in an hower, whiche with trueth, labour, & paine, hath bene gathered for, perhappes, xx. yeares, to the vtter vndoyng of some honest familie. Here thou seest gentle Marcellus, a miserable Tragedie, of a wicked shamelesse life. I nede not bring forth the example of the Prodigall childe. Luke. xvi. Chapter, whiche at length came to grace: It is I feare me in vaine to talke of him, whose ende was good, but a greate nomber of these, flee from grace, and come to endes moste vngracious, finished only life by this Hempe. Although sometime the innocente man dieth that way, through periurie for their one propper gooddes, as Naboth died for his owne Vineyarde, miserable in the eies of the worlde, but precious in the sight of God. This is one seruice whiche Hempe doeth.

Also this worthy noble herbe Hempe, called *Cannabis* in Latten, can not bee wanted in a common wealth, no Shippe can sayle without Hempe, ye sayle clothes, the shroudes, staies, tacles, yarde lines, warps & Cables can not be made. No Plowe, or Carte, can be without ropes
e.iiii. halcers

[side notes:]
A quicke medicene.

The misery of vnthriftes semeth pleasaunte, but shame & pain is the ende.

Th'innocent somtime dieth in the iyes of me̅ miserable

The consideracion of hēpe in Physicke.

The booke of Simples.

halters, trace. &c. The Fisher and Fouler muste haue Hempe, to make their nettes. And no Archer can wante his bowe string: and the Malt man for his sackes. With it the belle is rong, to seruice in the Church, with many mo thynges profitable: whiche are commonly knowen of euery man, be made of Hempe. Now furdermore, there be twoo kindes of Hempe, the wilde, whiche is hote and drie, in the second degree: and is called *Terminalem*, stamped with Oile of Wormewood, and warme applied to the bellie, it doeth asswage swellyng. And with swines greace thesame doe ripe apostumes of sores. This wilde Hempe, haue leaues like to the garden Hempe, but rootes and seedes, like vnto Mallawes.

Hempe will kill wormes.

The garden sowen Hempe, is also hote and drie: *Plini lib. xx. Cap. xxiij.* This herbe and seede sodden, and strongly pressed, or the iuce strained, and powred vpon the yearth, doe not onely bryng foorthe wormes for Fishers: but also dropped into the eare, do kil wormes, that be crept into them. And *Galen lib. 7. simplicium medicamen.* saith: that to eate moche of the sede, doe drie vp the seede of generacion, & is an aduersarie to the hedde, and bryng euill humours. *Simeon Sethi* saieth, it drieth seede, asmoche as doeth Camphire: And is harde of digestion, and hurteth as Coriander doeth

Hempe quēcheth natural seede.

that is immoderatly eaten, bryngeth madnesse. Howbeit, the seede or leaues sodden, and warme applied to the handes or feete: doe helpe against the contraxion, or shrinkyng of sinewes, whiche cometh of cold and is helped through the heate of this herbe. And all singyng birdes whiche be plentifull in laiyng of egges, thei reioyce greatly in Hempsede: as in their chief delicious foode. And thus I haue no more to saie but to answere to the next questiō, my deare felowe and frend *Marcellus.*

Marcellus.
Now I praie you, what is Barly of nature?

Hillarius.

Hordium Barley.

Ommonly knowen in all this Realme, it is the mother of the beste Malte, whereof bothe Bere and Ale is made of: there is Barly double, or with fower set, and single twoo set. The greatest and whitest is beste, and is colde and drie, in the first degree: and do not nuriche so moche as Wheate. Of this Barly beyng hulled, and clene from

Ptisan made of Barly, wil quenche choller.

the rinde, beaten or broken, is made the noble drinke, called *Ptisana*: a pounde put with tenne poundes of cleane water, sodden vnto halfe, into a stone potte, or Tinned vessel, close in the mouth, standyng vntill it be colde: and then let it run through a strainer, and so drinke simple of this, for it will quenche hote burnyng Choller aboue nature, in behement feuers. You maie put in the seedes of white Poppie, and Lettise not onely to coole: but also to reconsile sleape, to the afflicted with the

To helpe the lunges.

feuer, to clense corrupcion of the lunges, and horsnesse, with shortnesse of winde. Put in Figges, Liquoris, Aniseedes, Reisynges of the Son, and a little Hysope with Suger: seeth all, and let it stande close, vntill it be colde, and straine it with a strainer, and so drinke thereof, for the

foresaied

The booke of Simples.   Fol.xxix.

foresaied shortnesse of winde. Seeth Barly meale, Linte seede, and Fenigrece sede: and the iuce of Rewe with Malmesie, warme applied to the belly, it will put awaie swelling, & paines in the gutts. The meale therof sodden in Uineger, will asswage the hote burnyng Goute: and this is good againste all hote inflamacions of the bodie. And seeth barly in Honie, Rosen, and the iuce of Cheloden, and it will heale an olde rotten sore. With oile and Fenigrece meale, it will asswage the swellyng of the precordall or stomacke. Mellilot, Poppie and Honie, tempered together, do helpe the swellyng heate of the priuie mēbers: paines of the sides or fleshe, whiche is gone frō the bone, with many other goodly vertues, whiche Barly haue. As affirmeth *Dioscorides. lib. ij. Cap. lxxix. Galen lib. i. de alimentorium.* And *Thophrastus lib. viij. Cap de plantarum Historia.* Barly is the principall wine grape of Englande, that our Malt is made vpō. And mother of our Bere and Ale, whiche Malt, in the time of our extreme nede, haue been solde awaie, into forrain realmes: by certain old knowen theues, called Humber, and Lin hauen, with his braunches. Frō Cambrige, S. Iues, and Milden haule, Thetford, and Brandon ferie: and also Yermouth in Norffolke. I praie God amende the market, and staie soche practises, that for the priuate commoditie of a fewe, a great multitude should be famisshed. And now what haue you els to saie?   *Against inflamacion, heate or swellinges in the bodie.*

  The breade & drynke of the poore bee the life of the nedie: & he that take it awaie from them, is a murderer.

Marcellus.

IN the eight leafe of Simples, you spake but a little of Barly, and also of Beanes & Pease: but smally to the purpose, to myne instruccion. Therefore shewe me a little more of their natures, bicause I am a rurall man of the countrie: and loue Pease and Beanes, and as I heare tell, many good medicenes bee made of theim, to helpe in the tyme of sicknesse. I haue good plentie of them: more then any other Poticarie stuffe.

Hillarius.

FABA called Beanes, emong pulse bee very windie, and bringeth greuous dreames. *Pithagoras* would not suffer his scollers to eate them: belike terrible infernall dreames did folowe, whiche did hurte the witte, and the iye sight. Thei be colde and drie, in the firste degree, I nede not describe them: euery man knowe them. Beyng wel sodden with Mintes, thei doe stoppe vomites and the flixe: if the firste water, wherein thei be sodden, bee caste awaie, then seeth theim in the seconde, and so thei bee lesse windie and hurtfull. Beane meale called *lomentum* by it self, or with Barly meale and Uineger, doe quenche inflamacions: and molifie hote harde Apostumacions, and goute, sodden with swines greace. This meale drie vp woundes, and drieth vp milke in the pappes or breastes of women. Temper it with Fenigrece and Honie, then it will heale *Furunculum*, called a Fellon: and it doe the like to pusshes, in any parte of the bodie. Temper this meale with white frākinsence, the white of an egge, and Rose water: this helpeth sore swelled, or droppyng iyen. And this tempered with oile and Uineger, dooe

  A more larger discripciō of Beanes & Pease. Pithagoras saied thus: faba abstineto that is, abstain from benes Plini & Tulli saieth, because of the ingenderyng of grose humers he forbad thē: A nest oxenō and Empedocles affirmeth by abstaining from Benes: he meante lecherie, or filthy lustes: Plutarchus saieth, it was to beware, to be in office in a cōmō welth because it is so perillous.

asswage

The booke of Simples.

For coddes swelled.

asswage the swellyng of the coddes of men and boies, warme applied therunto. This meale do clense the face of women, washed therwith, tempered in cold milke at night: straine it through a clothe. xx. tymes, and let it drie on. And in the mornyng, with a hard linen clothe softly, wette in colde water and Milke, strike or wype the face therwith, and kepe the from the sonne: like good huswiues, spinnyng a thred of smal thrift vntill night for their labor: Mary then if thei will a mornings, take in. ii. or. iii. Reisinges, halfe a drame of yellow Flowes, then flusshyng will the soner departe from the face, by that meanes of openyng the liuer, and specially if it be in Sommer. I refarre the worthie consideracion of this Beanes to *Galen lib. vij. Simplice medicam.* Although hetherto I haue not onely alledged him: but other, as *Dioscorides lib. ij. Cap. xcvij.* which

Beanes in the old tyme, were vsed for lottes.

in Greke is called *Cyamos*, in deede thei will partly moue *Venus* lustes. And in thold time, the generall assent & consent: as in parlamentes, eleccions or questes, wer all declared by Beanes. The white Beanes did graunt, or affirme, and the blacke Beanes did denay, or refuse: And this maner doe still continue, in many places of Europe. As in that moste worthie riche, and noble citie called Venice: which began *Anno a partu virginis*, 154. Of

When Venice first began.

a fearfull nomber of people, whiche fled from the cruel handes of a famous tirant, called Attila the king of Hungarie, whiche brake into Italy, and destroied many places: emong all, the moste auncient citee, & chief marte of Europe, called *Aquileia*, whiche is now of no estimacion. Of this loste citee, be these Venecias come, whiche haue vsed hetherto to nomber with Beanes. The moste worthy, noble learned, & valiaunt *Famile* of the Romaines: whereof toke thei their names, I praie you? Of

The old Romaines were more humble then the new Romaines, & late Popes, in kepyng names of base titles.

any noble old citee, as Thebes, Troie. &c. Or of any valiaunt beast, as a Lion, Tiger, Panthar. &c. No forsoth. Thei toke their name onely of poore Beanes: As *Fabius Porcius*, & their worthy auncestours were sowers and sellers of Beanes, and kepers of swine, and for their vertues wer aduaunsed, and kept still their names. Although the sacred Vickar of Sathan, called the Pope, kepe not his old name: as example. If he be christened Marke, Laurance, Cornelis. &c. Well, when he is degenerated, or triple mitred, then he is newe named, Leo, Clemente, Paulus, Boniface. &c. A very Anabaptiste, or ashamed of his name, receiued in Baptisme. Welfare the olde Ethnicke Romaines, whiche excelled the newe counterfecte christian Romaines: whiche were not ashamed, to

The tyme of Cicero.

haue base names, as *Fabius* had: *Cicero* of a Fitche or Tare, tooke his name and for eloquence, his like was neuer: and was before Christes incarnacion fourtie yeres. *Piso* that auncient name, of a noble famile of the

Of base parentes, spryngeth noble children.

Romaines, tooke their name onely of Peson: whose parentes were Plowmen, and sellers of Pease.

Therefore of Pease, let vs saie some thyng of their properties, and vertues, more then we haue declared *Folio. vij. in libro Simplic.* And first from whence thei came: and why thei be called Pease, and in Greke *Pison*, in

Pease came first fro Piso in Grece.

Latine *Pisum*. The first spring of the was moste plentifull in Greke, in a countrie called *Pelopomensus*, in whiche was a noble citee named *Pisa*, by the

The booke of Simples. Fol.xxx.

the riuer of *Alpheus*. About whiche citee, euery fiue yeres, the nobles and moste worthy Grecians, did proue all maner of masteries: and made triumphes, pastimes and plaies, in the honour of Jupiter. *Ouid.ij.de arte:* Lo this Pease came from *Piso*, and be now in the moste parte of al Europe, aswell as emong the Grecians. And of nature bee of a meane temperament, cold and driyng, and is in al pointes like vnto Beanes, but not so windy: and more better for nourishing the bodie, and more clensing the bellie, saith *Galen*, & *Paulus* is of thesame minde. Let bothe Pease and Beanes bee well watred, hulled, and tenderly sodden, in shifte of waters, before you doe eate theim: and drawen through a colender, or strainer, with Onions, Mintes and Peper, sodden with theim. Then thei will not hurt the stomacke, or moue winde: but clense the raines, and make fatnesse increase with seede of generacion. The beste Pease potage

Tares doe thesame, and nourisheth milke, clenseth the liuer, gaule, splene, raines, and the mouthe of the bladder: sodden in wine, or with duritike, or openyng herbes, as Percely. &c. *Theophrastus* commendeth thē *lib.viij.Cap.v.de historia plantarum*, the white be the beste. There be, thankes bee giuen to God, no small plentie of Beanes, Pease, Fitches and Tares, growing in England: both white and graie Pease, the like of the Beanes, to the greate comfort of men, horse, and Swine. Although many Inkepers with their hostlers, through a cast of legerdemain: can make a pecke of draffe and Beanes, buye three bushelles of cleane Pease or Beanes. Wherby the poor Hackney horse, if he could speake, aswell as Balams Asse did: might call his hoste knaue for his labour, and wishe the Pillorie to be his ghostly father. For although an horse, doe bothe lacke money in his purse, and reasonable witte in his hedde. Yet without all doubt, he is the beste bonde slaue in the common wealthe, and least can be forborne, as it appereth in his seruice, bothe in warre and peace. &c. And seyng his drinke is so good chepe: it is a villonie to rob hym of his meate. For of all creatures, he suffereth moste paine in bodie: but I will meddle no furder in Stable matters, but ende of that, whiche I haue taken in hand, that is of Pease. *Anno salutis.1555.* In a place called Orford, in Suffolke, stones betwene the hauen, & the main sea: wheras neuer Plowe came, nor naturall yerth was, but stones onely, infinite thousande shippes loden in that place. There did Pease growe, whose rootes wer more then .ii. fadome long: and the coddes did grow vpō clusters, like the chattes or kaies of Asche trees, bigger then fitches and lesse then the field Peasō. Very swete to eate vpon, & serued many poore people, dwelling there at hand: whiche els should haue perished for hunger, the skace of bread that yere was so skāt. In somoche that the plain poor people, did make very moch of Akornes: and a sicknes of a strong feuer, did sore molest the cōmons that yere, as none was euer hard of there. Now, whether thoccasion of these peason, & prouidence of God, cam through some shipwrake, w moche miserie or els by miracle, I am not able to determine therof: but sowen by mans hand thei were not, nor like other Pease. And thus I doe ende of Pease, Beanes and

The booke of Simples.

<small>Of Otes called Auena, or Bromos.</small>

and Tares, which be good for man, horse, and swine, Geese & Hennes. And now I shall aunswere you of Otes, whiche in Grece is named *Bromos*, and *Auena* in Latine: thei be wilde and tame of nature, sowen in Marche, and ripe before midde August. And of temperamente be cold in medicenes: and is of the same vertue, that Barly haue in cleansynges, and in plasters it haue thesame effecte also. It partly warmeth and drieth inwardly: thus saieth *Galen lib.vij.simplicium medicamentorum*: And is

<small>Otes do clēse the lunges.</small>

of a bindyng vertue, againste the flowyng fluxe of the guttes: and is good against coughes, or foulnesse of the lunges. And *Plini* saieth *lib.xxij. Cap.xxv.* Otes sodden in Uineger, do take awaie molles, blaines, or spottes. And Otes is a good graine in the common wealth, for men, horse and foules: as thei haue little other bread, in many places of Wales, and Darbie shire. In Northumberlande, horse haue as greate plentie to eate of theim: as menne haue in moste places of this realme, either

<small>Plentie of Otes in North Humberland</small>

wheate or Rie, for their owne foode. And in the North it is called Hauer: the Southerne people Otes, the Italian *Vena*: the Frenche *auoine*, the Arabian *Cartamum*, or *Churtall*: and thus I haue ended of Beanes, Pease, Otes and Fitches, my friend *Marcellus*.

Marcellus.

What saie you of Wheate, whereof our bread is made, of whiche is our common foode, and best graine?

Hillarius.

<small>*Triticum* wheate, or our bread.</small>

The Grekes dooe call Wheate *Pyro*, many yeres before the name of *Triticum* was found: whiche is Latine for wheat *Triticum vero dicitur, quod tritum ex spicis sit*: It is called wheate, that is threshed, or broken from the Eires (wherein it grow) as saieth *Marcus Varro*. The kindes be well knowen, bothe red and white wheate: the tasseld or long eired wheate, and the naked or polled Wheate. The tyme, maner, and place of Sowyng, Reapyng, Thressyng, Grindyng, Bakyng, and eatyng, is naturally knowen throughout all this realme. Euen so is the ingrossyng, kepyng vntil it corrupt: and sellyng it into other forrain realmes, is knowen to thē, whiche neither feare God, obay their Prince, or loue their neighbour. And the naturall complexion of Wheat, is hote in the first degree, vsed in plaster. Wheat meale tēpered with the iuce of Henbane doe stoppe the fluxe of the senewes, and the inflamacion of the guttes saith *Dioscorides lib.ij.cap.lxxvij.* The bread that is leauened, is better to make plaster for the stomacke, then the meale. The iuce of Mintes, Rue, Sage, Wormwood. &c. bee good to mingle with meale, or crummes of bread for plaster, to pained stomackes, puttyng in Uineger. A plaster of the Branne with vineger, and the iuce of sowre Pomegranettes.

<small>To feede of bran, maketh a man leane, but flower bryngeth fatnesse.</small>

warme applied to the bellie, dooe stoppe the fluxe, and swellyng in the guttes. Many goodly vertues belongeth to Wheate, the Branne nourisheth little: and bread wherein moche Branne is left, shall make the common feeder therof leane. And the pure meale nourisheth, and maketh

The booke of Simples. Fol.xxxj.

keth fatnesse to incrsase: of fine meale, Starche is made. &c. The kingdome of Antichrist haue, not a little inriched theim selues, by meale and waxe: thei haue solde them deare. And many a man haue lost his life, by constantly affirmyng, that meale would onely be chaunged into bread, but not into fleshe. The determinacion therof, I leaue to the learned Diuines, but not to the Dunsmen: whose distinctions marreth all, in the chiefest poinct of our religion. &c.

Meale and waxe, haue made greate marchauntes at Rome.

The very diuines & Dusmen, did neuer agree generally.

And yet more of Wheate, this precious grain and corne. *Theophrastus lib. vij. cap. iiij.* dooe name many places, of the diuersitie of Wheate: as *Aphrica, Thracia, Pontus Assiria,* and *Egipt.* &c. And in all these places, wheate doe differ in shape, colour, greatnesse: he writeth meruellous of the kindes of Wheate. He obserueth the nature of euery soile and lande, and of the mancions vnder heauen, and the climates: and saieth in *Asia,* beyonde the countrie of the blacke Trions, the Wheate graines be as bigge as grene oliues, whiche be as bigge as Nutmegges. The Sonne and the soile is of soche vertue, and more *prodigius* wonders writeth he of Wheat. *Plini lib. xviij. cap. vij.* of all Wheate in the worlde, there is none to be compared in goodnesse, vnto the Wheat of Italie, for whitnesse and waight. In Spaine there is little Wheate, but the Wheate whiche thei haue is verie cleane, and their bread as white as the meane bread of Yorke. Well, I haue sufficiently written of breade in his place: Wheate will tourne, and degenerate out of his kinde, and bee chaunged into Darnell. Specially in weate yeres, so saieth *Mathiolus in Dioscorides lib. ij. cap. lxxviij.* I haue seen the like in a field named Helly, in a toune called Kelshall in Suffolke. There bee Tonges and Irons made accordingly, beyng made verie hote, doe presse forthe the oile of Wheate, whiche will heale vlcers and woundes, and all chappes: and open places in the handes, lippes, and feete, through the sharpnesse of the North winde in March plasters of Meale, Leauen, Salte, Vineger, Butter: and oile of Roses tempered together, warme made in a plaster, vpõ leather, and applied to the breast, or any place of hym, whiche haue fallen from some high place, if thei be curable, it healeth them: giuing theim *vnguentum patibile* to drinke, and roule the pacient with a longe roller or Towell. And thus I doe ende of wheate, the moste precious and beste grain, for the foode of mankinde, and is our daily bread.

The sondrie kinds & natures of wheat.

Wheate will degenerate out of kinde, that is from wheate to Darnell.

A plaster for a brosed bodie

Marcellus.

What be the *Lupines,* whiche the Grekes call *Thermos?*

Hillarius.

Hei be like Beanes, hauyng seuen leaues, somewhat like Beares foote: and are commonly knowen, whose meale mingled with Honie, and licked vp, or dronke, doe cast wormes out of the bellie. And made in plaster to the bellie, it doeth the like to children: sodden in Vinegar, to helpe the Kinges euill, made in plaster. And also doe breake a pestilẽce sore laied on warme: and seeth *Lupines* in rain water, vntill thei be wasted, straine

Lupines.

To kill wormes with Lupines.

f.i. this

The booke of Simples.

this water, and when it is colde, washe thy face, and it will cleanse it from foulnesse and spottes. Myrrhe, Honie, and *Lupines* incorporate together, and rolled in Wolle: make a Pessarie, and conueigh it into the place, and it will bryng forthe the dedde childe, and force the menstruall termes. This herbe and seede thereof, will kill Cancers, and skales in the hedde: tempered with Hogges grease, Uinegar and Brimstone. Seeth it in Percely, water, or whaie, and it will clense the bladder, and prouoke vrine: and drunke with Uinegar, it cleseth the stomacke, helpeth digestion, and expulse all noisomnesse, or abhorring of meate.

Diosco.lib.ii. Capi.ciii.

Lupines saith *Galen*, thei bee of an yearthly substaunce, and ingender euill humours: to be eaten as meate thei be hurtfull, but in medicen good. And be bitter, hote and drie.

Marcellus.

What is the goodnesse of *Staphis Agria*?

Hillarius.

Staphis agria Pedicularis. a seede that will kill lice in children, and haukes.

This herbe *Stauis Agria*, is also *Pedicularis*: for if it bee mingled with Oile, it will kill Lice, nothyng better for lousie children, and haukes. &c. The leaues bee like the wilde Uine, with blewe flowers, and is hotte and drie in the fowerth degree. If fowertene seedes stamped, or broken in swete water, bee dronke, it will purge grosse crude, rawe humours by vomite: but he whiche drinke it, ought to walke after it, saieth *Dioscorides lib. iiij. cap. ci*. And furder saieth he, the drinker thereof, must prouidently giue attendaunce, to drinke swete water, vnlesse, els he be strangled with the medicen. This seede with oile of Tartar, killeth tetters, itchyng and as thei terme it, manginesse: sodden in Uinegar, warme holden in the mouth, to helpe the paines in the teeth, and stoppe the reume. And with Hony healeth vlcers in the mouthe: but it is perilus to be taken doune, because it burneth. And is good to make an *Apophlegmatum* with, doe clense the matrix of women, made in plaster. Plentie of this do growe in the countries of Apulia, and Calabria in Italie: and this I ende of this. What haue you els to saie?

A plaster to bryng forthe a dedde child.

Marcellus.

What is that slepyng herbe, called *Solanum*, and his felowes, I praie you?

Hillarius.

Solanum, Nightshade, the slepyng Dwale.

It called *Solatrum, Solanum*, or *morrell*, in Englishe the greate sleping Nightshade, or Dwale. And of this there be thre kindes emong vs in Englande, as the greate Morelle, the little pettie Morell, or Nightshade, and Alkakengi, which is the Wisicke or bladder herbe, to clense thesame and open, skower, and purge the besselles of the vrine. The greate Nightshade, with blacke beries, like rounde Plummes, be venemous, when thei be eaten, bryngeth vtter madnesse or death: the lesser causeth moche slepe. These bee colde and drie of complexions, as

Galen

The booke of Simples.   Fol.xxxiij.

Galen saieth: *lib.v.cap.ix: Dioscorides* saieth, that pettie Morrell leaues, be cause of nature thei bee colde, and their iuce with Barly meale doe quenche *Sacra ignis*, or that we doe call sainct Anthonies fire, and by theim selues stamped, doe helpe the burnyng of the hed, or swellyng togerthe vnder the tongue, applied to them. This iuce drunke, dooe helpe the yellowe Iaunders, and burnyng of choller: but if you be euill at ease after the then drinke *Oximell simplex*, with warme hote water, and put your finger in your mouthe, and vomite. The madde greate Nightshade, is cold in the extreme degree, if one drinke one drame, saieth *Plini* thereof, then thei begin to plaie their pagiantes, past shame. But if thei drinke two dragmes, then thei shalbe starke madde: but if thei eate or drinke three dragmes, then presente death, and this venime is called *Doricnion*. The Ikathingi or Kengi, haue berries like Cheries in wrapped, in a close huske, with many singuler vertues to coole: to cause slepe, moderatly vsed or taken, their iuces in endiue of Ptisant. But chiefly it excelleth for the stone, with Parcele, Fenell, Asparagus, the fower lesse cold seedes, ana. ʒ.ii. and damaske Prunes. xvi. in nomber, stamped well together and put into cleane whaie, or Barly water, standyng. xii. howers, puttyng. ʒ.ii. of fine Reubarbe. Then straine it, and drawe into thesame pocion. ʒ.ß. of good *cassiafistula*, or Venice Turpentine, clene washed ʒ.ß then drinke thesame in the mornyng: this will breake the ston if any medicen can doe it. & clense the raines, and heale any sore in the same, anointe the backe with *vnguentum Scorpionis*. And thus I dooe ende of *Solanum Hortensis*, called pettie Morell, whiche is good in medicene, bothe inwardly to coole: and also outwardly to coole the hedde, to helpe the iyes from heate, tempered with the white of an egge. &c.

Drinke but a little, sodde in wine, of this Morell, ʒ.ii. will suffice.

A good medicene for the stone & raines

Marcellus.

What is the vertue of Henbane? I praie you tell me.

Hillarius.

Henbane is called of the Grekes *Hyoscyamus*, it is also called *Altercum* of the Arabians. This herbe doeth kill swine, excepte thei bee driuen in continently, through a greate streame of water, and is called the Swines bane: The nature thereof was first founde by Appollo. This Henbane is of three kindes: the blacke, the yelowe, and the white. The white is more better for medicen, then either the yellowe, or blacke. The seedes be as plentifully growyng, within the codde, as the seedes of Poppie, bothe in forme and bignes: it groweth vpon dūg hill sides, or els vpon old ruins, and about broken walles, and is ripe in the moneth of July. The temperamēt or complexion of the white seede, is cold in the third degree. The other twoo seedes be venemous, and full of poison. This white seede is good, with the ointment of Roses, to be laied vpon an hote goute, or swellyng of the priuie members or breastes of a womā, which swelleth or burneth. A halpeny weight of this seede beaten in pouder, with asmoche white Poppie sede, drōke

An herbe of veneme thorowe colde, called Henbane.

Three kindes of Henbane.

f.ii.

The booke of Simples.

The white Henbane is vsed in medicene.

in swete water, or the water of Plantan: doe not onely reconsile slepe but stoppes spittyng of blood, and helpeth the rednes of the iyes. The leaues of this white Henbane, Barly meale and vinegar, be good to make a plaster, to quenche the burnyng of the raines of the backe, or extreme hedde ache, whiche cometh of Choller, and also it helpeth all inflamacions. *Dioscorides* saith, this sede dronke in wine, doeth heale a feuer called *Hepyalas*: euen so doth the iuce of the leaues. But if this herbe be vsed, either in sallet, or in pottage, then doeth it bryng frensie and madnesse: the roote sodden in vinegar, dooeth helpe the paine in the teeth. *Galen* also doeth vtterly refuse, the blacke and the yellowe seede, as poison: but the white he doeth accept as medicene. *Plini* doeth commende the same white, saiyng: if it bee stamped with Honie, it healeth the bityng of a madde Dogge. And with wine, againste the bityng of Snakes. And against choughes and streightnes, through greate extreame filth of the lunges. The oile thereof helpes the deafnes in the eares, droppyng in but little. *Plini* would that none should vse more thā fower leaues of this herbe, the iuce thereof at ones. For who so vseth more, shalbe in daunger to slepe without wakyng. And thus I ende of Henbane, whiche is also called the poison, or bane for Hennes.

Marcellus.

What is the nature of Hemlocke, that stinkyng wede?

Hillarius.

The moste colde herbe, and a poison.

Hemlocke is called *Cicuta* in Latin: the Grekes cal *Koneion*, that is to saie, a tiraunt or killer of men, for it is cold aboue nature, if it be takē within the bodie. The cruell murtherers of *Athenes*, did moste traiterously, maliciously and falsly, poison their chief patrone, & well spryng of learnyng, called *Socrates*, an excellente Philosopher, soonne to *Sophroniscus* a Mason, and *Phanarista*, a midwife, whiche were his parentes. This man when he had beste the knowlege, of naturall Philosophie, gaue hymself to morall Philosophie: he was vertuous in liuyng, and disputed against thē, that were called *Sophistæ*. This mannes breastes of learnyng, gaue forthe the milke of knowlege, vnto the moste famous clarkes: *Plato*, *Xenephon*, and *Xenocrates*. And after he had taught a long tyme in *Athenes* he was by ye malice of *Anytus* & *Miletus* accused, to speake againste

The death of Socrates was with wine, and the iuce of Hemlocke.

their Gods: wherfore he was condempned to death, whose death was the iuce of this Hemloke, called *Cicuta*, mingled with wine. After which drink, he did expire the breath of life, before the yere of Christes incarnacion 367. *Dioscorides* saith, who so euer drinketh of this benemous iuce.

To help hym whiche haue drunke Hemlocke.

The remedy is onely to drinke, a great draft of clene newe wine alone without any other mixture put therunto with spede. The iuce of this saith he, doeth quench that disease, which we call S. Anthonis fire, applied to the burning place. It doeth extinguishe or quenche the heate, whiche is aboue nature: either in the breastes of women, or in the priuie members of boies or men, called the colt euil emong horses, but in men the aboundaunce of nature, with heate gathered vpon a lumpe.

And

The booke of Simples.   Fol.xxxiij.

And it doeth quenche and drie milke, in womens breastes. *Plini* writing of the nature of this, saieth it was the publike or common death, vsed emong the Athenians. The seede and the leaues, hath power through coldnes, to kill bothe inward, and outward partes of the bodie: the remeadie is this saieth he, before it come to the vital partes, is to drinke hote wine, but with wine it is incurable. But the iuce of this, dropped into the iye, doeth quenche the heate, and clense the sight, and healeth a disease called *Epiphora*, saieth *Anaxilaus*. And thus I ende of this venemous herbe, whiche here in Englande, women vse to bucke their clothes with: and Weauers doe make quilles vpon their stalkes, whiche be called Kexes.   *Humloke is a venemous herbe.*

Marcellus.

What is the nature of the Artichoke, whose heddes be sodden with Beeffe: and vsed emongest vs for meate.

Hillarius.

The Grekes call it *Scolimus*, it is called *Cinara*, bicause this herbe delighteth to growe in pearth, mingled with Asshes: Some suppose it to be named *Cinara*, of a maiden, whō the Poetes did fain, was transformed into a greate Thistell, or an Artichoke: this herbe is commonly knowen, and is of two kindes. That whiche is full of prickes, bothe in the fruicte and leaues is wilde, and of small effecte, and that is taken to be *Scolimus*. *Cinera* the tame or garden Artichocke is good. The roote or leaues beyng sodden, or dronke with wine, doe heale the stinkyng and filth, in the bladder or yarde of a mannes bodie: and maketh the vrine swete, and clenseth melancholy or fleume, whiche doth abaunde. This saith *Dioscorides* and *Galen*, in *lib.ii.de alimentorum facultatibus.* This fruicte doeth nourishe the bodie, and increaseth the seede of generacion, bothe of men and women: if it bee well sodden, in potage or wine, and is a prouidence of nature, and healeth. *Plini* doeth greatly commēd this herbe, saiyng: if the roote be sodden in wine, to the thirde parte, it is wholsome to be dronke, either after the bath, or after meate, and doeth cause vrine to be clensed aboundantly: through whiche the corrupciō of the raines and bladder, shalbe purged effectually. And thus I ende of the Artichocke, whiche is hotte and drie of nature: as appereth by the taste in the mouthe, whiche will burne, and is bitter in the mouthe.   *Scolymus. Cinara. Artichocke. A nourishing herbe.*

Marcellus.

What is the nature of *Trifolium*, called the three leaued grasse?   *Triple grasse*

Hillarius.

This herbe beareth a swete flower, and euery daie his nature is to leese .vii. tymes, his sauour or odour in a daie, and receiueth it seuen tymes againe, in thesame daie. But beyng dried, it kepeth still his sauour. Of this herbe there be twoo kindes, the one purple colour and swete, and the other white flowred, and not so sweete.   *Two kindes of Triple grasse.*

The booke of Simples.

Triple grasse hath many vertues, and excelleth against poison.

The rootes be long and white, this herbe groweth in euery meddowe, in June and Julie: and is hotte and drie, in the thirde degree. *Dioscorides* saieth, the seedes and leaues, sodden in water or wine, and so dronke, doe not onely helpe the diseases of the sides: but also the fallyng sickenesse, the dropsie, or water crepyng betwene the skinne and the fleshe, the strangurie, bothe in menne and women. And also purgeth the humours menstruall, three dragmes of this, stamped with Oximell, and dronke in wine : doeth helpe the bityng of all venemous beastes, and will not suffre no venime, to come within the bodie. Euen so it helpeth bothe Tersians and Quartens. *Galen* is of the same mynde, and *Plini* doeth affirme thesame: that it preuaileth againste poison and venime, drinkyng. xxv. grain waight, of the leafe, or the seede. And this saieth he, is a goodlie *Antidotari*, and also there is no Serpent dare come nere the triple grasse: it is wholsome to make warme, and heale woundes and cancer. And thus I ende thereof.

Marcellus.

Valerian.

What is the blessed goodnes, of that worthie herbe, called Ualerian: whiche some doe call the blessed herbe.

Hillarius.

It is named *Phu* in Greke, and *Nardus Syluestris* in Latine, or Ualeriā and be of twoo kindes, the great and the little, and this herbe of some learned men, is called *Triacle*, bicause it will cleanse venime, from the stomack and sides, and clense the stopping of the matrix, and the vrine, as *Plini* affirmeth dronke in wine. *Dioscordies* saieth, if you drie this herbe and drinke it, then it will moue the vrine, and helpeth the dolour in the sides, and forceth termes menstruall, & the best of this do growe in *Pontus*. We haue good Ualerian also, of good bertue, to helpe inwardly for the stone, and outwardly for woundes: and a goodly precious Balme maie bee made thereof, to heale woundes with all. The Spaniardes doe call it *Herba benedicta*, the blessed herbe, bicause it giueth soche health, to purge termes, and helpe the stomacke. It is not moche inferiour, to the *Nardo* of Inde: but for the stone, it is better. It is hote and drie in the seconde degree : and will growe in moiste places, of a greate heigth. Thei doe greatly erre, whiche doe take Calamus rootes, in the place of Ualerian: the roote haue many smal rootes, growyng vnto it, like vnto the Beares foote rootes, or the rootes of *Iuncus Odoratus*, somwhat yellowe and swete bee beste. And must bee gathered in Sommer, and dried for pessaris, and clensyng vrine: this herbe is commonly knowen, for his singuler vertue, emong Phisiciōs and Chirurgians, and also precious for women. And sodden in wine, with Fenell seede and Mastickc, it is diuritike, and moste beste for theim, whiche haue either the collike or stone.

For woundes
Ualerian maketh salues of greate goodnesse.

Marcellus.

What is the nature of Collumbine which beareth pleasant blewe flowers, some beareth white?

Hillarius.

The booke of Simples. Fol.xxxiiij.

Hillarius.

A Collumbine is called *Aquilegia* and is commonly knowne the flower of fiue heades, like vnto Egles, meetyng togetherin the neither parte of the saide flower, the vpper parte spredeth out with winges, & feete answeryng vnto the same, therfore it is called the Egles herbe, the leaues be like vnto the greater *Chelidon*, but somwhat rounder and softer, it florish in the mouthe of Maye, and is somwhat hot of nature, and doth drie vp Scabbes and Fistulaes if it be stampte & applied vnto them in ye manner of a plaster, it helpeth also to resolue clense and scoure Struma or painefull swellyng in the throate, called the Kinges Euill, receiued in Milke, swete wine or Oximell squillini either dronke or vsed in a Gargarisme warme, if it be mengled with wheat meale, the iuce therof and made warme this waye, it hath in plaster great vertu to drie vp moist humours in Biles or sores. Many doth affirme it to be *Ægilops*, wherin thei do greatly erre, for that is a kinde of Ottes or els *Iunccus odoratus* whereof is rehersed before. But this Collumbine may be vsed in his place. It also clenseth yonge children if it bee put in their drinke from a filthe growynge in their boddie through the aboundaunce of heate, called in the southe the Redgome: but in the North it is called the Fellon, and thus I ende of this herbe, what haue you else to say?

A: collumbin.

For swelling in the throate

A. h. medic?.

Marcellus.

What is then the nature of Chiledon, commonly called Cellenden.

Hillarius.

It is called in Greke *Chiledoneon. Mega* that is the great Chelidon, or if you wil the Swallowes herbe, for a Swallow in Greke is called *Chiledon*, and it agreeth well to the reason that *Plini* maketh mencion of this herbe, whiche obserued first ye nature of the same, saiyng it doth grow when Swallowes do breede, and if through the heate of the swallowes donge, their yonge ones loose their sight, eft soones nature hath taught the olde ones togather this herbe, through whose vertue the saied younge birdes receiue againe their sight, this herbe is hot and driein the thirde degree, and is commonly knowne of euerie reasonable man or woman. *Dioscorides. lib. ij. cap. clxxvj.* saith: if the iuce be streined into a brasen vessel, and mengled with Hony and so boiled into a thickenesse vppon a soft fire. This hath vertue to claresie the eies, and to lighten the sight. The leaues, stalke and roote, stamped & streined in sommer, and kept in a close vessell, and dried by littell and littell, of it self in a shadow place, this is good to make Trochis with al, to heale the eies. The roote therof sodden in white wine, with Aniseedes, and so strained, is good to be dronke against ye yellow Jaunders,

Chyledonion

Swallowes dunge will make blinde, example of Tobias.

For sore eies

f.iiii.

The booke of Simples.

ders, and stoppyng of the Gall. And also it driueth away all maner of Choler adhuste out of the bodie, if it bee sodden with vineger, Honye, white Rose leaues, and Swines greace, it clenseth the bodye from Scabbes, Biles, Soores, and Cankers. Many precious oyntmentes, waters, Salues, and balmes, be made of this herbe, as *Galen, Plinie.* And *Ramondus Lullus,* saith: it may rather be called *Celidonium* that is a gift of heauen for the singuler gifte and goodnesse thereof then *Chelidonium*, or the Swallowes herbe, and thus I ende of this most precious herbe called the great Chelidon. There is a nother lesser herbe of this name which is also called *Scrofularia minor*, hauing leaues muche like vnto Azarabacka or Iuie, hauing many small rootes white, in the forme of Peares, but very small, and this herbe hath yelow flowers, barnished within like gilte, whome the common people call Kynge Cuppes. *Theophrastus* saieth in *lib. vj. cap. xiiij.* this herbe banisheth away when Swallowes come in or beginne to breede *Galen* saith: that this herbe is hotte and drie in the fourth degree, *Dioscorides* saith it will exulcerate or blister the skinne, by whiche means it clenseth scoureth and casteth away foule scabbes, and leprose matter from the skinne. The iuce being tempered with Hony drawne vp into the nose, purgeth the head. After this maner vsed in a Gargarisme doth clense the throte and corruption of the stomacke and longes. This *Scrofularia* or small Cellenden is extreme hotter in Asia then it is in Spaine, and more hotter of nature in Spain then here in Englande. In Scotlande I haue sene the people eate of this small roote parboyled with other colde sallet herbes, with clean Oyle, Suger and vineger, for euery herbe flower and rote must be obserued according to the nature of the regent aswell as of their owne temperement. And thus I ende of these twoo herbes.

Marginalia: Dioscorides, lib. ii. cap. Clxxvii.
Marginalia: Scrofularia.

Marcellus.

What saie you then of an herbe called Pimpernell.

Hillarius.

Marginalia: Pimpinella is good againste the Pestilence.

It is called Pimpinella or Pampinula wherof bee two kindes the greater and the smaller. These herbes be commonly knowne with longe rootes, cornered stalkes, iagged leaues, white flowers and smalle seade, and dooeth growe in euery place, as fieldes, woddes, pastures and Meddowes, and it is hote and drie in the seconde degree, nerehande to the third, the iuce of this herbe is dronke against the biting of serpentes. If it be dronke in wine, it clenseth the raines and bladder. Nothing is better against the Strangurie, bothe in men and women. The distilled water of this herbe doeth drie vp moist humour in the eye, which we call blered watring eyes, it clenseth spottes from the face, and dronke with *Mythridatum*, ther is nothyng better against the pestilence, and thus I ende this herbe.

Marcellus.

What

What say you then of an herbe called Sheperdes purse?
Hillarius.

This herbe is called *Pera pastores*, because it is like a bagge which sheperdes do vse to weare. The seede is not vnlike vnto a little harte of a small birde. The leaues be like vnto Rocket, it is colde of nature, and stoppeth bloud or flixe, beinge dronke with small Red wine or Plantain water. A plaster made of this herbe with vineger and fresshe swines grece doth quenche all inflamacions, or heate of the body as the Shingels &c. The iuce alone doth heale a new wounde, and stoppe the bloud. Nothing is better to restraine the immoderate flixe menstruall, then to make a *fomentum*, and moist bathe of this herbe, and to sit ouer it close. And to drinke of the same clarified in Red wine, many greate learned men do affirme, that the only holdyng of this herbe in a mans hande, dothe stoppe the bloud flowyng at the nose, or any other parte of the body. Many meruels might be declared of the vertue of this herbe, but to the ignoraunte and incredible, to them it is but vaine to write any farther, and thus I ende of Shepards Purse, or bloud stoppyng herbe.

Sheperdes purse, to stop blood.

Marcellus.
What is the nature of Lyons foote, called *Pes Leonis*?
Hillarius.

IT is in forme like vnto a Lions foote, with brode iagged leaues with .viii. indented leaues together in one, smal flowers, yelow in couler, the stalke .vi. handfull longe, with a roote finger bignes, in couler somwhat red, in nature this herbe is drie in the seconde degre, the iuice therof doth ioyne new woundes together, and healeth them quickly, the decoction therof is holsome to wasshe all manner of woundes, new and olde, with warme linnen clothes, wasshed in the same, and the Decoction healeth womens soore breastes, if this bee dronke in wine, it healeth woundes inwardly, in the breast healy and guttes. And draweth vp the guttes in yonge children, that are slipped downe from the body, through occasion of weakenesse, coldenesse, or the flixe. This is an excellent herbe for Chirurgës, to heale woundes with all, and thus I ende of Lyons foote.

Lions foote. Pes Leonis.

To heale woundes and sores.

Marcellus.
What haue you els to say of the nature of an herbe called Knotgrasse, or cumber field?
Hillarius.

IT is called in Greke *Polygonon*, because it hath so many knottes, like knees or ioinctes, there is an herbe þ stoppeth bloud better then this doth, and it beareth an infinite number of small seedes. The leaues be like vnto Rue, somwhat longer, and by euery leafe the seede doth growe, and beareth a small white flower. This herbe is taken to be a weede of no estimacion, and is colde and drie in the seconde

Knotgrasse, Kneherbe, or Poligonon.

The booke of Simples.

conde degree, and in the beginning of the thirde. *Dioscorides* saith, it hath vertue to restraine and coole, if the iuce be dronke, either of them whiche spitteth bloud, pisseth bloud or els hath the blouddie flixe. Notwithstanding, it doth clense the raines, and doth preuent or put away the fit of a feauer, if it be dronke one houre before the acces of the same. It stoppeth the flixe menstrual, either in a vomet or a bathe, or to drink the same with wine. It doth the like against the distilling of the whittes of womē. Dropped into the eare, it fortifieth the hearing of theim which be dull or stopped. This herbe stamped with Hony, dothe heale soores, infectyng or corrupting the priuie or secret members, the leaues therof doth quenche the burning Shingles whote inflamacions and ioyneth healeth and clenseth new woundes. There is no better plaster then this against the heat of the stomacke, and thus affirmeth *Galen* and *Plini*, this muche of this herbe.

Marcellus.

What is the nature or vertue of *Stæchadus.*

Hillarius.

Stechadus or Siechas.

This is a noble herbe and of great vertue, leaued like vnto Time with knops in the toppe like Hoppes, whervpon groweth purple flowers, sweete of sauour, bitter of taste, the roote is small and harde, it beareth flowers in June, and it is of a restrainyng temperament, somwhat coolyng, the decoction therof helpeth the lunges euen as Hysop doth, and is put in many medicens of greate vertue, it doth extenuat or cleanse the inward partes of the body, the Lyuer, the Splene, the Reignes, Guttes, and priuie members: prouoketh termes menstruall and helpeth all the diseases of the stomacke, and thus affirmeth *Dioscorides, Galen* and *Plini*, this herbe groweth in Arabia, and is brought from Alexandria, euen so there is greate plentie growinge vpon the Mount Gargane in Italie. The Arabians do call it *Astochodos* the Italians call it *Stechade*, and thus I ende of this worthie straunge Herbe: whiche groweth not in Englande, but the Poticaries haue it.

Stichados good for the Splene. Dioscor. lib. 3. Cap. xxvi. Galen lib. 8. sim. medica.

Marcellus.

What is the nature of *Verbascum?*

Hillarius.

Verbascum

This herbe is of diuers kindes. The one is called *Mullen*, which is a longe herbe, like a waxe taper bearyng yelow flowers in the toppe with small seades, which is called the white male *Verbascum*, but the white female is in the same forme, and beareth white flowers. Then there is a kind of blacke *Verbascum* with great rootes, sondry braunches, and yellow flowers, & these herbes be called Lunge worte amonge the common people. The thirde kinde bee called Pagles, or Cowslips. These herbes are commonly knowne, and bee of a dryinge nature, and doe greately restraine or stoppe the bealy, in the time of a

Cowsloppes or Pagles.

blouddy

The booke of Simples. Fol.xxxvi.

blouddy flixe, and the decoction of them beinge dronke warme. The water of them quenche the inflamacion or burnyng of the eies. This herbe stamped with clarified Hony in a Leaden morter, puttyng therunto wine and Vineger, doth make a medicine to heale Vlsers withall. This same medecine is good against the stingynge of an Adder, Snake or Waspe. The iuce of their leaues tempered with wasshed Oyle of Lynseede, dothe heale scaldynge or burnynge of the skinne or fleshe. The pithe which is in the roote, is good to heale Fistulaes. And all the flowers sodden in vineger, doeth heale the Kynges Euill, applied to the place, or in gargarisme: the roote, seede, or leafe, sodden in wine, is good, not only to be dronke against all diseases of the lunges, breastes, sides, and reines, but also casteth out of the fleshe any thing therein fixed, as Naile, Thorne, or pricke. Of this herbe is there a singuler medecin made for beastes, Horse, Cowe, or swine, after this maner. Stampe this herbe, puttyng therin Fenicreke and Madder with warme ale, conuey it into the throte of the sicke beast, with a horne or tonnell, made for thesame purpose. and this wil heale and clense their lunges. For lacke of this, and many suche good liue medecines, do many beastes die. Therfore good *Marcellus* take here none occasiõ to dispise this my regement for men, although J here shewe a littell medecin for beastes, for we without thẽ should liue very beastly. Thei be the giftes of God, his creatures, and our seruauntes, and thus J do ende of this herbe called *Verbuscum, Mullen,* or Cowslip. Primerose is of thesame kinde.

Marcellus.
What is the nature of Tormentill?

Hillarius.

This herbe is called *Ceptaphillon, Tormentill* or of some *Bystorta,* this hath leaues like fiue fingers, but that it hath .vii. leaues in nomber, iaged or tothed like a Sawe, growyng aboute the stalke with yellowe golden flowers, with a greate roote, *Plini saith lib.xxv.Cap.ix.* that this herbe doth begin to grow, and banish whan the Vyne doe growe and wither: this herbe also growe vpon hilles, and in Heath grounde and in Woddes. The temperament or cõplection of this herbe is colde and drie in the thirde degree, saith the late wryters, but others affirme not the same, that it should be hot in the thirde degree, and that appereth by his facultie, it wanteth coldnes in the third degree. but rather is of the nature of *Quinq̃ folium,* and the roote is drie in the third degree & hot. *Paulus Ægineta* saith, if this herbe be stãped with oile, it will heale the sorenesse of the feete or scabbes, within three daies. The new wryters saith, it will close and heale newe woundes, and cleanse the iyes. The pouder of the roote, with the iuce of Planten, is dronke againste the stopping or scalding of the brine, it is good against poyson, pestilence, and bloudy flixe, Kinges euell, filth in the mouth, and sornes or swelling of the stomacke or spleane, Liuer and belly. and stoppeth bloud to be dronke in the decoction, the water or pouder. Shepe which feedeth there-

Tormentill do grow, and deminishe as the wine.

L. Fuchius in histo. strip.

Againste the Pestilence.

The booke of Simples:

Turmentill keepe Shepe from the rot.

therevpon shall not die on the rotte, and that I haue seene proued in sondry places in Norfolk, and in a place of Suffolke, called Blaxall, vpon a littell shepes walke, in the same towne, whereas Shepe liued many yeares without rottyng, through the vertue of this herbe, and Shepardes haue obserued the same. And thus I ende of Tormentyll.

Marcellus.

What is the vertue of Rocket Gentle?

Hillarius.

Eruca or Rocked. Dioscor.lib.2. Cap.xxiiii. Galen lib.2. de alement.

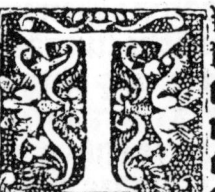His herbe is called *Eruca* for it doth erode and burne with heate, & biteth the tongue, it also smelleth like a Foxe, the seede groweth in a cod like to Rapes with a white roote, yellow flower, and iagged leaues, and is very hot of nature, and increaseth seede of generacion. And the people of Spayne saith *Dioscorides* did vse this Rocket seed in the place of Mustarde, it hath vertue to prouoke plentie of vrine. *Galen* saith, eaten alone, it hurteth the head: therfore his councell is to eate it with Lettis, to rebate the heate. The rootes sodden in water, will drawe foorth a broken bone. The seede is good against the stinge of Serpentes, and poyson of Spiders made in plaster: and dronke, it hath vertue to expulse wormes out of the bealy saith *Plini*.

Marcellus.

What is *Serpentaria*?

Hillarius.

Bistorta haue a crumpled roote, lyyng wrinkled like a serpent, but female rootes is black, without, and redde within, and a greate knotte in the ende.

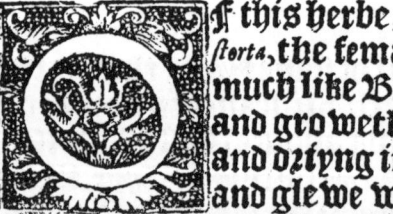F this herbe, there be twoo kindes, the male is called *Bistorta*, the female is name *Colubrina*, the leaues be fashioned much like Beates, a smal stalke with a bushe in the top and groweth in darke places, and is colde restrainyng and dryyng in the thirde degree. This roote doth heale and glewe woundes together in a plaster, & doth chifly stoppe the blouddy flixe, the pouder or decoction, and restraineth vomittes, & stablish the teeth, the decoction warme holden in the mouth. It hath the same vertue whiche *Britanicam* hath in stoppynge or restraynyng, it doth retaine the new conceiued seede without hurte in the Matrix of the mother, and thus I ende of Serpentary.

Marcellus.

Giloflowers are swete and pleasant, but are thei good for any medicen?

Hillarius.

Giloflowers Mathiol.in Dioscori.li.2. Capi.Clii.

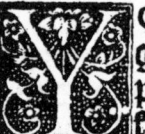E forsoothe, they are no lesse profitale, then pleasante, and greatly commended amonge the olde writers, for *Dioscorides* reporteth of them, they do not only preserue the bodies of men from corrupt heires, but also doth kepe the minde and spirituall

tuall partes, from tirable and fearefull dreames, through their heauenly sauour, and moste sweete pleasant odor, to fortifie the braine: there is no Apothicarie can by any naturall Arte, make any confection so pleasant as this is, which nature hath wrought most wonderous in pleasyng of the sences, both of seeyng and smellyng. If Gilleflouers be stamped they heale new woundes of the head, and draweth foorth broken bones. The decoction of thē be good to wasche the head withal. The Oyle of Gilleflouers doth heale the bityng of a mad dog, and woundes of the sinewes, and colde goutes. If this flower be sodden in white wine, it driueth away the terrour of a Tercian, and the horrour of a Quarten, beyng dronke warme before the fitte, by that means be wormes killed in the bealy. This herbe of nature is hot and drie, and of this there be sondrie kindes, some small and some greate, and of sondrie collours, as white, redde, carnacion &c. And is called *Garyophylum*, or a domestical flower, and in the olde time was vsed to be put in the gardens among ẏ Romayne virgens. The roote is good againſt the Pestilence and Fallyng sicknesse, and thus I ende of Gilleflouers. Gilloflowers will heale woundes.

Marcellus.
What is the naturall vertue of Houslyke?
Hillarius.

Y T is called Houslike in the Southe partes of England, but in the Northe it is called Sull, in Latten it is called *Sedum* or *Semper viuum*, that is euermore liuyng, and neuer dying: therfore the old writers do call it *Iouis barba*, Jupiters beard, and held an opinion supersticiously, that in what house so euer it groweth, no lightnyng or tēpest can take place to doe any harme. The leaues be like vnto tongues, this herbe is commonly knowen, and be of three kindes: thee greate, the meane and the lesse, and of temperement and complexiō, thei be somwhat dryyng, and vehemently colde, I meane the twoo first kindes. But the thirde, whiche is the least, called Stonecrope, is hote in the thirde degree, and will burne the tongue, if it bee bitten vpon, *Dioscorides* calleth it *Telethion*. The greate Houslike doeth quenche hote Apostimacions, Biles, painfull sores, Fellons, Rednes in the iyes, Scaldynges and burnynges, and the richemannes euill, called the Goute. Either stamped by it self or els mingled with Barly meale, oile of Roses and Vinegar: and this waie, it dooeth helpe the hedde, and reconsileth slepe. The iuce of this herbe drunke in wine, preuaileth again the bityng of venemous beastes, bloodie flixe, and womens termes, flowing immoderatly, and killeth wormes in the bellie: and thus affirmeth the said *Dioscorides, Galen*, and *Plini*. But the thirde kinde, called *Telethyon*, hath vertue to make hotte, to blister the skinne: and stamped with Hogges grease, it doeth heale the kinges euil, or paines in the throte. If it be warme anointed therwith oftentymes. And thus I doe ende of this Houslike, whiche is commōly knowen, growing vpon walles, or house toppes: and of the other.ti

Sedum.
Houslike.

Diosco.lib. 4.
Cap. lxxxvii.

Many goodly medicenes made of houslicke.

g.i. kindes

The booke of Simples.

kindes, growyng vpon ruines, rockes of the sea side, or broken walles.

Marcellus.

I Praie you, bee not Nettelles a noisome kinde of weedes, me thinke thei should be none other: as appereth by their spightful stingyng, for thei be fearfull, bothe to man, woman, and childe, and sondrie kindes of beastes.

Hillarius.

Vrtica the Nettle.

A Nettell is called *Vrtica ab vrendo*, of burnyng, blisteryng, or stingyng of the skinne. There be twoo kindes of Nettelles: the common Nettell, and the redde Nettell. There is also the thirde, though not commonly knowen in these parties: called *Vrtica Romana*, the Romaine Nettell, of the whiche, there groweth plentie, about the walles of Yarmouth. This Nettell beareth greate beries vpon it, and the other Nettles but sedes: and of nature thei be all very hot and drie. *Dioscorides* saith the vertue of them, is to heale the bityng of a madde Dogge, stamped with Salt, and so applied to the wounde. It doeth like vnto Cankers and to cold swelling Ipostumaciō: the iuce put into the nose, stoppeth bledyng. The iuce tempered with clarified Honie, clenseth the lunges stomacke, and sides: dronke with Ptisant, doeth clense the bellie, and matrix of a woman. The iuce also tempered with Mirrhe, will moue termes menstruall, if it be dronke warme. The seede therof finely beaten in pouder, and dronke in wine or brothe: doeth augmente and increase the seede of generacion. The seede of redde Nettelles, beyng gathered betwene the sainct Marie daies: maie serue poore men, in stede of Peper, and hath the verie taste of Peper, and is good to season pies, or what you will therwith. And of vertue is accompted, of no lesse valewe then Peper: the leaues of Nettelles sodden with Oisters, clenseth the raines of the back, scoureth the bladder, and prouoketh vrin. And is good againe obstruccion, and stoppyng of the liuer, vpon colde causes, and killeth wormes: the sirupe thereof is moste excellent, to be dronke of women, in their painfull trauaill of children, and causeth spedie deliueraunce. And thus I ende, of the nature of Nettelles.

Poore mennes Pepper.

Nettle sedes will serue in the place of Pepper.

Marcellus.

What is the nature of a *Paonia*?

Hillarius.

Paonia is called the chaste herbe.

T His is an herbe of an excellent vertue, and is called the chast herbe: the coddes therof is full of graines, in forme to the Pomgranet. There be twoo of them in kinde, the male and female. It is saied that the noble Clarke *Bias* was the first inuenter of this herbe: this is commonly knowen emongeste vs, here in Englande. The flowers, like vnto a Rose. The sede doeth growe in a codde, whiche be of colour redde and blacke, and florisheth in Maie: the roote is somewhat byndyng

dyng of nature, neither bitter nor swete, but betwene bothe. And is of a drying heate, in the seconde degree, and warmyng in vertue. *Galen* declareth, that a child did not fal, as long as she had this roote hanging about his necke. But we haue often tymes proued it contrary: but for the fallyng sicknes, the pouder thereof tempered with Mugwort water, and giuen vnto the sicke paciente: preuaileth greatly againe the fallyng euill. The iuce of this herbe or pouder, is good to be dronke againste the stoppyng of the gaule, liuer, or raines: if it bee sodden with olde redde wine, and drunken, it stoppeth the bloodie flire. The redde graines, doe stoppe the redde menstruall humour: the blacke graines, sodden in redde wine, doeth fortifie and strengthen the matrice, in thē whom the flure of blood doe abounde. The roote sodden in wine and drunke, purgeth the bellie, putteth awaie collike, maketh cleane the guttes: defendeth against freneses, and passions of the brain, strangurie, and bityng of serpentes. But there muste no more be taken in medicen at one tyme, but fower drames: and what is better then Pionie, againste the yellowe Jaunders, beyng drunke in white wine, with the pouder of Saffron. This and many moe vertues, haue this worthie herbe, and is beloued of the Spaniardes: and of theim it is called *Rosa Delmonthe*. And thus I conclude, of this vertuous Pionie, that the redde is better then the blacke.

A good medicen for the fallyng sicknes, and the yellowe Jaunders, made of Pionie.

Marcellus.

What is the nature of a straunge herbe, called *Asparagus*?

Hillarius.

This is an herbe of great vertue, and full of rootes, long stalkes, & full of braunches. The braunches that spryngeth first from the roote, be preuented of theim, whiche groweth after them. This is a garden herbe: but of his owne nature, it groweth in rockes, chiefly in Italie. Galen saieth, that this herbe of nature is marueilous: for it is sometyme coolyng, and sometyme warmyng or heatyng. And also clenseth and scoureth, if the tender braunches of these herbes, be sodden in wine and drunken, thei doe not onely molifie the bellie, but clēseth the raines. Nothyng is better to open the gall, and cleuse the yellowe Jaundes, then this herbe is: there is greate vertue in the roote, to be made in pouder, or sodden in medicen, for the same purpose. The beries be of a singular vertue, against the diseases of the teth: the water of this herbe, will clarifie the iyes: the sirupe doeth increase sede of generacion, the decoccion thereof in Uinegar, preuaileth againste the white leprosie. There is no herbe soner cōuerted into good blood then *Asparagus*, notwithstandyng the beries thereof, must be boiled and eaten with swete oile, Uinegar, & suger: and then it preuaileth against barrennes of women. *Plini* doeth commende this herbe, the .xx. boke, the .x. Chapiter. That it preuaileth againste the paines of the bones, called *spina*, and all these foresaied diseases, *Auecen* saieth in his last *Fen. lib. iiij.* that

Asparagus. haue many goodly vertues, specially to increase sede.

g.ii.   this

The booke of Simples.

To make the vrine swete. this herbe maketh a pleasant odour in meate, and bringeth swetenes to the whole bodie, clenseth stinkyng vrine, and causeth the bladder, and all the besselles to be swete. *Galen* doeth not a little commende it. *Lib. vij. de Alimen facultatibus.* And *Dioscorides lib.ij.Cap.cxvij.* do first begin the praise, and laude of this herbe, with all his vertues. And thus I ende of *Asparagus*.

Marcellus.

This same is an herbe, of incomperable vertues: and doeth excel all other, for his singuler goodnesse to mankinde, I truste to remember it therfor. Now I shall desire you, to shewe me the nature of the great Burre, which is more commonly knowen, then commended: notwithstandyng, I would bee glad to learne the vertue, for every manne dooeth knowe it, to bee an herbe of greate anoiaunce in pastures: and an vnpleasant atire, for the maines and tailes of horse.

Hillarius.

Bardana the great Burre This greate Burre is called *Personata, lappa maior*, or *Bardana* and is commonly knowen, whose Burres will cleaue to the apparaile of menne: the leaues be very broad, the roote greate, within white, without blacke, and doeth growe commonly in many places, and is drie, and byndyng of nature. *Dioscorides* saieth *lib.iiij.Cj.cap.* if one dragme weight of this be dronke, with the curnelles of the Pineaple: it doeth helpe the cough, and spittyng of blood, and filthinesse in the stomack, and is good againste the contraccion of the sinewes, and specially the Arteres. **Rotten sores helped.** If the leaues bee stamped, and applied plasterwaies, thei doe heale old rotten sores, and stinkyng filthie vlcers: euen so will the iuce of this herbe. *Galen* affirmeth thesame. The decoccion of the roote therof, is good to washe woundes withall: the roote stamped with Salte, doeth heale the bityng of a madde Dogge, applied to the wound. The iuce tempered with Honie, and so dronke, prouoketh vrin: and taketh awaie the paines of the bladder. The seede beaten in pouder, & dronke in wine, by the space of fortie daies: will take awaie the paines of the hucle bones, called *Ciatica*. **Scaldyng and burnyng helped.** The leaues stamped with the white of an egge, also heale Burnyng or Scaldyng: thus saieth *Apuleus*. The roote preuaileth against the bityng of Serpentes, either inwardly, or outwardly: thesame roote sodden in wine, doeth cleane deliuer a manne, from the horrour of the feuer quarten: If he drinke thereof, one houre before the commyng of the fit. And tempered with swines grease it maketh a goodly plaster, againste the swellyng of the throte, called *Angina*, and thus affirmeth *Columella*. And here I doe ende of Burres.

Marcellus.

What is the naturall bertue of an herbe, called *Gramen?* Or Stichewort.

Hillarius.

The booke of Simples.   Fol.xxxix.

This *Gramen* is called Spereworte, or Stitche grasse: It groweth in darke places, and an infinite nomber of stalkes groweth frõ one roote: the roote crepeth of a great length, within the groũd but not deepe. The flowers bee white, growyng vpon the toppe of the braunches, with a pretie round seede in the middes. This herbe is cõmonly knowen, cattell delite to eate thereof in pastures: thei doe greatly erre, whiche taketh this herbe for *Eufragium*. It florisheth in Aprill, moste swete, white, and pleasaunt. This herbe is cold and drie, with a little bitternesse, hauyng vertue to open: *Dioscorides* doeth saie, the roote hath vertue to close a newe wounde together. This herbe sodden in wine, dooeth breake the stone: it is good againste the hardenesse of the splene, stoppyng of the liuer and gall. It clenseth the raines, scoureth the bledder, and conduite of vrine. *Galen* doeth call this herbe *Pernasus*. For there grewe greate plentie vpon a mountain, in Greke so named: whiche had twoo high toppes, vnder whom did dwell the .ix. Muses, as Poetes faine. *Plini* saieth, the seede doeth vehemently purge the vrine, and stoppeth vomites, with many other goodly vertues. And thus I ende of Stitchworte.

Marcellus.

What is the nature of Sauine? That bitter bushe.

Hillarius.

This venemous herbe, is commonly knowen, from whom diuers Diuelishe drabbes, haue gathered venim: to destroie their bastardly children, to couer their filthie horedome withal. And yet oftymes it happeneth, that the mother is slain, and the child is deliuered: and by Gods prouidence, is helped and saued. Yet this herbe rightly vsed, is of a singuler vertue: I maie rather be nombred emong trees, then herbes, for no frost can kill it. It groweth very thicke, like vnto a bushe, the leaues doe neuer wither nor drie: it groweth in gardens, the beries are gathered in Harueste, and is hotte and drie in the third degree. *Dioscorides* saith, the first boke. 88. Chapi. There be .ii. kindes of Sauin: one hath leaues like vnto the Cipers tree, thother hath leaues like vnto the Tamarice tree: thei haue vertue being stamped, for to heale all painfull sores, Biles, and pusshes, applied vnto theim. This herbe is a good perfume againste the mother, to burne when women doe sownde: and receiuyng the smoke in at the nose. Tempered with Honie, it breaketh a Pestilente sore, made in plaster waies: Drunke in wine, it purgeth theim that pisseth blood. And by subfumigacion, it doeth drawe doune the dedde child, from the matrix of the mother. It is mingled in hotte ointmentes, againste coldnesse of the ioyntes and sinewes: and is good against the Palsie. *Plinie* doeth greatly commende this, in his. 42. boke. Chap. xi. It is good to put Sinamon to this, beyng vsed in medicen. ii. times the weight: It helpeth also the Kynges euill, or paines in the throte, made in the maner of plaster. The fume of this herbe doeth preuaile, againste the Frenche pockes: and thus I

g.iii.   doe

do cõclude of this herbe, called Sauin, whiche the Arabians call *Abell.*

Marcellus.

Daisies.

What be the natures of Daisies, double or single? I praie you tell me.

Hillarius.

Plini lib. 21. Capi. viii.

Neither did *Dioscordies*, nor *Galen* write of these herbes, nor any of the auncient Grekes: but *Plini* saith, that one *Bellius* was inuenter of this herbe, called *Bellis*. And this herbe hath .l. little braunches, or white beames growing round about the yellowe flower, whiche is in the middes, & some do call it *herba Paralysis*. What shall I saie any farder I nede no more discripcion therof: bicause this herbe is so commonly knowen, and groweth in euery field and pasture. Notwithstãding, the double Daisie doeth growe in gardens: & these greate Daisies doe florishe in Maie, and of nature be hot and drie, as we maie gather of *Plini*, whiche saith, this herbe doeth heale swellinges of the throte, and paines in the necke: therfore it must nedes be hote & drie, for no cold thing can help the swelling in the throte. This iuce is good for wounded mẽ to drinke: for it doeth resolue hard and cold thinges, Goute, and *Ciatica*, & is verie good against the resolucion of the members, whiche in Greke is called *Paralises*, whiche we call the Palsie, with this herbe *Bellis*, & other good medicenes. I Bullein did recouer one *Bellises*, not onely from a spice of the palsie, but also from the quarten. And afterward the same Bellises, more vnnaturall then a viper, sought diuers waies to haue murthered me: taking parte against me, with my mortall enemies, accompained with ruffins, for that bloody purpose, & dedly feede. Soche was his shamlesse ingratefull nature. Euill will stirreth vp strife: and a sedicious persone, seeketh mischief. This man beyng worshipfully borne, doe bare the name and title of a gentleman: rather then any cõdicions of one in deede. And incõplexion is more effeminate, then a feble pale woman: a dweller in the place, wheras holy Bede was borne but yet possessyng none of his vertues. And thus of *Bellis* the herbe, I make an ende: and of Bellises, whiche would haue ended me.

Paralyses.
Bellis.
Bellises.
Bullein.

Prouerb. 10.
Prouerb. 17.

R. Bellises of Jarowe, in the Bisshoprike.

Marcellus.

What is the nature of *Sene*, my gentle frende *Hillarius*: I praie you tell me.

Hillarius.

Sene of Alexander.

There be twoo kindes of thẽ: the one is called *Sene*, whiche beareth coddes like Brome. The other is a lesser kinde, bearyng his seede in a grosse codde. The codde is moche like an Almõd growyng on the tree, but as thinne as Perchement. The flowers be like the flowers of Brome, very yellowe. This herbe groweth in gardens, in the Monethe of Maie and June: and of nature is hot, in the first beginnyng of the second degree. And drie in the beginnyng of the firste degree, a dragme of the codde, saieth *Actuarius*, maie be dronke without any hurte: for it hath vertue to purge, bothe fleume and choller. The leaues and coddes be wholsome, to bee sodden in the brothe of an Henne: against olde paines in the hedde, scabbes, fallyng sickenes,

and

The booke of Simples. Fol.xl.

and the itche. The iuce in infusion or steped, is better to bee dronken, then the pouder, for all obstruccions in the body: and these be the wordes, of that greate learned man, Doctor *Actuarius*. This is vsed againste the aboundaunce of melancholly: and doeth open the instrumentes of the senses, and the partes bothe *Animall, vitall*, and *Neutrimentall*. There is of this growyng in Fraunce, but the beste commeth from Alexandria in Egipt: or els from Siria, whiche maie be giuen to women with child, and young children, without any hurte. Chiefly in infusion: it maie bee also mingled with *Cassia* or *Manna*: or els it maie bee beaten into fine pouder, and so tempered with Sirup of Roses solitiue, and so dronke: and this waie it is a gentle lenetiue purgacion. But the delutyng, stepyng, or puttyng these leaues in wine, colde whaie, or distilled water, with a pece of Suger, and some Aniseedes, standyng all the night in a close potte, and in the mornyng strein it. I assure you, this is more better to purge withall, then if it were in decoccion, or sodden in brothe: Note also, when you doe make a decoccion with sondrie herbes, let all your other herbes bee sodden softe, before you put in your *Sene*, for it is so thinne of substaunce, that els it will go awaie in a smoke.

Here wil I shewe you a moste excellent decoccion, whiche I purged sir Richard Alye, a knight of a singuler connyng: whiche knight hath been a profitable instrument, to our common wealth, in worthie ereccions and buildyngs, as of the strong, and famous toune of Barwick, whose walles are inuinsible, as presently appereth. Beside many of his other worthie workes. This manne beyng sicke, in whom diuers and sondrie purgacions and lectuaries, tooke small effecte: this onely did hym moche pleasure, the beste *Sene* leaues, dragmes, vi. white Ginger dragme one, the flowers of Buglosse, dragmes twoo, mingled together, in a newe cleane stone potte, with a narrowe mouthe: and one pinte of whaie, of Goates milke, this potte was closely couered in the mouthe, that no aire should go forthe of the mouth. Then it was sette in a vessell, with hote water, and so did seeth, by the space of twoo howers: and then was taken from the fire, and set in a close place till it was cold, and the vapour cleane delaied. Then it was strained, and giuen him to drinke, in the mornyng folowing, whiche did purge choler adust and melanchollie, whiche is his complexion. This whaie being dronke, preuaileth againste all passions of the braine, from the hedde doune to the bottome of the bladder. And helpeth all the senses, bothe of hearyng, seeyng, and smellyng, and will strengthen all the bodie: and it doeth exonerate, and vnburden the same of euery humour that doeth habounde as cholour, fleame, and melancholie. And this affirmeth *Mesue, Actuari, Ruellus, and Mathiolus* vpon *Dioscorides, lib.3, cap.lxx*.

Sir Richard Alye, his lenitiue, Mathiolus vseth the same in Dioscoridem. Lib.3.cap.70

Sene helpeth the hed, with al the sences.

Marcellus.

What is the vertue of Goose fote, whose leaues be like Geese feete: with iagged leaues.

Pes anseris

Hillarius.

g.iiii.   It

The booke of Simples.

Gosefoote, an euill herbe.

It is called *Pes anserinus*, leaued like Nightshade, but more iagged in the said leaues, bearyng small little red flowers, with great plētie of seede, like vnto Irage: it commonly groweth in eche place whereas plentie of dunge is caste, and is cold in the second degree, and it is venomous as *Solanum* is, and killeth Swine, if they doe eate of it, it maketh men to be madde, or die sleapyng, therefore beware of it.

Marcellus.

What is Fellon weede good for, which is named Sainct Iames weede?

Hillarius.

S. Iames worte, called Fellon wede

The olde writers made smale mencion thereof, it hath leaues like Rocket, many rootes, flowers like Chamamill, growynge by water sides, and in sandy places, and by pathe sides: it is hot and drie of nature, this will heale *Furunculi*, called Fellons and other sores and woundes, and fistulaes, and is holsom to make salues withall to drie, ripe, and heale, and wil not suffer any benomous scabbe, or sore to spreade any farther, therefore it should be good, bothe for *Sarpigo*, and the Canker, Ringwormes, &c.

Marcellus.

What will *Spatula Fœtida* doe?

Hillarius.

Spatula wil kill Lice.

It groweth by hegges, the Berries grow in coddes which codde openeth in three partes, like the *Peoni*, the leaues be long flagges this herbe is vehemently hotte, and hath vertue to kill lice, as *Staphisagriæ* hath, and to heale scabbes. &c.

Marcellus.

What can Orpyn do?

Hillarius.

Telephus. Crassula or Orpin.

This Orpin will longe hange in an house, after it be cutte, and grow still greene, we call it Orpin. *Telephus* the kynge of the Gothes, and *Myssæ*, sonne to *Hercules*, whiche warred vpon the Grekes before Christes birthe. *Anno. 1212.* This man slew a famous capitaine of Grekes, named *Thesandrus*, & his soldiours vanquished *Aiax*, and *Achilles*, but yet *Achilles* wounded him with a Darte, which wounde was healed by this *Crassula*, whiche he named *Telesphium*, and vntill this day, it is so called: wherof there be twoo kindes, the great with white flowers, and the smale with yellow, but these flowers be variable, and wil change their couller, the leafe is like Purslen, but grosser, and this doth grow in moist places, vnder the droppyng of houses in Gardens, and flourisheth in July, and August, and is drie in the seconde degree, and in the beginnyng of the thirde, and is very hotte. The iuce therfore is good **Orpin heleth the morphew** to anoint the place of the Morphew euery hower, so that it bee mingled

The booke of Simples. Fol.xlj.

gled with stronge white vineger, but *Galen* affirmeth that it doeth not onely clense the fainte Morphewe, whiche he calleth *Alphos*: but it also clenseth a foule corrupte stinkyng vlser, scoureth and dzieth the same. *Plini* saieth, this iuce will heale a filthy Leperous sore of diuers colers to be anointed therwith, euery hower, daie and night: iii. times in one moneth, & as you doe anoint thesame, to put vpon the same sore Barly meale. It maketh a plaster for *Hernia*, and healeth woundes, bothe olde and newe, and fistulas. And thus I do ende of Orpin, or herbe *Telephon*. To clense the Morphewe.

     Marcellus.

What is the goodnesse of Paunsis, or three faces in on hodde? Some call it Harteseale.

     Hillarius.

THis herbe is called *herba Trinitatis*: but I rede in an olde Monkeshe written Herball, wherein the aucthour write, that this herbe did signifie the holie Trinitie: and therefore was called the herbe of the trinitie, and thus he made his aligorie. This flower is but one, in whiche said he, is thre sondrie colours: and yet but one swete sauor. So God is three distinct persones, in one vndiuided Trinitie, vnited together in one eternalle glorie, and diuine Maiestie, &c. Well, although the three distincte persones be euē so, whose glorie is indifinable: yet this glory maie not be comprehended of mortall men, nor Angels. The maiestie thereof maie not with reuerence, be cōpared or likened, by any aligorie, to any base, vain, venerous flower: but maie rather be called, thre faces in a Monkes hodde: That this daie groweth in the Garden, and to morowe withered as duste. Moche more the offence & daunger is, for any christian man, to graue or painte any Image, callyng it the signe or Image of the Trinitie: whiche can not bee doen, of any liuyng creature, for God forbad thesame. God haue no man seen, but onely his soonne Christe, whiche is God of his substaunce, and of thesame deitie. Neither any mortall man maie se him, before he bee clensed by death, and transformed into an other life, saith the holy scripture: thus all glory be to the holie Trinitie. And now I will shew the right distinicio of this herbe, fitte and apt for thesame vain flower. It is called *herba Trinitatis*, that is, because it haue thre colours: yet the old Pagan writers, did cal it Iupiters herbe, because of the beautie of colours: is like a Violette in shape and sauour. And of temperament, is moche like Comphorie, hot and drie, and is good to bee dronke, bothe againste the fallyng euill in children, and also against all maner of rotten fleume, and filth in the stomacke, sides, and lunges. Thus it doeth inwardly helpe, in syrupe, decoccion, or the water inwardly drunke: no lesse it helpeth all wounded men, women, and children, and al thē whithe haue broken bones. Outwardly, it clenseth from the skin, all itche, skabbes, shingles, vlcers, and ringwormes: and healeth or closeth grene woūdes together, without the daunger of any apostumacion, if it be made in plaster, or Herba Trinitatis of.iii. colours so named.

An aligorie of an herbe.

Ihon.i.

Exodus.20.
i.Ihon.4.

els

The booke of Simples.

els the iuce preserued with oile. For herbes beyng stamped, strained, and clensed vpon the fire: and made colde, and kepte in a cleane glase, powre therevpon freshe cleane oile of Oliues, whiche wil conserue it, and kepe it from the corrupcion of aire, and so you maie preserue your iuce, as this and many other mo, for sirupps and salues, for the health of mankinde. And thus I do ende of the nature of Paunses, or the triple coloured Violettes, called *herba Trinitatis*.

Marcellus.

What goodnes is I praie you in the Iue, the womens christmas herbe, whose leaues be euer greene.

Hillarius.

Hedera or ye Iuie bushe.

The Iuie is like a freshe lusty yong plesanut body, still florishing and grene, the Grekes do call it *Cissos* of Bacchus, for they called him *Citton*, and this is Bacchus herbe or his winter Crowne, the Wine is his croune in summer. This is a very euil neighbor, for where as it doeth growe vpō any tree, the tree dekaieth, although the Iue do florishe still grene, wheras it is nourished. There be iii. kindes of Iuie

Iuie haue many goodlie vertues in medicene.

the white, whiche is the male, bringeth forth white beries: the second bareth blacke beries: the iii. is fruitles, or groūd Iuie so named, these be commonly knowen. Iuie is of a contrary compounded facultie, adstringing, binding, or stopping: whiche is cold & yerthly, it is also bitter and hote, if it be grene, but drie and cold. The beries sodden in wine & drunke, doe stoppe the bloody flire, drunke twoo tymes in the daie, and as moche in the night: the tender leaues sodden in sharpe vineger, tēpered with crommes of leauen bread, will helpe the liuer, made in plaster. Stamped with Roses, and temper it with oile of Roses, Vineger and womans milke, to make a good frontall, for his forehedde: that is pained in the hed. The iuce, with the oile of bitter Almondes, warme put into theares, to helpe the instrumēt of hearing: the leaues sodden in wine, be good to anoint or washe thē, whiche haue spots or scabbes in their face, skin, and priuie partes. Nothing preualeth more against the Cancer, then the iuce of Iuie, tempered with clarified Honie, and wine sodden together, & so vse thesame drinke. i.z. After the naturall purgacion of women, if it be drūke, it causeth sterilitie & barrenesse in them. The iuce warme, powred into the contrarie eare, doe helpe the teeth, on the other side, if thei doe ake, but if the beries of Iuie, called *Corymbi* be often times drunke, saieth *Dioscorides*, thei will vexe and trouble

To kill Lice

the minde. Honie and the beries of Iuie, will kille Lice in childrens heddes: the iuce put into the mouthe of the matrix, will drawe forthe the dedde childe. The grene leaues, sodden in wine, saieth *Galen*: doe knitte, heale, and ioine cuttes, and greate woundes together, and hea-

To heale woundes.

leth the bodie: But yet this iuce, often tymes dronke in wine, also it will heale the terrour of a Tercian, or horror of a quarten, dronke before the fitte. And also purgeth the hedde, putte into the nose: it will shorten the sicknes. The Gum of Iuie will blister, and is verie hotte,

and

The booke of Simples. Fol.xlij.

and thei whiche gather it, muste cut the barkes frō the Iuie: and euery morning, when the sap do ascende, thei shal find it in the nether cut of the barke. Euen so when it discende, in the upper barke or rinde, renue your cut euery morning, and washe your handes in vineger, and Rose water, and your face in like case, before you gather it. But whipe it not, and then your gum shall not blister, or hurte your skin: this gum tempered with ware, putto a pained tothe, will drawe it forthe without paine: this gum must be kept close in a glasse, or boxe of clene mettell, and to these foresaied vertues, affirmeth the beste learned, as *Dioscorides, Galen, Plinie.* &c. And thus I doe ende of this Iuie, whose gum, leaues, and beries, are wholsome for mankinde. Euen so thei are for beastes, as horse, or Oxe, againste the sickenesse of the lunges, sodden in Ale or wine, with Aniseedes and Baies.

To gather Iuie gum.

To drawe teeth without paine.
Dioscor.lib.1. Capi.Clxxv. Plini Lib.16. Cap.xxxiiii. Theophrastu. lib.iii.cap.18. Galen libri simp.medic.

Marcellus.

What is a weede, whiche haue leaues like Peres: growyng in Marris or moiste groude.

Hillarius.

This herbe haue broune spottes, in the midds of the leaues, and haue knottes in the ioyntes: stalkes redde, flowers like Lauender. First white, then purple, rootes yellowe, small seedes: many in nomber growyng on the braunche. This of nature is colde and drie, the taste doeth declare the same: this herbe sodden in Planten water, Ptisante or redde wine, doe stoppe the bloodie flire. And this same herbe, is good to heale fistulas, and clenseth rotten sores: and furdermore, healeth newe woundes. And thus I leaue of this herbe.

Persicaria or Pereleues growyng in marris groūd called Iasper

Marcellus.

What be Brakes good for?

Hillarius.

Commonly knowen, to lodge the Deare, to throude and couer the Conie withall. Drie Brakes be good fuell, wheras smal plētie of wood is, or cole. There be brakes male, without flower and seede. Growing frō one greater roote many braunches, with spots upon their leaues: the female Brake is common in Warreins and Parkes. And groweth long, if the roote be cutte ouerthwart, there wil appere the simslitude of an Egle spleid. iiii. ʒ. waight, of the male roote, dried and beaten into pouder, and dronke with swete water, doe kill broade wormes, in the cheste or bellie. But it is bitter, saieth *Dioscorides*, if sower halfpenie waight of prepared *Scamonie*, be dronke with the same: then it will worke accordyngly, or els as moche pouder of blacke *Elleborus*. The female Brake rootes. ʒ.iiii. dronke, sodden in wine, doe kil round wormes: it is perilous to giue to women, it maketh them barren. And if a woman with child drinke it, it maketh an obertiue or ded child come forthe: the meale or pouder of Brakes, healeth daungerous sores upō beastes bodies, as Swine, Kine. &c. The yong braunches of Brakes, eaten

Brakes called Filix, or Ferne.

To kil brode wormes in the cheste or bellie.

Dioscorides.

The booke of Simples.

Brake sedes were neuer seen emong chzisten people, but witches haue vsed practise of them, as foolishe writers affirmeth.

eaten, beyng tenderly sodden, doe molifie verie gently the bellie, *Galen,* *Theophrastus* and *Plini,* affirmeth thesame. This herbe beareth no seedes at any tyme, although Witches saine, that greate Secretes maie bee wrought with thesame: whiche must be gathered saie thei, vpon Midsomer night: As sure I warrante you, as the sea doe burne, it will doe no lesse. This herbe is hotte and drie, and is called *Thelepteris:* because it haue winges, or leaues like birdes fethers.

Marcellus.
What is the vertue of the dedde stinkyng Nettle?

Hillarius.

The dedde Nettle.

It maie bee called a dedde Nettle, it is like in shape, vnto the burnyng Nettle but stingeth not: it is called Archangell, with a stalke sower square, there be three kindes of Archangell. White, called *Lamium,* Yellowe, and Purple with Blacke seede, hote and drie of nature: the white flowers doe helpe the Shingles, stamped and applied to the sore places of the skinne: this herbe stamped with Salte maketh a plaster for the goute, swelling in the throte, and Dogges bityng. The rootes stamped with Salte, dooe drawe forthe thornes, or prickes from the bodie. And thus I ende of this dedde Nettle.

Marcellus.
What be the natures of Cresses?

Hillarius.

Nasturtium, Lepidion, or Cresses.

Cresses helpeth ye palsie.

Cresses be commonly knowen, there be bothe of the water, and also of the lande: Garden and Riuer, spring fro Marche, to the ende of Maie, and is nere hande hote in the .iiii. degree, not so moche dryng: the seede is chiefly vsed in medicen. The herbe is good grene, but nothyng worth drie: these seedes sodden in wine, in a linen bagge this seede holden vnder the tongue, or champed in the mouthe, to help a speachlesse man, or hym whiche haue the Palsie, through a longe or strong agewe. This will drie vp moiste humours, it prouoketh vrine, sodden in white wine: and stoppeth *Gomorrha passio,* or wastyng of nature. And this herbe so helped a gentilmanne of Suffolke, called Thomas Colby, whiche longe tyme was troubled with thesame: when other medicenes, did take in him smal effect. Duryng his seruice in the felde or warre, finally was recouered by this. (This herbe) specially saieth *Dioscorides,* the rootes stamped with freshe Hogges grease, dooe makean excellent plaster, against the paines of the iointes: laied vpon warme iiii. howers: but for women, but .ii. howers. And also thesame for *Ciatica,* and then quickly to sweate in the bath: then when the pacient haue sweate, to drie the bodie, and to anoint the bodie, with the oile of Cresses, and warme sodde wine. And to drinke of this wine, wherin Cresses be sodden: it is good againste paines in the iointes, Dropsie, Tim-

Cresses doe helpe many infirmities.

panie,

panie, Goute, swellyng Palsie, Pore, Apostumacions, Reumes, bloodie flires, broses, and moistnesse of the brain and iyes. &c. *Galen* commēd thesame *lib. i. de compos. medica secundum locus Cap. vij.*

Marcellus.

What is the vertue or nature of Horstaile?

Hillarius.

This is also called *Hippuris*, that is Horstaile, bicause it busheth like heere aboute the iointe: and is of twoo kindes, softe and long. And groweth in moiste grounde, and watrie places: it is called holie water sprinkle or bushe. It drieth, and restraineth, and is bitter: this herbe sodden, the wine or decoccion therof, is good against the blodie flire, stoppyng of the bladder. It mūdifieth the stomacke, sides, and clenseth the lunges: and if the guttes be hurte and wounded, nothyng is better to heale, then the syruppe or iuce of Horstaile, saieth *Dioscorides*: *Galen* affirmeth that thesame herbe, doe heale woundes, and stop blood in the nose, withall the deseases aforesaid, dronke with wine. Goodlie salues of healyng, maie be made with thesame: *Plini* saieth, and that I haue proued often times, that it healeth ruptures. And further saieth *Plini*, it stoppeth or defendeth *Enterocela*, whiche is a disease verie perilous, called *Cætum intestinum*, when the guttes are fallen into the coddes. Euen so it will heale theim, dronke often tymes. And a plaster of this, with warme Uineger, stamped together, and applied to the bellie, for the same purpose: the smoke or fume is good, to cause childrens guttes, to go backe into the bodie, when as through flire or colde, thei will hang forth. Euen so it will stoppe, the immoderate redde termes in women: and this shall suffice, of thesame herbe.

Horsetaile, *Cauda equina*.

To helpe the flire.

To helpe the guttes.

To stoppe the termes of women.

Marcellus.

What is that herbe Botris?

Hillarius.

This herbe *Botris* so named, because the seede is so plentifull: clustring with greate nomber on the braunches, it groweth by riuers, or water sides, & is ripe in Septēber. This herbe is swete, and when it is drie, it is good to caste into chestes: to preserue apparell from Mothes, and make bothe linen and wollen swete. This herbe is yellowe, wherof is plentie nere vnto Paris in Fraunce: It is hote and drie of nature. Dronke in wine, it helpeth the lunges, and clense them from cold coughes, and sorenesse in the breast: and helpeth against the shortnesse of wine, *Dioscorides*, *Paulus* and *Plini* affirmeth thesame.

Swete Botris.

Marcellus.

What saie you of Gentian?

Hillarius.

This was found by Gentian, a noble king of *Cillyrica*, which being wounded in battaill, had health by thesame herbe: it is leaued like Plantan, the rootes bee also not vnlike Aristodochia the long,

Gentian, a bitter herbe.

h.i.

The booke of Simples.

<small>Gentian a bitter herbe, hauing many vertues.</small>

long. This roote is grosse and bitter, with yellowe flowers, growyng vpon high Mountaines or Alpis: and we haue plentie therof emong our Apoticaries, it is hotte and drie, and moste bitter. Twoo dragmes dronke with Peper and Rewe in wine, dooeth defende poison, and bityng of serpentes, and is good for wounded men to drinke: and casteth dedde children from the matrix. This is against all opelaciō, and stoppyng of the liuer, gall, and splene, and wil purge choller: but it is perilous for women with childe, to drinke it. There is nothyng better for *Illiaca passio*, it strengtheneth the stomacke: This is not onely profitable to mankinde, against Dropsie, stoppyng of the bodie, venime, poison, and pestilence, to bee dronke in wine or water. But also it helpeth the dombe brute beastes, as horse, oxen. &c. for all diseases of the lunges: to be giuen them, as *Plini* saith. The roote sodden, is good against conuulsion, and shrinkyng of the sinewes. And thus I doe ende of Gentian.

Marcellus.

What is the propertie and vertue of Lauender?

Hillarius.

<small>Lauender the swete vertue thereof, wholsome for colde folkes.</small>

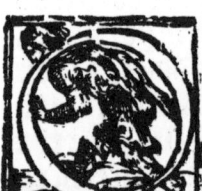F this kinde, there is Lauender Spica, whiche is the great Lauender: then there is the single Lauēder. This herbe is called the counterfet, or false *Nardus*, and is named *Lauendula*: because it is good in bathes and wasshyng, and giueth a swete odour. This herbe is commonly knowen and is hote and drie in the seconde degree: and is good against the coldnesse of the stomacke, hardnesse of the splene, and swellyng of the guttes, stoppyng of the liuer, and the raines, prouoketh vrine. Nothyng is better, against the diseases of the sinewes, the coldenesse of the braine, palsie, and fallyng euill: either to be dronke, or smel of this herbe: or also to be anointed with the goodly warme oile made thereof. Whiche oile hath vertue, againste all the diseases of the sinewes: And thus I ende of this herbe.

<small>Lauender helpeth the senewes. Oile of spike doe warme,</small>

Marcellus.

What is the nature of Mandragora?

Hillarius.

Any supersticious, and foolishe thinges haue been deuised, of this herbe: a verie inuension of Witches, and Hypocrites, through the sudgestion & mosion of the deuill, to delude the weake hart of mankinde withall. For thei doe affirme, that this herbe cometh of the seede, of some conuicted dedde menne: and also, without the death of some liuyng thing, it can not be drawen out of the yearth, to mannes vse. Therefore, thei did teye some Dogge, or other liuyng beaste, vnto the roote thereof with a corde: and digged the yearth, in cōpasse round about, and in the mean time, stopped their own eares, for feare of the tirrable shrieke, and crie of this Mandracke. In whiche crie, it dieth

<small>An old supersticion, inuented by witches, and a practise of Sathan.</small>

not

The booke of Simples. Fol.xliiij.

not onely die it self, but the feare thereof: killeth the Dogge or beaste, whiche pulled it out of the yearth. And this herbe is called also *Anthropomorphos*: because it beareth the Image of a man, and that is false. For no herbe haue the shape of man or woman, no truely, it is not naturall of his owne growyng: but by the craftie inuencion, of some false man, it is doen by arte. As many rootes maie bee made, in the formes of men, foules, and beastes, and secretly couered in the yearth: whiche when it is found, by the craftie hider thereof, the beholders be driuen into no smalle admiracion and wounder. Supposyng there by, that some straunge fearfull thing, shall quickly folowe the same. My frend *Marcellus*, the discripcion of this Mandrake, as I haue said, was nothing, but the imposterous subtiltie of wicked people. Perhaps of friers, or supersticious Monkes: which haue written therof at length, but as for *Dioscorides*, *Galen* and *Plini*. &c. thei haue not written therof so largely, for to haue hed, armes, fingers. &c. But there is an herbe called Mandracke, whose leaues be large and long, like vnto large Lettise: whose apples bee in the forme of Cheries, verie colde, properly giuen to helpe concepcion, some saie: as it appereth by the wiues, of the holie Patriarch Jacob. The one was fruictfull, the other did desire helpe, by the meanes of the Mandrack: brought out of the fieldes, by the handes of Ruben Leas sonne. This herbe haue a longe large roote, with twoo legges in forme, one wrapped about the other: and fine rootes like heere, growing vpon it. But no armes, feete, fingers, handes, hedde, nor stalkes, but the leaues crepe out of the grounde: whereof be twoo kindes, male, and female, the male greater then the female. This herbe is cold in the thirde degree, and haue vertue, to cause depe slepe: the strengthe is in the apple, and in rinde of the roote. The remenant, that is in the leaues, and inward partes of the roote, bee but weake saieth *Galen*: the seedes of the aple, saieth *Dioscorides*, beyng drunke, will purge the bellie. The iuce of this herbe pressed forthe, and kepte in a close pearthen vessel, accordyng to arte: this bryngeth slepe, & casteth men into a trauns on a depe tirrible dreame, vntill he be cutte of the stone. &c. This herbe sodden in wine, vnto the third parte, doe purge blacke choller as well, as *Elleborus niger* will do. This herbe stamped, and applied vpon a wound or vlcer, do heale the same, and so naturally, that it will suffre no skare or marke, called *Stigma* to remaine, the leaues be preserued in Salte, for the same purpose. The greene leaues stamped, and applied with the white of an Egge to the iyes, doe asswage swellyng, burnyng, or dropping of theim: if the roote bee cutte in sondrie places, there will come forthe a worthie iuce, to anoint the forehed, to bryng slepe. Pessaris be made of this, whiche will drawe foorthe dedde children, from the matrix: therefore rightly to saie, it rather hinder, then furder concepcion, the roote is vnpleasaunte to smell vpon, and pestiferous saieth *Plini*. The iuce must be gathered, when Grapes bee ripe, and clarified in the Sonne, and kept close. The aples must be dried in the Sonne, and the roote must be sodden in old darke coloured wine, whiche wine must be

h.ii. sodden

Mandrak is made like a man or woman by craft, for nature giueth no mannes shape to a beaste, moche lesse to an herbe.

Gene.xxx. This place proue not that Mandrake will helpe concepcion, but Mandrake wil clense the matrix, or cast forthe the ded child from the same, then it will kill the liuyng seede. Dioscorides is of y^t minde

The vertues of Mandrak, is to make one to slepe.

The booke of Simples.

sodden in the third part: the aples maie be bruſed and kepte, in vnripe oile Oliue in the Sonne. All theſe bee good to coole, to cauſe ſlepe, moderatly vſed. Two halfpenie waight of the pouder of the rinde therof, maie bee drunke in ſwete water, for the Kynges euill, or lacke of ſlepe. The iuce thereof with oile and Honie, healeth woundes: and thus I ende of Mandrack, whiche in the old tyme, it was called *Circæam*, of witches, whiche had vertue (ſaied thei) or craft to transforme, bothe man beaſte, and herbe out of kinde: Emong all other, thei wrought wounders by this herbe, to prouoke, bewitche, or caſt men into madde blind fantaſies, or frances, called Loue, whiche rather maie be termed, not ſome beaſtly luſte, and when it is wrought by herbes fooliſhnes.

Mandrake was called Circæ, & alſo Anthropomorphos.

Marcellus.
What is to be ſaied of Crowfoote: wherefore is it good?

Hillarius.

This herbe is called *Ranunculus*, or Frogworte: of this Crowfoote *Dioſcorides* founde fower kindes *lib. ij. capi. Clxxi.* But ſince his daies, three kindes more be founde: theſe bee herbes bothe of the water, wheras Frogges doe caſt their *Sperma* or ſeede, in whiche herbe, thei dooe greatly reioyce. And alſo of the lande, as garden, Medowe, and wood Crowfoote, this herbe is commonly knowen. Some haue white flowers, ſome yelowe, ſome purple: ſome haue leaues like Coriāder, ſome haue leaues like Beares foote, growyng vpon the toppe of the ſtalke, hauyng long rootes. And other haue broad iagged leaues, growing nere the grounde: but vpwarde ſmaller leaues like Crowfoote, doe growe vpon the braunches. Theſe herbes bee behemently hotte and drie, and doeth vlcerate and bliſter the ſkin: wherwith valiaunt beggers, doeth bliſter their legges and faces, whiche maketh them to ſeme Leperous and whoſoeuer doeth eate of theſe herbes, ſhall bee ſmitten into madneſſe. Their ſinewes ſhalbe ſhroke, and thei ſhall laugh them ſelues to death: if thei doe eate of the kinde of Crowfoote, called *Apium riſus* as *Plini* doeth teſtifie, the roote thereof dried, prouoketh neſyng. And is good to bee put in an hollowe tothe, to breake it, and drawe it forthe without paine. The iuce of this herbe, tempered with Beares greaſe: wil bring heer to the balde hedde. Alſo this iuce taketh awaie ſcabbes, and cruſtie ſcurfes from the legges and armes, of ſore people. And tempered with Swines greaſe, it helpeth the ſwellyng of the throte. And thus I ende of Crowe foote.

Of ſonderie kyndes of Crowe foote called Ranunculi, or little Frogges graſſe.

Dioſcorides lib. ij. cap. 171.

Marcellus.
What is the nature of *Aconitum*?

Hillarius.

This herbe is verie venemous, whereof be twoo kindes: the one is called *Pardalianches*, or Liberdes bane. The other is called *Licoſtonon*, or Wolfes poiſon. The firſt haue three or fower leaues, growyng

Aconitum Libardes bane.

The booke of Simples. Fol.xlv.

wyng in the toppe, with a rounde berie in the middes, and no leaues vpon the braunche: hauyng a long roote like a Serpent, very rugged. The seconde haue many leaues vpon the braunche or stalke, like vnto Crousfoote: with yellowe flowers in the toppe like Brome, with long deuided blacke rootes. This herbe groweth in Maie, and is accorisiue burnyng, poisonyng, and killyng. The pouder of this roote, put into peces or baites of flesh, poisoneth wilde beastes: as wolfes, Foxes, Grapes, Polcattes. &c. and is venemous for mankinde, and there is no remedie, but to drinke oile, and to prouoke voment, to expulse the poison. *(To poison wolues and Foxes.)*

Marcellus.

What is the vertue of *Ieranyum*: called Shepherdes nedell.

Hillarius.

This herbe is called the Storkes bille, or Cranes beake, for there groweth out of the flower, seedes like Bodkins or Nedelles, whereof there be sixe kindes. Some of their leaues be like Crowesfoote: and some like vnto Mugwort. Some haue purple flowers, and thei be the first kinde: and some white, with redde rootes, but some of them haue white rootes. And thei be all of nature stopping and dryng, the rootes be swete of the first kinde, and red also: *Dioscorides* saith, that if a dragme of the first kinde of the herbe, be dronke in wine, it doth aswage the swelling of the matrix, and belly, and healeth the cough of the lunges. *Paulus Ægenita* is of the same minde. But you must take the firste kinde, whose leaues bee in forme, betwene the leaues of Rocket and Mugwort: with the long redde roote, called *Geranium primum*. This roote will breake the stone, and clense the raines and bladder. This herbe and the third kind, with blew flowers, do heale woundes and sores: and the same third is called Doues foote, whiche if it be sodden, and applied on sores, it will heale them. The firste kinde with Mirrhe and Peper, sodden in wine, is good againste Dropsie, collike, winde, and woundes within the body, and crike in the necke. There is also a kinde of this *Geranium*, whiche is good for woundes, called herbe Robert: but rather I take it to be called *Rubertam, a rubro colore*, an herbe of a red colour. And thus I doe conclude of *Geranium*, called Storkes bille, or Shepherdes nedle: whereof the first kind, is the beste for the stone, and raines, and outward woundes. The Doues foote is good for sores and festers, so is herbe Robert: all the other be euil and venemous inwardly taken, but yet dryng for moiste sores outwardly, thei bee tolerable. And thus I make an ende of *Geranium*, called Crowe foote. *(Shepherdes Nedle. Geranium. Diosco.lib.3. Capi.Cxiiii. Doues foote. Herbe Robarte.)*

Marcellus.

What vertue is in *Angelica* that swete roote?

Hillarius.

This herbe *Angelica* is verie longe leaued indented, or with small teeth like Eldren, a greate stalke, and hollowe, a bigge sweete roote: Blacke without, and white within. Purple flowers with white spottes and greate brode seedes. This is called the *(Angelica or Angels blome.)*

h.iii. Angels

The booke of Simples.

Angels herbe, whiche is of .ii. kindes, of the garden & field: this herbe excelleth all other, to preuaile against poison, and is hote and drie. It doe open, warme, dissolue: and is good against the fearfull daungerus plague, called the pestilence, if it bee but bitten vpon, moche more it is effectuall being droke in the morning. The pouder dronke with wine, x. graine waight, or the water dronke. xx. droppes, in the mornyng in wine: is a goodly armour against poison, foule aire or plage, this clenseth the Lunges, Breast, guttes, Raines, and Bladder. This herbe sodden in wine & water, doe heale inward woundes: and this do strength the hart, and drieth superfluous moisture, as the Dropsie, Timpanie. And thei whiche can not kepe their meate, for weakenes, through bomittes, let theim drinke this: It deliuereth from bityng of serpentes, as Snakes, or els any pricke or wounde, if it bee sodden with Rewe, Honie, and wine. It haue one vertue, excellent for young lustie, single people, to quenche carnall rage, or youthfull luste: if one dooe bite or swallowe. ʒ. ß. of this, it will extinguishe the same, with many more vertues, the whiche fewe herbes, be compared to it.

Angelica defendeth the pestilence.

Angelica preserueth chastite.

Marcellus.

What is the vertue of *Lagopus*, with three leaues growyng vpon the stalke, and a rough flower, like an Hares foote, it groweth in Corne, in Haruest tyme.

Hillarius.

This is called *Lagopus*, or Hares foote, haue growing nere the flowers, three leaues together, in sondrie places: and is also called the triple Hares foote. And is of a driyng vertue, saith *Galen*, and sodden in wine and drunke, it do stoppe the bellie in a flixe: and to this affirmeth *Dioscordies* and *Plini*.

Hares foote Lagopus.

Marcellus.

What saie you of *Lunaria*: that increase and deminishe, in one monethe?

Hillarius.

This herbe spring in the ende of Maie, hauyng from the stalke xiiii. leaues, growing seuen againste seuen: in the forme of little hartes, but grene in colour, in the toppe it beareth seedes, like Beates seede, and is colde and drie of nature. Oh how this herbe preuaileth, or excelleth in healyng of woundes, knittyng theim vp, makyng no scarre. Goodly salues bee made therof, so there be balmes: this herbe in redde wine dronke, doe stop the whites and fluxe, whiche passeth from women vnnaturally.

Lunaria or the herbe of the Mone.

Lunaria healeth woundes.

Marcellus.

What saiest thou of *Lysimachus*, whiche is a long herbe, bearing a leafe like Sallowes, and is called Woodwaxen?

Hillarius.

The booke of Simples. Fol.xlvj.

Hillarius.

His herbe growe also emong Salowes, of twoo kindes, one beareth redde flowers: and the other yelowe or golden flowers. And was found by *Lysimachus*, it florish in June, and is of vertue dryyng, and bindyng vertue, it gleweth woundes together: stoppeth blood at the nose, applied to the same, it stoppeth the bloodie flixe, and termes menstruall, drunke in wine or Planten water. And the smoke thereof, killes Gnattes and Flies, this affirmeth *Dioscorides, Galen*, and *Plini*: it is so bitter, that no beaste wil fede therof. And it is in Englishe called Woodwax, it dieth grene.

Lysimachus stoppeth blod Lysimachus a king of Macedon, founde this herbe, he was scoler to Calisthenes, and one of Alexanders most worthie capitaines.

Marcellus.

What is that herbe, called Hartes horne?

Hillarius.

This herbe called *Cornu Ceruini*, Hartes horne: Some call it *Pes Cornicis*, Crowes foote. Some *herba Stella*, because it spreade abroade with iagged leaues, or beames like a Starre, growyng flat, nere the grounde, with flowers growyng, moche like smal Lauender, but yellowe. *Plini* writeth of this herbe *lib.xxiiij.Cap.xix*. this herbe helpeth the flix and is good in Sallettes. The rootes sodden and eaten, saieth *Dioscorides* and *Galen* doeth helpe the Ilias, and stoppeth blood in the newe woundes. &c.

Harts horne or the starres herbe.

Marcellus.

What saie you of Safron?

Hillarius.

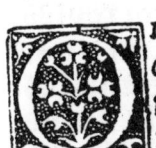Vid that pleasaunte Poet faineth, that a young man called *Crocus*, was transformed into Safron: for the loue of a virgin named *Smilax*, as it is written. *Crocus* with *Smilax* was tourned into small flowers.

Crocus Safron.

Et Crocum in paruos versum cum Smilace flores.

Ouid.

This Safron is commonly knowen here in Englande, bothe in Norffolke, Cambridge shire, and Essex. &c. with purple flowers, with yellowe small Chiues: and heddes growyng in the grounde, wherein be cloues of yerely increase. The beste Safron in all this worlde, dooe growe, saith sondrie writers, vpon a mountain called *Coricos* in *Sicele* the next from *Lycæ* in *Asia* the lesse. &c. But let vs go no furder, then this our natural realme: in whiche assuredly, there is no better safron in *Europe*. The flower do spring of this, before the leafe hote in the first degree, & drie in the second: it doe warme, make soft, digeste, prouoke vrin, make good colour in the face. It comforteth the hart, and defendeth dronkenes: moueth *venus*, and. ʒ.ij. is good againste poisone, and it will reconsile sleape tempered with Rose water and womans milke, droppe it into the iye, it will take awaie droppyng and dimnesse. Oile of bitter Almondes, and the pouder of Safron, warme powred into the deafe eare,

The beste Safron of this worlde, where it is.

Against dronkenesse, Safron helpeth.

h.iiij.

The booke of Simples.

A singulare medicene for the pestilence

eare, doe helpe the organ of hearyng. The pouder of Safron. x. graines walnuttes, twentie graines, Figges. ʒ. ii. and sixe Sage leaues stamped together, with. ʒ. i. of Pimpernel water, and three graines of Mithridatum: kepe this in a close glasse, and eate thereof in the mornyng twelue graines, and this will defende the receiuer thereof, from the Pestilence. Many goodly medicenes, be made of Safron, as *Diacurcuma* againste the Iaunders: and it is putte in many *Antidotaris*, and also plasters, as *Oxicroceum. &c.* with ointmentes againste Palsie and Goute. *Dioscorides, Galen,* and *Plini* affirmeth the same. *Simion Sethi* saith, Safron, milke Rose water, and *Opium* tempered together: doe make a goodly medicene againste the paines of the feete. Safrom stamped with Beate leaues, doe reconcile slepe, applied to the forehedde. Safron is good againste al

Safron haue many vertues.

maner of swellyng in the breaste, winde in the bellie and guttes: and stoppyng of the mothe of the matrix, either in ointment, or drinke. It is a good *cordiall*, to be vsed in meates, of melancholie persons: to reioice thee, and make glad a weake harte, And thus I dooe ende of this our Englishe spice, my deare *Marcellus.*

Marcellus.

What saie you of a Thistell, growyng nere the sea side, called *Eringium,* or *Cardus Marinus*: I haue seen moche thereof growyng, betwene Lestoffe rode, and Orforde nesse, by the Shore side in Suffolke.

Hillarius.

The sea Thistle, called Eringus, whiche is so called, because if the roote bee sodden & conserued with Honie & Cloues, it will preserue nature, or lifte hym vp, whiche is decaied it maie come of *Erigogis, erexi,* to lifte vp, or repaire. *Dioscor. lib. 3. Cap. lxxi. Galenus lib. 7. simp. medi.*

This in deede is called *Eringium*, but the true name is *Centum capita*, because of the number of the heddes: whiche is like a Thistell with thicke prickyng leaues, and long rootes, whose leaues beyng yet tēder, if thei be boiled, thei maie with salte and oile, bee trimly preserued for Sallettes. This herbe with the rootes, as *Plini* saieth, muste bee gathered, when the Sunne is in *Cancer*, in the middes of Somer. Thei bee blacke without, and white within: but some rootes of them, be white bothe within and without, very Aromatik and swete like spice. This roote or herbe, beyng made in pouder, infusion or decoccion, & drunke, doe clense the raines and bladder: and clenseth the matrixe, and cause the stopped termes to passe. And it greatly preuaileth against the collike, and turmente of the guttes, drunke, in, or with *Hydromel*. It is good against the falling sicknes, drinke a dragme at a time: the rootes must bee tenderly sodden, and preserued in Succate, to the vse of meate or medicen in Winter, as to restore nature, or helpe the concepcion of nature: *Plini* saith, this roote. ʒ. i. drunke in wine, healeth the pricke of any benemous beaste, or worme, or feuer. The iuce or oile of this, dooe cleane recouer any venome of the bodie, infected with a Spider. *Heraclydes* the Phisicion did affirme: that this herbe, the leafe or roote, beyng

Againste poison.

sodden and drunke, old preuaile and ouercome, the poisone of any benemous herbe, whiche any haue eaten ignorauntly. As *Aconitum* called

Leopardes

The booke of Simples.   Fol.xlvij.

Leopardes bane. &c. *Ætius* affirmeth, to drinke this. xvi. Euenynges to bedward, and as many morninges, doe heale all infeccions of the raines, stopping of the vrine, or stone. This *Eringium* is of nature somwhat warme, and verie drie.

    Marcellus.

There is a Thistell called *Chamælion*, wherefore is it good, and why is it so called?

    Hillarius.

Firste, to the vertue of this Thistell, it is ripe in August: and the roote is hotte in the seconde degree, and drie in the third. This roote sodden in Ale or wine, and drunke dooe kille the wormes in the chette and bellie. ʒ.i. of the pouder thereof, dronke in sharpe old wine, wherein Organ haue been sodden, will helpe the Dropsie: and also thesame will prouoke vrin, and breake the stone. It is drunke in wine in place of Triacle, saith *Dioscorides, lib.iiij.Cap.ix.* When Charles the Greate, his armie began to be deminished, through an horrible Pestilence. He was warned to vse none other medicen, but onely that euery soldiour should drinke. ʒ.i. in wine: whiche beyng doen, the saied Pestilence did cease presently. This roote sodden, thesame decoccion therof, holden in the mouthe, will lose rotten teeth and with little helpe, thei maie bee drawen. *Theophrastus lib.ix.Cap.xiij. de plantarum historia:* That there is distaunce, betwene the vertues of these twoo rootes. The one is blacke, the other white, whiche white is beste, to doe as is aforesaid. Furder, the iuce of these rootes, will kill dogges and swine: if it be put into their meates, *Plini* affirmeth thesame. Now to the name, whiche is called *Chamælion* not onely bicause it is diuers of colour: blew flowers, speckled leaues whiche is the blacke kind. &c. The white haue a long roote, no stalkes, leaues like wilde Artichokes: greate hedde, many sharpe prickes, with plumes shaken, or blowen awaie with winde. And to conclude, looke vpon what soile or yearth, so euer thei growe vpon: thei will chaunge their colours like thesame. As a little beast, whiche is in Inde, called *Chamælion*, spotted like a Libarde, which chaungeth into diuers colours: accordyng vnto the thing, whiche it seeth. This beaste neuer eate nor drinke, nor winke, but liueth by the aire onely: which little beastes, be yerely brought frō Barbarie, by the ships of London, into this realme.

    Marcellus.

What is to be spoken of Diars flowers, called *flos Tinctorum*?

    Hillarius.

This is a longe herbe, with yellowe flowers, hauyng small blacke Coddes, in whiche the seede is like Lintelles: the leaues be like Hisope, but moche larger and longer. This is hot and drie, in the second begree, and is of the nature of Brome and this herbe is good for a man ʒ i ß either the herbe or seede to drink

Margin notes:
- *Eringium* helpeth them whiche can not make water, or whiche haue eaten any venemous herbe. sateth *Aetius* and *Heraclides*.
- The Bore or carle Thistle called *Chamælion*.
- The Thistell healeth the Pestilence.
- Note that the black Thistle roote with swines grease and Brimstō wil heale scabbes and itche.
- Of the little beaste called *Chamælion*.
- *Flos tinctoris*
- To vomitte.

The booke of Simples.

to make vomite, to clense the stomacke, and purge the raines. Drinke twoo sondrie tymes, and it will prouoke vrine, when it is stopped.

Marcellus.

What saie you of *rubia Tinctorum*, called Madder?

Hillarius.

Madder & redde rootes,

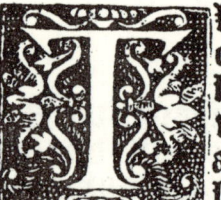Here be of them twoo kindes, the garden Madder, with quadrangle stalkes, and sharpe, and at euery iointe, the leaues growe rounde aboute the stalke: the berries bee rounde and grene, when thei are yong, beyng ripe, then are thei blacke: the rootes longe, small, and redde of colour. The wilde Madder is lesse, with stalkes fower square, leaues compassyng them like Starres: flowers white, but rootes not so rough. This herbe is called of the Greges *Erythrodanon*, with this Diars colour their wolle withall: it is hote in the second degree, and drie in the thirde. This will clense the bladder, breake the stone, and force vrine, saieth *Aueroïs*, and is good to bee dronke against bruses, and the Pestilence: dronke in swete water, helpeth kynges euill. The rootes or berries sodden, saieth *Galen lib. vi. simplic. medicamen*. will clense the liuer, splene, gall, vrine, matrix, drosynges: and the paines in the iointes, chiefly the huccle bones, called *Eschiades* or *Ciatics*.

Dioscorides lib. 3. cap. 143.

Againste the Pestilence.

Marcellus.

What is Paritorie of vertue?

Hillarius.

Parietaria that growe vpon stone walles.

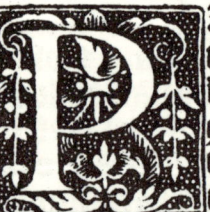Artriges doe delite to feede vpon, this herbe *Galen* saieth, it haue vertue to clense, stoppe, and coole: therefore it haue vertue to helpe flegmon. From the beginning, augmentyng, vnto the state of the saied flegmon: the hotter any apostumacion is the better, this herbe wil help thesame: if you make a plaster of this *Perietaria*, it is good to clense the lunges, when thei are stopped, for it haue vertue to scower or clense. No herbe is better to make cleane glasse, then this herbe as *Galen* affirmeth, if it be incorperate with Salte: then it will help the Hemeroides, and a Fistula. The iuce of this beyng dronke, clenseth the raines, and by little and little, doe breake the stone: and anoint Shingles, or sainct Anthonies fire therewith, and health will followe the same with spede. Thesame iuce with Waxe, and Goates tallowe melted together is a good plaster, for to take the paine of the goute awaie saieth *Plini*: this iuce also with the oile of Roses, powred warme into the eare, will take awaie the paine.

For the goute

Marcellus.

What saie you then to *Cartamus*?

Hillarius.

The booke of Simples. Fol.xlviij.

It is called wilde Safron of the garden, with indented leaues, sharpe endes: the flowers yelowe, and knoppes as bigge as Oliues. The seedes white and redde, longe and cornered: the seede is hotte in the thirde degree: the iuce of this seede pressed forthe, dronke with the brothe of a chicken, will purge the bellie. And to the stomacke it is noisome, the iuce tempered with Niter, Almondes, Honie, and Inisseedes, beaten together, is verie beneficial to clense the guttes. To eate thereof the third parte of a Walnutte, before supper it is very good for to conueigh excrementes, and superfluous humours, and fortifieth digestion.

Cartamus or wilde safrō

Cartamus clenseth humours.

Marcellus.
What is Spurge, or Purge of nature?
Hillarius.

There is one kind, called *Ricinus* or *palma Christi*: whereof there is Oile made for Lampes, and plasters called *oleum Riciminum*. *Dioscorides* saith if .xxx. sedes therof, be clene blaunched from the rind, and stamped, then drinke this saieth he, will purge fleume and choller, and water dounward. This seede will trouble the stomacke, and cause strong vomites: the iuce thereof will clense the face from pimples and spottes, and make smothe the skinne from wrattes, broken with Oile of Tartar, and anoint the place withall: this is hote in the third degree, and skowreth, warmeth, and clenseth, the leaues be like figge leaues. Then there bee seuen kindes of the *Tithymali*, saieth *Dioscorides lib. iiij. Capi. Clix.* and other old writers: whiche herbes bee called Goates Lettis, or the Milke herbe, for if you breake of a pece thereof, droppes of bitter milke will followe. But to our common *Catapucia* or Spurge, this is hotte in the thirde degree, and drie in the second: and is vsed to clense the bodie from fleume, choller, and melancholi, sodden in the brothe of a chiken with Polipodi, Damaske Prunes, and *Mirabolans*, and also the herbe called Marcurie. I doe hereby by occasion put to Marcurie, this woorde (herbe) because through the absence of a Coke, in the tyme when he should haue made his Lordes brothe in the Kichen: an ignoraunt fellowe, did put into his pot *Mercury Sublimated*, that is *Chalcantum*, Quicksiluer, Uineger, and Sal Armoniack together, whiche he sent for quickly to the Apothicaries shoppe: thinking it had been a pleasaunt, or els a verie wholsome confeccion, or at the least the same Marcurie, which the forsaid Coke, did put daily into the pot, for the health of his lorde and maister. But eftsones, contrarie to his purpose, or intente, this brothe in whom the lurkyng, slepyng, venome was spred, was receiued into the bodie, of the good Lorde Wharton, whiche if withall spede, medicene had not gotten the happie victorie by vomites. &c. This noble gentleman, had there lost his life, whose death had been no smal want vnto the publike wealth of his countrey. Nor yet no little comfort vnto the forrain enemie: soche I saie, would dedly poison haue doen in one hower by death, whiche fortune, wisedome, and honour had aduaunsed,

Great spurge called Ricinꝰ in Dioscorides daies. xxx. Seedes, but now. viii. will suffice bicause nature is weaker.
Dioscorides lib.4.cap.158.

Lathyris, or Cataputia minor, or the lesse Spurge

To purge choller.

Note.
Quid pro quo was giuen to the Lorde Wharton in his potage, of ignorance, to his greate perill of life.

The booke of Simples.

sed, and nourished many yeres with happie life. And now again to the matter *Marcellus*, I neither dooe abuse the tyme, nor yet vse to moche copie of wordes, when I speake of Marcurie, to put this woorde (herbe) therevnto. Vnlesse some should, or would, mistake the matter, as this good fellowe did. And furder note, that the pouder of this Spurge, supped vp with a little Sinamon, in the brothe of a Chiken, or els a reare Egge in the mornyng, will purge grosse fleume verie gently. Euen so it will doe, if it be taken with Honie of Roses: Seuen seedes eaten saieth *Dioscorides*, in a Figge, will purge melancholie and water. The said seedes seme swete, but thei purge by vomite behemently. *Plini* affirmeth that if one, whiche haue the dropsie, doe drinke twentie graines, of thē in pure swete water, thei shalbe deliuered from the dropsie. All the other Spurges as *Mirsenites*, hauynge leaues like Mirte, are perelous that grow by the sea side, *Cyparissas* like a Cipresse tree: *Helioscopius* that tourneth with the Sonne, from mornyng vntill night. And the reste of them, be all hote in the fowerth degree: and venemous, burning, as *Galen* saith, and what part of the bodie so euer it taketh, forthwith it do blister thesame, therefore it can not be taken without daunger. Howbeit, *Dioscorides*, *Galen*, and *Plini* affirmeth, it will helpe the tothe ache, tempered with waxe, and a dragme of the roote, dronken with *Hydromell*, wil purge fleume doune warde. &c. Thus I doe ende of Spurge.

Marginal notes:
Tithimalus Characias or Lathyris is good in medicen to purge melancholie, Choller and fleume.

Sondry kindes of spurge, but yet verie perilous, the great spurge and the secōd excepted, for thei be good.

Marcellus.

What is the yellowe walle Gilloflower, and the white and yellowe Gilloflower: called swete William: or hartes ease.

Hillarius.

This swete herbe is called *viola alba*, or *Cheirj*, the white Violette, that is one kinde: there is also purple, the thirde is yellowe, these be all swete, and verie pleasaunt. Thei florish in Maie and growe a cubite longe: and when their flowers doe fade, the sede doe growe in coddes, thei be garden flowers, and of nature be hote and clensyng. The yellowe saieth *Dioscordies*, is beste in medicen, the flowers maie bee kept drie to bee dronke, to purge the stopped termes. And the seede. ii. ʒ. sodden in wine, and drunke, doe quickly conueigh, or bryng forthe the dedde child, and the secondes. The rootes sodden in Vineger, be good to anoint flegmon, and the goute: and thesame root sodden softly with Vineger, and oile of Roses, will help the liuer and splene, to anoint theim, when thei be swelled, or hardened. This will the yellow Gilloflowers do, besides there is a precious oile made therof: whiche will helpe the raines and bladder, or paines in the iointes, or sinewes. As appereth in the compoundes. Folio. xx. and it is there called *Olium de violata alba*. Now to conclude of this herbe, the iuce thereof tempered with Honie, healeth sores in the mouthe and hed: And with waxe, the broken skinne fretted, with winde in Marche, called chappes, be made whole. And thus I ende of this herbe, which is commonly called Swete William, or Hartes ease: God sende thee hartes ease, deare

Marginal notes:
Viola Lutea the yellowe, Violette, the wall Gillow flower.

Flegmon, is a certain apostitinaciō, gathered of corrupted blood, into one place

The booke of Simples. Fol.xlix.

deare Marcellus, for it is moche better, with pouertie to haue thesame, then to be a kyng, with a miserable mynde. For, from thens springeth either felicitie, or aduersitie: an Image of heauen with ioie, or els hel with inward horrour of minde, and vexacion.

The greatest treasor of this worlde, is a quiet mynde,

Marcellus.

I Dooe hartely thanke you, for wisshyng to me so precious a iewell: so riche a treasure, and so heauenly a comforte. For what is more to be desired, then hartes ease, and who doe so sodainly slide or slippe awaie as hartes ease? Nothyng. For when aduersitie come in at the one doore, eftsones, hartes ease doee run out at the other. For thei can not dwell together, in one place. Why so? Thei be .ii. extreme contraries, & merueilous affeccions of the minde felt, & not seen, although oftentimes thinges, whiche are seen, maie be a meanes to bryng quietnes to the minde, and ease to the hart for a time. But rather my deare Hillarius, there be which affirmeth that hartes ease or reste, cometh by the eare. For saie thei, there is no rest in the harte of the Infidell, but in the beleuyng manne: and there can be no faithe, without hearyng, and not the sight of thinges worldly bryngeth faithe, whiche faithe giueth the true hartes ease, passyng all other iewels. And albeit Hillarius, thou art not without worldly hartes ease, whiche I graunt, doe please sometyme thy vaine delight. Yet I praie God giue you, but one handfull of heauenly hartes ease: whiche passeth all the pleasaunte flowers, that groweth in this worlde. Now what be the vertues of Harmodactulj? I praie you tell me then.

Hartes ease, or quietnesse of the minde.

Perfite hartes reste, and true quietnes of minde.

Hillarius.

HERMODACTILI, be of twoo kindes: the firste is *Colchicum wilde Bulbus*, or great wilde Safron, hauing great round heddes within the ground, like Oniõs, and with blacke rindes, and flowers like Safron. Redde seede, but shinyng white and redde chiues, but very greate, and a spã long: swete iuce, and doe florishe in the Spryng. The seconde is like a Lillie, with tender leaues, white flowers, bitter seede: one long roote, on the bignes of a finger. And bothe these *Hermodactilj* be called Mercuries fingers. *Colchium* is of nature hotte and drie, in the seconde degree. *Paulus Ægineta lib. vj.* saieth the roote of *Colchis*, sodden by it self, doe purge the bellie, and helpeth *morbus articularis*, whiche is the sicknes of the iointes: as the Goute, the *Sciatica*, and the paines in the iointes of the handes, called *Chyragra*. The rootes be perillous to be eaten, as other wholsome rootes are in meate, as a Sallette: for thei wil putte one in daunger of chokyng, or stranglyng. But thei will purge the superfluous of the humours, and blood dounwarde: and bee venemous saieth *Dioscorides lib iiij, cap. lxxix.* Yet saieth he, thei be swete, and somtime the ignoraunt doe eate them for *Bulbi*, a kinde of swete rootes: but the reamedie is, onely to drinke a greate draught of milke. Their rotes and flowers stamped, will kill Lice, to anoint childrens heddes therewith. The se-

hermodactili of .ii. kindes. Colchium & Ephemrum called the fingers of Hermis, or els of Mercurius, one is like Safron, the other like lilies.

Colchis rotes will strangle one, take hede thereof, although thei seme swete,

Hermodactilus will kille Lice.

conde

The booke of Simples.

conde *Harmodactilis* is called wilde *Irin*, or flowerdeluce of the field, or *Lillium conualium*, the rootes sodden, the decoccion of them, dooe clense the filthie teeth that stinketh: the leaues sodden in wine, doe dissolue humours, gathered into apostumacion, if it be warme washed, often times therwith, specially hote apostumes, or swellynges gathered of Choller. *Galen* dooe remember this *Hermodactilis*, callyng it *Ephemerum, colchium*, or *Irin*, describyng the same, as is aforesaied: with the same vertues, *lib. vij. simplicium medicamentorum.*

Marcellus.

Of Rumexe the Docke, Monkes Rubarbe, or bastarde Mercurie.

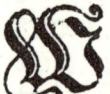Hat vertue is in the herbe *Rumex*, called the greate Docke, I meane not the Sorell, called *Acedula*, whereof you answered me, Folio. vii. in this booke.

Hillarius.

Monkes Rubarbe.

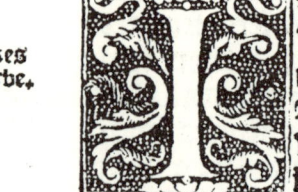Knowe your meanyng berie well, of that wilde herbe, which groweth commonly by pathes, hedges, and waters sides. And of this kind, there is one called Monkes *Rubarbe*, whiche growe in gardens, the other is wilde and with lesser leaues. *Marcellus*, the blinde ignoraunt people, haue of long tyme not a little erred, in one kinde of *Lappa* or *Rumex*. I meane neither Sorell, nor the common wilde Docke, or the bastarde Rubarbe: but that whiche is commonly called Mercurie,

Thei whiche call Rumexe with the golden Sande, Mercurie do greatly erre.

with golden sandes, vpon the backe sides of the leaues, greate rootes, clusters of seedes. Leaues like a brode speare hedde, not pursled aboute with tagges, or small teeth like a sawe, whiche in dede the very Marcurie haue, with one onely roote. Whereupon many small fine rootes dooe growe, like a bushe: and this Marcurie is moche like vnto wilde Hempe. But this bastarde Marcurie, wherof I haue now spoken, called *Rumex*, is none other but a kinde of Dockes, whiche beyng sodden, or vsed in glister, will moue the bellie to bee laxatiue. And is good to bee sodden in brothes for thē, whiche haue the yellowe Iaundes. And the roote of this Docke, whiche is yellowe, is also good for the same purpose, and for the Timpanie of water: a dragme of the pouder, of the

Of the great Docke, how it purgeth.

Munkes Rubarbe, called the greate garden Docke, drunke in wine, will purge fleume, water, and choller dounewarde. The herbes well sodden in wine, and applied to the swelling of the throte, wil spedelie helpe the same. And thus I doe ende of this *Rumex*, called the Docke, and also of the bastard Marcurie, whiche maister *Leonard Fuchius*, doe affirme to be *Rumex*, in his bookes of Plantes. Chapit. Clrriiii. And some there

Of the herbe called Atriplex or Arige.

be, whiche affirmeth this bastarde Marcurie, to be one kind of *Atriplex*, but dedde *Atriplex* is *Arage*, a garden herbe, whiche will quickly spryng forthe, to doe pleasure to mankinde. And is called the golden herbe, because of his yelowe flowers: and of nature is moiste in the second, and colde in the first degree. And this herbe rawe or sodden, will moue the bellie to be laxatiue: and is good in glisters, the seedes thereof drunke

The kynges euill.

with swete water, will very quickly helpe the kinges euill, saith *Dioscorides,*

The booke of Simples. Fol.l.

rides, Galen affirmeth the same. And furdermore, that it will open the gal, and purge choller: *Plini* would that the water, wherin *Atriplex* is sodden should be often tymes shifted: or els it will hurte the stomacke, and infecte the face with little spottes or pimples with Beates, saieth *Hippocrates*, it is good to washe, or clense the mouthe of the matrix with Honie and Vinegar tempered, it healeth the Shingles. This garden *Atriplex* is good for medicene: but the wilde *Atriplex*, or golden *Arage* is onely good to chaunge the colour, and make the heere yellowe, with Barberie barkes, and the flowers of *Calendula*, called the Marigolde. And thus I ende of *Atriplex*, called *Arage*, or *Chrysolochanon*, or the golden herbe.

Shift water often tymes, when Atriplex is sodden

To die the heere.

Chrysolochanon.

Marcellus.

What then of Germander, called *Quercula minor*, the little Oke?

Hillarius.

It is called *Quercula minor*, bicause the leaues thereof be like vnto Oken leaues, although verie small: It is euen so named *Chamædris*, of a verie lowe Oke of the grounde, it is named *Serrata*, for it was first founde by this Germander is commonly knowen, and dieth not in Winter the flowers bee Purple. And this will growe in rockie places, of his owne nature, although plentie growe in gardens: it florisheth in July, it is hote and drie, saieth *Galen*, in the third degree. But my frende *Marcellus*, vnderstande this, that although *Galen* saith so: yet for all that, the herbes here in Englande, be not so hote of nature, as thei be in the hotte countrey of Grece, where as *Galen* was borne, therefore, obserue the Climate and Region, and then you shall dooe verie well. Now to this herbe, whiche is skant so hote and drie, *Dioscorides* affirmeth that this herbe greene or drie, sodden in wine or water, and so dronke, haue all these vertues. It helpeth conuulcions, coughes, hardnes of the splene, stopping of vrine, dropsies: forceth the termes to passe. And in the tyme of perille, the Midwife maie giue it to the woman, whose childe is dedde, to come forthe. Drunke with Vineger, it doeth rebate the swellyng of the liuer, and preuaileth againste poison. And drunke with good wine: and swallowe pilles of this herbe, with Honie, and then it will purge sores and vlcers. It openeth the stoppyng of the iointes, and drieth grosse humours, thus saith *Galen*, *Theophrastus* affirmeth that the leaues stamped with Oile, will heale woundes: and the sedes draweth forthe yelowe choller, beyng dronke, and be good for the iyes. The iuce of the leaues, tempered with cleane oile Oliue, will clense the dimnes of the sore iyen, saieth *Plini*: and these be goodly vertues, which God haue giuen to this herbe, my frende *Marcellus*.

Quercula minor the little Oke, or Germander.

A good note of the nature of herbes.

Many good vertues of Germander.

Marcellus.

What is *Psyllium*?

Hillarius.

i.ii. *Psyllium*

The booke of Simples.

Psyllium called Fleworte.

PSyllium is called Flee worte, bicause ye sede is like to Flees, black and hard, which Flees in the North countrey, be called Loppes: or els as some doe saie, wheras this herbe is caste grene, into any house, no Flees will remaine there. It groweth in drie places, vnsowen, the seede is colde in the seconde degree: with oile of Roses, vinegar, and this seede stamped together, is good to anoint the iointes, swellyng, and hote burnyng paines in the forhedde. This herbe or sede, broken in a Ledden morter, with hogges grease, is good to heale, a foule, burnyng, rotten vlcer or sore. The iuce thereof with Honie, dropped into the eare, will kill wormes, or any Flee cropē therin: and thus moche affirmeth *Dioscarides* and *Plini*, of this herbe.

For paines in the hedde, comming of heate or burnyng.

Marcellus.

WHat saie you of Foxe Gloues, called commonly the Finger flowers: the flowers of some be yellowe, and there be Carnacion in colour. Thus I knowe theim by name and colour: but no furder, I can saie of them.

Digitales

Hillarius.

THou saiest well, I neede no furder discripcion of theim: it growe in mountaines, shadowe, or rockie places. It is bitter, and therefore it muste nedes bee hotte and drie, for *Galen lib:iiij. de simplic. medi. facul. cap. xvij.* those herbes saieth he, whiche be bitter of taste, dooe clense and purge: and dooe cutte awaie grosse matter in the vaines. Therfore with bitter thinges, the termes menstruall, and the filth from the breast, and lunges be clensed, what more? This herbe will dooe all, or asmoche as Gencian will dooe: in whose place, this herbe called yellowe or Purple or fingers, bee vsed, these be *Galen* his wordes of this herbe.

yellowe and Purple Fingers. Bitter herbes bee hotte and drie.

To clense the stomacke.

Marcellus.

ALthough you haue shewed me, the nature of common Gardein Mintes, I had almoste forgotten Calamintes, *Organ*, and *Marianus* I praie you shewe me some thynges of them.

Hillarius.

IT is called Calaminte, the profitable Minte, the vertue thereof, causeth Serpentes to flie from it: moche of this Calaminte doe growe vpon mountaines, and is called *Calamintha montana.* An other kinde is called *Nepeta*, or Neppe of the garden: an other is *Pulegium siluestris*, the wilde *Pulyall* roiall of the wood, with greater leaues then Peniroial, called *Pulyall*, growyng in Woodes, or moiste places. And Calaminte, is of essence, or beyng hotte and drie in the third degree: the rootes bee of none effect or profite, but the leaues be verie hotte, and eger to taste vpon. The vertues of Calaminte be many, as againste the poison and stingyng of Serpentes, either drunke, or anointed: againste the strangurie

Calamintha Montana Nepetam Pulegium Siluestris.

Dioscorides Lib.3.cap.36.

gurie, oꝛ the stoppyng of bꝛine, oꝛ stone, conuulcions, paines in the stomacke, *Orthopnæ*, whiche is a disease, that a man can not take his brethe but holding his necke vpꝛight, *Tormina*, oꝛ paines of the guttes, stopping of the termes in women: tercians, and the kinges euill. All these be clesed, opened, and healed, by, and thꝛough Calamintes, dꝛunke in wine: the pouder and siruppe, haue the like vertues, the water therof is but weake, except to stoppe vomites. What moꝛe of this herbe, it will kille greate woꝛmes, dꝛunke with Salte and Honie: euen so it will *Ascarides*, whiche be little rounde woꝛmes, bꝛedyng in the longe guttes of childꝛen. Who so haue *Elephanticus morbus*, whiche is a Lepꝛie, bꝛed of melancholie, with swelled fleshe, and blacke spottes: and vse to eate Calamintes soddē, oꝛ raw, and then dꝛinke their iuce in Whaie, shalbe healed of the same lepꝛosie. This sodden in wine, do take awaie blewe, oꝛ black spottes from the skin, made by a stripe of hand, wande, oꝛ rod: oꝛ stumbling against ones fist in the darke, applied to the same stripe, a plaster made thereof, oꝛ hote laied vpon the huccle bones, will asswage the paine of *Sciatica*, and it will dꝛaw doun humour. The iuce will kill woꝛmes that be in the eare. *Galen* doe wꝛite verie moche of Calaminte, *lib. vj. simplicium medicamen.* agreyng with *Dioscorides*, and doe moche commende the oile of the same, to anointe the bodie, saiyng: it will enter quickly, and that it is a pꝛesent remedie of the *Sciatica*. And thꝛough the bitternes of the same, it will skower, and cleanse the yellowe Jaunders, and open the galle: And to conclude, the mountaine Minte with the Purple flowers, hauyng leaues like to *Ocimum*, called Basill, *Nipotella*, called Neppe, is one of the Calamintes. So is an other called, S. Marie Mint, with flowers like to Chamamell. Some there be, that doe take *Organ*, to be a kinde of Calamintes: but it is not so, foꝛ *Organ* is a pꝛoper herbe of it self, in name and nature. And is distinguished in fower bye names, *Heracleoticum, Onitis, Syluestre,* and *Tragoriganum,* these bee swete herbes: Goates and other beastes, loue to feede of them. Some of them haue leaues like Hisope, but bꝛoder: Some like Sauerie, called *Satureia*, of increasyng of seede, whiche Sauoꝛie is nere kin in nature to *Organ*, so is *Amaracus*, called Maioꝛam, oꝛ *Samphuchion*. These all bee herbes verie swete, wholsome, and pleasaunte, good to mankinde, and enemies to venome, and poison of coꝛrupted woꝛmes oꝛ Serpentes: and of nature be hote and dꝛie in the third degree. These herbes will warme al the bodie, either in bathe, oꝛ to be anointed with the oile, against all cold sickenesses, oꝛ rigours of tremblyng. These herbes sodden grene in bꝛoth, oꝛ the pouder simplie of them: put into the same, oꝛ els dꝛunke in wine, oꝛ the siruppe thereof, will doe thus, as followeth. Helpe the dulnesse of sight, pꝛouoke nesyng, either in oile oꝛ pouder: openeth the raines, pꝛouoke vꝛine, foꝛce termes menstruall, kille woꝛmes in the bellie. Cleanse grosse fleume from the stomacke, maketh good digestion: helpeth the greene sickenesse, nothing better foꝛ melancholie, and paines in the left side. Good foꝛ the collike palsie, stinkyng bꝛeathe, shoꝛtnesse of winde, oꝛ vomites oꝛ swellyng with dꝛopsie. There is a foꝛgetfull sickenes, called *Lethargus*

The booke of Simples.

Lethargus helped with herbes, hotte and dry in the third degree.

or *Veternus*, whiche is placed in the hedde: in whiche the power of reason is contained, through a sicknes of fleume, as a quotidian not purged, or els of *Perripneumia*, whiche is a sicknesse of the lunges. When through heate, flegme is melted, or made thin eftsons, drawen to the hedde: the beste remedie is then, to purge the hedde, with *Hiria simplicis.* ʒ.i.ß. and to weare a garlande, or clothe full of these herbes, of *Organum, Mariarum*, or Sauerie, and health will folowe: and thus I doe ende of them.

Marcellus.

What is *Ormyn*? Whiche we doe call Clarie *Gallitricum*.

Hillarius.

Orminum Ormyn. Or Clarie.

Ormyn haue stalkes fower square, leaues grosser then Horhound flowers in forme like the Archangel: but purple coloured, growyng aboute the stalke, with blacke seedes in the coddes. This herbe is hote and drie: *Dioscorides* saieth, the seede drunke with wine, will moue *Venus*, with Honie it will cleanse the bloodie spottes in the iye, to this affirmeth *Paulus* and *Plini*, and is good for to cleanse the whites in women, sodden with Planten in redde wine, and drunke: stamped and put to a pricke, it will drawe it forthe of the fleshe.

Clarie, good for women.

Marcellus.

Ocimastrum wilde Basill

What is the vertue of wilde Basill, called *Ocimastrum*, hauyng stalkes fower square: flowers purple, seedes blacke, and leaues like vnto the kyng of herbes, for swetenes, called Bazill.

Hillarius.

This growe in sondry places, and florisheth in October: bearing the seedes and coddes, and is hotte and drie of nature, with bitternes. The seede sodden in Wine and drunke warme, helpeth the bityng of Serpentes: and drunke in Wine with Mirrhe and Peper, it healeth the *Sciatica*, saieth *Dioscorides*.

Marcellus.

What is the vertue of wilde water Peper, an herbe so named?

Hillarius.

Hydropiper water peper.

It is called *Hydropiper*, bicause it groweth in water, and the tast thereof burneth in the mouthe, as the spice Peper dooe. It haue a berie tough stalke, leaues like Mintes, but broader, thinner, and whiter, the seedes growe forthe by the leaues, vpon slender braunches, it florisheth in Auguste. It is hotte and drie, not so moche as Peper, *Dioscorides* saieth, this herbe with the seede stamped, anointe the blacke spotte, or harde knotte through a stripe therewith, and it shalbe healed. If this seede be dried, and beaten into pouder, mingled with Salte, it is good to with meate, or to season fleshe. The roote thereof is good for nothyng, of this herbe bee twoo kindes, the one hauyng leaues like Mintes: of the seconde speaketh *Mathiolus*, saiyng, he taketh it to bee *Percicaria*, whiche haue leaues like Peaches, with

Dioscorides lib.11.cap.155. Gale.lib.vii. Simp.medic.

Hydropiper one haue leaues like mintes: the other is Percicaria

The booke of Simples.   Fol.lij.

with colour spotted, somewhat like Puke. Of whiche *Percicaria*, I haue spoken of before. Folio.xlii.   *with leaues like Peches, and wil serue in the place of Peper.*

Marcellus.
What be the vertues of *Aristolochia rotunda*, and *Longa*?

Hillarius.

This herbe is good, to quicke the tyme of child birth, and expulse the secondes, whereof there be three kindes: one rounde with leaues like Iuie, but rounder, with round rootes, from whiche herbe cometh, a pleasaunte sharpe sauour. White flowers vpon pretie redde knoppes, this is *Rotunda*, or round, the female: an other is called *Longa*, or longe, with rootes and leaues, small braunches, purple flowers and stinkyng, when it dooe growe, and is of the fashion of a Peere. Bothe of them haue berries like Capers, very bitter, of colour like Boxe, and stinketh. Now to the third, whiche is swete, hauing small rootes, and flowers like Rue, or herbe Grace. The round rote is the best in medicē as salue, pouder, and oile. The fume or smoke thereof, put vnder beddes, or the Cradles of young children, is verie wholsome, and putteth awaie aire of infeccio̅: this herbe is moste bitter, and somwhat sharpe hotte and drie, in the seconde degree. This herbe haue vertues, to incarnate vlcers and woundes, with clensyng and mundifyng theim: And will extenuate and make thin grosse humour, and knitteth. The roote or curnelles thereof, dried and beaten into pouder, with peper and Mirrhe mingled together, is wholsome to rubbe the gummes and teeth, when thei bee foule and kancred. The pouder is good to take awaie dedde fleshe, to bee putte into a fistula, to clense it: euen so it will helpe the conduite of the vrine, conueighed in with a syryng, or instrument, when it is corrupted, with burnyng heate, or vlcered, a foment with Oile and wine, and this roote, will bryng foorthe a dedde childe. Gentian, *Aristochia*, and Honie, maketh a wholsome cōfeccion, for a stinkyng breath. The seconde twoo kindes, saieth *Plini*, drunke with wine, or water, be good to be giuen them, which haue the crampe: or els fallen doune from some high place, beyng sore brused. The seede drunke, is good against the pleuritie, and wormes, with Rosen and waxe, this roote, or rootes in pouder, withdrawe cornes from the feete, and also drawe prickes, nedles, arrowe heddes from the fleshe. With Vinegar, this pouder will heale a greene wounde: it is drunke againste the fallyng sicknes, and shortnesse of winde. And this roote must be gathered in Aprill.

Aristolochia Rotunda Longa. Clematis. Dioscorides lib.3.cap.iiii

Galen.lib.vi. simpl.medic.

Aristolochia helpeth Cācers and burnynges. Many good vertues of Aristolochia

Marcellus.

What is the vertue of that wilde climyng Vine, with the greate wighte roote: stinkyng berries, redde of colour, and leaues like vnto Hoppes, or wilde Figges?

Hillarius.

                           i.iiii.   This

The booke of Simples.

Brionia vitis alba, or the wilde runnyng Uine.

To heale sores with Brionia.

This is a hedge wede in euery place, commonly growing and crepeth aboute busshes, braunches, boughes, and trees, it florisheth vntill Haruest: the braunches be somwhat bitter and sharpe, a stopping of nature. The roote doe drie, with moderate warmnes, in the seconde degree it haue vertue to clense, skoure, with maturaciõ or ripenes. The roote of this Brion, or the pouder of the rootes, with Smalage, Mallowes, cleane Honie, Flaxe sede in pouder, and Barly meale clene *Terebinthin*, and a litle white wine, sodden softly togither, maketh a medicen, to heale fellons and vncomes withal, or pusshes. This herbe beyng yong and tender, maie be eaten as *Asparagus* maie be, saieth *Dioscorides* for then it moueth, or prouoke the bellie and vrine, the leaues, frute and rootes bee sharpe, and will bite the tongue, if thei taste of theim. Therefore thei will stampe it with Salte, to heale Cancers, filthe in handes or feete, or legges. &c. as sores, foule pusshes. &c. This roote wil clense all the filth from the bodie, and blacke spottes, blaines, blisters shingles, pimples, called good ale pearles, tempered with the pouder of Fenigreke, and the Oile of Tartar. Or els Briona sodden in white wine, from a quarte to a pinte, then straine thesame, puttyng some Campher, and washe the infected face, euery night with a sponge, and let it drie in. The rootes pressed in the spring, the iuce drõke with swete water, doe purge fleume: dronke daiely in the mornyng with wine, or ale well sodden, helpeth the falling euill, and *vertigo*. J. it. dronke against the poisone of Serpentes, or benome drinke. But yet it will kille a young child, in the mothers wombe. Mary, if the child be dedde, by any casualtie in the bellie, then it will bryng it forthe: by the waie of a foment, or aplicacion, by ingeccion into the mouth of the matrix. The berries of this broken, doe helpe to cleanse scurfe, and filthie leprosie from the skin. If nurces doe knede their wheate meale, with the iuce of the Brion berries, and bake it in bread: if thei eate thesame bread, it will increase milke in their breast. But to vse it moche, except cause of infirmitie, moue the pacient, it is hurtfull for memorie: it helpeth the lunges, liuer, and splene, to bee dronke, and drawe foorthe prickes, and heale woundes.

To clense the face with Brionia.

Brionia defẽdeth poison.

Brionia increseth Mylke.

Marcellus.

What is Pellitorie of Spain good for?

Hillarius.

Sternumentaria. Pyrethrum Ptermice Pellitorie.

Dioscorides lib. j. cap. 71.

THE flower thereof put into the nose, will prouoke moche nesyng: And therefore it is called *Ptermica*, it haue flowers like Chamamell, braunches moche like Sothernwoode. It will growe in harde stonie places, the roote must be digged in the ende of Haruest: it is hotte and drie, in the thirde degree, and in the beginnyng of the fowerth, specially if it bee dried. The leaues with the flowers stamped togither, will make a good ointmente, to take awaie markes, made with stripes, causyng blew or blacke spottes, in the face

The booke of Simples.

or any parte of the bodie. The rootes haue vertue, to drawe filthe and cold humour, from the corrupt pained teeth, saith *Galen lib: viij simplic. medica.* But if the said rootes, bee firste steped in strong vinegar, and beaten in a morter: and make small rounde pilles of them puttyng them into the mouth, thei will drawe moche filthe, from the pallet of the mouth and gummes. And finally, ease the tothe ache, that you made of Pellitorie rootes: or the said rootes or iuce of them, sodden in oile, will put awaie a cold feuer, if the bodie bee well anointed therewith, againste a feuer, before the fitte doe come, either in tercian, or quarten. And it is a good oile for a colde stomacke, that is swelled: and thus I doe ende of Pellitorie.

Pellitorie haue vertus to helpe the teeth.

Pellitorie will take awaie a cold feuer.

Marcellus.

What vertue is in a wede, which we cal Gosegrasse: some people call it Hare wede. It groweth in hedges, it haue rough leaues and berries, whiche berries hangeth by coples: and will cleue vnto menne or womens clothes, and therefore some doe call it Cleuer grasse, with white flowers, white round seedes, like nauelles.

Hillarius.

You haue rightly described this herbe, whiche in deede beare all those names, emong the people: it is called *Philanthropos*, for it loueth to hang vpon garmentes, and goe with men. This is a name of propertie, the verie true name is *Aparine*, it is drie and clensing: and this herbe and sede dronke in wine, preuaile against stinging of benemous thinges, and the iuce distilled in theare, helpeth them. This herbe tempered with freshe Swines grease, healeth *Struma*, or paines in the throte, applied to thesame place: the iuce thereof saith *Plini*, stoppeth blood in a freshe wounde, and heale thesame.

Philanthropos, Aperine commonly called gosegrasse & Harewede. Diosco lib. 3 cap. lxxxviii.

Marcellus.

What is the vertue of Missen, growyng vpon Thornes, Peretrees, and Okes, wherof I haue seen great plentie growing in the countrie of Suffolke, with many goodly herbes and flowers: as in these moste aunciēt Parkes, of Framingham, Kelshall, Netlestede, Lethryngham, Parham, Some, Henyngham, Westwood, Huntingfelde, Henham, little Glemham, and Benhal. &c. These Parkes bee old neighbours, God sende theim continuall frendshippe with eche other in vnitie, for where as vnitie is broken, the Parke pale will not holde, but fall into sodaine ruine and decaie, and the Dere will scatter.

Framinghā. Netlestede. Lethrynghā. Parham. Kelshall. Some. Heningham. Westwood. Huntpngfeld Henham. Glenham. Behall, these be Parkes in Suffolke, in whom florisheth sondrie kindes of herbes and flowers, & this Viscum.

Marcellus.

I knowe the places, whiche you haue named right well. Furdermore, I commende your good zeale, that you beare to that worthie countrie: wishyng their continuall vnitie and concorde, I desire thesame. For, thei be people of no lesse ciuilitie then of moste auncient good fame and worship: descended from houses

The booke of Simples.

A very gentleman, springeth not bi extorcion but by true scrapyng their Princes, and liuing of their own, hurting not their poor neighbor, preferryng the fauoure of the cositre, before luker, which is their chief treasure.

of fame, worthie of memorie, I meane no Parkes, but people, nor the whiche haue crept vnder a Gose wing, drawing forth a bastard sword, no lenger then a writyng penne. Fightyng their combate, vpon the backe side of a sheete of paper: to the hurte of many perhaps, and profite of none, but to theim selues onely. But of theim speake I, whose blood haue been shed, in the iuste quarell of their Princes: whose houses be builded vpon harde rockes, of true gotten gooddes. Whose dores be open, kepyng hospitalitie, accordyng to their callyng: whiche with the loue of the Countrie, garde theim selues, and with iustice defende causes of the poore. &c. These be thei, whiche be worthie of laude, that thus feareth God: these be the right gentlemen, otherwaies not. Now to our matter, from whiche we a little, haue lefte of. For this Mislen, whiche is called in Latin *viscum*, whiche is hotte and tarte, hauyng the

Diosco.lib.3. Cap.lxxxvii. Mislen healeth manye perilous sores.

Misteltowe, or Misle, wil make a good ripyng plaster and healeth Cornes. Galen.lib.6. Simpli.medi.

complexion, of aire and water. This herbe with Rosen and Waxe, boiled together, will make a medicen, to molifie, dissolue, drawe foorth the swellyng curnelles, distilled of foule humours, gathered behinde the eares: or any foule pushe, fester, or fellon, in any other place of the bodie, tempered with Rosen, it healeth an old vlcer. Take the berries of this Mislen, put therunto the pouder of Ieate, make it warme, apply it to the lefte side vpon Leather, when the splene swelleth, and it will help it. Temper it with *Auripigmentum*, or vnsleked Lime, and it will draw foorth the cornes. This Mislen, saieth *Galen*, is one of theim, whiche after the firste puttyng to in any medicene, will not be hotte, but requireth a tyme, by little and little, as *Thapsia* doeth: and this Mislen groweth of no seede, nor will growe vpon the yearth, but vpon the tree, through the dounge of birdes, that sitteth vpon them by night, which by little and little, breaketh through the barkes of the tree, into the sappe: fro whens at length, this *viscum* doe spryng, and groweth grene in Winter, when the poore naked Tree, seme withered and dedde. *Virgill* obseruyng his nature in the *Ænedos.lib.vj.*

Virgill.

> *Quale solet syluis brunmali frigore Viscum:*
> *Fronde virere noua, quod non sua seminat arbos.*

> The Misteldine by kinde, in stormes of Winter cold:
> Is neuer sowen yet grene doe growe on trees, both bare and old.

Misteltowe is not naturall in kinde, but a bastard braunches growyng vpō some other tree.

Plini the .xbi. booke, the laste Chapiter, saieth there be certain plantes, whiche can not be ingendered, or bred vpon the yearth: for whom nature haue prepared, to take their beginning and nutrimēt of trees. For when thei haue no places of their owne, then thei liue vpon other as this *Viscum* or Misteltow is wont. But now by the waie of protestacion: What benefite haue that tree, vpon whom this Misteltowe doe growe? No more then any member of the bodie, vpon whom a Cancer is placed: it will at length destroie all together, except it be pulled frō the tree, vnles it bee a mightie tree, stronge and full of humour, with plentifull incriment. Euen so, euen so, into what realme, or common wealth, Countrie, Borough, or Citee, that vnnaturall straungers, or

to sweare

The booke of Simples.   Fol.liiij.

forinars, be planted, placed, or as thei saie, made nailefast. Forthwith thei waxe high, I meane wealthie, lustie, and greene in winter: thei lacke nothyng in the tyme of darth and miserie. When as the natural people, vpon whom thei haue their gaine and profite: taste of sore labour, lacke, losse, hunger, and pouertie. And thus I doe conclude, both of miserie, and Mistleden, remembryng Plinis woordes, in the foresaied Chapiter: *Namq; cum suam sedem non habiant, in aliena viuunt, sicut Viscum.*

<small>Mistletowe, is like a stranger that waxe riche, and florisheth by the hurt and losse of a freeborne man of his naturall countrie or cicre.</small>

Marcellus.

What vertue is in *Ebulus*, called Wallworte, and in Suffolke thei call it Danes weede: it groweth like Elden, whiche leaues be like Walnutte leaues, and berries in the toppe?

Hillarius.

This herbe is of the nature of Elden, called *Sambucus*, of one *Sambix*, whiche first found out the vertue of this Elden: and of nature is hote and drie, resolueth, and drieth moist sores and vlcers but very hurtfull to the stomacke. Notwithstādyng, the tender leaues sodden, and eaten like a sallet, purgeth fleume and choller. And is good to heale the dropsie, and doe mollifie the mouthe of the matrix, to make a fomente therwith. The iuce of this *Ebulus*, or the berries stamped with fresh greas and Barly meale, will cleanse depe rotten sores: and coole the burnyng of a goute, and paines in the ioyntes. *Paulus Ægineta* saieth, these twoo kindes of Elders, doe glewe and heale: and either eaten or drunke, doe caste for the water by the bellie, and nether partes.

<small>Sambuchus, Ebulus, Elwerne, and Walworte.

Diosco lib.4. Cap.Clxviii.

Walworte maketh medicene for the goute, & paines in the iointes.</small>

Marcellus.

What is the vertue of *Epithymum*?

Hillarius.

This herbe doe wrappe and folde aboute Tyme, and is therefore so called: the flower is vsed moche in medicen, and is hotte and drie in the thirde degree. And purgeth Melancholie Fleume, and grosse humours from the hedde, and doe comfort the harte. *Cassutha* is hote in the firste, and drie in the seconde degree: and is of greate vertue to open the galle, clense the raines, deminishe the splene. Purgeth skoureth, fleume and Choller, and healeth the Iaundes: drunke in decoccions, posions, Syruppes. &c. And this *Cassutha* groweth grosser and larger, then *Epithimum*, with white flowers, no rootes: but groweth vpō other herbes, as Peritorie, young Flaxe, and other Plantes, as *Plini lib. xvj. Capitu vltimo.*

<small>Epithymum. Dioscorides lib.4.cap.172. Galen lib.6. Sim.medica.

Epithymum & Cassutha helpeth the Liuer, Gall, and Splene.</small>

Marcellus.

What saie you of *Vngula Caballina* or *Tussilago*?

Hillarius.

It is called *Vngula Caballina*, that is Horshoue, because no herbe is liker: but the Grekes call it *Bechion*, whiche is *Tussilago*, that is to help the cough. It is commonly knowen, some call it Clotte leaues:

<small>Vngula Caballina, Horshoue.</small>

white

The booke of Simples.

white on the one side, and grene on the other side. And growe nere waters, and in salowe landes: the flowers florishe in Maie onely, but the leaues all Somer, and of nature be cold and moiste. These leaues staped and strained, the iuce will heale shingles, skaldynges, burnynges, and hot inflamacions. *Dioscorides Galen*, and *Plini* affirmeth, that these haue leaues and rootes, beyng dried and cast vpon the coales, and to receiue the smoke thereof: through a reede or Trunke, into the mouthe, will clense the lunges, and helpe them, and quickly deliuer them, from old rottes, and cold coughes.

Dioscor. lib. 3. Capit. Cix. Galen lib. vi Sim. medica.

Marcellus.

What is *Apiastrum*?

Apiastrum.

Hillarius.

Apiastrum or *Melissa*, whiche we name Balme: be of twoo kindes, garden, and felde. Bees loue this herbe aboue all other, and it is called the Bees, or Honie herbe: and is drie in the firste, and warme in the second degree. The iuce of this herbe, healeth stinging of Bees, Serpentes, mad Dogges, and woundes, dronke in wine, and clenseth the termes menstruall. Nothyng doe more comfort the harte, then this herbe in decoccion, or the water thereof, Burage water, and fine Muske sodden in a clene vessel: and dronke when the hart is weake, or in a great hicket. This herbe will clense the lunges, and stop the bloodie flixe, and the paines of the throte, called *Anginæ* made in a warme plaster. It kepeth vomites, & helpeth collike, dronke in wine: Balme & Nutts staped with Honie, helpe to lighten, the dull blemished darke iyen and help the sight. It is like Horhoud saith *Galen*.

Mellissa Balme. Dioscorides lib. 3. cap. 101. Auicenæ qui libro medicinus.

Galen lib. 7. Simpl. medicamento. um

Marcellus.

What is *Caruj*, whiche we doe call Careawaies?

Hillarius.

This fine small seede, cometh from the countrie of *Cary*, in *Asia*, which is the place, where as thei growe very plentifull: this *Cary* sede is hot and drie, in the third degree. *Dioscorides* saith, this is the vertue of the seede, pleasaunt to the mouthe: and profitable to the stomach, prouoke vrine, helpeth digestion. It is good in medicen, & of the nature of Anisedes: the rootes be yelowe, and to eate vpon, bee better then the Pastnippe. The seede doeth not onely extinguishe hote swellyng, and moue vrine: but the plante also, saieth *Galen*, the decoccion of *Carj* wine, is best to be dronke, to clense the raines.

Caros.

Diosco. lib. 3. Capit. 57. Galen lib. 7. Sim. medica.

Marcellus.

What is *Cartafilago*?

Hillarius.

Cartafilago haue redde stalkes, twoo cubites longe, and hollowe long leaues, like Sallowe, and with small teeth like a sawe about them: yellowe flowers, many rootes, and redde without, it florisheth in August, it is drie, stoppyng, and bindyng.

Cartafilago vulneraria Herba.

This

The booke of Simples. Fol.lv.

This herbe is equall, to the beste healing wounde herbe: & it will incarnate and heale the saied wounde, and clense the same, stamped and put into it. You maie drie this herbe, and make pouder thereof, and caste into a freshe wounde, it will then heale spedely. What is better for a fistula? Proue it I pray you. *A goodlie wound herbe*

Marcellus.

What is Grummell seede?

Hillarius.

Grana Solis, or *Milium Solis*, is commonly knowen, these seedes bee good, to be finely beaten in pouder, and dronke, doe clense the raines, and cause vrine to passe, that is stopped: Fenell, Parcely, and this seede broken in white wine, and let it stande all one night, puttyng some Sene leaues to ye same. And in the mornyng seeth this in a stone vessell, put in Sugar, then straine it, & drinke the same, it will purge fleume, choler, and open the raines and bladder: and forse forthe vrine moste plentifully. *Grana Solis. To cause vrine to passe plentifully.*

Marcellus.

What is the vertue of Cichorie?

Hillarius.

This herbe is called in Greke *Serin*, in Latine *Intibum*, wherof are twoo kindes, the wilde and tame: these be the names of Endiue and Cichorie, that with broder leaues, somwhat like Beates is Endiue. The second with iagged leaues, like vnto Dandilion, is Cichorie, these haue hard stalkes, with trim blewe flowers like hattes, some haue white flowers. These bee cold and drie in the seconde degree: the Endiue is more colder then the Cichorie, & be bothe of a restringyng, or stoppyng, bindyng nature. These herbes greene, bothe rootes and leaues, haue vertue to coole the hot burnyng of the liuer, the stopping of the galle: the yellowe Iaunders, the heate of the harte, the lacke of slepe, the stoppyng of vrine, hote burnyng feuers, beyng first digested. The syruppe thereof, is excellent good against the saied sicknesses: the water can not bee missed, in all pocions & coolynges, or purgyng drinkes, to purge mankinde withall. The waters of Endiue, Planten, Roses, and stilled Milke, with fine Bole Armoniake, or seefe without Opium, is good to be caste with a Siring, in the filthie, burnt, swelled, or corrupted yardes, or Conduites, of vncleane persones. For the heate of the liuer. ℞. Endiue or Cichorie, whites of Egges, Barly flower, Sanders, cleane young freshe Swines greas, the oiles of Roses, Violettes, and water Lillies wrought together, in a Ledden morter, and applied to the side, spread vpon Leather. This plaster is verie good, against the hote burnyng goute in the feete: or the shingles, or burning in any parte of the bodie. Dandilion is of the same vertue. *Sponsa Solis. Intibus. Endiuia. Cichoria. Diosco.lib.2. Capi.Cxxv. A very good medicene for the vlcer in the yarde. A plaster for the liuer and goute.*

K.i. Marcellus.

Marcellus.

What is that roote *Napus,* **called the Naue?**

Hillarius.

Napus Bunias.

It is called *Napus Bunias*, becauſe of his owne nature, it groweth greate and round, whereof be twoo kindes: one beareth leaues like Rapes, the other like Rocket, but greater, and hau yellow flowers, the ſeedes groweth in coddes, and of nature be hote in the ſecond degree. The rootes of Napes increaſeth winde, and leſſe nouriſhe then Rapes: the ſeedes be good in many medicenes, and preuaileth againſt poiſon. The rootes ſodden and preſerued in Salt, be wholſome to eate vpon: in Egipt the people make moche oile of this herbe.

Marcellus.

What ſaie you of Rapes?

Hillarius.

Dioſco.lib.2. cap. Ciiii.

This Rape is a rurall common roote, and no leſſe knowē then common, of twoo kinds: the tame haue leaues like Radix, and yellowe flowers. The other haue blewe flowers, and ſmall ſharpe leaues, in the length of a finger with ſmall teeth like a Sawe, rounde about the ſaied leafe. The garden greate Rape doe nouriſhe, inflate, ingender, looſe, or weake fleſhe, moue carnall luſt. The roote ſodden, and warme applied, helpeth a kibed heele, and eaſeth the goute: make this roote hollowe, put therein oile of Roſes and waxe, then roſte it in hot aſhes. And this will heale kibes, whiche bee depely rotten, or feſtered within the heele. Seeth *Aſparagus* in the decoccion of Rapes: drinke the ſame to purge the bladder, clenſe the raines, and forſeth vrin. The ſede of Rapes is good in many medicenes, and in Triacle, and expulſeth poiſon: wilde Rapes be put in medicens, to clenſe the face, as with *Lupines* been meale. &c. *Plini* ſaieth, the ſeede being ſowen, within three monethes folowing, it will bee a greate roote: but it is very harde in decoccion, increaſeth winde and ſeede, ſaith *Galen lib. vj. ſimplicium medicamentorum.* There is greate plentie of the oile thereof made in Englande, as in Marſlande nere to Lin. &c. very profitable to our common wealth.

Goodly vertues of rapes

Plini libr. 17. Cap. xiii.

Marcellus.

What is the roote called *Rhoyda?*

Hillarius.

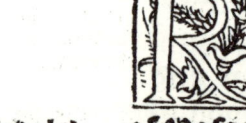

Roida helpeth the hed.

Roydis is a goodly roote, whereof is greate plentie in *Macedonia*, and now in many places of Germanie, growyng in gardens, and is hote and drie in the ſeconde degree, it ſmell moche like a Roſe, and theſe rotes ſtamped, and made warme with oile of Roſes, applied to the forehed, will aſſwage the grief: burnyng heat, lacke of ſlepe, & frenſie, that mankinde doe through weakeneſſe fall into. This herbe wil growe in Englande alſo, if idlenes wer not the let.

The booke of Simples.   Fol.lvj.

Marcellus.

What is the roote called *Doronike*?

Hillarius.

It is a precious roote, growyng in Egipte, and is called *Doronicus* *Actuarius* call it *Carnabadium*: it haue many knottes, and is no bigger then a mannes finger, and is putte into confeccion, for lacke of perfit digestion, and against poison, there is no better roote then this. *Ruellius* suppose it to be that, whiche the Grekes call *Arnabo*.

Doronicus of Alexandry

Doronicus dooe helpe digestion.

Marcellus.

What is the goodnes of Licorice rootes?

Liquoris.

Hillarius.

Licorice called *Glycirrhiza* of the sweetenesse, groweth greate plentie in hotte Countries. Euen so there is moche here in Englande, the yellower and moister the better: it is sweete warme, and moist of nature. Liquoris is wholsome against the exasperacion, or sharpnes in *Arterias*: to bite vpon this roote, or kepe it in the mouthe, for that purpose. For the burnyng heate in the stomacke, and sicknesse of the lunges, splene, and old rotten cough. Skabbes in the bladder, and sores in the raines: drunke in pocions or brothes, Liquoris healeth woundes, if it be anointed therwith. The pouder thereof put into the iye, will helpe *Ptergyus*, whiche is a little skinne growing from the corner, couering the sight. Liquoris, wine and Honie, healeth bothe woundes, without and within also.

Dioscorides
Licorice. helpeth the lunges, and woundes.

Marcellus.

I would as gladly learne, the vertue of Radishe rootes for medicen: as I haue been desirous to fede of them with meate.

Hillarius.

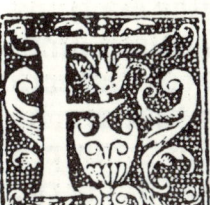

Firste, I shall declare vnto you, the name thereof. It is properly called *Raphanus*, because it springeth sodainly, and *Radix* is a name common to al rootes. But this Radishe beareth the chief name, emong other rootes, and therfore it is called *Radix. Plini* maketh mencion of Radish rootes. *lib.xix Cap.v.* that were as bigge as young infante children. Of Radishe rootes, there bee no small store growyng aboute the famous citee of London: thei bee more plentifull, then profitable, and more noisome, then nourishyng to mannes nature, ingenderyng of winde, enemie to the stomacke, saith *Dioscorides*. It is nombered rather emong rootes vsed for meate, then accompted of perfite wholsom nutrimente: good to bee eaten before meate, to vomite, and clense the stomacke. But wholsome in the ende of meales, for chollorike stomackes a little at ones, to helpe digestion, and to distribute the meate: but *Galen* affirmeth, that tender young Radishe with Uenigar, is good sause in

Raphanus Radix, or Radishe.

Diosco lib.2. Cap.Cvi.

k.ii.   the

The booke of Simples.

Galen lib. 2. de alemētoru̅ facultatibus

the beginnyng of meales, to loose the bellie. For the plaine people doe eate these rootes with breade, taught by nature, and not by arte: And so is *Organ* beyng greene, Cresses, Time, Sauerie, Peneroiall, Germander, Mintes, Calamintes, Peritorie and Rockette. These herbes and this roote, bee rather eaten of necessitie, then of will or fantasie. But

How to vse Radish rotes

sodden, and then prepared with sharpe vinegar, sugar and swete clere oile, is more profitable then crude, rawe herbes or rootes. Many learned and vnlearned, doe maruaile saith *Galen*, why men vse, to eate them rawe after supper, to helpe digestion: whiche answereth, long custome haue so taught them. Notwithstanding, the example of soche, are not to be folowed, without perill or hurte. *Plini* affirmeth, that Radish sodden in wine, drinke that wine in the mornyng, and it will diminishe and caste forthe the stone, openeth the galle, diminishe the splene, moueth Venus, clenseth spottes and bruses, made in the skinne by some

Radix helpe the bellie.

stripe. *Hyppocrates* saieth, that if women chafe their heddes, with Radishe rootes, the heare will fall: and applied to the nauell of women, it will quickly asswage the turmente of the bellie and matrixe. The iuce will helpe any paine within the eare, dropped in warme: with many mo vertues vsed in medicene, although abused in meates, through ignoraunce, in eatyng theim so rawe, and out of tyme. Of nature garden Radishe, is drie in the seconde, and hotte in the third degre. The wilde Radishe is hotter and drie of nature: the seede is good in medicene to clense vrine, and *Radix* loueth to growe in fatte groundes.

Marcellus.

what of Pastnips?

Hillarius.

Pastnips their rootes.

They be called *Pastinacæ a Pascendo*, that is of fedyng or nourishyng, or warming nature: pleasaunt taste, and moueth *Venus*, whereof be wilde growyng in stonie places, but the beste is sowen in gardens, and of nature be hote and clensing. The sedes of wilde Pastnips dronke, will prouoke termes menstruall and vrine: healeth dropsie, and *Pleuriticj*, and is good against venome, and stingyng of Serpentes, helpeth concepcion. But this herbe applied into the matrixe, by the hande of the Midwife, draweth foorthe the dedde child: Stamped with Honie, put vpon a spredyng vlcer, is healed there by. That of the garden is mroe apt in meate, then the wilde: and then the saied wilde, is more effectuall in medicene: one of these Persnips is called yellowe Caret. the other a Rape.

Dioscor. lib. 3. Capit. lii. Galen lib. vii Sim. medica.

Marcellus.

what is the *Sicer*, or swete white Carret good for?

Hillarius.

Dioscorides lib. 2. cap. 107 Galen lib. 8. Sim. medica.

This roote is commonly knowen, it is no lesse pleasaunte to the mouthe, then profitable in meate for the stomacke: prouoketh vrine, and helpeth appetite, and is hotte in the seconde degree.

And

The booke of Simples. Fol.lvij.

And is somewhat bitter, and is called white Pasnippe, with yellowe flowers, leaued like Pimpernell. The seede sodden in wine and drunke helpeth the collike, and winde in the stomacke, or hicket, whiche followeth after vomites, or weakenesse of the harte.

Marcellus.

What saie you of Rubarbe?

Hillarius.

Rhej *Barbaricj* or *Rhabarbe*, is a noble roote of great vertue, and doe differ from *Rhaponticum*, is better in purgyng, in sauor, in substance, compacte and heuie: golden coloured with graie Turkey coloured vaines, drie, and in taste bitter, whereas *Rhaponticum* is light, not heauie, not harde with drinesse, but soft with moistnes: not bitter, but tart, not compacte, but slender. And therefore *Rhabarbe* and *Rhapontike*, be not bothe one: as many haue more foolishly affirmed, then with good argumentes truely proued. And the beste *Rhabarbarj* commeth from *Troglotidæ*, whiche is a hote countrie, in the fardest part of *Africa*, beyond *Ethiopia*, whereas the people, to auoide the extreme heate of the Sonne, are constrained to inhabite in Caues, vnder the yearth : and feede on Dragons fleshe, whiche were called Barbarus people. From whens many precious gummes and spices be brought: as *Galen* saieth, *lib. vj. Simplicium medicamen.* and *lib. quarto Cap. vi. de tuenda sanitate.* Ginger is brought, saieth he, fro Barbari. Whom *Plini in lib. xii. Cap. xxi.* call it *Trogleditis*, whiche was Barbary. And in his .xix. booke saieth he, the cause why Sinamon is so scace, and of no plentie: the Irefull Barbarians, dooe burne the Spice trees. For Mirrhe cometh from thens, *Galen* and *Plini* agreeth, this to be that Barbaric, callyng it *Trogloditis*. *Pompeius Mela*, a greate writer, in his firste booke of the cituacion of the worlde saith, the vile people: wheras these precious spises, and rootes doe growe, doe rather grin like Dogges, then speake like menne, and dwell in holes, and feede on Serpentes fleshe. And *Strabo lib. xv.* in his *Geographia* doe testifie, that all kinde of spice and plates, beginneth in *Arabia Felix*, and in the Southe parte of Inde. For the Sonne taketh like forse in theim: But in *Arabia Felix*, whiche is betwene the sees *Arabicum* and *Persicum*, whiche is so fertile, that it haue twoo Haruest yerely, with all spices, fruites, and gummes. Whereas the people liue euer in peace, without warre, or walled tounes: out of these places cometh *Rhabarbe* to *Alexander*, and then to Venice, & so is dispersed into many paces. To the greate comfort, health, and helpe of mankinde, to purge choller, and humours, superfluous in the bodie: what is better to comforte the liuer, to clense the blood, and heales the kynges euill, called the Jaudes, then *Rubrabe*. How many goodly Electuaries, Pilles, Syrupes, and Purgacions, haue *Rubarbe* in them? Uery many. Simple by it self, by infusion, how maruelous dooe it purge, clense, skower, and expulse venemous filthe from the bodie. And asswageth timpanies, tercians, dropsies, reconcileth slepe, in drie collorike persones: by

k.iii. correctyng

Rhabarbe & Rhapontike.

The differéce betwene Rubarbe, and Rhapontike.

From where Rhabarbe doe come.

The crueltie of the Barbarians, is to burne the Spice trees, and plantes.

Pompeius Mela lib. i. de situ orbis.

The booke of Simples.

correcting hote choller in them, if it be sliced into clene Goates whaie Cichori or Buglosse water. ʒ.iii. and Spicknarde. ʒ.i. standyng al the night in the mornyng, strained and droke, it will clense the blood, and expulse Choller. *Mesue* affirmeth, that *Rhabarbari* excelleth all other *Rhaies*, bothe Turkeshe and Indiche. It is a purgacion hurtles, very gentle, and here is an infusion therof most excellent, to clense the blood: written by a famous man of this time, called *Leonelly Fauentinj*. ℞. *Rhabari* of the beste. ʒ.i. Spicknarde. Ʒ.iii. make an infusion, according to arte, in the waters of Borage, Violettes, Sorell, or Mallowes, almoche as shall suffice: after that it haue stand viii. howers, strain it hard, and put the same infusion *Diacatholicon*. ʒ. vi. and Electuarie *Succo Rosarum*, and *Diaphænicon* ana ʒ.ß. dissolue them in the decoccion of flowers and fruites: and this drinke will very gently purge all foule humours. If any man haue a bloodie flire, to helpe thesame, let the slice a peece of *Rhabarbe*, and toste it hard, and eate thesame, and crome it warme into red wine, and Planten water, and drinke it. In Italie there is *Rhabarbe*, whiche will purge choller, but not so good as I haue discribed aboue: *Rubarbe* must be preserued in waxe or Honie, flaxe seede, or the seede of *Spillium*, so it maie be kept. iii. or fower yeres. *Rhapontike* groweth by a famous citee called *Pontus Marcellellinus lib. xij.* saieth, it groweth by the riuer *Tanyes*, whiche seperate *Europe* from *Asia*. Of this saieth *Paulus Aegineta*, it is yearthly and colde, but the subtiller partes thereof, is moiste and warme: and but meanly tarte of taste. Therefore it will helpe fracturs, conuulcions, and shortnesse of winde, and stripes, it haue vertue to derecte, to drawe foorthe, and clense spittyng of blood, and paines in the guttes.

An excellent infusion of Laonellus Fauentinus to clense the blood.

Paulus Aegineta lib. 7. litera R.

Marcellus.

Of Agarici. what saie you of Agarike?

Hillarius.

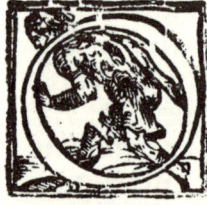

Dioscorides Lib. iii. Cap. i Howe to knowe good Agaricke.

F *Agarike* there is the male, whiche is compacted rounde, And the female beyng broke, haue derected straight vaines, and is flatte, these *Agarikes* be white: light compacte, thicke togither, and swete in the beginning of their tast and then very bitter in the ende of thesame, with biting on the tonge. It groweth in the region of *Sarmatia*, in a place called *Agaria*, wheras is a famous riuer and citee so named. Some saith that the roote thereof doe growe, and bring forthe this Agarike, other that it groweth like Musromps, on Ceder trees. There groweth Agaricke in Italie saith *Plini lib. xvi. Cap. vij*: But because it is a straunger vnto vs, it shall suffice to knowe the vertue thereof. It is hotte of nature, and is good against a tourment of the guttes, raunesse in the stomack, aboundaunce of flegme, ruptures, dropsies, broses or falles, stoppyng of vrine, strangurie, swellyng of the matrixe, fallyng euill, poisone or stingyng of any benemous worme. ʒ.i. steped in swete wine, or swete water, and strongly strained, and drunke before the commyng of a feuer quotidian, it putteth it cleane awaie. Drunke with Vinegar and Sugar

Agarick clenseth the guttes, & expulse raw humors

The booke of Simples. Fol.lviij.

Sugar sodden, and then well strained, it helpeth *Sciatica*, and the falling euill. This Agaricke is no lesse commended, then moche vsed in sondry electuaries and pilles. &c. to the greate helpe of mankinde. *Galeni lib.vj.sim-plice.medicamen.* doe remember Agaricke, emong some kinde of rootes, and that groweth on the trunke of a tree. Firste in taste swete, then bitter, and so forthe he declareth the vertue thereof, to purge the guttes, healeth Iaundes, and openeth the galle, and all viscus humors, who did euer commende any purgyng thyng, more then *Mesue* dooe Agaricke, saith he, it clenseth fleume and choller, and all the instrumentes of the sences: and the braines, backe bone, muskles, sinewes, lunges, breaste liuer, galle, splene. *Democrites* saieth, it is a familiar medicene, to all the principall partes of the bodie, and from them, to all the other partes: purgeth and do not weaken or decaie, any naturall or animall vertue, with many goodly commendacions, he giueth to the same Agaricke. And thus I ende, giuyng you warnyng, that it be very finely beaten, and close kept, and Spicknard put to it in medicen.

Agarick helpeth the fallyng sicknesse.

Agarick purgeth all the organes of the sences.

Marcellus.

What saie you of *Cassia*, and *Lignum Aloes*, and *Cassia fistula*?

Hillarius.

GALEN maketh mencion of *Cassia in lib.vij.Simplice.medica.* sayng it is drie, and hotte in the thirde degree: and doe warme the bodie, and doe strengthen the instrumentes thereof. This *Cassia* is of *Aromatike* nature, and is good for women to drinke, whose termes be suppressed: a goodly medicen of Sinamon, beaten in pouder, with *Lignum Cassia*, is thus made. ℞. Sinamon li.i. *Cassia*. ʒ.ii. water of Roses. li.iiii. clene white wine. li.vi. put these all together in a close potte couered: put this pot in a warme bessell, of leuke warme water, duryng. xxiiii. howers, that is a small fire, vnder the receiuyng bessell, wherin it is put. Then take it from the same bessell, and powre it into the pan of a common stillitorie, then set on the helmit close: and with a soft fire distill the same, kepe it in a close glasse, to giue it to theim, whiche haue any cold sickenes, as dropsie, quotidian, aboundaunce of fleume, stoppyng of galle, raines, or conduite of vrine, Colike, weaknes of the harte, dulnesse of spirite, moiste reume, or lacke of memorie. And if you cause this water to be distilled twoo tymes, it is the better, and of the greater strength. As for *Lignum Aloes*, whiche is hotte and drie in the second degree, it is called *Agallochum*, and groweth in Inde, and *Arabia Felix*, and is spotted, *Aromatike* smellyng sweete. And is a little bitter to taste vpon, with bindyng nature, and it haue a pleasaunte verdure in the mouthe: *Serapius* saieth the best is blacke, with variable or diuers colours, full of sappe. Heuie and harde, grosse and compacted together, with sharpe sweete smell. This wood cometh from a citee, called Mondell in Inde, and not from Paradise, as some doe foolishly fansie, it doeth, and so is conueied, by the Riuer Gangis. Well, to the vertue thereof. It will comforte the

Cassia Aromatike.

A precious water, made with Sinamon, Cassia, rose water, & white wine, for all colde causes.

Lignum Aloes called Agallochum whiche is Aromaticke.

Dioscorides Lib.1.cap.21.

Lignum Aloes cometh not from Paradise, but frō Mondell, a citee of Inde

k.iiii. brain

braine, when it is distempered with colde, through the swete sauour. The decoccion thereof, made with Barlie, Madder and Sugar, healeth vlcers, and woundes in the guttes: and it is good against bloodie flires, and hardnes of the splene, and is a very wholsome perfume. *Cassia solutiue* or *Fistula*, called the coddes of Egipt, can not be spared emong olde persones, and tender people: for the gentle purgyng of the bodie, clensyng of the raines, prouokyng brine. Either drawen with Endiue water, Goates whaie, or eaten newe from the Cane, tempered with Barly water, or Morell water. It maketh a good gargarisme for *Anginæ*, or paines in the throte, or apostumacions in the guttes. It is good in washyng or clensyng glisters, and it will make soft a harde apostumacion, applied thereunto, in any part of the bodie. It is good for the goute, to be made in plaster, for thesame purpose. Who so haue greate paines in the guttes, it is not good to giue *Cassia simple* a lone: but mingle it with the pouder of *Hiera picra*, and for the raines, to put it in the sirupe of Liquoris. It is hotte and moiste in the first degree, the heauier, the Ramishe in sauour: and shining blacke of colour, is beste *Cassiafistula*, and from *Memphis*, and *Alexandria* in Egipt cometh *Cassia*.

Cassiafistula cometh from Egipt.

Cassiafistula haue many vertues to help mankind it can not bee forborne.

Note.

Marcellus.

There is a berie swete Mosse, which groweth vpon trees, men saie it is good in medicen: what saie you to the matter?

Mosse.

Hillarius.

Dioscor.lib.1. Cap.xx.

THE beste Mosse that groweth vpon any Tree, is of the Ceder: the seconde of the Popular tree, the thirde of the Oke. The white is good, but the blackishe is to be refused. It is swete and odoriferus, and haue vertue to stop: the decoccion thereof is good to washe, and helpe al the paines of the mouthe of the matrix. This white Mosse is good in bathes, and in comfortable ointmentes, for the weakenesse of the cold feble stomacke. *Plini* doe commende it, *lib.xij Cap.xxiij.* callyng it *Sphagnos* or *Brion*: saiyng, it groweth in the Prouince of *Cyrenaica*, whiche is a countrie in *Affrike.&c.* In other places, as *Cyprus*, Egipte, and *Phœnicis*, there groweth very good in Fraunce and Italie, bothe sweete, and will mollifie. *Galen lib.vj.simplici.medica.* saieth, *Brion*, whiche is *Splanchnon*, is found emong Okes, Pine trees, and white Populars: it haue power to stop or binde but very weakely, it is neither hotte nor cold, but meane. It haue vertue to derecte and molifie, chiefly that, whiche come from the Ceder trees: *Auicen* saith, it will make a wholsome Cordiall medicen. And also the sauour is good for the brain, and spirites or sences, that be weake. Of sweete Muske *Serapius* saieth, it cometh from a beaste, moche like a Goate, that feedeth vpon *Aromatike* trees: *Ruellus*, and *Simion Sethi* affirmeth, that Muske cometh from a citee in the Easte, called *Chorasa*, the Barbarians call it *Pat*, and of colour is somewhat yellowe. In other Muske cometh from Inde, not comparable in vertue to the firste: and this is blacke of colour, and this cometh from a beaste like a Goate, armed with

To comforte the spirites.

Swete Muske.

The booke of Simples.   Fol.lix.

with one horne in his forehedde: And this cometh from betwene their legges: and also is gathered in the clere aire, and bright shinyng daies from the dunge, and closely preserued in vesselles: and sold to the marchauntes, bothe this pure dunge, swete, and coddes, and or it commeth to our vses, it is adulterated by the Ipothicaries, by many craftie wayes, as with Mouse doung, Charcoles. &c. But of the own nature it is moste pleasaunt and comfortable, to the weake spirites of mankinde: against fransie, collike, Cardiace, Pallsie, lacke of memorie, heauinesse of minde, dropsie, lacke of digestion. &c. And what is pleasaunter in swete water, to washe handes, hedde, and beard, and good in apparell and maie bee rightly vsed, it is Goddes gifte, to adorne and garnishe mankinde with, although light, wanton, lecherous people, doe make it an instrument of prouocacion to naughtines withall. Yet the good vse therof, emong the honest, is no more to be forborne: then the abuse is worthie to be suffered emong the harlottes. Precious Balmes and perfumes, are not forbidden by Goddes woorde: although Judas did murmure, when the woman did anoint Jesus, with the precious *Nardus*. And Isaac beyng blinde, did reioice in the precious smell, whiche came from the garmentes, of his soonne Jacob, when he blessed hym, saiyng: behold the smell of my sonne, is as the smell of a felde, whiche the Lorde haue blessed. And thus I doe ende of Muske, whiche is hote in the seconde, and drie in the thirde degree. Some affirmeth, that if Muske dooe swim in water, then it is good, but the contrary of it sinketh. As for *Zibetto*, called Siuet, is a beaste like a Catte, whiche beaste cometh from *Syria*, and somtime there be seen of them here in England brought from Venis: and betwene the *testicles* of this beaste, cometh the swete zeuit, or Siuet, whiche is hotte and moiste of nature, if women bee stopped in the matrixe, put some of this anointed vpon a pessarie, into the mouthe of the matrix, and she shall be sone helped. *Mathiolus*, reporteth more thereof *Lib.i.Dioscorid.Cap.xx*. whiche I will not name, it is so venerus. As for Amber Grice, or Amber Cane, whiche is moste swete mingled with other swete things: some saith it cometh fro the rockes of the Sea. Other saie it springeth out of the yearth, in *Arabia Felix*, or Inde, vpon thynges that swell like Mosrumes, and so is pressed forth and preserued. Some saie it is gotten by a Fishe, called *Azelum*, whiche fedeth vpon Amber Grece, & dieth, which is taken by cunning fishers and the bellie opened, and this precious Amber found in him. Other doe saie, it is found swiming vpon a fountain of pure water: and that is thought to be the beste inuection. For *Symion Sethj* saith *Amper* called Amber, is increasyng, or found in diuers places: and is gathered in fountaines swimmyng aboue, as *Bitumen* is, or Brimstone, whereof be three kindes, the first is *Fuluus*, whiche mixt of grene and red, a darke yellowe whiche is brought from Inde. An other kinde cometh from *Arabia Felix*, whiche is darke, white, or graie. in colour: the thirde is blackishe, and is the worste, a very counterfecte Amber. This Amber Grice is of nature hotte and drie, the sauour thereof doe greatly comforte the harte
and

Sidenotes:

The beaste which giueth Muske, is like a Goate: that whiche bringeth Ziuette, is like a Catte.

The blaunchynge of Muske.

Swete thinges bee good for mankinde but yet abused of youthfull wantons it is not to be suffred in thē

Marc.xiiii.

Gene.xxvi.

Muske.

Of the Ziuet Catte.

Diuers opinions, howe Amber grice is founde.

Amber grice of three kinds.

and brain of old people, or weake women, and to comfort the harte, it is equall to any other odoriferous treasure. It is put into many precious *Cordials*, & wholsome medicens: and nothyng is more better to quicken the spirites and comforte memorie, then this riche Amber Grice. Gloues swetely perfumed, with Muske, ziuet, Amber Grice, and oile de Ben, be very wholsome for Citizeins, that dwell in close, currepted foule aire. Indeede, it can not bee forborne of noble Princes, Lordes, Ladies, and gentle folkes: God giue them grace, to knowe it to be his gift, to pleasure the Sence of smellyng, and to defende euill aires, and not to (moue or to) be an instrument of vngodlines. Whereas to vse it well, it is of no smal profite to nature, as example. ℞. *Storax Calamite* ʒ. iii. Beniamin. ʒ. ß. Cloues. ʒ. ß. *Lignum Aloes*. ʒ. ii. *Gallia Muschata*. ʒ. iii. ß. Amber Grice. ʒ. i. ß. Muske. ℈. rbi. zeuet. ℈. rii. a little swete Terebinthin, all putte into a warme morter, and strongly beaten with the pestell: pouryng in sweete Rose, or Damaske water. Of this is made a precious Pomamber, to be worne against foule stinkyng aire: weakenes of the braine, commyng of cold. And thus I doe ende of this moste swete oders.

Marcellus.

What saie you of the wood, called *Ebenus*?

Hillarius.

The best *Ebenus* cometh frō *Ethiopia*, and is very blacke, it haue no vaines in it, but abiting sharpe taste: yet very swete in perfume, and is gummie, this is the best. There is another darcke yellowe, and spotted, and this haue a bindyng vertue, and is good to bee put in Collires, for sore iyen. And *Galen lib. v simpli. Ebenus* is one of the woodes, beaten into pouder, and resolued in water, to be dronke to helpe the stone: and of nature is hotte and scouryng. And for that cause, it is good to bee put in medicens, for to helpe the sight of the iye, or blisters in them. If *Ebenus* be fine ground, vpon a whette stone, and with a knife taken frō it ℈. iiii. and the pouder of *Lapis Calaminaris*. ℈. ii. See f ℈. iii. Chamfer ℈. i. ß. the white of an Egge, Rose water, and womans milke ana. ʒ. ß. mingled together: this will moste effectually, clense and scoure sore darkened iyes. *Theophrastus lib 4. cap. vi. de historia plantarum*, saieth in Inde the wood is common, and of twoo kindes: the one is precious, and doe seruice, and the other is of estimaciō. The Princes of Inde doe esteme *Ebenus*, richer then gold, for of that wood, thei doe not onely make their drinkyng vessels, against poison: but also the Scepters of regall honour. And finallie, their Idols of their Gods, whō thei doe worship. Thus the Indians do bothe vse and abuse this riche woode, whiche will sincke like mettall, and not swim When *Pompey* did triumph ouer *Mythridatū* the king of *Pontus*, one of the greatest glorie the Romaines had, was in this strange wood whereupon the Scepters and besselles were made. This *Ebenus* also though it bee good, yet it haue been an instrument of Idolatrie, in many places of Englande: whereof beades haue been made, not onely

The booke of Simples. Fol.lx.

of *Ebenus*, but of Corrall, Jette, Amber, Jasper, Granites, Glasse, Amill, Golde and Siluer: whiche creatures were ordained for mannes bodily health, and not for their contemplacion, and Spirituall praiers. I did knowe within these fewe yeres, a false Witche, called M. Line, in a toune of Suffolke, called Perham: whiche with a paire of *Ebene* Beades, and certain charmes, had no small resort of foolishe women, whē their children wer sick. To this same Witche thei resorted, to haue the fairie charmed, and the Spirite coniured awaie: through the praiers of the *Ebene* beades, whiche she saied, came from the holy lande, and wer sanctified at Rome. Through whō many goodly cures had been doen, but my chaunse was to burne the saied Beades. Oh: That damnable Witches be suffred to liue vnpunished, & so many blessed men burned: Witches be more hurtfull in this realme, then either quarten, Por, or pestilēce. I knew in a toune called Kelshal, in Suffolk a Witch, whose name was M. Didge, with certain *Aue Maris* vpon her *Ebene* Beades, and a waxe cādle, vsed this charme folowing for S. Anthonis fire, hauing the sicke bodie before her, holding vp her hande, saiyng: there came .ii. Angels out of the North East, one brought fire, thother brought frost: out fire, and in frost *In nomine patris, &c.* I could reherse an. C. of soche knackes, of these holy gossips, the fire take thē al, for thei be Gods enemies

Twoo Witches in Suffolke, Charmed & Ebeni Beades.

A witches blessyng for saincte Anthonies fire.

Marcellus.

This is wod of great vertue, and excellent goodnes, few woddes maie bee compared to it, for the estimacion: yet for the Frenche disease, there is an other riche wodde, called *Guaicum*, I pray you speake some thing of that wood.

Hillarius.

GVAICVM, or *Guaiacanum*, called *Lignum sanctum*, or the holy wodde or wodde of life, is of a kinde of *Ebenus*. And as almightie God prepared a tree of great vertue, for Moyses to caste into the water called *Mara* or bitternesse, through whiche tree, the same water was made pleasant and sweet, for the children of Israell to drinke vpon, in the wildernes, whan as they murmored against God and his holy Prophet Moyses. Euen so it hath also pleased him to ordein & prepare this *Guiacum*: wherby, through his ministers knowledge, it might be a meane to make whole, and clense the filthy stinking corrupted boddies, of his disobedient children, which haue liued in most shamles lust & lechery, among painted stinkyng harlots, for which offence, they be smitten with the plague, called the Frenche Pockes, an euill most noysome to nature, cosin iarman to thincurable Leprosie. This *Guiacum* I say wil not onely make a Pockie body clene, but also is good to clense any of the principall humours, whan thei do abound, wherby there shalbe a tempraūs moste perfite in nature, it will clennse the raines, itche, and skabbes. And nothing may be compared to the same, to rebate, aswage, clense, consume, and waste, without hurt greate fatty grose bellies of idle mē

Of the wood of life, called Guaicum.

Exod.xv.d.

The Poxe of Fraunce.

and

The booke of Simples.

and women, which be puffed vp with eating, drinking, sleapyng & sittyng in the house all the day without labour, the tables, cardes, & Pot excepted, which causeth thē but litle to sweat, & lesse to thriue, for such folkes *Guiacum* drinke is incomperable to all others for the goodnes, to renew them & make them appere yong againe: for the Goute, Dropsie, *Sciatica*, Cancer, & Timpany. This is equal to the best medicēs, therfore it may be called *Lignum vitæ*, the wodde of life, because it hath vertue to renew. This worthy wod of life God hath geuen to the christian people, in these last daies, whiche wodde was vnknowen to the olde Fathers, as *Dioscorides, Thophrastus, Plinius, Galen, Paulus, Aetius. &c.* And that is no maruell, for that parte of the worlde wheras this wodde doth growe, was neuer founde forthe by the famous Cosmographer *Ptolemeus, Pomponius,* and others, but of late yeres. This wodde was founde by the saylers into the new Ilandes, called *Corterali, Hispaniola*, distant somewhat frō the *Equinoctial* line, and in many other partes there about, whereas the people of those landes be often infected, with sores, biles, and a sicknesse muche like the Pore, or els the very same in deed, to recouer the same: the sicke folkes doo eate of the fruite of *Guiacum*, and are made whole: this fruit will sone rotte, but whereas the fruites can not bee gotten, then they do make a decoctiō of the wood or barkes of the same which bringeth the like health, the Spaniard perseuing the same, did bring this woodde into Europe, not only for to heale their owne Por, but also for Fraunce, Italy, Germany, & for England, in whome this woodde taketh no small effecte for the forsaide Por: of this *Guiacum* are three kindes, the first is blacke within, in the harte, pale coullerid, hauing in it russet lines, very hard and heauie. The other blacke within but white without and is hard & heauie, and not so great as the first. The third is all right white within and without hauyng very small lines, and the harte of this woodde is the best, the arme of the tree is better then the body: the bowes nerer the fruites hath more vertue, warmnes and drinesse, then the lower partes of the tree, which is groser and more earthly of nature, and the more vnctious the wood is, it is the better, the sappe is not so good as the harte, neither the barke as good as the sappe. But the white wood is sweet and most excellent in operacion, and is *Lignum sanctum*, the holy wood. The barke of the straight yong braunches or bowghes, being heauy and whit, moist and without lines hard cōpacted, be the best barkes for the Por. All these woddes called *Guaiaci*, hath a rosin or matter like Beniamen or plesant gum within the wodde, which is the sprite or liuely helpynge humer in decoction for the Por. For the extreme paines in the ioyntes, senewes, baines, muskels, head, handes, feete, and the bones: no sicknesse is so sharpe and cruell to nature, but this precious wod, will bothe quickly and gently, asswage the paine and grief of the same, if it bee ministred accordyngly in decoction, namely to them whome either the Por hath turmēted or els the goute hath torne or racked, with intolerable grief: Among al mortall infirmites, who is more greuous to nature, then ÿ

Strangurie,

Antoni Musa exam. omnium Simpl. de lignis.

Thre kindes of Guaiacum but the white is mooste excellent.

The consideracion of Guaicum.

The booke of Simples. Fol.lxj.

Strangury, pissyng of bloud, or stopping of the stone: what againe be more enemies to mannes nature, then swellyng of the belly, Hydrops, putrifaction of humours, opilacions, hedache, *Vertigo*, feuers, through heate aboue nature, with fier in the arteris, shingles & horrible apostimacions, with a great number of plagues more, which be all mortall enemies to nature, as a continuall fier to burne him, or els a merciles drownyng water of vtter destruction, or finally a deadly earthly graue to swallow him vp, through the corrupcion & infection of ayre. Thus the .iiii. elimentes or humours in mankinde, through euell mixture, or one aboundyng the other, growing to corrupciō. The cases of deadly peril, and to bring the body againe into good order or perfit healthfull estate. As I haue saied, what is better then *Guaicum*, called the wod of life: whiche wodde was not a litle abused of a great number of ingnorante, murdering, shameles practisioners, whiche haue taken vpon them, to binde sicke men to a law, obseruyng the new diet, onely with *Guaiacum*, wherin thei haue sodden in the decoctiō therof many drugges *Colocynthites*, *Briony*, *Turbith*, *Diacridium*, with an hundreth sondrie more such like simples sodden or brewed with this *Guaicum*: this they do vse one generall rule, to euery complexion a like, to euery age the same, and to the man, woman, and childe all a like, neither obseruynge the quantitie, place, or time: But as I haue saied, one only generall rule. Close chāber like a Bee in a boxe, bread by the ounce, a few Raysons, and sometime a chickens legge, with many such folish serimonies, muche cost & small good cheare, if one be healed by chance medlie, a hūdred are slain through this diat wilfully, or els very folishly, and who so go to borde to such an hoost, first let him make his last wil and testament, perhaps he shall not die the soner, but liue the wiselier. For this diat with close ayre, Raysons and Chickens legges, is very good victail for mareners that purpose to saile through the dangerous rockes, and sandes of the fearfull passage betwene *Scilla* and *Caribdes*. Experiens hath learned vs sufficiently, by the deathes of many which haue ben slain in this purgatorie of this folishe Phisicke, ignorantly vsed, or this *Guaicum* rather folishly abused for money: as many goodly creatures, by, and through mony, are changed, transformed and altered out of kinde, for money is a meruelous instrument, a chaunger, a transformer, or a bewitcher of mankind, and an instrument wherupon the couetous man doth continually play his infernall discordes vpon: as example, if lawers take wrong matters in hande. If deuines desire many spirituall promosions, and be carelesse of their heauenly duetie, if Phisicions prolong or abuse their times, with their miserable sicke pacientes, then what is the cause? nothing but couetous hartes and money. Couetousnesse is the mother of all the euils of this worlde, and golde and siluer is euer disceitfull, and begileth mankind. Gold is the prince of euill, the shortner of tyme, the waster and consumer of vertue, loue, liberalite, reste, peace, and quietnes, the instrument of treason, warre, theeft, horedom slaughter, bloudshedyng, and perilous pariurie, this wretched money

L.i. should

Mannes nature is subiect to many euils for wante of perfite temperament.

what euill haue happened through the abusing of Guaicum emong the imperikes.

Beware of the newe diat excepte you haue twoo liues, or els a wise minister of the same.

Couetousnesse and money, do make blind, bothe Diuines, Lawers, and Phisicions, & trāsforme thē from the nature of menne into infernall monsters.

The booke of Simples.

should not thus be abused of the christians, seing one of the Heathen wise men moste behemently doe counte it a vice moste hurtfull and intollerable in any common wealth, accordyng to my wordes aforesaid, cryng out against couetousnesse, with her instrumentes (golde and siluer) whiche is abused, saiyng.

Nummus dolosus.
$\begin{cases} Auaratiæ\ mater\ est\ vniuersæ\ malitiæ, \\ Aurum\ argentum\ q̃\ semper\ insidias\ struunt\ hominibus. \\ O\ aurum\ malorum\ princeps, vitã\ distruens\ õia\ deniq̃\ minuens. \\ V\ tinam\ non\ esses\ amabile\ nocumentum\ mortalibus. \\ Tua\ enim\ culpa\ pugnæ, prædæ, cædes\ q̃\ humanũ\ pturbant.\ &c, \end{cases}$

(Three moste notable and best instrumentes of the cõmon welth The Deuine the Lawer & the Phisicion)

Therefore God graunt of his mercie to three kindes of callynges in this worlde, that thei maie walke truely, obediently, and charitable, in the sight of God and man, whereby that Christe maie be chiefly honoured, and his people profited. First, to theim of the Churche whiche should be the mouthe betwene God and his flocke. Secondly the Magistrate, or Lawer, that rightuousnesse maie be ministred, and Justice obserued, and no man wrongfully oppressed. Thirdly, for the preseruacion of the bodie, that the Phisicion, marre not, or caste awaie that, whiche God hath so richely garnished, with the giftes of nature, whiche is mankinde. And now let vs retourne againe vnto our *Guaiacum* or *Lignum vitæ,* called the woode of life, whiche through couetousnesse, haue been rather made the woodde of death, through longe newe diates, to small effecte to many, though fortunate to fewe. *Marcellus* my brother, when your frende *Senior F. Neopolitani* was smitten with the Pox, his heere fell awaie, he could not slepe for boneache, his breath did stincke, Lorde how pale he looked, his muskles consumed the skabbes appered, vnder whom where deepe hooles grauen with putrified matter, &c. but now his hedde is couered with heere, his skinne cleane, rose coulered in his cheekes, full of strength, he sleapeth verie well, and is in health.

Marcellus.

I am not a littell glad of that good tidinges, but gladder I wold be to learne how he was healed, and with what medicen. For a man may through chaunce medly faule into this perill: then a present remedie for a mischief would doe well for that purpose.

Hillarius.

March and Aprill is the best time to help the Pox

Dioscorides, lib.3.cap.xci. Atractylis is Cardus Benedictus.

Thus he made his drinke for him self and one of his companions in the monthe of Marche and Aprill last paste. ℞. The best *Guaicum,* moste heauie, and full of gum. li. iiii. let it be well rased with a rape or turned into fine chips by a Turner, and of the same barkes. li. ii. *Cardus Benedictus,* which is called the blessed Thistell, which Thistell *Dioscorides* calleth *Atractylis,* with prickes like *Carthamus,* with many leaues which Thistell is good against pricking of Serpentes, and among herbes it excel-

The booke of Simples. Fol.lxij.

excelleth all other against poyson. And in decoction with *Guaicum*, saieth *Petrus, Andrias, Matthiolus*, it will helpe the French pox. Therfore of the said Thistell, put. li.ß. Maiden heere *Cetrach*, the flowers of the wilde, & garden Buglosse, ana. li.i. sweet *Cassia*. ʒ. vi. Aniseede. ʒ. i. ß. white Sugar li.v. cast all these into a wine vessell, cleane and apte for the same purpose, vpõ which, powre on the cleanest and best white wine, that may be got, very hot, in quantitie. li. one hundreth and fiftie, couer this vessell close three daies, then straine it through an heere clothe, then kepe this in a cleane vessell, for the patient at dinner and supper, but not to drinke in the mornyng, and euenyng: like vnto *Sirupus*, or medicens as mani men rashely haue vsed. Besides the drinkyng of this *Guaicum* at dinner and supper, the pacient may betwene the times, as one hower before and after dinner and supper drinke. ʒ. iiii. or. v. also your foresaied receites may be put in cleane new white or claret wine, beyng fined, and made in the prescribed maner. Furthermore the paciēt which hath the por, dropsie, or goute, may drinke amonge: this worthy medicen folowynge, the dosse or quantitie is. ʒ. ii. or more, accordyng to the age and complexion of the pacient. Take Mayden heere, cleane freshe Hoppes, Femitory, Sitrach, called *Asplenum*, Sene of Alexander, of eche. ℥. iii. great Sētauri rootes, Liquorice, Polipodi wilde and garden Buglosse, ana. ʒ. iiii. Aniseedes, *Nigella Roma*, the flowers of Buglosse, the three Saders, Sinamom, añ. ʒ. v. put this into. li. xxiiii of the *Guaicum* water, sodden after the discription in the compoundes folowyng folio. xlvii. then put it in a close vessel, & stoppe the mouth, and whan that is done, set the saied vessel in an other seethyng kettell vpõ the fier, so let it stande and seeth for. xx. howers fayre and softly, then straine it, and kepe it in a cleane close vessel, for the vse aforesaied. But if the pacient be very full of humours, then do thus. Take Sene of Alexander. li. ii. *Succorosarum solutiue*. li. vi. white Sugar. li. vii. Rhabarbe elected. ʒ. iii. finely cut, Turpit of the best. ʒ. i. put these in a cleane stone pot with a narow mouthe, poure into this potte. li. xxiiii. of the common *Guaicum* water, made in maner in the cõpoundes folowyng, stoppe your pot mouthe, seeth it in the foresaied maner vpon a soft fier. xxiiii howers vntill it come to a thin syrup, called a Julep, then straine it & kepe this precious pourging drinke for mornynges, the dose. ʒ. i. ß. accordyng to the age, complexion and strengthe, the pacient must also eate bread. ʒ. iii. well baken like Bisquet, and the fleshe of Chicken, Hen, Capon, Partrige Fesant, small birdes of the wod rosted, excelleth sodden meates, and if the common drinke be to stronge, then the pacient may poure some smale cleane wine or beere, let the pacient be mery, kepte in a faire cleane chamber with sweet perfumes, not much fedyng, but litle and fine, & cleane warme apparell, with a fier of charcoles, eschewyng venery, wines, fruites, fishe, grose flesh, potage, and white meates. Care, anger, colde, much heate, and thus I doo ende of this precious wod *Guaicum* called *Lignum sanctum*.

A good way to seeth Guaicum for the Pox.

The most excellent & best manner to seeth Guaicū in composicions with other simples, to clense the Pox from all the members of the body.

The diat for the pox shortly declared.

L.ii. *Marcellus*

The booke of Simples.

Marcellus.

I pray you what is the nature of *Mumia, Bytumen, Sperma ceti, Tartar, Terra sigillata,* and Dragons bloud?

Hillarius.

Mumia, or Mumme.

MVMIA, is of nature hotte and drie, in the seconde degree, and cometh from *Arabia*, and is made of dead bodies, of some of the noble people: because the saied dead is richly embalmed with precious oyntementes and spices, chiefly Myrrhe, Saffron, and Aloes. This *Mumia* hath vertue to staunche bloud, to incarnat woundes, to help the Fauling sickenesse: beaten into pouder and squirted with a syring with *Mariarum* water into the nostrilles. Tempered with *Cassia fistula* and dronke with Planten water, it is very good against bruses: but Dragons bloud, Planten water, Madder, *Terra sigillata*, and *Mumia*, tempered together and dronke, helpeth greate bruses, bloudy flixes, and stauncheth woudes applied to the place. *Bitumen*, which is a fome of the dead sea, and turneth into a matter like Rosen, and is hot in the second degree, it hath vertue like vnto *Mumia*, to straunche bloud, to heale woundes &c. The Grekes call *Asphaltos*. *Sperma Ceti*, the seede of the generacion of the monstrous whale, hath vertue beyng dronke with Planten water, Ale, or olde cleane wine, to helpe bruses of greate faules. *Tartare*, is made of wine lies, hot and drie in the thirde degree, it is most excellent against itche and skabbes, put in oyntmentes whan it is beaten into pouder, it clenseth the Morfew. A litle Sene, Mastick and *Tartaria*, sodden in a Chickens brothe, is beneficiall to purge the belly. *Terra sigillata*, is stipticke and will cleeue to the tongue, of nature hotte and drie, and is put to ointmentes to stoppe bloudy flixes, new bloudy woundes, & hath vertue of *Bitumen*. *Sanguis draconis*, is colde and drie in the thirde degree stipticke of nature, therfore it stauncheth bloud, and bloudy flixes: If it be stamped with Mouseare and Planten, it will stoppe bloud, applied to the place. But mingle the pouder of Dragons bloud with Teribintine, and Frankensence, whiche is good for to stoppe a newe blouddy wounde.

Against running of bloud or bruses.

Bitumen of the dead sea.

Sperma ceti of the whale.

Tartar, made of wine lies.

Terra sigillata stoppeth bloud.

Dragons bloud.

Marcellus.

What vertue is in Masticke, Rosen, Frankensence, *Beniamen, Storax,* and *Mirrh* calde Stact. &c.

Hillarius.

Mastik, is holso to chap vpon for the rume.

Masticke is a fine sweet dropping gum, from a tree of great vertue, and his hotte and drie in the seconde degree, and is good for the Rume to champe vpon, and plesant against corrupted ayre in perfume. The pilles be of singuler vertue for the saied rumes. The Oile will much comforte the sinewes, and also wil incarnate the flesh. Masticke with Stauesager prouoketh humours, by retraction from the braine to the mouth, champed vpon. Myrrhe, a noble

The booke of Simples. Fol.lxiij.

a noble gum of most singular vertue, which is hot and drie in the secōd degree, and preserueth against rotte and putrifaction, and is of great vertue in fresh woundes to defende them from apostimacions or rotten matter, to heale a wounde quickly, nothinge is better, in balmes artificiall, Mirrhe is principall. In wounde waters, Mirrhe taketh the chief force. In the pilles of Ruffy, against the pestilence, Myrrhe, Aloes, & Saffron, do resist the poyson of the same pestilens, for woundes in the head, Mirrhe is of great vertue. The bodies of princes are longe preserued after death through Myrrhe. The sauour of the same and daily drinking in Betony water, ʒ. vi. of Mirrhe defendeth the fallyng Euil, and sorenesse of the longues. *Thus*, called Frankensence is hotte in the seconde and drie in the first degree, and droppeth frō trees of the same name, which we do call Furre trees, it hath vertu to nurish and ingender flesh, in the tender bodies of men or womē, and this Frankensence is vsed in many salues, to help mankinde, and is more profitable for mankinde in medicen. Then commendable to be wasted in Churches, in parfumyng the insencible images. Frankensence is good to parfume the clothes, for them which haue the bloudy flix, and thus I ende of *Thus* called Frankensence, *Olibanum* is not much vnlike in nature to this Frankensence, but ye very same in grece. Gum *Sarcacoll*, is drie in the first degree and hot in the second, it is a sanatiue gum to incarnat woundes & sores, and nothing excelleth this Gum to put into Colyries for sore eyen, as whan ye sight is couered with white spots. Rosen, called *Resina pini*, hath warmyng, mundifiynge, & dissoluyng nature. This Rosen no ship, or Chirurgin can want. Rosen drieth and warmeth colde Melancholy, sores, Apostimacions, and vlsers: and furthermore it will produce flesh in the woundes of stronge persons: therebe sondry kindes of Rosen, as droppynge from the Ceder &c. but all of one nature. Also a litle I shall put you in remembrance of *Pix*, commonly called *Pix nauallis*, of nature hotte and drie, and hath vertue to dissolue, consume, and is put into plasters, against colde diseases, it is also put in, inwarde medicines to be dronke against bruses, as Mume is. There is another Pix called *Liquida* whiche is more hotter and thinner, euer moiste commonly called *Terre*, whiche hath vertue to spreade, consume and waste humours, put into sondrie goodly oyntmentes against colde sores, and also to heale skabbes. Tarre is not onely holsome for mankinde to kill sondrie skabbes and sores, and scaules (as take *Pix Nauallis*, Tarre, *Letarge* of Siluer, Hony, ana. ʒ.ß. sharpe Vineger, Planten water, Beane meale, a litle Salte, boyle all these in a littel close vessell, sturre it, and shaue the head, and make a plaster, and lay it on hot. xxiiii. houers & then teare it of, and put on another, and so doo vntill the skabbe be rooted foorth). But also Tarre, greese, and Frenche Sope, tempered together, is good to anoynte skabbed sheep, horse. &c. with a tente of Baken and Tarre, I haue healed the fistula often times: and thus I do ende of Tarre.

There is a goodly gumme called *Galbanum* whiche commeth from the

l.iii. *Galbanum*

Myrrhe preserueth the bodie from putrifaction, or rottyng.

Thus called Frankensēce or Olibanum Dioscor. lib.1. lxx.

Gum Sarcocole.

Resina. Rosen. Diosco. lib.1. capi. lxxiiii.

Picea. Pix nauallis. and Tarre.

A goodli plaster for a skaule in the head

Galbanum, is a holsome gumme.

The booke of Simples.

Galbanum will drawe foorth dead children.

Galbanum trees in Syria, which is put in sondrie plasters, and is hot in the beginning of the thirde degree, & drie in the second, and it hath vertue to molifie and spreade. Dioscorides affirmeth that if it be applied plaister waies or in subfumigacion, it will not only draw foorth the stopped Termes, but also a dead abortiue childe: The smoke thereof maketh venomous thinges to flee. It preuaileth against poyson. And a littell Galbanum with Myrrhe dronke, clenseth the lunges, cough, and stopping of winde, but yet it is very noysome to sauour vpon: therefore it helpeth the Mother.

To clense Galbanum.

To clense Galbanum, put it in very hotte water, and by litle and litle the filth therof will seperate from the cleane parte, and so you may vse the said clene parte for your plasters, as it is writtē in the booke of Compoundes. You may also resolue Galbanum all the night in Vineger, and in the mornyng boyle it: and in water or vineger you may doo so to other gummes, and some other hard gummes you may breake into pouder in a morter, or vpon a stone.

Euphorbiū of Lybica.

Euphorbium commeth from a tree that doth growe in Lybica. The best Euphorbium is that is cleane, like vnto glasse, and is sharpe of taste, this is hotte and drie in the fourth degree, and is very good for woundes in the head dropped into them. It is holsome in Linamētes and Cerots.

To helpe the prickinge of synewes.

If it be sodden with Oyle of Elder, Beane flower & earth wormes, is good against the pricking of the sinewes. In plasters and Cerots, for the Frenche Pox it is profitable. Plinius affirmeth that Iuba the kynge of Libye did first finde this Euphorbium vpon the montan Atlante beyonde Hercules pillers, and called it by the name of his Phisicion which healed Agustus the Emperour, it will not only drawe foorth rawe fleame, but water aboundynge as in Dropsie, but it is euell for a drie cholorike body to drinke in medicen, it is so hot of nature.

Amoniacū of Ammon.

Ammonicacum commeth from Afrikke, by the place where as the Oracle of the false God Ammon was. This gumme Amoniacum is much like Frankensence, bitter in tast, and smelleth like to Castorium, it molifieth warmeth and draweth. It is good in any Linamentes. And being dronke doeth lose the belly, and casteth forth the dead childe: helpeth the Splen, and Sciatica, one dragme beyng dronke. And thus I do ende of Amoniak, whiche is hotte in the thirde, and drie in the first degree.

Assafetida doth stinke, yet it helpeth the mother & Lunges.

Assafetida, stinketh, and is good for women to smel vpon, that be commonly sicke of the Mother, it is hotte and drie in the seconde degree, some do affirme in the thirde. It hath vertue to drie, to consume, to clense, and spreade. Fiue pilles of Assa, taken in a reare Egge at midnight, doeth cleanse the lunges, and helpeth a shorte winded man or woman. Oyle of Spike, Mastike, Saffron, Wax, Castor, and Assafetida, stāped and sodden together, maketh an excellent medicen for the goute, or paines in the ioinctes: and thus I do ende of stinkyng Assafetida.

Sagapen, or Serapinum, a goodly gū.

Sagapenum or Serapinum is a precious gum, runnyng from a smal tree, like a Kir or a Reede, and is hot in operacion. The best of this gumme is that which shineth through, and in couler is darke yelow without, & white within. This gumme is good in many Linatiues, and also inwarde

The booke of Simples. Fol.lxiiij.

warde medicens, as to pourge fleame, to helpe the fallyng sicknes, to cleanse the Lunges, helpeth the swellyng or hardnesse of the Splene, and is good against the resolucion of the sinewes, conuulsion, ruptures, first steeped in wyne or *Hydromell*, then drunke.

Bdellium is a goodly tree, growing in *Arabie*, from whiche tree distilleth a worthy gum like war, but cleare shining, vnctuus, and sweet of sauour, and bitter in tast, it is hot in the seconde degree, and is putte in many ointementes, resolueth consumeth and disperseth apostimacions that be harde.

Boras, is hot and drie of complexion, whose vertu is to knit, and glew woundes together by a traction.

Glaucium, or *Memitha*, so called, is colde and drie in the firste degree, and cometh from *Syria*: *Plini* affirmeth this to be the lesser *Celidon*, & that can not be, for *Celidon* is hotte, and *glaucium* is colde: therefore they can not be one, seing they be of twoo sondrie natures, yet in couller it is yellow, and meruelous good for to make Syef, for to clense and helpe sore iyen *Dioscorides* doth commende this iuce, *lib.3.cap.lxxxiiij.*

Gumme *Arabyk*, is hotte and moyst, of vertue will staunche bloud in woundes, because it is slimy, it will also molifie & make thinges softe that be hardened, as apostimacions, and it will stoppe the bloudy flix, resolued in Red wine and drunke.

Glew, called *Glutinum*, of nature is hotte and drie, and is made of the skinnes of beastes, the best is made of the strongest beastes, as Bulles, Oxen, red Deare. &c. that which is whitist, and cleare shinyng, is very good. Resolued in Uineger all the night, the same wil clense Leprous filth, and Marmols from the skinne, the place beyng warme anointed therwith. And sodden in warme water, with Oile of water Lilles or Flax, it will helpe skaldyng and burnyng of the body, to anoint the sore place therwith. Woundes be helped with Glewe resolued in Uiniger, and tempered with Hony, and put into the said woudes, or els with vineger resolued for the same purpose. And thus I do conclude of Glew, made of skins, which cannot be forborne, neither of bowers, or fletchers. There is a Glew made of Fishes, as of the bellies of whales, and other greate fisshes, which wil quickely be resolued. And this is very good for to make *Emplastrum* for the head, or clense the filthe or red spottes from the face. Ther is another Glew made of corne, as Wheat &c. good for Paste, for Stacioners whiche *Galen* doth remember *libro.vij. simplic.medic.*

Gum *Opoponax*, is a gum commyng from an herbe called *Panax*, and of nature is hot and drie, and of vertue resoluyng, warmyng, & makinge softe thinges whiche be grose, colde and harde, and is vsed in sundrie Oyles and Lynamentes.

Tragacantha cometh from *Mons Gargano*, and is a noble gumme of greate vertue, and helpeth woundes inwardly in Linamentes: and resolued in fenell water. And dronke helpeth the raines of the backe & bladder And with cleane clarified Hony. z. s. doth clense lunges, and will clere

l.iiij. the

The booke of Simples.

Diosco. lib.3. Cap.20. the voice from cough, and is of great effect to helpe sore iyen. Many good Pilles, and mixtures to be put vnder the tongue be made of this gum, against *Anginæ* and all the paines of the mouthe and throate.

Laudanum. Laudanum, is a precious gum, hauing vertue to heate and humecte or moist in the seconde degree: the best cometh from *Cyprus*, and is sweete of sauour, *Galen* doth commende it *lib. 7. simplic. medica.* because it putteth away colde, and geueth heate, and is good against the coldnesse of the braine, or colde rume. And *Laudanum* melted with Beeres grece, wil kepe the heere from fallyng, to anoint or emplaster the naked or bare pallet. It maketh goodly Pessaries for to cõfort the Matrix that is colde and openeth the mouth of the vaines. Melted in hotte Oyle of bitter Almondes, it maketh a singuler oyntment for deafe stopped eares: in subfumigation close vnder the secrete clothes of women, whiche be newly deliuered of childe, it will eiecte or cast quickly forth the secondes, it moueth vrine. If it be dronke in olde Redwine, it will stop the guttes in a bloudy flixe. Masticke and *Laudanum*, incorporate together, doth faste lose teeth; and this *Laudanum* is vsed both inwardly & outwardly, for the health of mankinde, & hath a sweet sauor of singuler vertue.

Laudanum, doth help the heere from fallyng, sayth Paulus.

Lycium cometh from Lycia. Lycium or *Pixacantham*, so called of *Dioscorides. lib.j. cap. Cxiiij.* which cometh from a sharve thorny bushe or tree, leaued like Box, fruit like Pepper black and [bit]ter, it groeth in *Cappadocia* and *Lycia*. The braunches beinge cutte, stamped and sodden, and so strained, from which cometh a iuce, which is as thicke as Hony, which is sophisticat with sundrie substance: as the iuce of Wormewood, Oxe gaules &c. This *Lycium* is yellow & bitter driyng and percing, of substance very earthly, and stiptik, it hath vertue to helpe the eyes, drieth moyst skabbes, and is good to be geuen thẽ which be bitten with a mad Dog, and haue *Tenasmus* or the bloudy flixe.

For yellow heere. It will make one haue a yellow heere, & stoppeth the immoderat flix, either Red or white abounding in women. And thus I ende of *Lycium*.

Acacia stoppeth ý bloudy flix. Acacia cometh from a thorne in *Egipt*, whiche hath coddes growynge vpon it like a Broume, out of which coddes, leaues, and seede, is pressed forth the gumme *Acatiæ*, whiche wil restraine and stoppe most effectually, and is colde and drie. This *Acatia* aboue al gummes hath vertue to coule and stoppe bloud, and bloudy flixes, and coole the burning of the eyes, and in the commendacion therof rede *Dioscorides, lib.j. cap. xxv. Theophrastus lib.4.cap. de plant. historia. Galen lib. 7 simplicium medicamentorum. &c.*

Terebinthus or Terebintine hath great vertu. Galen lib.8. Sim.medica. Terebinthus, is a goodly tree, hard and blacke, and groweth in *Arabia*, frõ which droppeth a precious liquor, or thinne gumme called Terebẽtin although from euery Rosen tree a kinde of Terebentin doth droppe. Terebentine is hot and drie of nature in the seconde degree, and is vsed in many outwarde partes or paines of the body, and is put in sondrie oyntementes and Cerots, &c. It will helpe the senewes and muskels, it stoppeth *Tenasmus*, which is a running of the guttes or flix, made in a subiumigation vpon the cooles. Clere venis Terebentin washed and tempered with Hony, will clense the Lunges. Taken with suger in Pilles, it will clense the raynes, open the bladder, purge grauell, cause

The booke of Simples. Fol.lxv.

cause much vrine, and helpe the yarde, and also mollifie the belly. Terebentine.ʒ.ii. often washed in Fenill or Time water, then put in the pouder of new Saffron, and *Hyria simplex*, an̄.ʒ.ſs. and kepe this in a boxe & who so feeleth grief within their guttes or raynes, let them eate of this.ʒ.ii. euery mornyng, during.iiii. daies. Ther is a fine Terebētin comyng from the tree *Larex*, vsed much: and thus I leaue of Terebentin which is sweet, and shinyng cleare, yet somewhat noysome to the stomacke. There is much counterfet Terebentin, made of Rosen & Oyle &c. which the Chirurgians can craftly *Sophisticate*.

<small>The vertue of terebentin</small>

<small>Gum *Larex* is equall to ÿ *Terebinthin* reede in *Aetius*.</small>

Styrax Calamitie and *Styrax liquide*, be both hot and drie, the best of this saith *Galen* is brought from *Pamphilia*, it is good to be incorporat with *Laudanum*, clene new wax, Muske, Seuit, it will make a pleasant Pomambre against stinkyng ayre, or coldenesse of the braine or melancholy. *Syrax calamite*, or of the Reede so called, maketh good Parfumes. The blacke is worst, the gum vᵈ shinyng couller is best: but to say the truth, the Apothicaries can so well Sophisticate the same with waxe.&c. that we can haue but litle true *Styrax*, as Myrrhe, Amber, Muske.&c. the Poticaries do geue them al their blessynges with adulterat baggage with a cast of legerdemaine, to fill their purse, but if we had them in their right kinde, litle ware were worthe much money: and now in sondrie places, much ware is worth litle money, or nothing at all. This very *Styrax calamite* doth mollifie, warme, and dronke with wine, helpeth the greatest griefes in the stomacke and reume, and let the termes slip naturally: and helpeth stinking breath. Tempered with Oyle, maketh a precious oyntment for the head, of thē which be ouercome with colde. *Styrax liquid* is good in oyntmentes for skales, skabbes, and French Pox, and is good to be burnt in Parfume against a pestilent ayre.

<small>Styrax calamitie, and liquid *Styrax*, be sweet and holsome.</small>

<small>The iuell craft of subtil Apoticaries, doo muche harme.</small>

Diacridium is hotte and drie in the fourthe degree, and is pressed out of an herbe to purge with al, the best is shining in substance, and black, there is good which is whitish, but much is sophisticated with spurge *Colophoni*.&c. but that is not good, if it be brittell and bitter in sauour: and if you licke *Diacridon* with your tongue, so that white some doth remaine after it, then it is good to purge choler, flegme and melancholy beware you receiue not *Scammoniæ*, before it be wel prepared as you may se in *Fol.l.* of *Compoundes*: for this *Scammoniæ* is very benomous before it be prepared, and expulseth good matter, and retaineth still the euill or hurtfull humers to the great perill of the receiuer, and will put the bodye in daunger of a blouddy flixe incurable: therefore prepare I say your said *Scammoniæ* in Quinces made hollow, or in gray Costardes, after the same maner, put in your *Scammoniæ*, sprinkled with Oyle of Violettes and bake it in paste, that the benim may passe away, when it is colde: then it is *Diacridion* fit to purge, being corrected with *Mastik*: and why shal *Mastik* be put in? because it will abate the violence therof, and kepe the stomacke and hart from daunger, and the guttes from the bloudy flix. Gum *Arabyk* is also holsome therwith. Cholorike persons may be purged with lesser prepared *Scammoniæ* or *Diagridi*, then the flegmatike or Melancholy

<small>*Diacridij.*</small>

<small>To knowe good *Diacridon*.</small>

<small>Scamonie is perillous, except it be first prepared.</small>

The booke of Simples.

lancholy, and it may not be occupied .xv. daies after it be prepared as with *Myrobolans. &c.* It is vsed in sondry electuaries, pouders, and pilles. And vndiscretly ministered it anoieth the hart, drieth good humers, washeth nature, yea disolueth and finally killeth the body. Reede in *Valerio cordo*, which is a good Pothicary, not only to prepare this, but also all other thinges profitable for nature.

Marcellus.

I Thanke you with all my harte, I haue conceiued no lesse pleasure, to heare you al this long day, then you haue taken paines of your part to teache me, the vertues of so many thinges without many questions moued, yet I had almost forgotten to moue you, what vertue is in *Myrobalans*, which euen lately you haue named to be good with prepared *Scammoniæ*.

Hillarius.

Myrobolans of .v. kindes.

To seme yōg how to do it.

MYRABOLANVM is a noble fruit of Inde like Plummes, whiche hath vertue to purge superfluous humers, and comforteth nature, and who so vse to eate often of *Myrobalans* beyng condite, shall not seme olde saieth *Mesuæ*, and maketh pure couler. There be .v. kindes of them, as *Flaua Chepula, Indica*, or *Nigra, Empelica, & Bellerica*, which doth differ one from the other, for the *Flaua*, and *Chepula*, do grow both of one tree, for the *Flaua* is gathered vnripe, and the *Chepula* hath his ful nature and ripenes *Myrobolans, Flaua, Indica, Chepula*, and *Belerica*, be colde in the first, and drie in the seconde: *Empelica* is colde and drie in the first degree, and be good for the lyuer, gaule, splene, raines and bladder, and put in infusion of the iuce of Quinces, standing .xxiiii. houres, and then strained, then put in prepared *Scammoniæ*, it will purge choller, as for example: Take *Myrobalans, Flaua*, ʒ.i. the iuce or syrup, simple of Quinces. ʒ. iiii. stampe your *Myrobalans*, and then mingle them with the saied iuce, the iuce beynge made warme, and let it stande in a close stone vessel .xxiiii. houers, thē straine it forthe, whan this is done, beate your prepared *Scammoniæ*, fine into pouder. ʒ.iiii. and temper it together, putting it in a close warm place, to drie it by litle and litle, and of this .ʒ.i. or litle more wil purge choler, and humours superfluous without hurte. *Myrobalans* may be staped with the Syrup of Wormewood, and then sodden with the infusion of *Agarice*, and *Rhabarbe*, to purge flegme and choller, it may be drawē with *Cassiafistula* and *Manna*, for noble persons or people of tender nature. This fruit defendeth the body from corrupcion, trimbling of the hart heauines, Melancholy, and bringeth to nature, clenlinesse, fauour, myrthe. And drawen with Fenill water and Suger, it wil clense the sight to be dropped into them morning and euenyng. The pouder of them with Rosen, wil heale sore vlcers. And thus I do ende of Myrobalans, which will draw backe the venomous force of euery purgacion that will abounde in operacion.

To purge tēder parsons.

To clēse sore eyne.

what

The booke of Simples. Fol.lxpi

Marcellus.

What is the bertue of Gaules, called *Galla?*

Hillarius.

Gaules will binde, and nothinge will clense the mouthe from filth better, applied to any sore therin. Whan the intolerable paines of the teeth doeth rage on still, a pece of a Gaule aplied to the place, will sone aswage the same. Gaules sodden and stamped, applie them to the Matrix whan through weakenes it is displased or faule doune, and it will go backe to his naturall place againe. Gaules will stanche bloud, and make heere blacke, and stop the bloudie flixe in glisters. *Galen lib. vij. simplic. medic.* saieth Gaules be cold, stopping, and yearthly of nature, drie in the thirde, and cold in the seconde degree. The cuppes wherein they doe growe bee of the same nature. And thus I doe ende of Gaules whiche is good also to make Inke withall.

Gaules grow like Thornes. Diosco. lib. cap. cxxiii.

Gaules will stoppe the flix

Marcellus.

What say you of Acornes of the Oke tree?

Hillarius.

The Oke tree of all noble trees for strength excelleth all other for substanciall buildinges, whiche tree shall be ones in no smale estimacion in this realme of England to vpholde houses, dwellinges, and the royall Naues: although the Oke be of litle price, yet for the age strength and vertue, few other trees excelleth the Oke, the barke can not be forborne of Tanners to make Leather, to serue the common wealth. The timber as I haue saied is principall in buildinges. The Acrons hath vertue to stop *Dysenteria,* and *Tenasmus,* whiche be extreme flixes. Of all trees that be *glandiferus* or bearing nuttes or Mast, nothing doth restraine more then the Oke and Acorns, as *Dioscorides, lib. j. cap. Cxxi. Thophrastus, lib. iij. cap. viij.* and, *ix de plantis historia, Fagus* the Beeche tree, and *Ilix* doe beare mast, not only good for Swine to feede vpon, but also in medicen doth stoppe termes imoderat, or restraineth or driueth backe guttes, that be ralaxed, or the precipitacion or comyng foorth of the Matrixes of women, if either the barkes, leaues, buddes, Acrons cuppes be sodden in red wine, running water, to sit close ouer it warme, and to drinke the decoction therof in cleane Red wine, Synamon, & Suger. *Suber* the Corke tree with his frute, hath the forsaied vertue to stop the flix or bloud. Reade *Plini. lib xi.*

The Quarce or Oke tree, will stoppe the bloudy flix or bloud so will the barke Acorns, or leaues with the cuppes.

The Beeche tree with his frute will stop flixes.

Suber the Corke, will stop bloud & flixe.

Marcellus.

What then of *Castian* the Chest nut?

Hillarius.

Chestnuttes be commonly knowen, whiche of nature will stoppe flixes and restraine, make fatte, & indurate the Splene. In many places

Castana the Chestnut.

The booke of Simples.

Chest nuttes helpe the bityng of a dog. places of Italie and Fraunce, the people doth liue by these Chestnuttes in winter, whan they want other fruites. Stampe Chestnuttes, Hony, and Salt together, and applie it to the biting of a mad Dogge and it will heale it. Chestnuttes moueth venous or carnall lust being roosted and eaten. But customable eaten, thei do offende the head and splene, because thei doe inflate and stoppe, thei be called *Iouis glandes*, that is Jupiters Nuttes saieth *Dioscorides, lib.j.Cap.cxxij.*

Marcellus.

What say you of *Myrtus*?

Hillarius.

Myrtus haue vertue to restraine. MYRTVS the blacke, that grow in the gardens be of more vertue to restaine, then they whiche growe vpon the Monnates which be white, the seed hath great vertue to restraine. The seede is good to be geuē to them which haue the bloudy flix and spit bloud, and it openeth the brin. The iuce of Myrts dronke in wine, doeth stop the flire, and healeth filthe, breading aboute the preuie members, beinge washed therwith, and it doth clense the iyen. Myrtes haue vertue, restrainyng both inwardly and outwardly, and drieth *Galen* affirmeth, *lib.7.simplic.medic.* it is partly ouercome with coldnes and pearthly nature, yet it hath also a thinne substance of warmnes, whiche giueth it drinesse. And thus I doe ende of *Myrtus*, called so of the Latens: and of the **To stop the flixe, called *Dysenteria* & *Tenasmus* with Myrts** *Arabians* it is called *Alas*, whereof bee three kindes, *Saliua, tarentina*, and *Exolica*, and all be of vertue good to helpe the bloudy flire.

Marcellus.

What say you to *Coloquintida*?

Hillarius.

Colocīthis, or Coloquītida Diosco.lib.4. cap.171. IT is most bitter, white like a baule, full of seedes, leaues like to Cucummers, hot in the seconde, drie in the thirde degree. Good in glisters, against the collike, resolucion of sinewes, & purgeth flegme, choler, and rawe humours, it openeth the mouthe of the baines, yet it is perilous to be giuen to women with childe, or weake people. A peece of *Coloquintida* knit in a cloute, and steped in a draught of white wine all a night, with. iiij. or. v. braunches of Hisop, strained in the morninge, and so dronke, will purge a stronge bodie from muche filth and *Ilyac*: euen so it will beyng sodden in swete **To kill wormes in the bellie, with *Coloquintida*** water, clense al the body. *Coloquintida*, Ore gaule, Hony, mele of *Lupins*, and Oile of Wormewod, and Aloes, ana. ʒ.i.ß, stamped together, & warme applied to the belly, eftsones a lax will followe, with wormes if any be within the guttes. *Sandarak.* ʒ.ij. vineger. ʒ.ij. *Coloquintida*. ʒ.i. in pouder incorporat and sodden together, put into sore teeth, taketh away the **To helpe the teeth with *Coloquītida*** paines, if the paines cometh of colde, the Oile of *Coloquintida* wil kil wormes, helpe *Sciatica*, and put into the eares will take away the sounde or tingling

The booke of Simples. Fol.lxvij.

tingling in them: and thus I do ende of *Coloquintida* which is moſt bitter and muſt be taken with diſcreſion, the *Arabians* do call it *Chandel*.

Marcellus.

what is Turbit?

Hillarius.

Turbit is to purge flegme, but as for the very Turpit, moſte men be vncertein what it is. *Actuarij* ſaieth it is the roote of *Pytiuſa*, *Manardus* and *Meſue*, affirmeth it to be ſecond kinde of *Tithymalus* whiche is called *Mircyniles*, but *Dioſcorides* plainly doeth affirme it to be *Tripolium*, as ſome ſuppoſe by the minde of *Serapio*, *Antonius Muſæ* ſuppoſe it to be the ſeconde kinde of Spurge agreeynge with *Manardus*, and *Meſue*.

Turpit whiche purge flegme.

Much varitie of Turpit what it is.

Marcellus.

what is *Tamarinds*?

Hillarius.

Tamirinds is a ſower fruite of Inde, which be wilde Dates, called *Tamardactylos*, and be colde and drie ſaith *Meſue* in the ſecond degree. This fruite will aſſwage the heate of choler, open the Gaule, & purge the belly. A decoction of *Tamarinds* with Ptiſant, and the iuce of Pomgranets, will quenche hotte Apoſtimacions in the throate: whā humers be to ſharpe, and bitter in the increaſinge or augmenting of the ſaied Apoſtimations. The very pure garden Dates, be fruites of greate vertue. This Date is the verie fruit of that tree whiche is called the Palme tree, whiche fruite maketh precious wine in the lande of *Syria*, theſe Dates be commonly knowen here in England. Sodden Dates in old wine, will helpe the Emeroides. A Date ſtamped with Hony of Roſes, will glewe and knit a new wound. But muche eaten vpon, beyng rawe, is vnfrendly to the head, and maketh groſe bloud, and ſtoppeth the Liuer. Notwithſtãding cleane pared Dates be good in ſtewed brothe, as we do comonly obſerue by cuſtome. *Galen* doeth remember Dates, *lib.7.ſimplic.medicamentorum*, ſaiyng thei be ſwete and warme and vſed muche in meates. &c.

Tamarinds, or Tamardactylos. Dioſcorides, lib.i.cap.116.

Dates of the beſt kinde.

To helpe Emeroydes.

Dates good in ſtewed brothe.

Marcellus.

What ſay you of *Tamariſcus*, or *Tamarix*?

Hillarius.

Tamariſcus, is a wodde muche like *Quickbene*, whereof there is plentie in one parte of Germanie, within a certaine Iſlande, belonging to one of the Germaine Biſhops: and this *Tamariſcus*, is the better knowen here in England by the famous learned man Williã Turner Phiſiciõ: not onely this, but many other ſimples, by the ſame doctor, whiche Doctor is a ieuell among vs Engliſh men, as well as among

Tamariſcus is a litle tree, like quickben

Doctor William Turner

m.i. the

the Germaines, as *Conradus Gesnerus* reporteth of him: for his synguler learning, knowledge and iudgement. The wine of the decoction of *Tamarix*, is holsome to drinke against the hardnes of the Splene, & stopping of the vrin or strangury, because it doth open so much. The pouder therof in bread is holsome for them to eate which haue the quarten or Dropsie. it is as good as *Asplenum* for the Splene. *Galen* affirmeth that *Tamarix* or *Myricæ, lib. 7. simplic. medic.* that it hath vertue to clense & open, and is hotte and drie. Sodden in vineger, it also helpeth the Splene, and also the tothe ake. *Dioscorides, lib. j. cap. xcix.* doeth commende *Tamarix*, and saith it is vsed often times in the place of *Galles*, and is good to be dronk against spitting of bloud, and flixes. &c.

Tamarix doe helpe the Splene.
Tamarix against the flixe.

Marcellus.

What say you of the Nutte called *Pistacia*, whiche is a Nutte of Italie. The *Iuglans* called a Wall nutte, the Hasell Nutte, Nutmegges, Almondes, and the vomitinge Nutte.

Hillarius.

Pistacia a nut of Siria, or Italie.

PLinius affirmeth that the *Pistacia* is a fruit of *Syria*, and was first brought into Italy by the famous *Censor* called *Lucius Vitellius*, in the time of *Tyberius Cæsars* daies, and now there be great plentie of these Nuttes in Italy. *Galen* reporteth of them *lib. 2. de alementorum facultatibus*, that thei be but litle profitable to nutriment, notwithstanding good to the liuer clensyng euill humours from thesame. But whether good or euill to the stomacke profitable or no to the belly, relaxing or bindyng he doth not affirme. *Auicen* saith thus, one saith he affirmeth that the *Pistate* doth not profit the stomacke: but I saith *Auicen*, saie, that the saied *Pistate*, doth not only preuaile against the noysomnesse of the stomacke, but also will coroborate and make stronge the ventricles. And to conclude *Dioscorides, lib. j. cap. cxl.* saieth that *Pistates* of *Syria* be friendes to the stomacke, stamped and teperid with wine: either eaten or dronke doth preuaile against the stinging of Serpentes. *Nux Iuglans* the Walnut. *Quasi iouis glandis* as Jupiters nuttes, with whiche fruites the people liued by, before thei knewe Tillage, and called theim the great Gods nuttes. These be commonly knowen, sweet within and bitter without. And this tree, with all parteining to thesame is adstrictiue of nature, and good oile is made thereof, and is bitter, and soner digested then the Filbirde or Hasel nut, and is vsed in medicens against poisons. Thei be hot in the first and drie in the seconde degree: and holsome cleane picked & washed in wine, to be eaten after fishe, and best new. *Plini* reporteth that when *Mythridatus* the king of *Pontus* was ded, there was founde in a chest of his, his own hand writing, in the laud of Walnuttes, against poison. ℞ Walnuts, in nūber. ii. Figges. ii. Rue leaues. xx. stamped together with a litle salt, & eaten fastyng doth defende that day from the Pestilence or poison: put Honie to it, and it helpeth the bityng of Dogges, laied vpō the wound. The oile of nuttes with Hony, or the grene nut rindes

The vertue of the Pistace Nuttes.

Walnuttes against poison, as Mithridatus reporteth

rindes will kill the Canker, to anoint the place, and also bringe heere and defende baldenesse.

Filberdes be good of digestiō, not good to be eaten before meate, for then they be not litle noysome to the lunges and head. Notwithstandyng if they be rosted and eaten with a litle Pepper or *After*, then they shalbe comfortable to helpe a most rume. Stamped with Hony & Hysop water, then thei be good for old coughes. Theris a good ointment made of small nuttes, and Beeres greece, for to anoint a balde head to bringe heere. *Galen* affirmeth that they be more colde and earthly then the Walnuttes. *Diocles* saith they do lesse nourishe then the Almondes, how be it the greene be more holsome then the drie. There is a comen medicen made of Hassell nuttes or Filberdes, the iuce of Dittany and blacke Sope stamped together, and this wil draw forth a pricke fixed within the flesh. And these Nuttes be tolorable after fishe, to drie vp moiste matter, and the Greekes call them *Karia pontica*, because they came first from *Pontus*, and now be almost in all the places of this worlde.

Almondes: the bitter Almondes, their rootes sodden, the decoction of them will clense the face from spottes. Bitter Almondes stamped with oyle of Roses and Vineger, wil asswage the paines of the forhed to anointe the head temples or forhead therwith. Tepered with Hony and Rue, it maketh a good plaster for the biting of a mad Dogge, and the reason is this, the plaster is very hotte, and the bitte of the Dogge is colde with Melancholie. The oyle of bitter Almondes is holsome for many thinges, as to warme the body, stomacke, Matrix &c. and to poure into the eare to helpe them which be defe, if it be curable. Bitter Almondes be hotter then the sweet, they wil clense the guttes, the liuer, stomacke, and draw foule homours from the lunges saieth *Galen libro. vj. simplic. medic.* Almonde milke will clense, scower, and cut grose humers, and may be made in the decoction of Hennes, Partrige or Chicken, to strengthen nature, or with colde herbes, as Sichory, Endiue, Violets &c. to quenche choller, to reconcile sleape. To clense the raines stampe Almondes in cleane washed Venis Terebentine, and eate it, bothe for the Collike, Strangurie and the Stone: eate Almondes before meate and drinke, if you be afraide of dronkenesse: quench Golde Siluer, Steele, Flinte, or any of them in Almonde milke, wherein is put the pouder of Ryce, and it will stoppe a flixe to drinke the same. Many greate vertues be written of Almondes, as *Dioscorides libro primo cap. cxxxix. &c.* The gumme of Almondes steped in wine and drunke, helpeth the flix or spitting of bloud, so will the gumme of Cheries.

Thereis a Nutte called *Nux vomica*, whiche if it be stamped and eaten by it selfe, or els with a litle Salte, or *Oximell simplex*. ʒ.i. it prouoketh vomittes of choller and flegme. And mingled with Hony, the seed of Fenell, Dill, and warme water, it maketh a most holsome vomitte for a foule stomacke, but beware ye take no more then. ʒ. i. for then it is most perillous to nature or life. With this Nut and *Helleborus Albus*, many dogge leches do put the ignorant people in daunger of their liues. As

The booke of Simples.

Edwardes the imperike. Cutbert Blunt. of late one called *Edwardus*, a doltish impericke, came to Newcastell, and had like to haue killed Cutberte Blunte, a Gentle man of the same towne, which through drinking of the syruppes of Violets, Quinces and Mintes, was happely recouered, and after through infortune finished his carefull life in London, being prisoner in the Fleete. *An.* 1560

Nutmeg, or muske nutte, haue many singuler vertues againste colde. The Nutmegge or Muske Nut moste odoriferous, pleasaunt, and sweet, vsed in many Cordials and holsome reseites against coldnesse, and cometh from the hotte countrey of Inde, from an Ilande called *Badan*, and is inclosed with his Maces, as with a nut, which Maces is a spice most holsome, the cloue is not the stalke wherupō this worthy Nut doth growe, the *Mauritanians* affirmeth that they be hot in the secōd degree. The olde writers speaketh but litle of this Nut, it is proued to be good against winde, collike, flegme, weake digestion, vomittes, hed ache, coldenesse of the liuer, cardiakes, stopping of the splene, dropsie, swellynges, bloudy flixes, comforteth the senewes, muskles, & veynes of colde, or olde people, maketh sweet breath, putteth away trimbling of the harte, and is holsome to be beaten in pouder, & tempered with oyle of Mintes, and to anointe the forhead and temples against coldnesse of the head, or dulnesse of memorie, and holsome in plasters for the stomacke, twilted in Leather and Silke: good in stewed brothes, for them whiche be longe sicke, and the oyles comfortable for colde stomackes: but *Auicen* speaking a litle of the Nutmeg saith, it is euel for **Nutmegges not good for hote complexioned men.** a Sanguen man to vse it, because it will adust the bloud, (and make one appere with a face as though he had a visor of Currall,) because of the drinesse: so to conclude, the Nutmegge is the fruite, the Mace the flower, or Rose that doth enclose it, the Cloue is the smale stalke that bare it they say: But Sinamon is a nother maner of barke. **Sinamon.** *Dioscorides* saith there be diuers kindes of Sinamon which ar hot and drie of nature in the thirde degree, and helpeth the stopping of the Liuer, Dropsie, Flixes, and all the paines of the guttes, lunges, and breast, & causeth a sweete breath, and is holsome in blanche pouder or soppes. **Cloues.** Cloues cometh from Inde, and growe like nailes vpon trees, and bee hotte and drie, and odoriferous, and be good against colde.

Marcellus.

What say you of *Fraxinus* the Ashe tree?

Hillarius.

Fraxinus the Ashe tre. This tree is commonly knowen, whose leaues being stāped or sodden in wine, doth heale the stinging of serpētes. *Plini* saith the leaues of Ashe trees be deadly to beastes, but that should seme to eronioussly spokē of *Plini*, because we se the contrarie: but there is an herbe **Ditten.** whiche hath leaues like Ashe leaues called Ditten. Which *Mathiolus* maketh mencion in his comment vpon *Dioscorides*, whiche herbe is good for mā against poison, wormes and swellings, but no best dare eate therof. And I suppose *Plini* ment this Dittany, which I haue proued to be good against the Tympanie of water. I haue proued it at Tinmouth castle, where plentie doe growe vpon the rockes. But to cōclude of the

Fraxi̅

Fraxin or Asshe tree, the leaues beeyng sodde̅ with the Oyle of S. Jhons grasse and Terebentin againste Cuttes, sores, and open woundes to glewe or drawe theim together againe: thei also bee good with *Consolida Camphori*, Bene meale, & oyle of Mirtes, to lay vpon broken bones. And the kayes of the Asshe tree sodden in wine, Citrach, fresh Capers and Sugar, is good to drinke to diminish ye swelled Spleue, and of nature is colde and and drie in the seconde degree.

To help broken bones.

To helpe the Splene.

Marcellus.

What say you of *Populus* called the Popler tree.

Hillarius.

Here is the white and the blacke Popler, whiche be colde and drie in the thirde degree. Of the Popler is made the goodly *vnguent* called the *Populion*. The iuce of the leaues bee wholsome to be dropped into the hotte stopped eares. The Popler young buddes, incorporate with cleane Hony and Rosewater, be wholsome to asswage the paines of the iyen, commyng of heate. And the iuce of the barke, or the barke in red wine wil stoppe a bloody flixe, *Sciatica*, reade further *lib. primo Dioscorides. cap. xciij.*

Populus the Popler tree.

Marcellus.

What say you of brome called *Genesta*?

Hillarius.

The Brome and the Whin or Furre busshe be hot and drie in the seconde degree: and the seede will prouoke vomittes, clense filthe in the stomacke, and kil wormes. The iuce tempered with Staphisagrie, oile of Wormewod and Aloes, will kill lice. The oyle of Brome will heale a Tetter.

Brome.

To kill Lice

Marcellus.

What is the vertue of the Jenuper?

Hillarius.

DIOSCORIDES in his first booke *Cap. lxxxvij.* saith there are twoo kindes of Jenupers, one bigger then the other bothe sower or tarte of taste, hot of nature, mouyng the vrine, Sarpentes will flee from the smoke thereof. Jenuper beries be holsome to clense the stomacke, help the coughe, inflacions, and the turme̅tes of the belly. There is a precious oyle made of Jenuper to warme the senewes and comfort the head, being ouercome with colde. Jenuper berries be holsom to put in medicen against the Pestilence, and biting of serpe̅tes. *Plini* in the laude of Jenuper saith that the beames in the riche temple of *Diana* of *Ephesus*, had the beames made of Jenuper, the which remained many hundred yeres vnperished, vntill the burning of the same. The *Chymistes* or Distillars of waters, make their ardente hotte fiers of Jenuper.

Jenuper

Jenuner wil driue awaie Serpentes.

Jenuper was the beames of Dianas temple. Plini. lib. 16. Cap. 40.

m.iii.   *Marcellus.*

The booke of Simples.

Marcellus.

What vertue is in *Hypocistis*.

Hillarius.

Hiposistis.

Hipocistea wil stop blod.

Ypocistis is cold and drie in the seconde degree. *Galen* saieth, *lib.7. simplice medicamentorum. Cistus* is a bindyng fruite, the leaues and small buddes doe drie and binde, and glewe woundes together: but the flowers bee of moste effecte. Dronke in wine againste the bloodie flire, or weakenes of the bellie: and is good for women, that haue to moche redde fluxe menstruall. And with *Sanguis Draconis* and Bole armen, with the white of an Egge, it will stoppe a bloodie wounde.

Marcellus.

What saie you of the Pomgranet, and *Balastia*, Limondes and Oringes?

Hillarius.

Malum Punicum the Pomegranet

Balaustica the flower of Pomgranete whiche will stoppe a fluxe.

Limondes Oringes.

Emplaster made of Pomgranetes, be good against hotte feuers: the wine of Pomgranetes, is good to comforte the stomack after meate. There is twoo kindes of them, the sower and the swete: the sower be colde, drie in the seconde degree, but the swete bee colde and moiste in *primo*. And this fruict is called *Malum punicum*, the flowers bee called *Balaustium*, of the wilde Pomegranette, whiche flower haue vertue to stoppe flixes, by the reason thei be colde and drie, and verie stipticke of nature, and is good to be put in clisters and in the drinke of them, which haue *Disenteria*, or *Tenasmus*. The sower Limondes are cold and drie, but the swete are warme, the rindes are all drie. And Limondes are good in wine, and doe resiste poison: Oringes are weaker of nature, and are cold and drie.

Marcellus.

What is *Cubebes*, I praie you of nature?

Hillarius.

Cubebes haue goodlie vertue agaist melancholie.

Thei bee hotte in the beginnyng of the thirde degree, and bee good to cleanse the breastes and bellies, of rawe flegmatike persones, whiche bee full of grosse humours. Helpeth the splene, and coolnes of the guttes: with Mastike it wil draw filthe from the hedde. And with Balme water, there is nothyng better against Melancholie trembling of the harte, and the fallyng euil. And these *Cubebes* be vsed in many goodly medicenes.

Marcellus.

What saie you of Figges?

Hillarius.

Figges will ripe apostumes, best of al fruictes, and is wholsome to be eaten.

Figges bee of diuers sortes, but hotte in the firste degree, and drie inthe seconde: and be full of maturitie or ripenesse, and will open the pores, cause sweate, breede Lise, by the reason foule humour, is clensed through the skin by theim. Relaxe

the

The booke of Simples. Fol.lxx.

the bellie, and sodden in wine with Hysoppe, strained and dronke, helpeth the throte, lunges, and olde rotten coughes. Figges bee good against Melancholie, and the fallyng euill, to be eaten. Figges, nuttes and herbe Grace, doe make a sufferent medicen against poyson, or the pestilence. Figges maketh a good gargarisme, to clense the throte, and stamped with Shomakers waxe, it will heale an vlcer. Figges will ripe hard apostumacions, of the plague sore: Snailes, Swines grease and Figges, with Bene flower stamped together, and warme applied to a sore, swelled throate, will ripe it, and helpe *Anginæ*. The wine of the decoction of Figges, are wholsome to be dronke against bruses, or falles. Figges be fruict moste worthie and commendable to mannes nature, bothe inwardly in meate, to clense the blood, beyng also a goodly medicen. And outwardly in wholsome plaster, to ripe an hard apostumacion or sore: by the reason it will warme, and make the skin thinne And thus I doe ende of Figges. *Figges healeth vlcers. Figges bee bothe meate and medicen.*

Marcellus.

What saie you of the Mulberie?

Hillarius.

GALEN *lib.7. simplicium medicamentorum* saieth the ripe sweete Mulberies will somwhat relax, but the tarte vnripe will restraine and stoppe the belly: so it is then of nature relaxinge & binding. The barke of the Mulberie tree roote sodden in water to drinke that water doth resolue the belly, saith *Dioscorides, lib.cap.cxliij*. the leaues staped with vineger, to heale scalding, or burnyng, to anointe the place therwith. *Tricoctus* called the Medler, or *Mespilus* haue vertue also to restrain, stoppe, and coole. *Morus the Mulberie. Mespilus.*

Marcellus.

What is *Sebesten* **good for?**

Hillarius.

Sebesten and *Iuiubes* be good to helpe the grief in the throte called *Struma* if thei be sodden in swete water, Meede or in the decoccion of Liquores and Figges. And thei bee bothe of a temperate heate and moistenesse, vsed in many medicenes. *Sebesten will helpe Struma.*

Marcellus.

What saie you of Leuen?

Hillarius.

Leuen called *Frumentum*, is hote and moiste, and will quickly dissolue a hard apostumacion: and if it be stamped with Figges it wil spedly ripe & drawe. And Leuen is wholsome to help the pricke within the fleshe or sinewes, made like a Cerote. *Leuen dissolueth harde thynges, and make the soft*

Marcellus.

What saie you of Ceruse?

Hillarius.

The booke of Simples.

Ceruse cooleth inflamed sores.

It will scoure, & is vsed emong the Chirurgians, for to quenche hote vlcers: it haue vertue to drie, and is colde and drie in the seconde degree.

Marcellus.

What then of *Licium*?

Hillarius.

Licium.

Licium is verie subtle, driyng and penitratyng: and of nature is cold and stiptike.

Marcellus.

Wherefore is Litarge good for?

Hillarius.

Gale. lib. ix. simp. medica.
Litarge.

GALEN remembryng *Spuma argenti*: saieth *Lythargyrus* doe drie, as other medicenes doe, that bee made of mettall, stone, or any other yearthly thyng, of a stronge facultie, and is vsed in sondrie linimentes, againste hotte burnyng vlcers. And is naturally colde and drie, and is tried out of Sande, called *Molybditim*. Looke *Dioscorides lib. v. Capt. lxiij.*

Marcellus.

What saie you of *Galanga* and Cost?

Hillarius.

Galanga.

GALANGA is hotte and drie in the thirde degree, and bite as Ginger doe vpon the tongue, with burnyng like Peper, and will take awaie coldnes from the breast, harte, guttes, matrice and raines: dronke with Planten water, stoppeth the bloodie flixe, strengthen nature. Comforteth the braines, and trembling of the hart, Ciperus, which is called *Aspalathum*, is very swete, and of the nature of *Galanga*, and is called wilde *Galanga*. but that it dooe more vehemently expell the termes beyng droke: the rootes be like Ginger. Coste is duritike, hotte and warme, and resiste venime.

Ciperus.

Marcellus.

What saie you of *Iris*, called Ireos?

Hillarius.

Ireos.
To resolue.

IRIS so called, because of similitude of the Rainbowe, and is commonly knowen: it is called the flower Delice, hotte and drie in the ende of the thirde degree. And is of twoo kindes, garden and field Ireos: and it will resolue, soften, and open and is put in molifiyng Cerotes, with the grease of Duckes, Capons, Hennes and Gese, and the pouder of Flaxe, Beane meale, Holioke, and waxe accordingly. Ireos pouder tempered with Honie, make therewith a conueniente Pessarie, to drawe foorthe the dedde childe. It is wholsome for *Struma*, or swelling in the throate, in linamentes. And the pouder thereof will heale a fistula, or a rotten vlcer. Vinegar, oile of

Roses

The booke of Simples. Fol.lxxj.

Roses and Ireos, sodden and strained, put thereunto Honie of Roses, and it will couer a naked place: whereas the fleshe is gone from the bone, and will quikly couer it again. The whiter it is, and the meaner it is, the better: *Plini* doe not a little commende it *libro.xx.* for ointmentes, so doe *Ætius lib.xiiij.Cap.iiij.* but not in inward medicenes.

<small>To couer a bone with fleshe.</small>

Marcellus.
what saie you of Peper?
Hillarius.

PEper cometh from Inde, the blacke groweth vpon clusters, like to little blacke Ienuper beries: Some growe in huskes, and bothe the white Peper, longe Peper, and blacke Peper, be all hotte in *quarto*, and drie in the seconde: the long is moste bityng, because it is gathered before it bee ripe, therefore it haue still the hotte humour. The blacke is perfite ripe, and is wholsome: the white is swetest, but weakest of theim three. Peper is vsed in sonderie medicenes, and in meate againste coldnes: it draweth, dissolueth, and consumeth moiste humours, and drieth them, and helpeth an Agewe, beyng dronke many tymes, specially before the fitte. Grose Peper wil helpe digestion, and neuer hurt the liuer. There is a goodly Dia made of the three Pepers, called *Dia trion Piperion*, whiche haue greate vertue against horsnesse, stoppyng of the lunges, and cold reumes.

<small>Peper.</small>

<small>Peper dissolueth, and consume moiste humours.</small>

Marcellus.
What saie you then of the three Sanders: haue not thei the samt vertue, that the three Pepers haue?
Hillarius.

NO sir, for the Saunders be wodde, or a Tree called *Santalum*, of three kindes: the pale, the white, and the redde, cold in the seconde degree. And all these be wholsome to stoppe flixes and woundes: and with Rose water, Saunders be wholsome, to be applied to the forehedde in a clothe, with a pece of a Rose cake, to aswage the hotte burnyng paines in the forehedde. Sanders be wholsome in drinkes, to be giuen, to quenche a hotte feuer. Temper the iuce of *Solanum*, and Purslen, with Saunders, and the oile of water Lillies, and anointe the raging goute therewith: and the paines will banish awaie, through the vertue thereof. *Auicen in libro de veribus Cordis*, affirmeth Sanders be put in sondrie good medicenes, against the tremblyng of the harte. A noble *Dia* is made thereof, called *Diatrion Santalj*.

<small>The three kindes of Sanders.</small>

<small>Sanders doe coole the head and reconsile slepe and helpeth the gout.</small>

Marcellus.
What saie you of *Cardamonis*?
Hillarius.

CARDAMOMVM, is a precious spice, called the grain of Paradice, growyng in *Arabia Felix*: the beste be the heauiest and sharpeste, bitter taste in the mouthe, with a pleasaunte verdure, stening vp into the hedde, or pallet of the mouthe: these bee hotte

<small>Graines of Paradice, called Cardamū</small>

The booke of Simples.

Cardamom, helpeth the falling sicknesse.

hotte of nature, and to bee dronke againste the fallyng sicknes, Sciatica, cough, resolucion of the Sinewes, ruptures, paines in the bellie, and killeth wormes in the bellie, and prouoke vrine. A dragme dronke in wine, with as moche of the barke of Laurus, breaketh the stone: the common graines be nigh hande as good, and are hotte and drie.

Marcellus.

What saie you of Laurus, called the Baie?

Hillarius.

Laurus called the Bay. Against the stone.

IT haue been in greate estimacion, since Tyberius Cæsers tyme, whiche was crouned with Baies: it signifie victorie, and is of a fierie nature. For example, case twoo drie Baie stickes ouer eche other, and cast a little pouder of Brimstone betwen them, and eftsones fire will flame forth. Merueilous thinges be written of the Baie tree: reade Thephrastus lib.iiij.Cap.viij. Galen libro.vij.simplice medicamen. saith, the Baie tree leaues & berries, doe drie and warme vehemently: the more thei be bitter, the more thei are adstructiue. It will breake y stone, and is good for a colde liuer, dronke in strong wine. ʒ.i. yet it is euill for women with childe. The berrie is hotter then the leafe, and the oile is holsome against cold agues, goodly plasters be made therof.

Marcellus.

THE children of Israell, in their hunger had Manna fallyng from heauen, during their passage in the wildernesse: and after their commyng ouer the riuer of Jordan, thei were fedde no more therewith. And as I doe heare saie, there is a certaine Manna, whiche our Apothicaries doe sell, to delicate persones, to quenche the heate of choller, and purge their blood withall.

Hillarius.

Manna. Exodi.xvi. Sape.xvi. Psal.78. Iohn.6.

THE children of Abraham, Isaac, and Jacob, were fedde by the prouidence of God: because he was their God, and thei his owne people. He prouided for them by miracle, because thei should loue hym, and honour hym aboue all yearthly thinges: for feedyng theim with heauenly breade, called Manna, whiche as the holie writers affirmeth, was the Spirituall foode, euen Jesus Christe: whiche the true faithfull Christians, are most comfortable nourished within the blessed sacramēt of Christes body, which is our redēpcion, ones bodily offered on the crosse. And daily in y congregaciō of the faithfull, spiritually ministered in y holy Sacramentes, vntill thende of the world accordyng to his promise. But this Manna, whiche we doe vse in bodily medicene, is a swete liquour: doe still from the aire, in the tyme of the Caniculer daies, fallyng vpon Trees, Braunches, Herbes, Flowers, and Stones. &c. Some Manna cometh from the Orient, and other from Calabria, whiche is swete, light, and in smalle graines, moche like vnto Masticke.

Manna of Calabria.

There

The booke of Simples. Fol.lxviij.xii

There is a Citee in *Calabria* called *Coßentia*, that the Ashe trees aboute the same, ones a yere in the *Caniculer* daies, haue greate plentie of *Manna* hangyng vpon theim. There is but little diuersitie, betwene *Manna* and *Teryniaben*: but that it is like droppes of Honie, and will quenche heate, purge blood, and relaxe the bellie, and *Manna* will doe thesame, and is white and cleare like gumme. And yet these twoo doe descende from heauen. *Galen, Plini*, and *Theophrastus*, remembring *Manna*, saiyng: in one tyme of Sommer, there is Honie rainyng from heauen vpon trees. &c. At whiche tyme, the Husbande men plaieth and singeth, saiyng: Jupiter raineth Honie, *Iupiter Mella pluit*. This *Manna* is wholsome for to clense the breast, lunges, raines. &c. And of nature is hote, temperate, and moiste and the more it is to be lamented, by false crafte it is sophisticated, or it cometh hether. And when it cometh into Englande, it is but little helped, emong some Apoticaries, and this *Manna* with *Caßia* is wholesome to purge: and you maie receiue *Manna* Simple. ʒ. ii. in your drinke, or eate it like bread in the mornyng, or at noone, it is moste delicious, and pleasaunt to tender folkes. Children maie eate, ʒ. i. atons and young babes in their milke, maie receiue. ʒ. ii. ß.

Manna of the Ashe tree in Italie.

The greate vertue of Manna for mankinde.

Marcellus.

What saie you of Suger of the Cane?

Hillarius.

DIOSCORIDES remembryng Suger *libro. ij. cap. lxxv.* saiyng, there be Redes in *Arabia*, in whiche is a thing contained like Salte, and breaketh in the mouthe like Salte, and is bothe pleasaunt, and good to the bellie & stomacke, deluted or steped in water, if it bee dronke, it helpeth the raines. And Suger is good to clense the darkenes of the iyen. Suger is vsed in moste Sirupes, and Juleppes, *Manus christi. &c.* Suger can not be spared in bankettes, or garnishmente of feastes: Although Suger can not bee simply made, from the panell, or sande, whiche cometh from the Cane, without some art yet there is moche crafte in it, by the sophistacion, to make it trim to the sale: swete and pleasaunte, like Muske to the mouthe, more pleasaunte then profitable. But the cleane clarified Honie, dooe excell for health: the Suger specially, the Hony of *Athenes*, where as the Bees feedeth most vpon time, Suger Candie is good for the lunges.

Suger of the Cane.

Hony is more excellent then Suger to preserue.

Marcellus.

What say you of Spiknard?

Hillarius.

Spiknard is odoriferous, plesant and sweet, comfortable to braine and sinewes, and warmeth eche parte of the body, beyng colde and is good to bee dronke against the falyng euill Collicke, Flix, Caradacis, Dropsies, and Hickit, and it will increace heare, the pouder being tempered with Hony to anointe the place.

Spicknarde of Spain helpeth the brain

The booke of Simples.

For sore eien to help them. place. Spicknarde beaten into pouder, tempered with the waters of Fenell, Roses, and Iyebright, puttyng a little *Lapis tutia* and *Aloes Epatike*, standyng all the night together, and strained in the mornyng, thus dropped into dimme iyes, will comforte, scoure, and strengthen the sight. And of nature is hotte in the first degree, and drie in the second. And thus I doe ende of *Spica Nardi*, wherof there be twoo kindes, one of Syria, and the other of *Inde*. Rede more thereof *Dioscorides lib. i. Capit. vi.*

Marcellus.

What is the nature of *Caphuræ*, commonly called Campher.

Hillarius.

Caphuræ, called Campher, a gum of a greate tree of Inde. It is a gum of a tree of Inde, whose bignes, and bredth of the branches be so large, that a .C. men or more, maie bee shadowed vnder the same: this tree groweth nere the sea side, and the people of Inde doeth couer them selues from the heate of the Sunne vnder the shadowe of the same. There was a certain king amōg them called *Riach*, **Riach founde first Capher.** whiche founde out the worthie vertue of this gumme, and from the base cullour therof did by arte chāge it into shinyng whitnesse which is the best Campher, all the other is but base and of small estimacion. **Sondri opinions of campher.** Some also saieth that Campher is a heauenly influence, caste downe by the violence of thunder and lightning, and is gathered out of the earth like vnto Sulpher or Brimstone, although it be by the tugemētes of *Serapio* and *Auicen* colde and drie in the thirde degree, and commeth from the Meridian parte of the worlde: but there is muche craft and sophistication of the Campher, through the craft & subteltie of strangers before it is brought into the Realme. But if you will know good **How to know good Campher.** Campher, do this, take a new Manchet hot from the ouen, and cut it a sonder in the middes, then put in the Campher & close the loof loose together, then if the Campher do caste a moistnesse, it is the best argument to proue it to be good Campher, but if it remayne drie like vnto earth, then it is false and counterfet, good Campher will burne vpon Snowe, and also in water, it ought to bee kept close, couered aboute with flax seede, Pepper, or such like, for by it selfe it will waste away quickly, it is put in many goodly ointmentes to quench the heat that **Campher will quenche nature.** is aboue nature and to extinguish carnall lust, as to temper it with the iuice of Nightshade, Vineger, and water Lilles, then to anoynte **To cause sleape.** the Testicles or priuie partes, and this shall quenche the heate of nature, it will also reconsile sleape, to make oyntment with Rose water Oyle of water Lilles and womans Milke, and to annoynt therwith the temples and forhed. Planten water and Campher, wil stoppe the bledyng at the nose, it is put in goodly oyntmentes to clense the spottes from the face, and the filthe from the skinne: it preserueth the e- **To stop the whites and runing of the Raines.** yes from blindenesse tempered with medicine accordyngely. It stoppeth the runnyng of the Raynes and white flures passing from women, dronke with the iuce of water Lilles: it is good agaynst the Pestilence

The booke of Simples.   Fol.lxxiij.

stilence, and finally it will preserue a dead body from stincking, putri-
faction. And thus I ende of Campher called *Capburæ*, Vitex called *Agnus castus* is also of the nature of Campher to drie vp the seede of generacion, but in complexion as *Galen* saieth, it is hot and drie in the thirde degree bitter of taste and bynding, Rede *Galen* therof. *lib.xxiiij. cap.ix.* and *Dioscorides* the first booke the. Cxvi. chapter of the nature of *Angnus castus* doth greatly laude it for the singuler vertue, beinge so goodly an instruuent for chastitie. And how the women of Athens that professed chastitie did strawe the leaues therof aboute their beddes. And thus I doo ende of *Angnus Castus*, that is to saie chaste.

<small>*Agnus Castus, or vitex for chastitee.*</small>

Marcellus.

What is the nature of *Sulpher* called Brimstone?

Hillarius.

SVLPHER called Brimstone, is hot and drie in the fourth degree, with this Sulpher & fyre, God plaged the people of Sodom and Gomor, for their abhominable sinnes against nature. Sulpher is one of the simples put into the recept of Gunnepouder, wherwith God by his instrumentes, plaged y proude world with all, through merciles gunnes. Sulpher is founde in diuers partes of the worlde, as in vaines of the earth, welles, and pittes, aswell in the cold partes of Iselande, as in the hot partes of Inde. Of a sulpherus humour it is presupposed that the waters of the Bathes here in Englande haue their continually warmenesse of. Also in Italy in the fieldes *Senensis*, vpon the mountaines not farre from the warme Bathes of S. Philip, is muche Bristone founde, therefore it is none errour to saie that the hot Bathes haue their originall spring of Brimstone. Sulpher hath vertue to drie vp Scabbes being tempred with fastyng spittle, Wineger and Swines greece. It also helpeth Leprous Scabbes & Pores, being sodden in Oyle Debay and sharpe Wineger. And *Galen* saith that it doth resist the venum of Serpentes. Notwithstanding through the heate therof it will exulcerat, if it be not corrected. And thus I ende of Brimstone, the whitest and clearest is the best.

<small>*Sulpher or Brimstone.*</small>

<small>*Bath spryng came from a vaine of Brimstone.*</small>

<small>*To clense skabbes.*</small>

Marcellus.

Hetherto haue I not remembred the noble Rose, with his singuler vertues, I pray you shew me the nature of the same.

Hillarius.

DIOSCORIDES writyng vpon the Rose. *lib.j. Cap.Cxij.* saieth that the Rose is colde and bindyng, and is friendly vnto the eyes. Roses beyng fyrst dried in the shaddow and sodden in wine, the same liquor is good for the paines in the heade, iyes, and eares, the places to be washed or annoynted therewith. The Oyle of Roses is of a syn-

<small>*The Rose, a friende to the brain & iyen.*</small>

n.i.   guler

The booke of Simples.

Oyle of Roses for ye head

guler vertue to be put Linementes, for to coule hot burnyng ulsers, inflamacions, and such like, because it will resolue, & also extinguish and comfort woundes in the head, through any stripe or fall. And of this *Galen* doth remembre, *lib. x. simplic. medic. de sanguine.* Ther is precious ointment of Roses called *Vnguentum Rosarum,* whose vertue is to extinguish the heate of the Raynes of the backe, and reconsileth slepe, for to haue the temples and forheads noynted therwith, if it be made sweet & white accordyng to arte. There is fewe Cordials can wante the helpe of Roses, and Rose water. And as *Dioscorides* saieth when the Rose is pulled from the Busche, the whitest must be cut away from the redde with a payre of sheres, whiche redde leaues must be dried, preserued or stilled, to the vse of medicen.

Sondry kindes of Roses all of greate vertue.

There be diuers and sondrie kindes of Roses, as the redde Rose, the white Rose, and the prouince Rose, which is excellent in medicine, and most pleasant to be smelled vpon, comfortable to the braine and harte, amonge all flouers none excelleth ye prouince Rose for his manifolde vertues: as against the trembling of the hart, dimnesse of sight, fransies, lacke of sleape, corrupcion of the ayre, heate aboue nature, flixes. &c. Of *Succo rosarum* is made the moste excellent electuarie to purge choller with all. The waters of Roses excelleth all other waters, if they be purely stilled. Rede *Plini* the .xxi. *lib. cap. iiij.* whiche writeth most copiously of the natures, shapes, and vertues of Roses.

The best Roses be in Italy.

The more leaues that Roses haue, the preciouser they bee. The best Roses of the worlde doth growe in Italy and Fraunce. The Roses of England be not much inferiour vnto them. The littell yellow tuftes growyng within the Roses, finely beaten into pouder, be holsome to stanche bloud, to kil wormes, the clense the Canker in the mouth, and to take Pollipus from the Nose. There be also many wilde stinkynge Roses, as *Theophrastus* maketh mencion. *lib. 6. cap. 6. de historia Plantarum.* There is also *Rosa Solis* which is distilled to make a water compounded to preserue nature withall, and thus I do ende of this precious flower called the Rose, whiche the *Arabians* for the excellent sweetnesse, doth call it *Narde.*

Marcellus.

What is the nature of Alum?

Hillarius.

Alum.

DIOSCORIDES doeth remember the same in his .5. booke, the xcii. chap. saying it cometh out of Egipt, founde where as mettals do growe, and in many other places, as in *Melo* and in *Macedonia,* also there is great plentie therof in Italy, which is most whit and cleare, it is hot and drie in the fourth degree, and is

Alum for the Canker.

very holsom in the cure of Cankers, and if it be sodden with Planten water, it helpeth vlsers that seeme incurable, sodden with Hony and Uineger alone, will stablish and make fast teeth. Alum doth clense & scoure, and is vsed in many medicens: burnt alone, maketh Corosiues

Burnt Alū, consumeth flesh.

to corode, consume, & take away dead flesh: you may reade more therof

The booke of Simples. Fol.lxxiiij.

in *Galen lib.iiij.simpli.medica.* of the vertue of the clensing, and the scoweryng: Alum is profitable in every common wealth, where as good clothes be made.

Marcellus.

What is the nature of Quickesiluer?

Hillarius.

There is moche varietie whether it should be hot or colde in the .iiii. degree, but it should seme rather to be hot, by reason it doth dissolue and perce, it hath vertue to consume: and it is perelous to be vsed in oyntmentes to kill scabbes with al for it is so persinge and subtill, at lengthe it will come into the inwarde partes, where as finally it will mortifie and kill. It is founde in Minerals of Siluer, and is a distroier of other mettals. With this Quickesiluer and *Sal Armoniake*, is made Marcurie sublemmat, whiche muste bee kepte in a cloose vessell, athusted in the Ouen, or burnte vntil it come to the couller of white Suger, which Marcurie sublemmat, is vsed of Cherurgians for to clense foule vlcers and sores, and is a poyson inwardly to be taken, except with all speede after the same a boment be také of oyle or *Azarabaccha*. If Quickesiluer be taken inwardly, it is also perilous, and nothing better to helpe it, then to drinke Wormewood wine with the seede of Clarie boiled therin. Maruaylous thinges be done by the means of Quickesiluer: as the Chimistes doth know, and yet for all that we see littell Golde multiplied therby. Thus to conclude, Quickesiluer maye bee conueniently ministred in ointmentes, to heale the Pox.

Quicksiluer or Mercury.

Marcurie sublemate.

Marcellus.

I pray you what is the nature of *Atramentum* of the Minerall?

Hillarius.

It is a naturall Corosiue, and hot and drie in the third degree. *A.ramental.*

Marcellus.

What say you of vnslecked Lime called *Calx viua*?

Hillarius.

It is hot and drie in the thirde degree: vnslecked Lime, oyle of Roses, the iuce of *Enulacampana* and Vineger, strongly beten together in a leden Morter with puttinge in Turpentine, maketh an oyntment which will heale scabbes, infecting the thighes, or legges, and all rotten vlcers.

Calx viua. Lime helpe rotten sores.

Marcellus.

What is the nature of Verthigreace?

Hillarius.

It hath vertue to consume superfluous flesh, and doth mondefie rotten humours, filthy vlcers, depe stinking sores, and rebateth and consumeth proude flesh, and is the chief thing in *Vnguentum Egipsiacum*

Vertegrece.

n.ii.

The booke of Simples.

Vnguentum Egipsiacum. — gipsiacum, for Verdigrece, Hony, Roche Alum, Wax, Oyle, and Veniger, sodden together in a conuenient vessell, sturred together with a sticke till it come to a thicknesse, this oyntment is good *Egipsiacum* which hath the foresaied vertues, and is hot and drie of nature.

Marcellus.
What is the nature of *Spodium*?
Hillarius.

Spodium. — Spodium is colde and drie, and tempered with Roche Alum, it wil heale vlcers, and Cankered matter in the mouthe.

Marcellus.
What is the nature of *Minium*?
Hillarius.

Minium and Serus. — MINIVM is vsed in diuers linementes, and Cerotes, and by burnyng in the furnis, it is made of *Serus*, & of nature is cold and drie.

Marcellus.
What is the nature of Varnish?
Hillarius.

Varnish. — It is good for Armorers, it hath vertue also to scower & clense sores and woundes, and is hot and drie in the seconde degree.

Marcellus.
What is the vertue of Sope?
Hillarius.

Smigma or Sope. — SMigma is called Sope. Sope can not bee forborne in any common wealth, for washyng of linnen, and clensing of the bodies of men and women, whiche be defiled with sweate and filthe, through trauell and labour. But it is perillous to be put into woundes, becaule it maketh seperacion: notwithstandyng, it is hotte and drie, yet it doeth neither burne, nor athuste. Frenche Sope, *Nighter*, common Salte, ana. ʒ. i. put in a little close stone vessell, *French sope.* with three sponfulles of Vineger: let it stande in the fournes, vntill it be dried. This is good to washe the hedde, in a little Walmesie, wherein *Azarabaccha* hath been sodden, againste al coldnesse and dulnesse of the braine. Frenche Sope mingled in the pouder of *Elleborus niger*, called the roote of Beares foote, Verdegreace, Litarge of Siluer and Gold, Tartar, and quicksiluer corrected, beaten all together in a Leaden morter *Sope will kill Tetters.* with the iuce of Houselike, and Stone croppe, maketh a goodly oyntment to kill Tetters, blacke morphew, Ringwormes, spottes, and melancholie, infecting the skinne. Frenche Sope, Oile of Roses, and the white of an Egge beaten together, are good against scalding, or foule stinking scabbes, or itche. If Sope bee applied in a Walnutte shell to the nauell of a childe, foorthwith it will cause the vrine spedely, to purge. Sope is vsed also among the emperickes, or vnlerned practisioners to be taken inwardely, to prouoke vrine and stoole: but this practise is not to be comended. And thus I ende of Sope, called *Smigma*.

Marcellus.

The booke of Simples. Fol.lxxv.

Marcellus.
What say you of Leade?
Hillarius.

GALEN *lib.ix.simplicium medicamentorum*, saith Leade to refrigerat and coole, it hath also humidite, and is a litle earthly of nature, cold and moiste in the seconde degree, & is good against foule cankred sores, & filthy vlcers, fistulaes, Emeroides, &c. thus washed. White or redde Lead beaten with an Iron pestill in a Leaden Morter, poring in Oyle of Roses, or *Vnguentum Rosarum*, labour it well, and then it will make a good oyntment for hot burnyng sores, and wil resolue the hardnesse of them. A plate of Leade is good to coole the burning of the raines, *Plumbum vstum* burnt Leade with Brimston, hath vertue to corode and wast superfluous flesh.   *Leade will coole, and helpe sores. Burnt ledde*

Iron doth mundifie much, and is colde and drie in the seconde degree, so is *Scoria* or *Rubigo*, called the skales or rust of Iron, but more drier: stamped in a Leaden morter, with Vineger and oyle of Roses, it maketh a good cooling and drying ointmēt. And the rust of Yron beaten fine and sodden with strong vineger is holsom to be dropped into sore runnyng eares, reade *Galen. lib.ix.simplici.medicam. Calebs*, or Steele made hotte, quenched in Redwine and dronke, doeth stoppe the flire.   *Iron doe mundifie and clense.*

Spodium is cold and drie of nature, blackish and heauy, tempered with *Olibanum, sanguis draconis*, and Benemeale beaten in a Leaden morter, it will stoppe bloud. *Spodium* with Roche Alum, and strong vineger, beaten together, will kill the Canker in the mouthe. *Spodium* cometh from Furnaces of Brasse, or Copper, Reade of this *Dioscorides, lib.iiij. Cap.xlvj.* and *Galen, lib.ix.simp.medica.* Of *Spodium* and *Pompholix*, it is rather a kinde of *Cadmæ* then *Tutia* and is tolorable to put into Colyres for sore eyne.   *Spodium stoppe bloud. Cadmæ.*

Golde, the moste pure & vndefiled mettell, not leprosse whiche Sol hath digested by heauenly influens. This mettell is most riche. This golde is not more profitable to our worldly businesse, thē holsome for medicens, specially as *Auicen* saith, for to put away Melancholy, and to make burning actual cauteres of Gold is holsom, as if any filth be in the mouth, to burne ye same with Golde is most best, so it is whan the *vvala* is fallen, a Cauterie of Golde is best, in medicens of Cordials. Golde is holsome to deaurate or gilde Losinges. And for ye dimnesse of sore iyen, Golde is tolorable for thē in some Coloris, & is good for Leproses, al mettals wil corrupt, when as Golde wil remaine vndefiled. God graunt we vse Golde as a seruaunt, but not as a maister, for thē we are bonde slaues: for Golde wil not helpe in the day of vengance.   *Golde the moste vndefiled and pure mettall. Gold put into Cordials.*

Marcellus.
What say you of Salte?
Hillarius.

Without Salte we liue not, it is vsed comonly in our meates. With Salt, Flesh, Fish, and many fruites be preserued. The greate Ocian sea is Salt, through which Saltnesse the earth   *Salte, what it is.*

n.iii.   is

The booke of Simples.

is kept from poyson, through the exalacions, or vaupur comyng from this. Salt is of nature hot and drie, and hath vertue saith *Diosco.lib.5.cap 85.* to scouer, stop, warme, drie, and mundifie, and defendeth from putrifaction, and is put into suppositors and Clisters to clense, with Hony and vineger, with Orgā, and Hisop, it maketh a good medicen against stingyng or bityng of Dogges, Snakes, Adders, &c. Salt vineger and Suger sodden together, maketh a good wholsome drinke against the drinking of *Opium* or eatyng of the Moisron called *Fungus*. Salte is good against the vlcers of the mouth, to burue salt, & make it white, wash it ones in water, poore foorth the water, and gather the Salte in the bottom, and put into a stone vessell couered, and put into the Ouen, & couer it with coales, and drie it, and so it may be vsed in medicen. *Oribasius* affirmeth salte to be compounded of matter Abstersiue and stiptike, which is matter bindyng and driyng moyste humers: but salte is not good for leane persons, it will make them seme olde, and moueth anger to the Cholorike. Much salt is made in England, as of Sand and Salte water in pittes, in Hollande, in Lincolneshere, and onely by a maruelous humer of water, at the Witch, far from the sea, and in the North there is salt made, at the Shiles by Tinmouth castle, I Bullein the author hereof, haue a pan of salte vpon the same water. At Blith in Northumberland is good salte made, and also at sir Jhon Delauals Panes, which syr Jhon Delauall knight hath been a patron of worship, and hospitalite, most like a famous gētilmā, during many yeres: and powdreth no man by the salt, of extorciō, or oppressing his neighbour, but liberally spendeth, his Salte, Wheat, and his Maulte, like a gentilman: J neede not put his name in remēbraunce, in my booke for it shal liue by immortall good fame, when my poore booke shal be rotten, deare brother *Marcellus*.

Therebe also sondrie kindes of Salte, among which there is a salt flowing about the brinkes of that famous Riuer Nilus called *Flos salis*, the flower of salte, of a Saffron couller, of tast and sauour vnplesant whiche *Flos salis* is put into sondrie oyntmentes to heale soores aboute the priuie partes, or other places of the skin. In colliris it is tolerable for to clense sore eyen. And tēpered with *Vnguentum Rosarum*, or other ointmentes, it moueth sweat to all the body, well rubbed with the same.

Sal gemma, is a Salt of the earth, plentie is digged therof in *Calabria* in a place called *Altomonte*, and is cut foorthe like stones moste cleare *Translucens*, or through shinyng like to Christall, which if this salt be cast into the fier, it will not cracke nor breake, but kepe still whole, burnynge like Jron. *Plini* maketh large mencion of Salte, *lib.21.cap.7.* saiyng that Salt is either growyng naturall in the yearth, or in vaines of hilles, &c. or els made of Salte water sodden in Pannes, vnto a thicknesse: where of white common Salt is made.

Salt *Armoniac* whiche is hot and drie in the fourth degree, saith the *Pandact*, saiyng it cometh from *Armoniac*, and is made of Camels vrine, but it is called of the best writers *Sal Ammoniacus*, that is founde vnder the sands

in

The booke of Simples. Fol.lxxvj.

in Aphrike nere vnto the the Oracle of the God Ammon, and also in the region called *Cyrenaica*, which salt is blacke without & white within like Alum, but not very bright, noisome to the mouth, but holsome in medicen, to clense the skinne, mingled with Campher and Rosewater tempered together and made warme: Many and sondry Losyons for Apostimacions and soores, be made with these saltes, and they muste be mingled with other simples. — *Sal amoniac doe clense the skinne.*

Sal Indus groweth in Inde, through the heate of sunne, vpon Reedes, whiche salt is much lyke Suger. With Suger and common salte, the Apothicaries do sophisticat and craftely counterfet this salt. — *Salt of Inde.*

Sal Nitrum, or saltepeter, is digged in vaultes, flowers of houses, or walles, whiche salte is white, whan this is prepared, therof with other resettes, as Cooles, Brimstone &c. is Gunpouder made, whiche doeth shote of Gunnes, whiche are the instrumentes of Gods wrath. And *Spuma nitri*, is called *Barach* of the *Arabians* of these saltes Rede *Dioscorides. lib 5, cap. 86. Galen lib xi. simplicium medicamentorū*: further saith *Galen* in the same boke, there is salte made of the water of *Mari mortuum*, the ded sea, wheras Sodome and Gomor was, called *Asphaltum*. — *Sal Niter or Peter, for Gun pouder.* *Spuma nitri or Barach.* *Salt of Mari Mortuum wheras Sodome was.* *Asphaltum*

Salt of the yearth is grosser, and more colder adstring, then the salt of salt water: but there is a salt called salte vpon salte, whiche is very good to the vse of manne, so is Baie salt, whiche through the Marche winde is so made and finished, which will continue for euer like stone, beyng kept close: but yet Salt peter will growe therein at length, and thus I ende of salt, whiche the Arabians call *Melba*.

Marcellus.

I Haue seen sondrie saltes, for before this time: as white salt and Baie, whiche we doe vse to pouder fleshe, and fishe withall. I would your salt Peter had neuer been knowen, whereby Gunnes dooe so muche mischief, and the noble state of mankinde, through them are decaied, yea through a very bile coward or boie, often the baliaunt man is slaine and caste awaie. But *Hillarius*, I will a little more procede in simples, and leaue Gunning matters, to the man of warre or seruitors to the noble princes: now I praie you what is the nature of *Spuma maris*, and *Fumus terre*. — *Baie Salte.* *Boies cā kill the strongest menne with Gunnes.*

Hillarius.

These are twoo cleane contrary simples, of twoo sondry natures, the one of the lande called *Fumaria*, an herbe ingendred of the Fume or vaupur of the earth, *Dioscorides lib 4 Cap. cv.* in forme much like Coriander & couller like ashes, purple flowers, bitter of tast, the iuce will make cleane sore iyen, and this herbe dronke, the decoction thereof will purge choler by vrine. *Fumus terre*, or *Fumaria*, is good against the stopyng of the Splene, Liuer, Gaule, or Raines, and doth make stronge ye ventricles, through the drinesse, warmnesse, sharpenesse and bitternes sodden in wine, stilled, or in syrup, and so dronke. And so I do ende of — *Spumamaris Fumus terre.* *Against stoppyng of the Splene, Fumitorie dooe preuaile.*

n.iiii. this

The booke of Simples.

Spuma maris dooe make clene ỹ teeth.

this *Fumus* called *Capnos*, but as for *Spuma maris*, the fome of the sea, it hath vertue to clense, scower, and drie, and is cold and drie in the thirde degree, it is good to rubbe the teeth, to clense them, and the fine pouder therof with the white of an Egge, Rose water and Sief beaten together, put into the eye, doth clense them, and taketh away the webbe:

To clense sore eien.

And thus I do ende of *Spuma maris*, or the stone which the scriueners doo rub, and make cleane their parchement withall. what haue you els to say?

Marcellus.

What say you of *Spongia*, the sea Sponge.

Hillarius.

Sponge of the sea.

GALEN *lib. xj. simplic medic.* saith that they did use sponges to be a manuell instrument to receiue bloud, wherwith they used to wipe and drie up bloud in woūdes: and also they do receiue thinges to stoppe bloud. A sponge is hotte in the first degree, and drie in the second, it is of a resoluing vertue. A sponge adust, or burnt not muche, the pouder therof will consume flesh, whiche is superfluous, and may be put in woundes of the head. With a sponge whiche is softe, Tentes for the head may be made. With sponges sodden in wine, and oyle of Capers it is good to washe and chafe the left side, nothing is better to anoint the stomacke for a Pleurasie, then with a sponge in warme Oyles, as of Mintes Chamamel, Roses, the greace of Hens, Capons & Duckes. New sponges are holsome of them selues, will heale woundes, without any thing put to them. Olde sponges be euil. Pitche & the Asshes of sponges together, will stoppe bloud. A sponge sodden in Hony, will heale and resolue woundes, and harde Apostimacions, Reade more therof *Dioscorides, lib. v. cap. xcvi.* and of *Aristotle* of the nature of spōges, which grow among the rockes of the sea, and hath stones in them, beaten in pouder and dronke, will breake the stone in the bladder.

Spong good for woundes.

Sponges newe ar good but old are euill.

Sponge stones do breake the stone.

Marcellus.

What say you of Currall?

Hillarius.

Corall grow in the sea.

The Indians hath Coral in no lesse estimacion, then we haue their Diamondes and great Perles. *Diosco lib. 5. cap. 97.* calleth Corall *Lethrodendron*, whiche is a braunche growing in the bottome of the sea. which by certain meanes is drawen foorth, and soone turned into hardnesse, and eftsones into a stone: we do se of this Coral greate plentie of beades, more vain glorious, then religious godly. Of Corall be twoo kindes, the red whiche is beste, and the white, whiche of nature be colde and drie in the second degree, and be restrictiue and stoppyng. Corall beaten in pouder, mingled with Dragons bloud, whites of egges, *Bole armeni* and the iuce of Sheperdes purce, Knot grasse, and Rabbettes

Coral of two kindes.

To stoppe bloud.

The booke of Simples. Fol.lxxvij.

bettes woll beaten in a Lead morter will stop bloud. The pouder of Corall dronke with wine, prouoketh vrine, and will rebate the swellyng of the Spleane, and finally as *Auicen* saith, doth comforte the hart and helpeth digestion. The pouder of Corall will clense woundes, in whom flesh superfluous doth remaine, and also heale the same. what is better to stop a blouddy flir, called *Dysenteria*, it stoppeth bothe the flir of men, running from them in their sleape. And also the whites from women. Reade more in *Matthiolus* vpon *Dioscorides, lib 5.*

<small>Corall prouoketh vrine.</small>

Marcellus.

What say you of Pearle called the Margarit?

Hillarius.

The Pearle is not only riche and pleasant to beholde, but also holsome and good in medicen. *Plini. lib 9. cap. 35.* saith that there be plentie of Pearles in *Arabia*, in the mouthe of the Red sea, growyng within their shelles, called the mother of Pearle, in whiche they are conceiued, the vnion which is cleane, bright, white, rounde, and heauy, is the richest. The pouder of Pearle is good to be put in cordial as *Manus Christi*, and the same pouder with the white of an Egge, will clense ye eye. Aboute this Realme many Pearles be gathered in Mustels, and other shell fish, but not the most orient.

<small>The Margarit or Perle, good in Cordials.</small>

Marcellus.

Is there any vertue in *Lapide lasule?*

Hillarius.

There is nothing better to purge Melancholy. There be Pilles called *Pilule de Lapide Lazule*, against olde Quartens, or Madnesse, this stone is colde and moyst.

<small>Lapis lazule</small>

Marcellus.

What say you of *Saphyrus?*

Hillarius.

DIOSCORIDES affirmeth this heauely coloured precious stone is wholsome to be dronke against the sting of Serpentes, to resist the poyson: and being dronke it helpeth all exulceracion of the gutties, and also is holsome for sore eyen, to cleare the sight. Many goodly vertues belonging to the Sapher, as chastitie &c. Yet it is not cold inough for the quenching of venus. They say the Turkis will kepe a man frõ fallyng, but it is a lie. The riche Hemerald, some sayth, will declare whan the knot of Mariage is vndone, then it will seperate & breake a sonder, and that were a perilous case to lose a good iewel for an euell wife, with many such folish olde fables gathered out of some writers which hath rather vnwittily reported, then truly proued the nature of stones so farre passing their natures, although they bee of great

<small>Saphyrus resist poyson.</small>

<small>Fables gathered.</small>

The booke of Simples.

great vertue, and both pleasant and profitable to mankinde, and nothing vnder heauen more riche or costly.

Marcellus.

If the Emeraldes wolde so quickly breake or cracke whan suche partes be plaied I assure you there would be great losse in costly iewels and some seperaciō of freendship, but they be of much vertue and patiens when such offenses be committed: that they will tell no tales by breaking them selues, well let this matter passe, it is but to feare folkes withal, and I pray you what say you of *Lapis Naxius* and the *Iasper*.

Hillarius.

Lapis naxinus, helpeth to increase heere.

Iasper doeth comfort digestion.

The pouder therof with Beares greace will increace heare and kepe one from baldnesse. This stone will make small a maidēs breastes, & defend them frō growing: if the pouder therof with Vineger be dronke, it wil consume the greatnesse of the Splean. And this stone is good against the Fallyng sicknesse. The Iasper is holsom to be hanged about the necke, downe to the mouthe of the stomacke, for it is comfortable to the same saith *Galen, lib.ix.simplic.medicamentorum.*

Marcellus.

What then of *Lapis Tucia*, and *Lincis*?

Hillarius.

Lapis Tutia and lapis Lincis.

It is vsed in many vlcers, and foole stinkyng Cankers, for through the coldenesse and drinesse, it clense and incarnat foule soores: and this *Tucia* is most excellent, if it be prepared, to be put into Colíries to clense the eyne. What is better with Planten water to clése the yarde. *Lapis Lincis*, is hot and drie, ingendred of the brin of Lynx, and is good in pouder. Э.iii. to be dronke attons, or put into *Cassia fistula*. ʒ.i. to consume the stone, and clense the Raynes.

Marcellus.

What say you of the stone called *Byzahar*?

Hillarius.

Bizabar a precious stone against poyson.

The *Arabians* doth call it *Bizahar*, whiche stone is precious, & resisteth poison, & is put into precious *Antidotaris* which preuaileth against al foule ayre, pestilence & benim. This stone is yellow without oder or smell: if it be hanged vpon the left arme, touching the flesh, it wil preuaile against the foresaied euils, looke *Matthiolus lib.5.Diosco.cap.73.*

Marcellus.

What then of *Lapis Phrygius*?

Hillarius.

Lapis frugiꝰ for sore eyne.

GALEN *lib.ix.simplic.medic.* with this stone *Conbust* saith he, iuce to help or clense stinking vlcers, and it hath the same vertue that *Lapis Pyrites* hath. And of this stone, medicens be made for sore eyen, mingled

The booke of Simples. Fol.lxxviij.

mingled with Coliries accordingly. And this stone called *Pyrites* loketh like Brasse, and wrapped in Hony, then put it in a small earthen pot such as Goldesmithes doth vse, and set it in the fiar blowyng vntill it be Red so coule it: and this stone in pouder will clense scower, and consume flesh superfluous. — *Pirites lape against proud flesh.*

Marcellus.
What say you of the *Hæmatist?*

Hillarius.

It is colde and bindinge of nature. *Alixander Tralianus* saith, I haue often times without any *Thyriaca* or any precious medicen, hath cured many, namely by ye *Hæmatist* stone, for then ye had the blouddy flix: and with the pouder of this stone, the iuces of Pomgranets, and knot grasse, mingled together, of this. ℈.iiii. was his dose in this iuce for the flix. — *Alixander Tralianus vpō the Hematist for the flix.*

Marcellus.
What say you of Iette?

Hillarius.

Therof is great plentie in England and Irelande, and at Whitbe in the North: it hath vertue beyng dronke to clense the bladder, and burnte, the smoke doeth helpe theim whiche swelleth and are in perill with the mother. — *Ieta for the Mother.*

Marcellus.
What say you of *Lapis magnis?*

Hillarius.

The best is that which will draw Iron or Steel to him: geue three halfe peny weight in pouder tempered with swet water, it will cast foorth filth and groose matter out of the bodie. *Plini* sheweth, *lib.xxxiiii. Cap.xiiij.* that one builded a Temple, couered with this *Magnus* stone, wherein his ymage with pompe was brought in, which was made of Iron, whiche assended by attraccion, and did hang in the roffe, his name was *Arsion.* The *Arabians* and *Mahmetans* did in like case bring in the steel Toumbe of maister Mahumet (their iugling false Prophet) into a Teple of Magnit stones, whose nature was to draw the saied Toumbe vp. But the best seruis that the *Magnis* doth, is in the Shippe, for the Compasse of salyng in true settyng the needle. Also in plasters the pouder thereof, to drawe foorth the Iron or pricke, from the fleshe. — *The magnit stone.*

Marcellus.
What is the vertue of the flesh of Oxen, Steeres or Bulles, and Calues?

Hillarius.

I will not vndertake to show mine opinion at your request only, but I wil also declare the mindes of some wise and learned men: and first of *Simeon Sethi*, which saith that the flesh of Oxen, that be yonge — *Of the flesh of Oxen, steres, Bulles, and Calues.*

The booke of Simples.

Beefe good for the cholorike, but euill for tender stomackes.

yong doth much norish and make them strong, that be fed with Beefe: but it bredeth choler adust, and melancholious diseases, it is cold and drie of nature, and hard to digest, except it be eaten of chollericke persons, but being tenderly sodden, it norisheth muche: Beefe customably eaten of idell persons, and nice folke that laboureth not, bringeth many diseases, as *Rasis* saith, and *Auicen* saith, that the flesh of Oxen, or Kine, be very grose, ingendring ill iuce in the body, wherof oftentime commeth scabbes, Cakers, and Biles, but vnto hot strong chollerike stomackes, it is tollerable, and may be vsed as wee haue the dayly experience therof.

Beefe brothe, againste the flixe.

The brothe wherin the Beefe hath ben sodde, is good to be supped or dronke halfe a pinte euery morning against the flix of the belly, and runnyng foorth of yellow choller, if the saied brothe be tempered with Salt, Mustarde, Vinegar, or Garlike, commonly vsed for the saied sauces to digest Beefe with all, for the said sauces doe not only helpe digestion, but also defendeth the body from sondrie inconueniences, and diuers sicknesses, as Dropsies, Quartens, Leprosies, and such like.

Oxe Gaule clense the eyes.

The Gaule of an Oxe, or a Cowe, distilled in the month of June, and kept in a close glasse, doeth helpe to clense the eyes from spottes, if you put a drop of this water with a feather into the eyes when ye go to bedde:

Oxe Milte stop the flixe.

the Melte of a Bull dried, and the pouder therof dronke with Red wine, wil stoppe the bloudy flixe, light poudred yong Beefe is better, thē either fresh or much poudred, in specially of those cattell that be fed in faire and drie pastures, & not in stinking Fennes

Gesnerᵒ writeth moche of braftes, the male better then the female.

the great learned man *Gesnerus* in his discription of beastes, doth write more of the vertues of Bulles, Oxen, Kine, and Calues, thē any other hath done: and thus to conclude, the flesh of the Male beastes, is more better then the female, and the gelded beastes, be more commodious to nature then any of them, and the yonge flesh, more commendable then the olde, for it is moister, and a frende to the bloud. *Haliabas* saieth, rosted flesh doth greatly norish the body, for it is warme and moist, baken meates be very drie, cleane boiled meates with holsome herbes, & frutes, be exellent in vertue to cōforte the bodie, if thei be nutrimentall flesh.

Calues flesh the profite thereof.

Calues flesh doeth greatly increace, norish, and make good bloud. Specially the brawne or Muskels of the thigh, is best, saieth Maister *Conrade Gesner*, and further saieth he, if a man be wounded, then lay Calues flesh newly slaine to it, & this will defende the wound frō apostumacion or swellyng: and sodden in vineger, and warme applied to any part, as armeholes, breast of them that stinke like a Rāme or Goate, it will take awaie the saied stinke:

Against Rammishenes vnder ȳ armes.

also helpeth the biting of a man or a madde Dogge, so that this fleshe remianeth vpon the said wound, during fiue daies, and .v. nightes close, and not taken awaie.

Celsus for a vomitte.

Celsus in his medicens against the biting of Serpentes, if nothing cā sucke it foorth by medicen or boxing saith he, then drinke the broathe wherein Geese or Veale hath ben sodden, and then prouoke vomit. Great is the goodnesse of this flesh, both in meate and medicen: Take the knuckel or sinew parte of a Calfe, seeth it in white Wine & water,

put-

puttyng in Dates, Prunes, Reisynges of the Sunne, grated breade, Maces, Cloues, Fenell rootes, Liuerworte, Planten, Purslen, freshe Capers, Borage, and Rosemarie flowers, sodden all together in a siluer, iron, or stone pot, close boiled, that no aire can go forthe. You maie put in halfe a Cocke: this fleshe and brothe giue health to theim, that are in consumpcion, weake bodies, or them, whiche be euill complexioned, or colde of nature, ouercome by Melancholi. &c.

Marcelles.

What is the goodnes of Porke, or of gelded swine, Pigges, and Bores fleshe. &c.

Hillarius.

Most of thauncient, and wisest Phisicians, that euer wer in this worlde, did consent, that of all fleshe, the fleshe of yong gelded swine, partly salted or poudered: was euer meate of the best nourishing, moister, and colder then other fleshe. For *Isaac* saith, it is a fleshe moste moist, except it be the fleshe of Lambes, as *Galen* reporteth: yet it is not good to euery complexion, nor to euery age, but vnto youth and middle age. And whereas almightie God, did prohibite the Jewes, to eate swines fleshe: it was a figure to abstain frō vncleane thinges, whiche I leaue to the deuines. The Mahumites abhorre swines flesh, because their dronken false Prophete, and *Pseudo* Apostle was torne, and rent in peces with hogges: beyng dronken, and fallen into the mire, and now we must giue credence to tyme, and to learned Phisicions. The blood of swine doeth nourishe moche, as it is seen in Puddinges, made with greate Otemeale, Peper, swete suet, and Fenell, or Aniseedes. Young Pigges be verie moiste, therefore Sage, Peper and salt, do drie vp the superfluous humors of thē, when thei be rosted. Thei be not wholsom to be eaten, before thei be three weekes old: the Tripes and Guttes be wholsomer, and doeth nourishe better, then any other beastes guttes. Bacon is very hard of digestion, and moche discommēded of some men and is hurtfull onely, vnto a hotte Cholerike labouryng bodie: but a tēder gammon of Bacon is tolerable, and very good fleshe with wine, as custome doe proue it.

Agatharsides saieth, that the swine in *Æthiopia*, hath hornes growyng vpon their heddes, there bee diuers kindes of swine, bothe wilde, and tame: whose inwarde partes, be not moche vnlike vnto mankind, and for that cause, *Galen* began to make *Anatomies* of theim, in the beginnyng of his practise, teaching the *Chyrurgians* to doe the like. These kind of beastes, doe heare verie easely, and bee giuen moche to slepe, and will eate their owne Pigges, and feede vpō moste vile thinges, for whiche cause thei haue moste vile diseases, as *Anginæ* in the throate, sores, botches, and biles. If thei bee letten blood, in the veine vnder the tongue, and giue theim Madder, and an herbe called Pancis, otherwise named in Latine *herba Trinitatis*, it helpeth theim, if it bee sodden in Whey. Those

Margin notes: Porke the commendacion thereof. Swines blood. Pigges. Tripes. Bacon. Swine of Inde haue hornes. Why hogges are diseased.

The booke of Simples.

swine that vse to feede by the sea side, and eateth of yong Crabbes, be deliuered of many diseases, if thei doe feede vpon *Polipodi*, thei shalbe deliuered of the Pestilence. Emong the christen men, Bores fleshe is had in greate estimacion, to bee eaten in winter: and chiefly vpon Christmas daie. *Galen* doeth greatly commende thesame fleshe, or braune, to be eaten in winter: and also this Bores fleshe is proued in the tyme of Pestilence, to breake a plague sore. Bores greace, and his stones, or any parte of theim, stamped together, and warme applied to thesame sore, woorketh this effecte. And thus I dooe ende of swine, whiche in their liues be moste vile, noisome, and neuer good vntill thei die.

Marcellus.
What is the vertues of Lambes, and Weathers fleshe?
Hillarius.

Lābes fleshe

Simeon Sethi saith, Lambes fleshe is partly warme, but superfluous moiste, and euill for flegmatike persones, & doeth moche harme, to them that haue the Dropsie, boneach, or a disease called *Epialus*, whiche is spittyng of flegme, shinyng like glasse.

Lābes fleshe good rosted, euill sodden.

Therefore, if Lambes fleshe were sodden, as it is rosted, it would bring many diseases vnto the bodies of theim, without it were sodden in wine, and some hotte Grosseries, herbes, or rootes. When a Weather is twoo yere olde, whiche is fedde vpon a good ground: the fleshe therof shall bee temperate, and nourisheth moche. *Hyppocrates* saieth, that the Lambe of a yere old, doeth nourishe moche. *Galen* semeth not greatly to commende Mutton, but that whiche is tender, swete, and not olde, is verie profitable, as experience and custome, doe daiely teache vs: The doung, Tallowe, and Wolle, bee verie profitable in medicenes, as *Plini* saieth, and *Conradus Gesnerus, de animalibus*, and *Galen* in his third booke *de Alementis*.

Mutton.

Marcellus.
What be the vertues of Goates, or Kiddes fleshe?
Hillarius.

Kiddes flesh verie good.

These be beastes verie hurtfull, vnto yong trees and plātes, but *Simeon Sethi* saieth, that Kiddes fleshe is easie of digestion, in health and sicknesse, thei be very good meate thei be verie drie of nature. *Hyppocrates* saieth, it behoueth that the conseruers and kepers of health, should studie,

Fleshe good for sicke persones.

that his meate be soche, as the flesh of Kiddes, yong calues, that be sucking, and lābes of one yere olde, for thei be good for thē that be sicke, or haue euill complexions. *Haliabas* saith, that the fleshe of Kiddes, doeth engender good blood, and is not so flegmatike, waterie, and moiste, as the fleshe of Lambes, thei remain Kiddes for sixe monethes, and afterward cometh into grosser, and hotter nature, & then be called Gotes: the fleshe of thē that be gelded, are wholsome to eate. The lunges of them eaten, before a man doeth drinke, doeth defende him ȳ daie from dronkenes, as I haue heard, by the reportes of learned men:

Gotes fleshe. but the fleshe of olde male Goates be euill, and engendereth Agues, or Feuers,

The booke of Simples.   Fol.lxxx.

feuers. If the vrine of Goates be distilled in May, with Sorell, the water distilled is not hurtfull, nor noysome, but whosoeuer vseth to drinke therof. z.ii. mornynge and euenyng, it will preserue him from the Pestilence. The Milke of Goates I wil describe in ye proper place. *Conradus Gesnerus, de animalibus. Mathiolus super Disco.*

Marcellus.
What is the vertue of Redde and fallow Deare?

Hillarius.

Thei ar more pleasant to some, then profitable to many, as appereth once a yere in the corne feldes, the more it is to be lamented. *Hipocrates & Simeon Sethi*, doth playnly affirme the flesh of them doth engender euill iuce, and Melancholie, cold diseases, and Quartens, the fleshe of winter Deare, doeth lesse hurte the body, then that whiche is eaten in sommer, for in winter mans digestion is more stronger, and the inwarde partes of the body warmer, and maye easelier consume grosse meates, then in sommer, as we se by experience, in cold weather & frostes, healthfull people be most hongrest. The lunges of a Deare sodden in Barly water, and stamped with *Penedice*, and Hony, of equall quantitie, to the saied lunges, and eaten amorninges, doeth greatly helpe the olde coughes, & drinesse in the Lunges, therbe many goodly vertues of their hornes, bones, bloud, and tallow. Looke *Conradus Gesnerus de animalibus.*

Dere red and fallowe, bee spoilers of corne.

The winter Dere, better then the sommer.

The lunges of the Dere.

Marcellus.
What is the vertue of Hares and Conies?

Hillarius.

AVICEN saieth, the fleshe of Hares, is hot and drie, an engenderer of Melancholy, not praised in Phisicke for meate, but rather for medicen: for in deede if a Hare bee dried in the monthe of Marche, in an Ouen or Furnice and beaten into pouder, and kept close, and droke amorninges in Beare, Ale, or white wine, it will breake the stone in the bladder, if the pacient be not old: if childrens gummes be anoynted with the braines of an Harte, their teeth will easely come, and growe. The gaule of an Hare mingled with cleane Honie, doeth clense watery iyes, or redde bloudy iyes. The flesh of Hares must be tenderly rosted, and wel larded, and spiced, because of the grosenesse, but it is better sodden. The fleshe of Conies, are better then Hares flesshe, and easier of digestion, but Rabets be holsome, for meate of sicke people: and thus to conclude of Conies, experience teacheth vs, that thei are good, thei be colde and drie of nature, and small mension is made of them emong the auncient Phisicions, as *Galen* saieth, I nede not to speake very long of euery kinde of beastes, as some of the beastes that be *Hiberia*, like little Hares, whiche be called Conies.

Of Hares fleshe and Conies.

The pouder of the Hare, for the stone.

Galeni de simp.medica:

Marcellus.

The booke of Simples.

What is the nature of a beast called *Erinaceus*, called the Porpintine and *Echinus* called the Hedghog, which be ful of prickes?

Hillarius.

Erinaceus, or Porpintin for baldnesse, to increase heare.

DIOSCORIDES *lib.2.cap.2.* saith, the skinnes of them combust or burnt, and beaten in fine pouder, and tempered with Terre, is a good oyntment for to increace heare, and kepe of baldnesse. The dried flesh of them sodden in Winiger and Suger, is good to be dronke against the stopping of the raynes, couulsions, Leproses, of flegme or an euill complexion. The pouder of this Purpentine must be kept close in a vessell for medicen. The pouder of the Hare whiche is dried in Marche, must be vsed for the purging of the Raines, & clensynge of the bladder, the saied pouder is to be dronke with white wine, and *Casciafistula*. Also the greace of the Porpintine, or Hedghogge, with Beares greace and *Laudanum*, anna. ʒ.i. beaten in a Leaden morter, this is a good oyntment against baldnesse or losse of heere, to rubbe ye place daily therwith. The Liuers of Purpentines dried & beaten into pouder are good for the Raines or *Morbus Elephanticus*. These beastes be of cold nature, better for medicē then meate, and be vermen or beastes of the night, armed against Dogges, with longe prickes, and hedded much like a Hare, with teeth accordyng, and eares like an Ape. &c. The Urchin or Hedghogge is commonly knowen, and headded like a Swine or yonge Pigge. The pouder of them as *Plini* affirmeth, beyng dronke will helpe and defende consumption, and thus I do ende of this beast called *Echinus*, which the *Arabians* cal *Caufed*. The Urchin of the Sea is good for the belly, stomacke and vrin. *Dioscorides lib.2.cap.j.*

Hares pouder for the Raines.

The Urchin or Hedhog.

Marcellus.

What say you of the Fiber, Beuer or Castor?

Hillarius.

Castor or Beuer.

This Castor liueth by water and lande, he loueth to feede vpon Crabbes and Cankers of the Sea. The stones of a Castor is a warme medicen, and preuayleth against poyson, to be dronke, or in oyntment. And the pouder of the same stones be good to moue starnutacion or nesyng, blowen into the noose. Of the pouder. ʒ.ii. w Penyroyall, called Pulial. ʒ.ii.ſ. tempered together in wine & dronke wil cause a womā in her trauel, sone to be deliuered & the secondes to folow, and finally to clēse the body, and helpeth swellinges, collickes Iliaces, sighinges, Cordiaces, Lytharges and poyson dronke with Wineger, and in fine it is so warme, that it helpeth all the passions or sickenesses in the brest, belly, liuer, and sinewes, commyng of colde: the Beuer stones be best, that be most graue and strong of sauour, & hath a liquor much like Cerose within the codde, and couered with a naturall coueryng. *Plini.xxxj cap.iij.* Castor is good to helpe the Comitiall or fallyng sicknesse, to be dronke. The oyle of them be also good for the teeth

Castor stones do help al colde infirmites both in men and women.

The booke of Simples. Fol.lxxxj.

teeth, raynes, belly, brest, and to be dropped into the eares.

Marcellus.

What say you of the littel beast *Mustela*, called the Weesell or Wezell whiche is commonly knowen.

Hillarius.

This *Mustela* called the Weesell, is commonly knowen: and this Weesell, the flesh therof sodden in Wine, and dronke, is a preset remedie againſt all benim, poyson, and the fallyng sicknesse. With vineger, the greace of the Weesell sodden, is a goodly medicen to anoynte the goute with all. The bloud of Weesels is good to anoynte the neckes, throates, and stomackes of them, which haue *Struma* that is the swellyng of the throate, or the fallynge sicknesse, or Palsie. The donge of the Weesell with Hony, Fenigrece, and Lupins beaten together is good to anoynt warme ye throte, for ye sicknesse called *Struma*: the gaule of the Weesell tempered with the water of Fenill, is a presente remedie for the dimnesse of the eye, to be put therin: and al the spottes as Morphew of the skinne, is clensed therwith. The Lunges of the Weesell is good in pouder, to be dronke againſt all the infirmities of the Lunges, with many other vertues of the Weesell, and properties as to kill Mise and Rattes, to serue in the house like Cattes, but the sauour of the saied Weesell is mortiferous and deadly. *Plini lib. 8. cap. 22.*

The weesell good againſt the falinge sicknes and Struma. Ingine or swellyng of the throte.

For to heale ye Morphew.

Marcellus.

What say you of Raynard the Fox, and the Beare?

Hillarius.

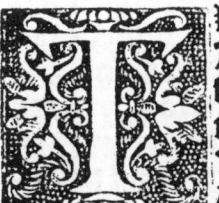
The Lunges of the Fox is good in medicen, for the sicke Lunges of mākinde. The greace of the Fox is also good for all Coldnesse, Palsey, and the contrarion of the sinewes, and trembling of the body. The Beare is a beast whose flesh is good for mankinde: his fat is good with *Laudanum*, to make anointment to heale balde headded mē to receiue the heere againe. The greace of the Beare, the fatte of a Lambe and the oyntmente of the Fox, maketh a good oyntment to anoint the feete againſt the paine of trauell or labour of footemen. All the partes of the Foxe, the Badgar, and the Beare are good in medicē, or meate againſt the Palsey, trembling or coldnesse of the flesh, or any of theim. There is a common fable emong the people, that is to saie a Beare hath a disformed whelpe in the time of deliueraunce, without members, whiche is not true, for the Beare in the birthe, hath all the members, as other beaſtes hath. Reade *Matthiolus* in *Dioscorides lib. iij. cap. supra.*

The Fox the Beare, the Badgarde.

To help baldnes.

Beare, Fox, and Brocke are good to helpe the Palsey.

Marcellus.

What is the vertue of a birde, called the Ospraie?

Hillarius.

O.iij. The

The booke of Simples.

Halæetus the Ospray, a water Egle.

Like as the Egle, and all kindes of Haukes, dooe praie and fede vpon the fleshe of birdes: euen so God haue ordained the water Egle, called *Halæetus* the Osprale, to feare the Fishes, and fede vpon them. And all Haukes, or birdes of the nature of Egles, with harde croked billes, are compted vncleane fleshe. *Leui.xi.* are not vsed cōmon emong vs, vnto this daie. Howbeeit, the Oile or grease of the Ospraie, is had in greate estimacion, to take fishe with all: and the hedde thereof dried and beaten into pouder, maketh a good medicene for young infant children, to bee put into the nosthrilles, to breake winde verie gentle. And the Gaule is wholsome for sore iyen, to bee dropped with the white of an Egge into theim: And the grease and Gaule, will heale the stingyng and bityng of serpentes, and also is good to be dropped into the eare to clense them, and helpe hearyng. Rede *Gesneras lib.iij.de Auibus.*

Ospraies oile good to put in water to gather fishe redy to be taken.

Medicens made of the Ospray.

Marcellus.

what say you of Iuery.

Hillarius.

Iuery.

A drinke for the Iaūders

It is good to astring or binde & to race it with: *Turnerace* & Saffrō puttyng in *Diacurcuma in Tabulis,* sodden in ẏ water of Endiue, wher with many people are helped of a perilous hot and dry sicknes called *Regius morbus,* or the yellow Iaunders.

Marcellus.

what is the vertue of Chickens and Hennes?

Hillarius.

Of House Cockes, Capons and Chickens. Their flesh much cōmended.

All foules, whiche haue harde pennes, be strong of nature, as Chekens or Hennes, saieth *Auenzoer,* whiche bee moste commended, and laudable of any other fleshe, and nourisheth good blood, & are light of digestion, & doeth also comfort the appetite. Cocke chickens be better then Hennes, the Capon is better then the Cocke, thei do augment good blood and seede, as *Rasis* reporteth, and experience proueth in men, bothe whole and sicke. An olde Cocke whiche is well beaten, after his feathers be pulled of, vntill he be all blouddy, and then cutte of his hedde, and drawe hym, and seeth hym in a close potte with faire water, and white wine, Fenell rootes, Burrage rootes, violettes, Planten, Suckerie, and Buglosse leaues, Dates, Prunes, greate Reisons, Maces, and Sugar, and put in the Marie of a Calfe, and Saunders, this is a verie good brothe, to theim that bee sicke, weake, or consumed: the braines of Hennes, Capons, or Chickens, be wholsome to eate, to comfort the brain and memorie: and will cause young childrens teethe to growe quickly. And thus to conclude, these foresated fowles bee better for idell folkes, that labour not, then for theim that vse exercise, or trauell, to whom grose meates ar more profitable. The Cocke is the best clocke, to kepe the tyme. *Gesneras lib.iij.de Auibus.*

A good broth for a body which hath bene longe sicke.

Marcellus.

The booke of Simples. Fol.lxxxij.

Marcellus.
What is the vertue of Geese?
Hillarius.

The fleshe of wilde Geese and tame, are very grose and harde of digestion, as *Auicen* saieth: the fleshe of greate fowles, as of Geese be slowe and harde of digestion, for their humidite, theidoe brede feuers quickly, but their Goselinges, or yong ones, beyng fat, are good, and muche commended in meates, and *Galen* saieth, of the fleshe of Beastes, and Birdes. But vndoubtedly, Geese, Mallardes, Pecockes, Swannes, and euery foule hauyng a longe necke, be all harde of digestion, and of no good complexions: but if these be well roosted, and stuffed with Salt, Sage, Peper, and Onions, thei will not hurt the eaters of them. There be greate Geese in Scotland, whiche bredeth vpon a place called the Basse, there be also Bernacles, whiche hath a straunge generacion, as *Gesnerus* saith, whiche neuer laie Egges, as the people of the North partes of Scotlande knoweth, and because it should seme incredible to many, I will geue none occasion to any, either to mocke, or to maruell, & thus I geue warning to them whiche loue their healthe, to haue these foresaied fowles, somwhat poudered, or stopped with Salte, all the night before thei be roosted.

Of Geese & Goslinges.

Goose flesh bredeth Melancholie.

The Barnakle of Scotlande, neuer lay Egges, but are bred only of the Ocean Sea, reade Gesnerus de auibus, lib. 3.

Marcellus.
What is the vertue of Cranes fleshe?
Hillarius.

Simeon Sethi saith, their fleshe are hotte and drie, the yonger be good but the old encrease Melancholy, thei doe engender seede of generation, and beyng tenderly rosted, dooeth helpe to cleare the voice, and clense the pipe of the Lunges. Cranes be birdes of a wounderfull prouidence, *Gesnerus de Auibus.*

Cranes, are hot, and encrease seede.

Marcellus.
What is the vertue of Duckes flesh?
Hillarius.

Hey be the hottest of all domesticall or yarde fowles, and vncleane of feeding: notwithstandyng though thei be harde of digestion, and maruelous hote, yet thei will norish the body, and maketh it fatte. *Hipocrates* saieth, that thei that be fedde in puddels, and foule places, be hurtefull, but thei that be fedde in Houses, Pennes, or Coopes, are nutriue, but verie grose, as *Isaacke* affirmeth. There are sondrie kindes of Duckes. *Gesnerus de Auibus.*

Duckes are very hotte of nature and Melancholi.

Marcellus.
What is the vertue of Pigeons, Turtles, or Doues?
Hillarius.

The fleshe of Turtles be meruelous good, and equall to the beste birdes: and *Auicen* saieth, thei bee beste when thei bee young, and wholsome for flegmatike people. *Simeon Sethi* affirmeth, the house

Doues are very hot.

O.iiii. Doue

The booke of Simples.

Of Doues

Doue is hotter then the fielde Doue, and doeth engender grose bloud the common eatyng of them bee euill for cholorike persones, with red faces, for feare of Leprosie, therfore cutte of the feete, winges, and hed of your Pigions or Doues, for their bloud is that, whiche is so venemous through heate, thei bee beste in the Spring time, and Harueste, and *Isaack* saieth, because thei are so lightly conuerted into choller, thei did commaunde in the olde time, that thei should be eaten with sharpe

Doues flesh must be eaten with Uineger.

Uineger, Purselen, Cucumbers, or Citron. Roosted Pigions be beste, the bloud that commeth out of the right winge, dropped in ones iye, will sone helpe the iye, if it swelleth, or pricketh: and thus muche haue I spoken of Pigeons, or Doues.

Marcellus.

What is the vertue of Pecockes?

Hillarius.

Pecocks flesh is hot & moyst in the first degree.
Gesnerus lib 3, de auibus.

THE Pecocke, his voice feareth Serpentes: *Aristotle de natura ani.* and is hotte and moiste, in the first degree, But *Simeon Sethi* saeith, it is a rawe fleshe, and harde of digestion, vnles it bee very fatte, but if it be fatte, it healpeth the Plurasie. *Haliabas* saith, that bothe Swannes, Craines, Pecockes, and any greate fowles, muste after thei bee killed, bee hanged vp by the neckes, twoo or three daies, with a stone waying at their feete, as the weather will serue, and then dressed and eaten, prouided that good wine be drunken after theim. Their Egges are noisome to be eaten, *Dioscorides.*

Marcellus.

What is the vertue of Swannes flesh?

Hillarius.

Swannes flesh, cholorik

Swans sing

EVery grose fowle is Chollerike, and harde of digestion: The Swanne is grose, therfore slowe of digestion. But the Signettes bee better then the olde Swannes, if their galentines bee well made, it helpeth to digest their fleshe. The Swanne is numbred emong the vncleane birdes, *Leuiticus. xi.* and will singe a litle before his death, *Plini Gesnerus de auibus.*

Marcellus.

What is the vertue of Hernes, Bittures, and Shouelers?

Hillarius.

Bitters. ... ...ars.
... meate ... ...plex̄o.

THese fowles be fishers, and be very rawe and flegmatike, like vnto the meate whereof thei are fedde, the young are beste, and ought to be eaten with Peper, Sinomon, Sugar, and Ginger and to drinke wine after them, for good digestion, and thus doe for all water fowles.

Marcellus.

What is the vertue of Partriches, Fesantes, Quales, Larkes, Sparowes, Plouers, and Blacke byrdes?

Hillarius.

Partiches

The booke of Simples. Fol.lxxxiii

PArtriches will binde the belly, and doeth noriṡhe muche, the Cockes be better then the Hēne birdes, thei do drie vp fleume and corruption in the stomacke. Fesantes be the best of al flesṡhe, for their sweetnesse is equal, vnto the Capon, or Partriche, but thei are somwhat drier: & *Rasis* saith, Fesantes flesṡhe is good for them that hath the feuer Ethicke, for it is not onely a meate, but a medicen, and doeth clense corrupte humours in the stomacke. Quales although thei be eaten of many, yet thei are not to be commended, for thei do engender Agues, & be euell for the Faulyng sicknesse, for as *Conciliator* saith: of all fowles ẏ be vsed for meates, a Quaile is the worst, *Dioscorides* saith, Larkes roosted be wholsome to be eaten of them that be troubled with the Collike. Blacke birdes taken in the time of Froste, be holsome, and good of digestion. The donge of Blackebirdes, tempered with vinegar, and applied to the place of any that hath the black Morphew, or blacke Leprosie, oftentimes anoynted with a Sponge doth helpe them. The flesh of Plouers, doth engender Melancholie. Sparowes be hotte and prouoketh Venus, or lust. *Plini* doeth describe their properties: the Braines be the best parte of them. Woodcockes be of good digestion, and temperate to feede vpon. All small birdes of the fielde, as Robin Redbrest, Linnets, Finches, Redde Sparrowes, Goldewinges, and such like: if they be fat, they be meruelous good, & do greatly comfort nature, either roosted, or boyled, and thus do I cōclude with thee of birdes: that the small field birdes are most holsom for sicke folkes, Rede *Gesnerus lib.j.de auibus.*

Partriges.
Fesantes
Quales.
Larkes help the cholicke, blacke birdes Plouers, Sparowes, wodcockes, small birdes.

Marcellus.

What is the vertue of Fisshes?

Hillarius.

IN many Ilandes of this worlde, placed nere vnto the Ocean seas, the people liue there most chiefly by Fisshe, and be right stronge and sounde people of complexion, as *Aristotel* saieth, *consuetudo est tanquam altera natura*, custome is like vnto another nature, but because I speake of fish, I will deuide thē in three partes. First of the Fisshes of the Sea. Secondly the fish, of the fresh running riuers. Thirdly of the Fisshes in Pooles, and standyng waters. The Sea hath many groose, and fatte fisshes, which be noysome to the stomacke, but the small kinde of Fisshes, ẏ feede aboute Rockes, and cleare stony places, be more drier, and lesse of moistnes thē the fresh water fish, and doth engender lesse flegme, and winde, by reson of their salte feedyng, as *Galen* saieth, they be the best fisshes, that feede in the pure sea, and chefest of all Fisshes, for the vse of mankind, & *Halias* saith, new fish lately taken, is colde & moiste, and flegmatike, thē the best of al next ẏ sea fish, is ẏ which swimeth in fresh cleare riuers or stonie places, where as the water is sweete, being fisshes that beare scales, be meruelous good, but if they feede neare vnto places where much filth is daily cast out, ther ẏ fisshes be very corrupt, & vnholsom

Thre things considered in fish.
Sea fish holsomer then ẏ of the fresh water.

as

The booke of Simples.

Muddy fishe not wholsom. as the saied *Haliabas* saith, Fish that feedeth in Fennes, Marshes, diches and muddy puddels, be very vnholsome, and doeth corrupt the bloud, they be groose and slimie, corrupt and windie: but those that be fed in faire pondes, wherunto running water may ensue, & where as swete water, herbes, rootes, and weedes, that growe about the bankes, doe feede the fish, those fisshes be holsome. *Galen* saieth, Fishe that is white scaled and harde, as Perches, Bremes, Cheuiens, Ruffes, Carpes, Roches, Troutes &c. be all good, but vnscaled fisshes, as Eeles, Tenches, Lampres, and such like, be daungerous, vnlesse they be well baked or roosted: and eaten with Pepper and Ginger, and Vineger. And note this, that it is not holsome traualing, or laboringe, immediatly after the eating of Fishe, for it doth greatly corrupte the stomacke, & as *Galen* saith, the norishmentes of Flesh is better, then the norishementes of Fishe: and thusmuch generally I haue spoken of Fishe. Of the natures of fishes, rede *Rondoletius*, and *Conradus Gesnerus de Piss*.

Fishe that haue skales be good, but fishe without skales are not wholsom.

Marcellus.

VVHat, it semeth by these wordes, that greate Fisshes, whiche be deuourers in the Sea, as Sele, Purpose, and suche like, be vnholsome, & that the small Fishes, as Coddes, Whityngs, Place, Smeltes, Buttes, Soole, Pike, Breme, Roche, Carpe & suche as feede in cleane stonie waters, thou saist thei be very wholsom. Eeles Lampers, and other muddie Fisshes, thou doest not greatly comende: There be some kindes of Fishe softe, and some harde, but whiche be the beste?

Hillarius.

Fishe soft and hard. IF fishe be softe theldest fish is best: if Fishe be harde, the yongest Fish is best, for it is either soft or harde, of harde Fishe take the smallest, of soft Fish take the greatest: prouided that your Fishe be not very slimie, and thus saith *Auicen* in his booke of Fishes.

Marcellus.

What is the vertue of Shell fisshes?

Hillarius.

Shell fishes. CRauises, & Crabbes, be very good Fishes, the meate of them doth helpe the Lunges, but they be hurtfull for the bladder, yet they will engender seede. If Crabbes of the fresh water, be sodden in pure greene Oile Oliue: this Oile dropped into the eare luke warm, doth heale of burning obstructions, & stopping matter, that hindereth the hearyng. As for Limpetes, Cockels, Scallapes, as *Galen* saieth, thei be harde of digestion. Muskels, and Oisters, woulde be well boyled, roosted, or baked with Onions, Wine, Butter, Sugar, Ginger, and Peper, or els thei be windie, and flegmatike: cholorike stomackes maie well digest rawe Oysters, but they haue caste many one awaie, yet rawe Oisters will clense the raines.

For deafnes.

Oisters.

Marcellus.

What saie you of Milke, Butter, and Cheese?

Hillarius.

Hillarius.

WOmens Milke is the moste gentle nutrament for yong children, which milke is of the decoction of pure blood by naturall heate, and drawen foorth by the Nibles frō the breastes or Pappes, this is the first foode of man-kinde: for like as breade is a blessing of God for men, euen so is Milke one of the great blessinges as appereth in the promise which God made to Israell. Without Milke it is not possible to bring vp man or beast. The best Milke is of womē and most temperate, for it preserueth against consumption. The seconde is Goates Milke, which doth nurish and is hotter then womens milke, Sheepes Milke, is not so much nourishing, and not pleasaunt to the stamacke. Yonge Cowes Milke is thicker, and full of Butter. Note also that iiii. thinges must bee considered in milke, the withnesse of collour, the sweetnesse of sauour, the plesantnesse of tast, the substance neither thicke nor thinne, it is good Milke, whan a drop will stande whole vpon your thum nayle without sheding. There be thre essences of Milke, Cheese, Butter and Whaie, the best Milke is of the yongest and fattest Kine, or Goates, that be fed in the clenest, driest & sweetest Pastures, wheras plentie of sweet flowers are growinge, and purest Claie or Chalke water, with holsome laier. The best time of Milke is in Aprill, May, and June. The new Milke is most holsom for them to drinke, whiche hath cleane stomackes, to drinke it with Suger as it cometh from the Cowe, three houres before all other meate or drinke, and then it wil not coagulate nor crude in the stomacke, but quēcheth Choler. More ouer milke is not onely good to yong children & health full people: but if it be sower, then beware the stone in the raines and bladder through the same, and to thē which haue feuers or head ache Milke doth much harme, as *Hippocrates* saith: *Lac dare caput dolentibus, malum: malum vero febricantibus & quibus hypochondria suspensa murmurant & siticulosis: malum autem in quibus infebris acutis, biliosæ sunt deiectiones, & quibus sanguinis multi deiectio facta est, conuenit autem tabidis qui non multum febricitant & in febribus longis & paruis, si nullum supradictis signis affuerit, &c.* That is, Milke saieth he, is very vnholsom to such as haue paines in their heddes, or that be sicke of any feuer, & also to them whiche haue any noyse or winde in the vpper parte of their belly called *Hypochondria*, & that hath choloricke decoction in hot feuers, or hath lost much bloud notwithstanding, milke is good to suche as haue a consumptiō without a Feuer, and may be geuen to thē whiche haue Feuers long time if none of the forsaid tokens doe appere &c. And to conclude of Mylke, seing oftentimes it is very euell, and will through the coldenesse, and winde, offende the whole bodies of men, what harme doeth it then to sickly persones? how be it we do se that milke is a goodly staie in a comon wealth, and the feders thereof are people of a good temperamēt, or cōplexion, as in Wales, Suffolke, Essex, and in a place in the mountaines in the North called Alsten Moore, whereas little tillage is but bringing vp of cattell, in this coūtrie the people be al chiefly nurished

Milke of women, is the beste of all milkes.

Milke of Goates.

Milke of Kine.
Milke foure thynges considered in it.

Milke hurtfull to whom

Hyppocrates of the hurt of Milke, and the vtilitie thereof.

Milke is a good thing in a common wealthe.

Alsten moore in the North.

with

The booke of Simples.

Sir Thomas the Baron Hilton, his lande.

with milke, little other drinke thei vse, milke excepted. This countrey was somtime the land of a worthy knight, called sir Thomas the Baron of Hilton, to whom I dedicated my little boke, intituled the *Gouernment of health*, promising in the same boke, to set forth an other boke, wherof the copie perished with my bokes, in shipwrack, and when I came to London, to haue reuiued my dedde booke: one William Hilton gentleman, brother to the said sir Thomas Hiltō, accused me of no lesse crime

William Hilton letted Willyā Bullein, to finishe his booke of healthful medicenes.

then of moste cruell murder, of his own brother, which died of a feuer, (sent onely of God) emong his owne friendes: finishyng his life in the christen faith. But this William Hilton, causing me to be arained before that noble Prince, the Dukes grace of Norffolke, for the same: to this ende, to haue had me died shamefully: That with the coueteous Ahab, he might haue through false witnesse and periurie, obtained by the counsaill of Iezabell, a Vine yarde, by the price of blood. But it is written, *Testis mendax peribit*, a false witnesse shall come to nought, his wicked practise, was wisely espied, his folie derided, his bloodie purpose letted, and finally, I was with iustice deliuered. Notwithstāding, yet by the same William Hilton still molested & troubled asmoche as lieth in him, to shorten my daies, by some meanes or accidence. Which with neither lawfull policie, nor false testimonie, could hetherto accōplishe his wicked intent. Now therfore blame me not my dere friend *Marcellus*, though this man be remembred in my boke here of health, and preseruing of life, seing I was somtyme in his boke of a false indightment, conspiring my death. This man hath letted me, in so moche that I cā not run to the marke, that I did set before myne iyen, therfore I must make a shorter course, finishing with fewer thinges, trustyng not vnprofitable for the common wealth: whose profite I doe seke, and more would haue dooen, this his malicious factes excepted, whose malice doeth the lesse molest me, being a straunger to him. Seing he haue vered a lady, whiche was his own brothers wife, whose shame, losse, yea and blood he hath sought which brothers wife, redemed muche of his lande, from losse, in lending him a greate somme of money. And when this man should thankfully haue repaied this lady her money, then he

A bloodie practise against the ladie Hilton.

gratified her as he did me. And so to cōclude, you that are gentlemen, beware of shamefull ingratitude, wheras you haue reaped cōmoditie. For it is the most leprous sicknes against nature, to do euill for good, prefarryng a little lucre, before honestie, worldly worship, shame: & finally, Gods wrath or vengeaunce, due for suche wickednes, against cōsciēce, & nature. For ingratitude do degenerate mankind, & transforme him moste monstruous, into an euill vile nature. Frō gentlenes into

What a very gētilman is.

churlishnes, for like as gentlenes vs vertues, maketh a very gentlemā although somtime obscury borne. So do ingratitude blemishe & defile thē, whiche can bring nothing els for thē selues, but petigrees, lines, cotes and standerdes, moste aunciently descended, yet thē selues voide of all goodnes. Thus I leaue to molest thine eares with him: whiche hath thus molested me, profitable to fewe, and noisome to hymself.

The booke of Simples. Fol.lxxxv.

A louer of fewe, a flatterer of many, a vessell of ignoraunce, full of ingratitude, vnnaturall to his childrē, in that he spoileth in law which should be their relief: and thus I commende hym to this cataplasma, to his mortified conscience. Faithlesse and fruitlesse he is.

   Butter of nature is hot and moist, and hath vertue to molifie hard Apostimacions that are aboue nature, as *Galen* saith, fresh Butter do ripe, clense, and warme the inwarde partes in meates: ointementes or drinkes. Fresh Butter is holsome for to anoynt the swellyng of the *Hypochondrion* or bellie, and for the *Phlegmon* and *bubo*. Furder, to cause young children their teeth to growe, through the anointing of the place: and it is good to make an ointment for the *Pleurici*. And to be dronk in wine or Beare, for the stopping of the Lunges. Butter, Hony, and bitter Almondes, be wholsome for to clense the breast, and beyng put in Suppositors, and Glisters doe molifie the belly. Newe Butter meanly salted, is good with Bread, Fleshe, and Fishe. The olde Butter changyng with many colours is the worste, it is noisome to the stomacke. Butter is good in the mornyng, but not holsome at night: yet Butter preuaileth against poison in woundes, it will purge clense, and increase fleshe. When the Butter is first made, there is a Milke commyng from the same somwhat sharpe, sower, and colde, very holsome to be dronke in the mornyng or euenyng, against hotte burnyng choler, it openeth the liuer, clenseth the gaule, prouoke vrin, cause slepe, and nourisheth muche, if it be eaten with Sugar, and newe white bread.

   Cheese which is a parte of Milke of the groser substance, throughe the coagulacion or cruddes, beinge gathered and pressed together, from the moyste Whaye, the same Cheese is finished, and if it be made of cleane Milke, and the Creame therewith, then it is beneficiall to the stomacke, specially if it bee freshe and good, it nourisheth the fleshe moche, and for greene woundes to knitte them, and will also quenche heate, or clense a spotte in the iye, beyng laied thereon. xxiiii. howers. Chese meanly salted, nourisheth but littell, by the reason of the Salt. Olde Chese stoppeth the flix of the belly, but it is harde to digest, hurtyng the stomacke, gaule, raines, and will breedd the stone in the bladder, and cause the increase of Melancholie with moche coldnesse and drinesse. *Galen lib.4.de alimentorum* commendeth the Chese of his owne natiue countrey, because of the purenesse of the Milke, and sweetnesse of the Cheese, but in his. *x. lib.* of Simples, he refuseth Cheese for the sowernesse. &c. whan stone pottes be broken, what is better to glew them againe or make them fast, nothing like the Symunt made of Cheese, know therfore it will quickly build a stone in a drie body, which is ful of choler adust. And here in Englande be diuers kindes of Cheeses, as Suff. Esser, Banburie. &c. accordyng to their places & feeding of their cattel, time of y yere, layre of their Kine, clenlinesse of their Dayres, quantitie of their Butter, for the more Butter, the worse Cheese. And thus I conclude of Cheese, like as the Welchmen loueth it rosted, euē so doth Fleminges loue Butter at all times, and of all makinges refusing

Cataplasme for M. Hilton of Birdick, of the Bishoprike of Duresme.

Butter the vertue of it.

Butter Milke called Charme Milke is good.

Cheese fresh is beste.

Grene Chese help woūdes

Cheese olde, stoppeth the flux, but bleedeth the stone

Sondry kindes of Chese.

Much good Butter, litle good Cheese.

p.i.

The booke of Simples.

fusing non, what coullour so euer it hath, and from whence so euer it cometh their stomackes are such.

Whaye, the vertue therof
Whay is the thinnest parte of Milke. Whay with Femitory sodden in May, and dronke colde in the mornyng and Euening, hath vertue to scower, clense, and open the partes of the body that are stopped prouoketh vrin and maketh cleane the bladder, and is good to quenche choler, helpeth the belly, asswageth thirst, yet it inflameth and bringeth wind to the guttes, but recocted or two times soddē whay, is the best whay, and will bring sleape, and also is good in Glisters to coole, scower, and quenche choller in the guttes or helpe the excoriacion in them, made by blouddy flix, *Galen* commended Whay *lib. x. simplic. medic.* and *Mesue* doth not a litle praise the Whay of blacke goates, and how it is

Gotes whaie
hot and drie in the first degree vnto the seconde: this whay is good to be giuen to them which hath much Melancholie, or frensies, and cleseth the water betwene the skinne and the flesh openeth the gaule, & molifieth the Splene in sharpe acute Tertian Feuers, or stopping of the vessels with yellow choler, this whay doth much helpe, to drinke the same, and nothing is better to be drōke against a hot Leprose thē whay, it maketh a cleane skinne. Whay is vsed in many decoctions, & infusions, for Linatiues to purge the belly, and thus I doo ende of Whay, whiche is a good drinke in Sommer in the common wealth, whereas good Dayres be, as in Suffolke, the best countrey of Milke, as aboute Lethrigham, Stratebroke, Larfeld, Kelshall. &c.

Egges of birdes.
Egges be commended of the moste excellent writers, as *Dioscorides* and *Galen* that thei do excell all other noriching meates, & also good in medicen, *Isach* the *Arabian*, in his diates doth praise Henes Egges, for that thei be plesant to the mouth, and profitable to the stomacke, and that thei nourishe more then any other meates, and are sonest turned into good bloud, and eftsones into seede of generacion, specially Egges that bee newe and white, but old Egges be most filthy and noisome to the stomacke. Furthermore Egges be no partes of the Fowle saith *Galen simplic. medi.*,

Egges, three thinges in them.
but a porcion of the thing from whens thei come: and *Symeon* saith iii. thinges must be considered in Egges, the first of the substance and clenes of nature, the second is their age, either new or old: the third is of the maner of their dressing, as potching, sething or rosting. Potched Egges be holsom to be supped vp in the morning vpon an emptie stomacke. To clense the Lunges, brest, and the raines, harde Egges doth binde: fried Egges hurtefull, to the stomacke, next in goodnes vnto them are the Egges of Fesantes, & Partriges, and the Egges of smal birdes of the wood, whose Egges are white, but the Egges of water foules, as Swanes, Geese, Duckes, with al their kindes, be grose and not pleasannte to nature, although good to stronge stomacked labourers. Doues Egges, because of their greate heate, are more better for medicen, then meate. Pecockes and Estrige egges, bee not good: of an

Egges of great foules be not good.
euill nature, and enemie to mankinde: In foode, the yellowe parte of egges be warme, and nourishe the blood, and the white of the egge, is

cold

The booke of Simples. Fol.lxxxvj.

cold and flegmatike. *Galen* doe commende the white of Egges, because thei frete not, but coole: and therefore thei are good for medicenes for the iyes, and vlcers, and woundes of the hed, and other places, whereas blood doe flowe. Rawe egges, with oile of Roses, beaten together, are good for flegmon, in the eares, breastes, armes, legges, or priuie members. The white of an egge, the iuice of Pomgranettes, vineger and the oile of water Lillies, are good beaten together, to anointe the forehedde to cause slepe. Egges sodden in strong sharpe vineger, vntill thei bee harde, eate theim, and thei will stoppe the flixe in the bellie. Whites of egges, the pouder of the flowers of Pomgranetes, Planten water, and *Hypocistes*, with oile of Roses, and Alume, beaten in a leaden Morter, will heale a burnyng or skaldyng in the fleshe, coueryng the place with a Launde clothe, and anointe the saied Launde with this ointment. Oile of Egges are good, to heale *Serpigo*, the breakyng or cramis of the lippes, handes, skaldyng, burnyng, paines of the eares, stomacke, raines, bellie, and the priuy members: whiche haue great burnyng, filthe, or heate, and finally, all the paines of the iointes.

Of Egges cometh all foules, saue Barnacles, whiche are ingendered of the marueilous worke of Occian sea: Rede *Gesnerus* of the nature of foules. The horrible Serpente called the Cockatrise, is bred in the Egge: so is Crocodili, and many mo Serpentes, and many fisches of the sea, and little wormes, as the Antes. And thus I doe ende of Egges, whose yokes or reddes be firste, brede within the foule bodies, as it doeth appere when thei be killed, greate plentie of the saied yolkes and no whites, of whiche yolkes, the birde is bredde and nourished of the white: So is mankinde ingendered and formed of one parte, and nourished of an other. Rede *Hyppocrates in libro de natura pueri.*

Marcellus.

What vertue is in *Coagulo Leporis?*

Hillarius.

Three halfe penie waight, after the olde waight of the Apoticaries, tempered in wine, and drunke, doe preuaile againste benim, or prickyng of Serpentes, bloodie flixes, and paines of the matrix, after the tyme that the termes menstruall bee paste: it helpeth conscepcion, but to drinke it, it will drie the seede, and letteth conscepcion. *Aristotle* doe remember *Coagulum lib.iiij.Cap.xxj. de historia animalium,* saiyng: it is the substaunce of Milke, of those beastes, whiche cheweth the cudde, and sucketh, of a curdie substaunce, as Calfe, Lambe, Kidde, &c. And of nature is sower and driyng: and drunke with vineger, it helpeth the fallyng sicknes, as *Galen* affirmeth *lib.x.simpli.medica.*

Marcellus.

What saie you of *Sepum* called Tallowe, and *Adeps*, whiche is fat, or the grease of beastes and foules. I praie you tell me?

Hillarius.

y.ii. first

The booke of Simples.

Tallow of male best are hotter then the femall.

Irst of Tallowe, vnderstãde that of nature it is warm and therefore it haue vertue to resolue, and make softe: and is vsed in sondrie medicenes, among the Chyrurgians notwithstandyng. You must vnderstande, that one beaste beareth more warmer Tallowe, then an other: and the Male hotter then the female. As example, the Harte hotter then ye Hinde: the Rãme more warmer then the Ewe. &c.

But for the fattes of beastes & birdes, thei be all warme and moyst: some more, and some lesse, accordyng to the ages, fatnesse, and natures as example, folowyng shortly saied.

The fat or grease of ye {
Swannes, Gese, Duckes, Bustardes, Hennes and Capons, beyng freshe, doe comfort the matrice, breastes and iointes, and are warme.

Gelded Swine not salted, is moche like oile and moist good against the pleurisie, and vsed in many ointments.

Goates is harder then the Swines, and is also drier, and is good againste the paines of the greate guttes, in Clisters or Supositers.

Beares is warme, and melted with *Laudanum*, maketh an ointment to increase heere.

Foxes, is good against colde and palsie, and paines of the eares.

Purpentine against baldnes, as the Beares grease is

Bulles and Calues doe warme, and are good to binde and stoppe flire, put in glisters, oyntmentes, &c.

Male beastes hotter and drier, then the female.

Lions is moste subtill and hotte of all fattes.

Cattes hotte, and good to anointe ache and goutes.

Seles, or other Sea fishe, clarified with Honie, will clense the iyen that are dimme.

Snales clense the iyen, helpe the eares, and wholsome for bone ache.

Vipers good to anoint the dim sight, dropped into the young lustie creatures, not salted and cleane clarified is best kept close.

Rauenyng beastes hotter then theim, whiche eateth Grasse: and the water foule, hotter then the lande birdes

Wolles called *Oesypus*, will resolue hard apostumacions and *Struma* in the throate.
}

Marcellus.

What saie you of Mary, whiche in some place is called Marthe: contained within the bones of beastes?

Hillarius.

The booke of Simples. Fol.lxxxvij.

It haue power to molifie, and make harde thynges softe, and of nature is hotte and moiste, as Galen saith *lib.xj.simplicium medicamentorum.* Example.

The mary or *Medulla* of the {
- Stagge or Hart, is the best of all beastes, to molifie muskles, ligamentes, tendontes, and the guttes.
- Calues or young Steres is next in goodnes, vsed in sondrie ointmentes and linamentes.
- Bulle and Goates, whiche are verie warme, and good in pessaris for women.
- Oxe, is good for the stomacke, the Lunges, and increaseth seede of generacion.
- Foxe, for the palsie, and trembling of the members.
- Backe bone of beastes, is drier then other Marie, and vnpleasaunt to the stomacke, drunke with Aligante, stoppeth the whites in women.
}

All these must be kept in cleane besselles, a lofte in a chamber, with windowes towardes the Northe. For ye South winde, or standyng in besselles nere to the grounde, will sone corrupte Marie, excepted thei bee clarified vpon the fire, and preserued in cleane close stone or glasse besselles. *To preserue fatte.*

Marcellus.
What saie you of the Gaules of beastes or fishe?
Hillarius.

The Gaule is the moste hottest and bitterest parte of all beastes, the place of Choller, and Choller it self and drie Specially in hotte beastes, as Lions, Wolues, Foxes, Dogs. &c. more then of ye other beastes, whiche diuideth the houes. Euen so it is emong foules, the croked billed birdes, hottest of all next them whiche feedeth vpon weedes or seedes: and the water foule, more then the fielde birdes, as *Dioscorides* affirmeth *lib.ij. Cap.lxxj.* and are vsed in medicen, as example. *Gaules of beastes.*

The Gaule or fell of the {
- Scorpion of the sea, the Sea Snale, or loche like of the sea, for sore iyen.
- White Cocke, a Capon, Hen, Fesant, Partrige, Doue, against sore iyen, dropped into them.
- Crane, Ospraie, for paines in the eares, with oile of bitter Almondes, dropped into them.
- Swanne, Malarde, will kill wormes.
- Bul, oxe, Cowe, Goate, Rame, good for woundes or swellynges, & to kill wormes in ye belly made in plaster.
- Swine for vlcers in the eares.
- Beares, to anoint the heddes and nosetrelles, of the whiche haue the fallyng sicknes.
}

Also Gaules with Honie, and the iuice of Rue, maketh a good ointment, to anoint the bellie: to kille wormes, and helpeth collike, and is

p.iij.   vsed

The booke of Simples.

Stones of Oxe bladder. vsed in inward medicenes. There are stones founde within the Gaules of Oxen and Bulles, the pouder of theim drunke, will cleanse the raines and bladder. As you maie see, *Mathiolus in Coment. Diosco. lib. ij. Cap. lxxj.*

Marcellus.

What saie you of Braines?

Hillarius.

Braines of beastes. 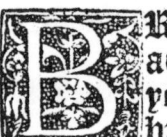Raines are colde, and moiste of nature, euery beaste or foule, accordyng to their kindes. Some not so moiste as other, as you haue had example, of hotte and colde beastes: and their braines are vsed in medicen. As Example.

The braines of the
- Hare sodden or rosted, is good to make young childrens teeth to growe.
- Hennes, Capons, or Fesantes, to bee drunke in wine against poison, saieth *Dioscorides.*
- Weesell or Ferit dried, and drunke in Wineger, againste the fallyng sicknes.
- Swallowe mingled with Honie, against the dimnesse of the iyes.
- Shepe prepared, good to cause teeth to growe, and mollifieth apostumacions.
- Fielde birdes rosted, are all good to nourishe the brain of manne, when it is weake.
- Calfe and Pigge, not good for flegmatike people.

Marcellus.

What saie you of Liuers?

Hillarius.

Liuers of beastes. The Liuer is the nutrimentall part, and the fountain of blood, a spongie matter: whereas the vaines doe begin, and is warme and moiste, accordyng to the nature animall or beaste, and is vsed in medicene. As example.

The liuer of the
- Madde Dogge, rosted and eaten, helpeth hym, whiche is bitten with a madde Dogge.
- Goates beyng cleane, dooe comforte the sight, applied rawe or distilled, and is eaten to help the fallyng sicknes
- Wolfe, with Liuerworte dried, maketh a goodly pouder, to helpe the liuer and lunges.
- Fore, clene washed and dried, doe the same.
- Asse or horse broiled & eaté, against the falling sicknes
- Bore, bothe in meate and medicene, against the styng and bityng of Serpentes.
- More Henne, or water Henne, againste the stone, or grauell in the raines.
- Henne, Capons, Chickens, Partrige, Fesante, and all field birdes, doe nourishe and comfort nature.

Marcellus.

The booke of Simples. Fol.lxxxviij.

Hillarius.

What saie you of the Horne?

Hillarius.

Not moche, I assure you, although many thynges, maie bee saied thereof, bothe for nature and propertie: I commende the descripcion to theim, that couet to bee merie. And thus moche will I saie with *Aristotle in libro de natura animalium*, saieth: all beastes wantyng their vpper teethe, haue naturally hornes, for their defense: as we doe see the Bulle, the Harte, &c. and thei are good in medicenes, as example.

Hornes their nature.

The horne of
- Unicorne is moste excellente, to be drunke againste venime and poison, and helpeth the yelowe iaunders.
- Harte rased and drunke, againste Collike, or Iliac, Iaunders, and the bloodie flixe.
- Goates maketh good pouder to cleanse the teethe, and stablishe them, so doe Hartes horne.
- Bulles in pouder, drunke with wine, helpeth to heale the Hemeroides, burnt in pouder.
- The Elephantes tothe, wil help the yellowe Iaunders, rased and drunke in Endiue water.
- Sondrie monsters of the sea, are good against poison.

Marcellus.

What saie you to the Houes of beastes?

Hillarius.

Thei are their naturall Shooes, keppyng still their old fashion, whiche God haue prepared for them. For neither Horse nor Oxe should bee profitable for mankinde, but for the Houe: without whiche, he could not go or trauell, or haue any Shoe made fast. Thei are also good for mankinde in medicen, as example.

Houes of beastes.

The houes of
- Horses rased are drunke in wine, and good to helpe the fallyng sicknes.
- Asses will doe the same, and help the mother: burnt in perfume sodden in oile, it will helpe *Struma*.
- Goates, with Uineger and *Laudanum*. will increase heare, anointyng the place.
- Any beast burned, ye smoke thereof helpeth the mother, and killeth Gnattes that trouble your chamber.
- Any beast drunke in pouder, maketh women baren and fruitlesse.
- Mule, will retaine moste stronge poison, or deadlie venime.
- Them, which are deuided in twoo partes, are clene beastes, Leuiticus, Chapiter, xi.

p.iiii. *Marcellus.*

The booke of Simples.

Marcellus.

What saie you of bones?

Hillarius.

BOnes is the timber and strong postes, which coupleth the bodie of euery liuyng man, beaste, fisshe, and foule together: without which we might not be perfite. If any of them are broken, then are we lame. Thus bones bee not onely good to nature, when we are liuyng: but *ossa humana*, mannes bones, are good in medicen. As example.

The bones of
- Man beaten into pouder, doe greatly drie moist humours and sores. &c.
- Lions strongly smitten together, will bryng light fire, and are moste drie of nature.
- Hogges beaten into pouder, and drunke against the fallyng sickenesse.
- Hennes burnt with Eggshelles, made in pouder, maketh a frettyng pouder.
- Pigges are good for wrytyng Tables, and to kille wormes in the stomake, dronke in wormewood wine.
- Many sea fisshes ar holsome in medicen, against poisō
- *Sepia*, or Cuttle, colde and drie, wil cleanse the skinne, and the iyen.

Marcellus.

What saie you of vrine?

Hillarius.

IT is the whaie of the blood, conuaighed by the raines, into the bladder: hot and drie of nature, verie salt, accordyng to the complexion of the bodie that make it, as man and beast. Foule pisse not, for the moister is tourned into feathers. *Aristotle de natura animalibuus*. Vrine is vsed in medicen. As example.

The vrin of ye
- Man is weakest, except gelded swine, and is wholsome to be drunke against venime.
- Younge boie, to be distilled with Letarges of mettal, a water to wash against Leprosie, is made therof.
- Mule, to wasshe handes and feete, and againste the goute, and paines of the iointes.
- Goates or Camelles, to be dronke againste dropsie, or swellyng of the bellie.
- Bore, with oile of Wormewood, anointe the bellie, and kill wormes.
- Dogges will kill Wartes, and ringwormes.
- Vrine, will corode and frette, clense and skower corrupted humers.

Marcellus.

The booke of Simples. Fol.lxxxix.

what saie you of blood?
Hillarius.

THE life of euery liuyng thyng, consisteth in the vitall blood, **Bloud.**
without whiche, the soule can not remaine within the bodie:
and is vsed often tymes in medicen. As example.

The bloud of the {
Geese, Duckes, and Kiddes, are in sondrie *Antidotaris.*
Stocke Doues, Turtle Doues, House Doues, and Partriges, are good for sore iyen, and newe woundes.
Hare, for the stone and bloodie flixe.
Dere, for the flixe, or termes immoderate runnyng in women.
Goates, whiche are fedde with opening herbes, killed in June, for the stone.
Calfe fedde so for the same stone, and also the flixe.
Dragons is declared before.
Swine is colde blood: yet it is vsed in puddynges, but not commendable.
Beares, and Bulles are horrible, not good.
Shepe helpeth the Emerodes,
Hennes, Cockes, and Capons, stoppeth blood and woundes.
Duckes, kepeth a goodly colour long tyme: the Idolatours did practise therewith, deceiuyng the people at Hailes, with a bloud which thei called holy.
}

Marcellus.
what saie you to the nature of ordure, the dunge of beastes.
Hillarius.

ORdure or dunge, is the corrupcion or filthe excremente, **Ordure or**
whiche nature expulseth to the yearth, by the office of the **dunge.**
guttes, without which no creature should liue, if the dong
were still retained, in the saied guttes: and yet it is good in
sondrie salues, plasters, and medicenes. As example. And
thei are hot and drie of complexion, according to the nature of beasts.

The dung of {
Oxen and Kine, doe mitigate inflamacion of woundes: and helpeth stingyng of Bees.
Calfe sodden with vineger, helpeth *Struma* in the throte, or swellynges of ioyntes.
Goates doe resolue, and make soft: a plaster thereof applied to the matrixe, forseth the child to the birthe.
Horse or Mule, sodden in wine, strained and drunke helpeth the Jaunders.
Shepe, sodden in vineger, and oile of Roses, resolue quencheth, and healeth burnyng and skalding.
Dogges fedde with bones, helpeth the bloody flixe,
}
drunke

The booke of Simples.

The dung of {
dronke in milke, with Honie, helpeth *Anginæ*, to anoint the place of the throte withall.

Mile dooe cleanse, and with Honie tempered together, doe increase heere in ointement for the hedde.

Swine cleseth, it stoppeth blood in flowing woundes

Curlue dronke in wine, helpeth the faling sicknes.

Crocodilus of *Nilus*, cleseth the skin, the best of this is white

Mannes is beste in medicen, although moste abhominable to the sence of smellyng: yet there is arte to make oile for the goute, swellyng of the throate, and to helpe flegmon, of this ordour of mankinde, and a water to be dronke against the falling sicknesse, stone, and the water betwene the fleshe and skin: And finally, helpe euil complexion. Reade *Galen lib. x simplic. medica.* and *Diosco. lib. ij. Cap. lxxiiij.*
}

Marcellus.

What saie of the Scorpion, Frogge, Mouse, Lasarde, Cantharides, Horslech and yearth wormes?

Hillarius.

Scorpion. THE Scorpion is a cruell worme, whose stynge will pricke to death, except the oile of Scorpions be gotten, whiche reconsile the hurt, anointyng the place therewith. Also this oile is good to anoint the raines, to breake the stone, and prouoketh vrine.

Frogge. The Frogge sodden with Salte, and cleane Oile, and so eaten, helpeth against all benime of serpentes. *Dioscorides lib. ij. Cap. xxv.*

Mouse. The Mouse beyng rosted, is good to be giuen to children, that pisse their bedde, to helpe them. Furder it will drie vp the fome and spattle in their mouthes. There are sondrie kindes of Mice, *Aristotle, lib. vj. de Hystoria Animalium.*

Lacert. *Lacerta* with legges, a longe taile an earth Serpente. The head broken and applied to any place on the bodie where as either pricke or nayle is fired, foorth with it shall be drawen foorth. This worme is much vsed of Chyrurgens.

Canthard. *Cantharides* are flies hot, drie, and burning of nature, & hath power to blister and make issue, and draweth for the water: there be that write in their bookes of Phisicke, how these flies may be dronke inwardely against the Dropsie and the stone, but I dare not here commende the same, for feare of no small perill that might folowe.

Horsleche. Horsleches are wholsome to drawe foorthe foule blood, if thei are put into a hollowe Rede, and one of their endes cutte of, whereby the blood maie run forthe.

Snaile. Snayles broken from the shelles & sodden in white wine with oyle and Suger is very holsom, becaufe thei be hot & moist for the straightnes of the lunges and colde coughe. Snayles stamped with Comphori and leuen will drawe foorth prickes in the fleshe.

Earth

The booke of Simples. Fol.xc.

Earth wormes are hot of nature and of thē are a pressious ointmēt made to close woundes, and if thei be sodden in goose greece and strained it is a good oyntment for to drop into a dull hearing eare, poringe it in the contrarie side. Earth wormes stamped are good for payned teeth. The Oyle of wormes be greatly commended for the comforting of ẏ sinewes, iointes, vaines, and goute, thei must be washed in white wine, and the Oiles of *Verbascum* or Cowslops, of Roses of Lilles of Dil, of Chamamill all sodden together, whan it is colde put in your earth wormes, stoppe your glasse, let it stande. xl. daies in the Sunne then straine it, it will make an excellent oile against ache, *Sciatica*, goute. &c. Reade more of them *Plini lib.xxx.cap.ix.* And thus I do ende of Earth wormes, whiche are the bowels of the grounde or earth, whiche earth is colde & drie of nature, yet the mother of eche liuing wight, fostereth and geueth fode to euery creature, both sensible and insēcible and remaineth still firme and stable, and eche creature hath his originall spring, and first life vpon the earth, whan thei haue runne their race, some in pleasure and other some in wretchednes, the earth doeth deuoure them againe at length and swallow them, as though thei had neuer bene: and thus is generacion turned into corruption as Aristotle affirmeth. But how mightie is that Lorde God, whiche with his blessed worde did for our sakes make therth to be our owne free dwellyng place during this our mortall life, to what ende to abuse ẏ same, as the olde worlde did, for whose sakes he did destroy al flesh, his smale chosen people excepted. Now forseth to vse the earth with diligent trauell, in tillage sowing, cherishing herbe, plant, grasse.&c. whiche be Gods giftes, both for our medicen and meate: not to dispise the sweet creatures of God, whiche spring in sōdrie times of the yere, as flowers fruites, seedes, barkes, rootes, with conning to be preserued for mans vse, against the dayly danger of cruell sicknesse, whiche assalteth eche man, woman, and child, through the corruption of humer, and other euill accidentes of our life. And for as muche as we can not make one flower, neither can giue to any of them his proper beutiful shape, vertue, or sauoure: whiche Salomon, whan he was florishinge in his regall estate, was not comperable to any of these flowers for their excellent beutie: Therfore let vs dayly beholde the earth wherbnto wee must once come: and also in the meane time, humblie laude & prayse the high diuine prouidence of the almightie our Lord and God which hath layde the foundations of the earth, that it should not moue at any time, and hath couered it with the deepe, like as with a garment, the waters do stande betwene the hilles, yea he sendeth his springes to the riuers, whiche runne among the hilles: all beastes of the fielde drinke therof: and the wilde Asses do queche their thrist: besides them all the fowles of the ayre haue their habitacion, and sing among the braunches, and watreth the Lilles from the cloudes. The earth is filled with the frute of his workes: he bringeth foorth grasse for the cattel, and greene herbes for the seruis of mankinde, that he might bring

y earth wormes.

Oyle of wormes.

Earth the mother of euery liuing creature.

Generation faule into corruption.

Math.6.

The prouidence of God.

Spal.ciii.
Spa.ciiii.
Iob.xxvi.
Ier.v.
Gen.iii.

foode

The booke of Simples.

Wine, Oile, and Bread, Gods giftes. The trees of the Lord are full of sappe.

foode out of the yearth, and wine that maketh glad the harte of man, and oile to make him a cherfull countenans: and bread to strengthen his hart withal. The trees of the lorde are also full of sappe, euen the trees of Libanus whiche he hath planted. Therin the birdes do make their nestes: & the firre trees are a dwelling for the Storke. The high hilles are a refuge for the wilde Goates, and so are the stonie rockes for the Conies. He appointeth the Moone for certain seasons and the Sunne doth know his going doune, he maketh darknes, that it maie be night, wherin all the beastes of the Forest doeth moue. The Lions roring after their praie doeth seke their meate at God, the Sunne ariseth, and then thei get theim awaie together, and lurke theim close in the dennes. Then man ariseth, and goeth forthe to his worke, and laboureth vntill euenyng: O Lorde how manifolde are thy woorkes, in wisedome haste thou made theim all. The yearth is full of thy riches: so is the greate and wide Sea also, wherin are thinges innumerable bothe small and greate beastes: there saile the Shippes, and there are greate Whales, whom thou hast made to plaie therein: all these creatures waite vpon thee, that thou maiest giue them meate in due time when thou giuest them, thei gather it, & when thou openest thy hand thei are filled with good thinges: when thou hidest thy face, thei are troubled, when thou takest awaie their breathe thei die, and thei are tourned againe to their dust. &c.

Spal. 92.

Esa. 27. Iob. xi. Spal. lxii.

Euery thing tourne to the duste.

Lo here my dere brother *Marcellus* I do ende simplie of Simples, praiyng thee in the meane time to take them in good parte. wayinge my present case disquietnesse, and trouble, good will euer was with me & shalbe to my small power althoughe leasour lacked, and time woulde not serue for the purpose: but whan it shall please God that we shall talke together againe, I will make amendes for all faultes escaped, GOD willing, who euer kepe thee, thine owne *Hillarius*. Moreouer, beholde two old frendes aproche at hand, the one is called Sornes, and the other Chirurgerie. Let vs heare what thei wil saie, a little while.

Trouble haue so hindered me, that I am constrained, presently to staie.

¶ *The ende of the Simples.*

A horned still.   Bagpipe still.

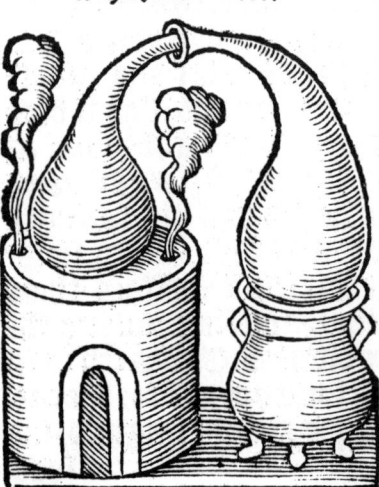 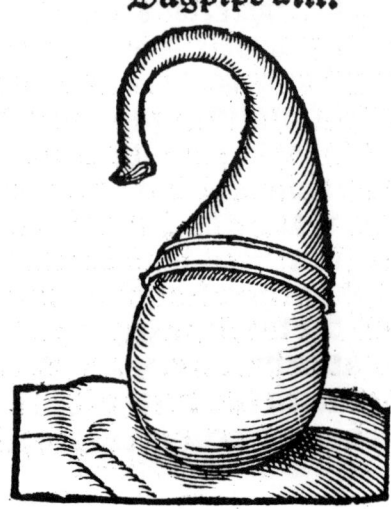

An index of the booke of Simples.

Chicken wede.   **Radiche.**   **Twoo heddes.**

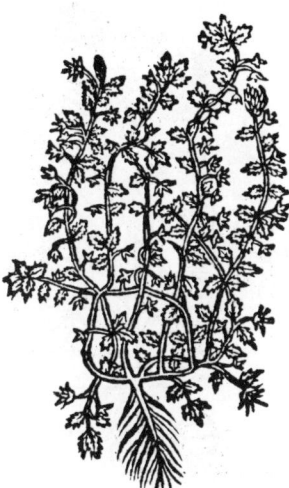 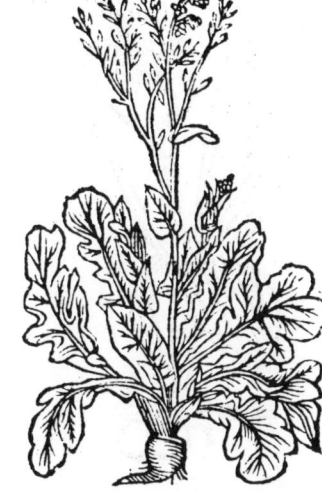 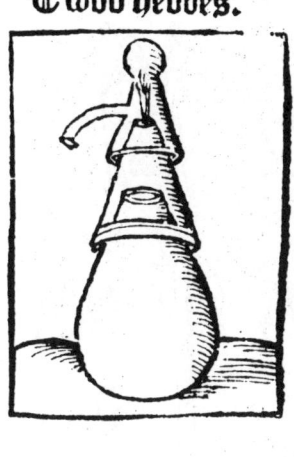

Straberie.   Solanū ẏ **great nightshade**   **Pelican still.**

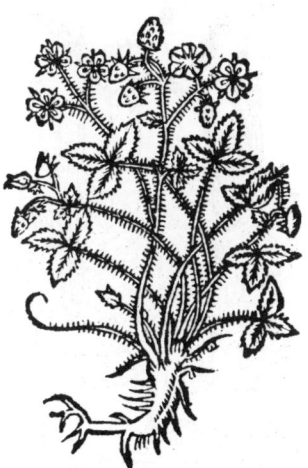 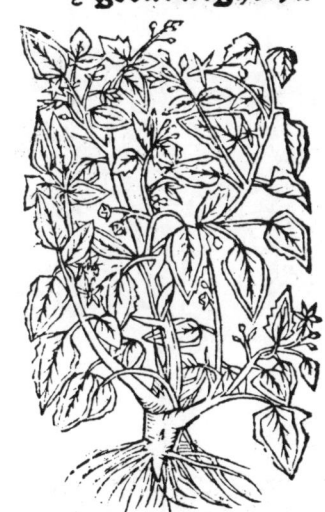 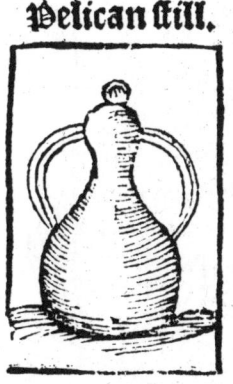

Cherie.   **Hyssope.**   **The little glasse still.**

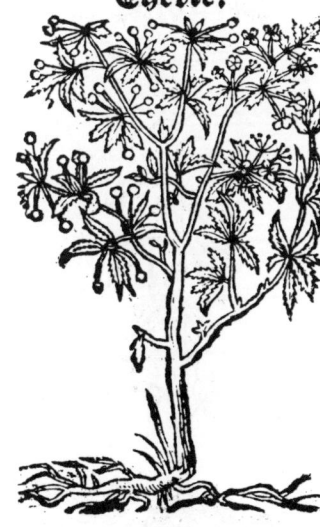 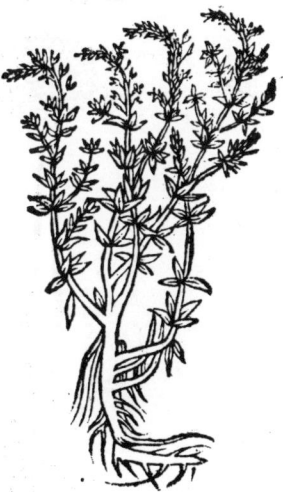 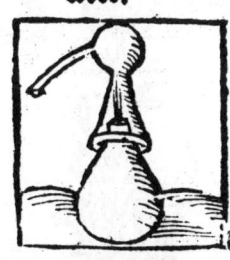

These stilles are verie good, to destille, cleanse, and rectifie all waters.

q.i.

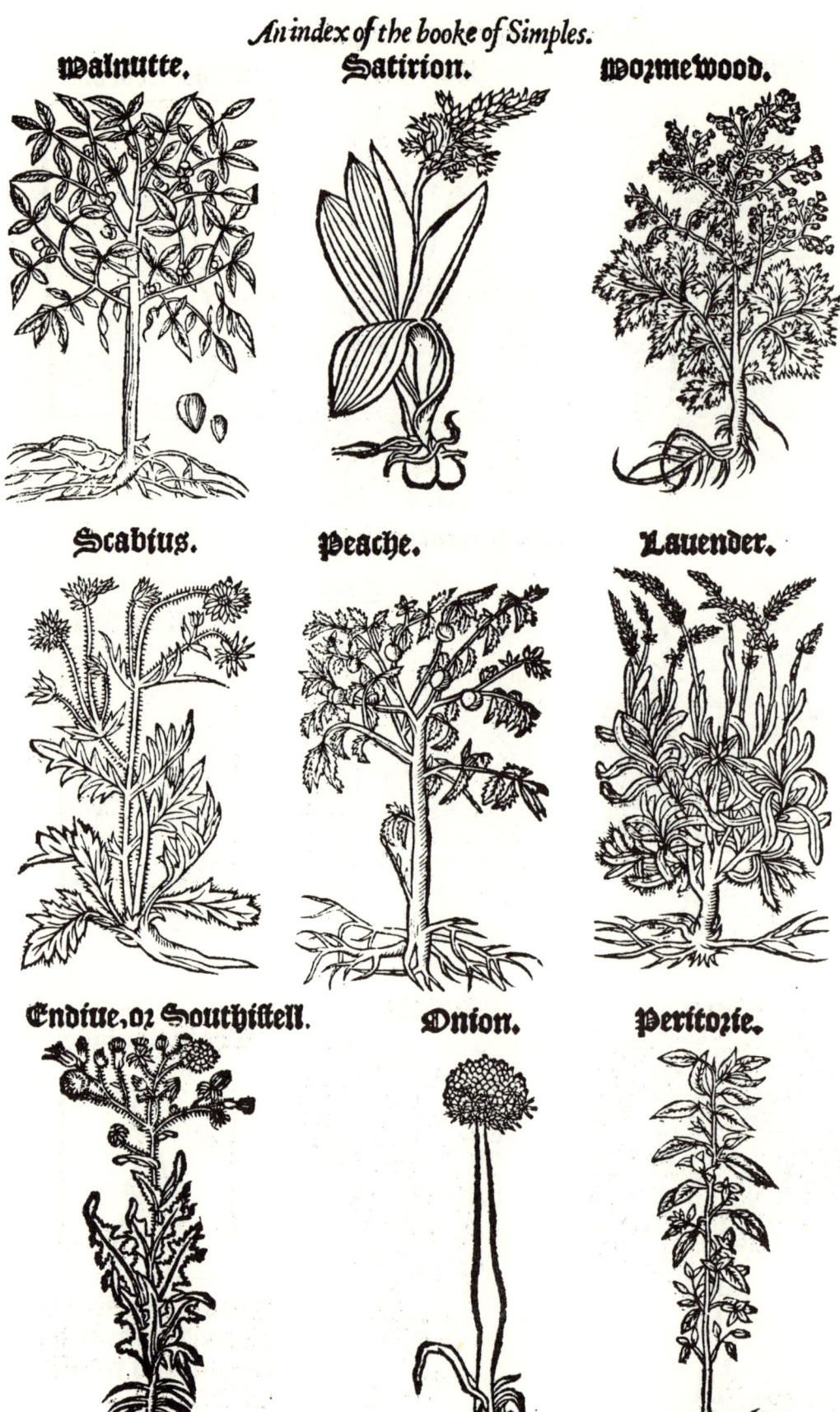

An index of the booke of Simples.

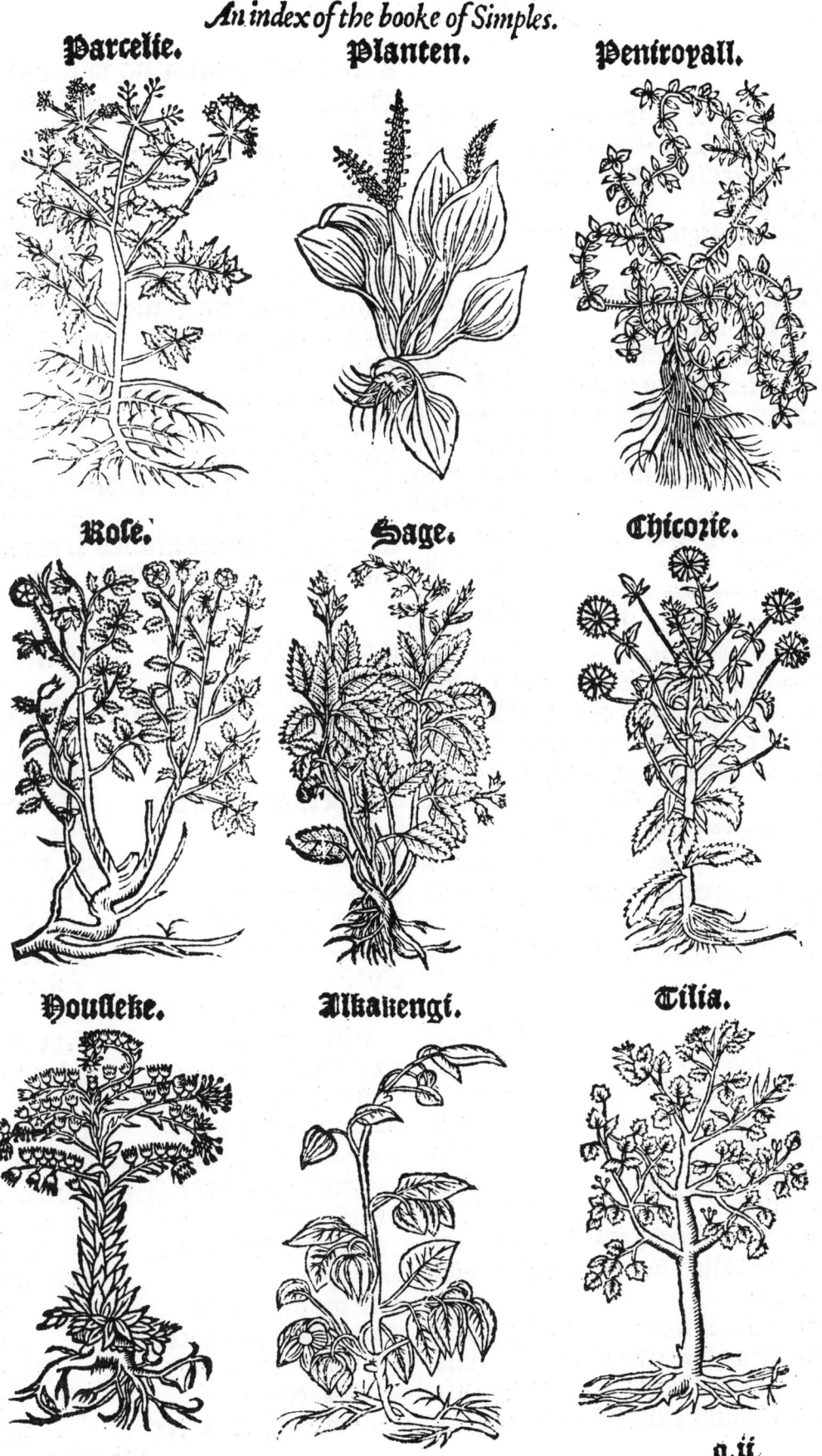

q.ii.

An index of the booke of Simples.

A.

Azarabaccha or wilde *Nardus.* fol.i.
Asplenon called *Scolopendrion* or *Citrach* idē.
Absinthium called Wormewood. fo.ii.
Aniseedes Ibidem.
Anagallus called Chickenwede. fo.vii
Aples fol.xiiii.
Aloes of twoo kindes fol.xv.
Agrimonie fol.xvii.
Apium called Smalage fol.xxii.
Aron called Coko pricke fol.xxx.
Artichocke called *Scolimus* or *Cinaria.* 303
Asparagus fol.xxxviii.
Aconitum twoo kindes, *Pardalianches*, and *Licoctonon* fol.xliiii.
Angelica Angelles flower, or *radix sancti spiritus* fol.xlv.
Aristolochia rotunda & longa. fol.lii.
Apiastrum Mellissa or Balme fol.liiii.
Agaricj or Agaricke fol.lviii.
Amoniacum, of God Ammon. fol.lxiii.
Assafetida a stinkyng Gum. Ibidem.
Amber Grice moste swete. fol.lix.
Acacia a fruite of a Thorne in Egipt xviii fol.lxiii.
Almondes swete and bitter. lxviii.
Agnus Castus or *Vitrex* fol.lxxii.
Alum, or roche Alum. Ibidem.
Atramentum fol.lxxiiii.
Alston more in the North. lxxxiiii.

B.

xiii
Beates fol.viii.
Betonie. Ibidem.
Beare and Ale fol.xii.
Barbaries xiiii.
Buglosse xvi.
Basill or *Ozimum* xvii.
Burnet Ibidem.
Bell Woodbinde called *Smilax* xxi.
Barlie called *Hordium* fol.xxviii.
Beanes xxix.
Bardana the Burre fol.xxxviii.
Brackes or *Felix* the Ferne xlii.
Botris a swete herbe of Fraunce. liii.
Basill wilde called *Ocimastrum* fol.li.

Brionia vitis alba y running wild vin. 52
Boras fol.lxiiii.
Bdellium Ibidem.
Balastia the flowers of Pomgranet.
Baie or Laurell fol.lxxi.
Brimstone fol.lxxiii.
Barach fol.lxxvi.
Baie salte Ibidem.
Bores flesh and Bakon. fol.lxxix.
Beare and Badgard fol.lxxxi.
Blacke birde fol.lxxii.
Barnacle wonderous fol.lxxxii.
Bitter the birde Ibidem.
Butter the vertue fol.lxxxv.
Braines of sondrie kindes lxxxvii.
Byzahar the stone. Ibidem.
Bones of sondrie kindes lxxxviii.
Blood of sondrie beastes lxxxix.

C.

Camamill fol.vii.
Cucumers x
Cabage or *Brassica,* wortes fol.ix.
Claret wine fol.xi.
Cheris fol.xiiii.
Caphers and Oliues fol.xv.
Scabius fol.xvii.
Calamus Aromaticus fol.xviii.
Centaurj or *fel terre* fol.xix.
Cumphorie called *Simphitum* fol.xxv
Consolida minor Daises Ibidem.
Coriander fol.xxvi
Chelidon the great or *Chelidonion mega* Collumbin. fol.xxxiii.
Cresses or *Nasturtium* fol.xliii.
Crowfoote or *Ranunculj* fol.xliiii.
Crocus or Safron fol.xlvi.
Cartamus or wilde Safron fol.xlviii.
Calamintes of the Mountain, l.
Clarie called *Orminum* fol.li.
Carawaies of *Carintha,* liiii.
Cartasilago Ibidem
Chicori or *Speusa solis* lv.
Carrettes the rootes lvi.
Cassia ligni a swete wodde lviii.
Cassiafistula to purge Ibidem
Castian the Chest nutte lxi
Colocinthida

An index of the booke of Simples.

Colocynthida — Ibidem
Cutbert Blunt — fol. lxviii.
Cloues — Ibidem.
Cucubes — fol. lxix.
Ceruse — fol. lxx.
Ciperus — Ibidem
Cardamon — fol. lxxi.
Campher or *Capher* — lxxiii.
Cadmie — lxxv.
Corrall — ——
Calues flesche — lxxviii.
Cockes flesche — lxxxi.
Chese fresche and Salt — lxxxv.
Coagola leporis. &c. — lxxxvi.
Cantharides the flie — lxxxix.
— lxxxii

D.

Dragons — fol. vi.
Dandelion — x.
Dictamnum — xv
Diapentia the great fiue leaued grasse — fol. xxiiii
Dogges tong or *Cynoglossum* — fol. xxiii.
Darnell — fol. xxxi.
Daises called *Bellis* — Ibidem
Diars flowers called *flos Tinctoris*. 47.
Dockes the great called *Rumex* ——
Digitalis called fingers or fore gloues — fol. l.
Doronike a precious roote of Alexandria — fol. lvi.
Dragons blood — fol. lxii.
Diacridij called *Diagredium* — fol. lxv.
Dattes — fol. lxxviii
Ditten —
Duckes flesche — fol. lxxxii
Doues flesche — Ibidem

E.

Enula Campana — fol. xv.
Eleborus albus & niger — xix.
Ebulus or Walwort — liiii
Epithimum — Ibidem
Eringium of the sea — xlvi.
Ebenus wodde — lix.
Euphorbium — lxiii.

F.

Fenill or Fincle — fol. vi.
Filipendula — Ibidem
Fenum Grecj Fenicrike — xxvii
Flare or Lint — Ibidem
Felonwede, or S. James wort — xl.
Flos tinctoris for Diars — xlvii
Fore gloues, called *Digitalis* — l.
Frankincense, or thus — lxii.
Filberde nuttes — lxviii.
Fraxinus the Ashe tree — Ibidem
Figges — lxix
Frenche Sope — lxxiiii
Fumus terre — lxvi.
Falowe Dere — lxx
Fiber — Ibidem
For — lxxxi.
Fesant — lxxxii.
Fische — lxxxiii.
Fatnesse of beastes — lxxxvi.
Frogges — lxxxix.

G.

— lx.
Garlike — fol. iii.
Groundsill — ix.
Grapes — xiiii.
Ginger — xviii.
Gallowgrasse or Hempe — xxviii.
Giloflowers — xxxvii.
Gramen — xxxix.
Goose foote — xl.
Gentian — xliii.
Germander — l.
Goose grasse — liii.
Grummell — lv.
Gum Sarcocole — lxiii.
Galbanum — lxiiii.
Glaucium — lxiiii.
Gum Arabicke — Ibidem
Gum Tragacanthe — Ibidem
Gum Lak — lxv.
Gaulles — lxvi.
Gum of Almondes — lxviii.
Galanga — lxxi.
Goates — lxxix
Beese — lxxxii.
Grene

q.iii.

An index of the booke of Simples.

Grene Chese	lxxxv.	Lapide Lasula	lxxvii.
Goates w.	lxxxvi.	Lapis Tutia	lxxviii.
		Lapis Phrygius	
H.		Lapis magnis	Ibidem
Honie	fol. iiii.	Lambes wolle	lxxx.
Hoppes	viii.		
Horehounds	Ibidem	**M.**	
Hysope	xi.	Mouse eare	iii.
Helenium.	xvi.	Mustarde	x.
Henbane	xxxiii.	Minttes	x.
Humlocke	Ibidem	Mellilote	xviii.
Houslike	xxxvii.	Mugworte	xix.
Horstaile	xliii.	Mallowes	xxi.
Hartes Horne.	xlvi.	Marigolde	xxvi.
Hermodactilis	xlix.	Mandragora	xliiii.
Hypocistis	lxx.	Mislen, or Viscum	liii.
Hæmatiste	lxx.	Mosse	lx.
Hernes B S	lxxii.	Mumia	lxiii.
Hippoglossum	xxiii.	Mirabolans	lxv.
Hypiricon	xvi.	Mirtus	lxvii.
Hempe	xxvii.	Mulberie	lxx.
Hilton of Bidick.	lxxxiiii.	Minium	lxxv.
		Margarit	lxxvii.
I.		Milke B, C,	lxxxiiii.
Jenuper	lxix.	Maidenheare	xxv.
Ireos	lxxi.	Masticke R, F, B, S,	lxiii.
Jette	lxviii.	Mustela	lxxxi.
Iuerie	lxxxi.		
		N.	
K.		Nettles	xlii.
Knotgrasse	xxxv.	Nigilla Romana	xxvi.
		Napus the roote	lvi.
L.			
Lilles	vii.	**O.**	
Lettes	x.	Onions	vi.
Liuerworte	xx.	Oile	xix.
Lunges		Orpin that liue so long	xlvi.
Ligusticum	xxiii.	Oke tree	Ibidem.
Lupines	xxxi.	Osperey the sea Egle	lxxxi.
Lions foote	xxxv.	Otes	xxxi.
Lauender	xliiii.	Oile of wormes	
Lagopus	xlvi.	Otter that liue by fishe	xc.
Licorice	lvi.		
Leauen	lxx.	**P.**	
Licinum	lxxi.	Philitis or Hartes toungue.	i.
Litharge		Purslein or Portulace.	vi.
Laurus	lxxiii.	Planten, or Plantago, Lambes	
Lime	lxxiiii.	tongue.	Ibidem.
Leade	lxxv.		Pease

An index of the booke of Simples.

Peafe or Beanes	viii.
Peares	xiii.
Peaches, or *Persica*	xiiii.
Prunes, or *Pruna*	Ibidem
Polipodi of the Oke	xvii.
Peneroiall, or *Pulegium*	xix.
Poppie, or *Papauer*	xxvi.
Peafe of *Pisum*	xxix.
Pimpernell	xxxiiii.
Pæonia or Pionie	xxxvii.
Paunfis, or *herba Trinitatis*	xli.
Paritarie Perietarie.	xlvii
Purge, or fpurge, called *ricinus*.	xlviii
Psyllium or flewoꝛte.	l.
Peper of the water	li.
Pellitoꝛie, or *Sternumentaria*	lii.
Phylanthropos, that will hang vpon mennes apparell, called Goofe grafle.	liii.
Paftnippes, or *Pastinacia*	lvii.
Pix naualis, or Pitche of the fhip.	lxiii.
Pistacia a kinde of nuttes	lxvii.
Populus or Popple tree.	lxix.
Pomegranet, or *Malum punicum*	Ibidē
Pepper, or Piper	lxxi.
Pearles, or Margarite ftones	77.
Poꝛke or Bakon.	lxxix.
Pigges.	Ibidem.
Poꝛpintine, or *Erenaceus*	lxxx.
Pecocke, their flefhe.	lxxxii.
Partriches, their flefhe	Ibidem.
Pluuers	Ibidem.
Plaice the fifhe	lxxxiii.

Q

Quinces.	xiiii.
Quercula minor.	l.
Quales.	lxxxii.
Quickfiluer	lxxxiiii.

R.

Rice	viii.
Rue, or herbe Grace	x.
Raifens	xiiii.
Rofemarie	xviii.
Rufhes	xxi.
Rocket gentill.	xxxvi.
Rumer called redde Docke.	xlix.
Rapes	lb.
Roides	Ibidem.
Radifhe rootes	lvi.
Rubarbe	lvii.
Rofline	lxii.
Rofe	lxxiii.
Roche	xciii.

S.

Sage.	v.
Soꝛrell	vii.
Sauerie.	viii.
Sencion, or Gronfell	ix.
Scabious	xvi.
Spinage	xvii.
Setwall	Ibidem.
Senturion	xxii.
Smallage	xxxiii.
Simphitum or Comferie	xxv.
Scilla or Skilla or the fea oniō.	Ibi.
Stauefaker	xxxi.
Solanum	Ibidem.
Shepherdes purfe	xxxv.
Sticados	Ibidem.
Serpentaria	Ibidem.
Stichewoꝛte	xxxviii.
Sauin	xxxix.
Sene Alexan.	Ibidem.
Spatula fetida	fl.
Shepherdes nedle	xlv.
Saffron	xlvi.
Spermā Ceti	lxii.
Stoꝛax	Ibidem.
Stact	Ibidem.
Sirax Calamite	lxv.
Sanders	lxxi.
Suger of the Cane	lxxiii.
Sulpher, called Brimfton	Ibidem
Spodium	lxxiiii.
Sope	Ibidem.
Salte	lxxv.
Spongea, the fea Sponge	lxxvi.
Saphirus	lxxvii.
Sparrous	lxxxii.
Shelfifhe	lxxxiii.

An index of the booke of Simples.

Sepum called Tallowe.	lxxxvi.
Scorpion	lxxxix.

T.

Tasill, *Labrum veneris*	xvi.
Tyme	xvii.
Triple grasse	xxxiii.
Tartar of wine lies	lxii.
Terra Sigillata.	Ibidem.
Turbit	lxvii.
Tamarindes.	Ibidem.
Tamarisces, or Tamarix	Ibidem.

V.

Violettes	vi.
Veruen	viii.
Valerian	xxxiii.
Verbascum	xxxv.
Vngula caballina or *Tussilago*. horsehoue	xliii.
Verdegrece	lxxiii.
Varnishe	lxxiiii.

Wormewood	Fol. ii.
Wine	xi.
Woodbinde	xxii.
Wheate	xxx.
Wilde water Peper.	li.
Wesell	lxxxi.
William Hilton.	lxxxiiii.

Azarabaccya called *Vulgago*, hote and drie in the thirde degree: prouoketh vrine, helpeth the liuer, and purgeth termes menstruall. &c.   Fol. i.

Azaron is good against Feuer, dropsie, and frensie   Ibidem

Asplenum is good for the splen   ii.

Absinthium, helpeth sore eares, iyes, splene, and the dropsie. Ibidem.

Anisedes openeth the raines. Ide.

A good remedie for the running of the raines.   Ibidem.

Against the bloody flix   Ibidem.

Against poison.   iii.

A medicen for the fistula. Ibidem

An healthfull drinke for Sommer   Ibidem.

An excellente pille, whiche helped W. Bullein, thauethour of this booke, for the reume   v.

A medicen of Fenill for the raines and bladder.   vi.

An example of Purslen   Ibidem.

An encreaser of the seede of generacion   x.

Against the bityng of dogges and serpentes   Ibidem.

A glasse for a drunkarde.   xi.

Ale and Bere   xiii.

Asshes made of wilde Peretree, their vertue   Ibidem.

Apples their vertues   xiii.

A medicen for the smal pox Ibide.

Against stinkyng breath. Ibidem.

Against drunkenes   Ibidem.

Against hotte choller   Ibidem.

Against the Pestilence   xv.

A cause of the Emeroides Ibidem

A marueilous worke of *Dictamnū*. ib.

A pained stomacke   xix.

A present helpe to be deliuered of a dedde childe   Ibidem.

A medicen for womens breastes. xx

Althos doe signifie medicen,   xxi.

A good Gargarisme to washe the throate   xxiiii.

Against poison   xxvi.

A good medicen for sore iyes. Ibi.

A quicke medicene for a stale ruffen.   xxviii.

Against hote inflamacion, or swellyng of the bodie   xxix.

A more larger discripcion of Beanes and Pease

A knauishe practise of Inholders and their Hostlers   xxx.

A horse is a good seruaunt. Ibidē.

A plaster for a brused bodie.   xxxi.

A plaster to bryng forthe a dedde childe.   Ibidem.

A good medicene for the stone and raines.   xxxiii.

An index of the booke of Simples.

An herbe venime, called Henbane or *Altercum*　　Ibidem.
Againſt the Peſtilence　　xxxviii.
Aſparagus haue many vertues, as to encreaſe the ſeede. &c.　Ibidem
A good medicen for the fallyng ſickeneſſe.　　Ibidem.
An aligorie of an herbe, an old ſuperſticion, inuented by Witches a practiſe of Sathan　　xli.
Angelica defendeth poiſon, and preſerueth chaſtitie　　xlv.
Againſt dronkenes, Saffron doe helpe　　xlvi.
Againſt poiſon　　Ibidem.
Againſt the peſtilence　　xlvii.
A good note of the nature of herbes
Againſte euill ſight, Sauerie preuaileth　　li.
Ariſtolochia helpeth Cancers　　lii.
A very good medicen for the vlcere of the yarde.　　Ib.
A plaſter for the liuer or goute ibi.
A good wounde herbe　Ibidem.
An excellent infuſion of *Leonellus Fauentius* to clenſe the blood　lvii.
Agaricke clenſe the guttes, and expulſe rawe humours. Ibidem.
Agaricke helpeth the fallyng ſickeneſſe　　lviii.
Agarice purgeth all the Organes of the ſences　　Ibidem.
A precious water with Sinamon Caſſia. &c.　　Ibidem.
Amber grece of thre kindes
A good Pomeamber againſt coldnes of the braine　　lix.
A witches bleſſyng for ſainct Anthonies fire.　　lx.
A good plaſter for a ſore ſkabbed pate　　Ibidem.
Ammoniacum commeth from the Oracle of God Ammon　lxiii.
Aſſafetida do ſtinke, yet it helpeth the mother and lunges.　ibidem.

Acatia ſtoppeth the blodie flix. lxiiii.
B.
Bityng of a Snake　　fol. iii.
Bees be an example vnto vs, both for loue, and woorkyng in the common wealthe.　Ibidem.
Bees maintain no ſtraungers, for thei be not profitable.　iiii.
Bread of a daie olde　　xiii.
Blacke Friers preachers in Norwiche.　　Ibidem.
Bees in the olde tyme, were vſed for lottes　　xxix.
Biſtorta haue a crompled roote, lyyng wrinkled like a ſerpent, but the female roote is blacke without, and redde within, and a greate knot in the ende.　xxxvi.
Brake ſeedes were neuer ſeen emong chriſtian people, but witches haue vſed practiſe with thē as foliſh writers affirmeth. xlii.
Bitter herbes be hotte and drie. l.
Brionia vitis alba or the wilde runnyng vine.　　lii.
Brionia defendeth poiſon　Ibidem.
Brionia increaſeth milke　Ibidem.
Bitumen and *Caſſutha* helpeth the liuer, gaule, and ſplene　liiii.
Beware of the newe diate, excepte you haue two liues, or els a wiſe miniſter of the ſame.　lxi.
Bitumen of the dedde ſea.　lxii.
Balauſtaca the flower of Pomgranet, whiche will ſtop a flixe　lxix.
Bathe ſpryng come from a vaine of Brimſtone　　lxxiii.
Burnt leade good for *Chyrurgians*, 76.
Boies can kill the ſtrongeſt men with gunnes.　　lxxvi.
Bizabar a precious ſtone againſt poiſon and bloodie flixe · lxxvii.
Beefe good for the Cholorick, but for tender ſtomackes. lxxviii.
Beefe brothe againſt the flix. ibidē
Beare and Badgard, haue vertue

iii

An index of the booke of Simples.

in medicene. Fol. lxxxi.
Beare, Foxe, and Brocke, are good to helpe the palsey Ibidem.
Butter, the vertue of it lxxxv.

C.

Coughes, how to helpe it iii.
Corrupt fleume, to helpe it. Ibidē.
Colde coughes, to helpe it. viii.
Coloquintida is perilous ix.
Comforte against hotte choller in the stomacke. x.
Claret wine, warmeth ý body. xi.
Capers and Oliues, good for the Splene xv.
Cousleppes, or Pagles xxxv.
Cresses helpe the palsey xlii.
Cresses dooe helpe many infirmities. Ibidem.
Cartamus clenseth humours xlviii.
Clarie good for women li.
Cassiafistula cometh from Egipt. lvii.
Cassiafistula haue many vertues to helpe mankinde, it can not bee forborne emong vs. Ibidem.
Couetousnes and money, do make blinde, bothe Diuines, Lawers and Phisicions, and transforme them, from the natures of men, into infernall monsters. lxi.
Cubibes haue goodly vertur againste melancholie. lxix.
Ceruse cooleth inflamed sores. lxx.
Cardamon helpeth the fallyng sickenesse. Fol. lxxi.
Caphur called *Camphera*, of a greate tree in Inde. lxxii.
Campher will quench nature ibi.
Corall groweth in the sea. lxxvi.
Corall of twoo kindes Ibidem.
Calues flesche, the profite therof. 78
Celsus for a vomite Ibidem.
Castor stones doe helpe all cold infirmities, bothe men & women. 80.
Cranes are hotte, & increse sede 82.

D.

Dioscorides was an Heathen man, yet was he moste cunnyng in the natures of Simples. Fol. xxv.
Drinke but two dragmes of night shade in wine. xxxii.
Doronicus helpe digestion. lvi.
Dates good for nature lxvii.
Duckes flesche is verie hotte, and corrupted & vnholsome flesh. 82.
Doues flesche nourisheth colde folkes, and is verie hot it self. ibidē
Diuerse opinions, how Ambergrice is founde. xlix.
Dragons blood is verie good to stoppe the bloodie flixe. lxii.
Doctour William Turner, founde the verie *Tamarix* in Germanie, which is best for the splen. lxvii.

E.

Epithimum & *Cassia* helpeth the gaule 54
Edwardes, a foolishe imperik, had almoste killed Cuthbert Blunt, with *Elleborus albus*, at newcastle 67.
Egges of birdes, thre speciall thinges considered in them. lxxxv.
Egges of great foules, are noisom to the stomacke Ibidem.
Egges their whites helpe the iyen and quenche heate. Ibidem.
Eringium maris, to increase seede. xlvi.
Erth is the mother of euery thing and into yearthe eche creature shall retourne lxxxix.
Earth wormes are very wholsom for mankinde, so is their oile ib.
Euery thyng shall tourne to duste in the ende. Ibidem.

F.

For to helpe the biting of a dog. v.
For the braine Charte, a good medicene. xvi.
For the Stomacke, Liuer, and the Splen, a good medicen. xvii.
Fragaria haue vertue to coole. xxiiii.
For to helpe the Emeroides. Ibidē

From

An index of the booke of Simples.

From eating of Beanes, what Pithagoras ment. Fol. xxix.
For coddes, when thei are swelled a remedie. Ibidem
For grene woundes, vse Valarian to heale them xxxiii.
For to helpe the swellyng of the throate Ibidem.
For sore iyen, to helpe them. Ibidē
Flegmon is an apostumacion, gathered of corrupted bloode, into one place xlviii.
Framyngham, Netlestede, and Lethryngham, auncient Parks. liii.
For paines of the hedde, commyng of heate, a remedie. l.
From whence *Rhabarbe* do come. lvii
Filberdes are good after meate, & also for moiste reumes. lxviii.
Figges are bothe meate and medicene. lxx.

G.

Garlike will prouoke vrine, but it is not good for Collorike persones. Fol. iii.
Grene sichenes. vi.
Guaicum is of greater vertue, then the Bathe, or Burtons well, against the nosegaie of Naples 62
Good for the shortnes of wind vii.
Goodly Syruppe to clense the stomacke, is made of *Squilla* xxv.
Gose foote is a perilous herbe. xl.
Genesis. xxx. dooe not proue, that Mandrake helpeth concepciō. 44
Greate Spurge or *Ricinus* maketh strong vomites xlviii.
Goodly are the vertue of Rapes. 55
Galbanum is a Gum of greate vertue, to bryng forthe a ded child. xlii.
Gaules dooe growe like Acornes, and haue vertue to stop flixes. Folie. lxi.
Guaicum will clense the iyes. lxiii.
Gum Arabicke will restrain flixe, and blood in woundes lxiiii.

Glewe wil heale woundes. Ibidē
Gum Larix is equal, with the best Teribentin. Ib.
Golde the moste vndefiled mettall is good in Cordialles lxxv.
Generacion come again into corrupcion lxxxviii.
Gillowflowers are good for the harte, and helpeth woundes. 37.
Gose flesshe brede Melancholi. 82.

H.

How to correcte *Elleborus albus* that it shall not hurte. xix.
Honie is not good for hotte people for it will tourne moste soneste into Choller iii.
Honie is an heauenly dewe. Ibid.
Here how to preserue it. vi.
Hydropiper maie bee vsed in the place of Pepper. Ibidem.
How to knowe good Agarick. lvii
How to vse Radishe rootes lvi.
Hempe will kill wormes in the belie, and destroie seede of generacion. xxviii.

I.

If Harpe stringes were of one degree: vnpleasaunte were that hermonie. xxi.

L.

Lekes Fol. vi.
Letha a floodde, whose water did cause men to forget them selues when thei drinke of it. xi.
Lungworte so called, because it is like the lunges of man. xx.
Liguria, is a parte of Italie, from the hille Apeninus, vnto the Tuscan sea xxiii.
Lauender the swete vertue therof wholsome for colde folkes. xliii.
Lauēder healeth the sinewes. ibi.
Lunaria healeth woundes. xlv.
Lisimachus stoppeth bloodde, Lisimachus a king of Macedonia, foūd this herbe, when he was scholer

An index of the booke of Simples.

ler to *Calisthenes*, and one of Alexāders worthie captaines xlvi.
Lathiris or *Cataputia minor*, or the lesse Spurge. xlviii.
Lethargus helped with herbes, hotte and drie in the third degree. li.
Liquoris helpeth the kynges euill folio. lvi.
Lignum Aloes called *Agallachum*, whiche is Aromatike. lviii.
Lignum Aloes cometh not from Paradice, as fooles affirmeth, but frō Mondell, a citee of Inde. Ibidē.
Laudanum doeth helpe the heere frō fallyng, saith Paulus. lxiii.
Licium cometh from Licia. lxiiii.
Leuen dissolueth harde thynges, and make them soft. lxx.
Laurus called the Baie, againste the stone. lxxi.
Lead will coole and helpe sores. 75
Lapis naxius helpeth to increase heere. lxxvii.
Lambes fleshe is good rosted, euill sodden. lxxix.
Larkes helpe the chollicke, blacke birdes, Plouers, Sparrowes, Woodcockes, small birdes. 85
Lime helpe rotten sores. lxxiiii.
Liuers of beastes. lxxxvii.

M.

Mouseare is good for the fallinge sickenes. fol.ii.
Mouseare helpeth the throte. ibi.
Michell the *Chyrurgian* of Newe Castell. Ibidem.
Maister Roger Straunges medicene, brought frō Venice, written by a learned Italian doctor for runnyng of the raines. xiiii.
Markes of stripes in the skin. xv.
Marcurie helpeth concepcion. xx.
Maister Luke of London xxvii.
Many good medicenes made of Hempe seede. Ibidem.

Meale & Waxe, hath made greate marchauntes at Rome. xxxi.
Many good medicenes made of Houseleke. xxxvi.
Mandrake is moche like a manne or a womā, by crafte, for natur giueth none mannes shape to a beast, moche lesse to an herbe. 4
Mandrake was called *Circæ*, and also *Anthropomorphos*. Ibidem.
Madder with red rootes, against the pestilence. xlvii.
Many good vertues of Germander. xlix.
Many good vertues of *Aristolochia, longa, & rotunda*, lii.
Millen healeth many perilous sores. liii.
Misseltowe or Mislen, will make a good rippyng plaster, to heale the cornes in the feete. Ibidem.
Misseltow is not naturall in kind but a bastard branched, & growyng vpon some other tree. Ibid
Misseltowe is like to a straunger that increaseth & florisheth, by the hurte and losse of a fre borne man of his own naturall countrey or citee. liiii.
Mannes natures subiecte to many euilles, for wante of perfecte temperament. lxi.
Marche & Aprill are the best time to heale the poxe Ibidem.
Mirrhe preserueth the bodie from putrifaccion or rottyng. lxiii.
Mirtes haue vertue to restraine. folio. lxvi.
Manna of the Ashe trees in Italie. lxxii.
Medicenes made of the Ospraie. folio. lxxxi.
Muddie fish not wholsom. lxxxiii

N.

Nettle sedes wil serue in the place of Peper. xxxvii.

Note

An index of the booke of Simples.

Note, that the blacke Thistle rote with Swines greace and Brimstone, will heale Scabbes and iche. Fol. xlvii.

Note, Quid pro quo was giuen to the Lorde Wharton in his potage of ignoraunce, to his greate perill of life. xlviii.

Nutmegge, or Muske nutte, haue many singuler vertues against colde. lxviii.

Nutmegges, not good for hotte complexioned men Ibidem.

O.

Onions prouoke slepe. v.
Oile of Oliues best. xviii.
Olde sores Ibidem.
Oile of Roses Ibidem.
Olde Rushes, and old Curtiers be past pleasure. xxi.
Of the healyng comfortable herbe so named. xxv.
Of Poppie wilde and tame. xxvi.
Otes doe clense the Lunges. xxx.
Orpin healeth the morphue. xl.
Oile of Spicke doe warme. xliii.
Of sondery kindes of Crowe foote called *Ranunculi*, or little frogges grasse. xliiii.
Of the little beaste called Chamelion. xlvii.
Of Rumex the Docke, called Mōkes Rubarbe, or bastarde Mercurie. lxix.
Of the greate Docke, how it purgeth. Ibidem.
Of the herbe called Atripler, or Arige. Ibidem.
Orthopnæ is difficultie of winde. li.
Of the woodd of life, called Guaicum. lx.
Opponar doeth resolue lxiiii.
Oile of Roses for the hedde. lxxiii.
Of the fleshe of Oxen, Steres, Bulles and Calfes. lxxviii.

Oxe gaule clense the iyes. Ibidem
Oxe milte stoppe the flixe. Ibidem
Ospraies oile, good to put in water, to gather fishe readie to bee taken. lxxxi.
Of house Cockes, Capons, Chickens, their fleshe moche commended. Ibidem.
Of Dragons, whiche helpeth against the pestilence. vi.

P.

Pouertie is better emōg the common people, then aboundaunce of riches. xxi.
Perilous practicioners be here discribed. xxvii.
Ptisan made of Barley, wil quēch Choller. xxviii.
Pithagoras saied this *Faba abstinete.* that is, abstaine from Beanes, Plini and Tulli saieth, because of the ingenderyng of grosse humours, he forbad them. xxix.
Plutarcus saieth, it was to beware, to bee in office in a common wealth, because it is so perillous. Ibidem.
Pease came firste from Piso in Grece. Ibidem.
Pease growyng on the owne accorde, without Sowyng, where no yearth but stones be. xxx.
Plentie of Otes in Northe Humberlande. Ibidem.
Pimpinella is good againste the Pestilence. xxxiiii.
Poore mennes Peper. xxxvii.
Pæonia is called the chaste herbe. ibi.
Paralises, or Palsey xxxix.
Persicaria, or Peche leaues, growyng in marris grounde xlii.
Parietarie that groweth vppon stone walles. xlvii.
Perfect hartes reste, and true quietnesse of minde. xlix.

v.i. Psyllium

An index of the booke of Simples.

Psyllium called Flewort. l.
Purple fingers. Ibidem.
Pellitorie haue vertue to help the teeth. liiii.
Pellitorie will take awaie a colde feuer Ibidem
Philanthropos, Aperine, commonlie called Gosegrasse, and Harewede. Ibi.
Pistacia, a nutte of Siria, or Italia. lxvii.
Peper dissolueth, and consume moiste humours. lxxi.
Pirites lape, against proude fleshe. 78.
Porke. the commendacion therof. lxxix.
Pigges. Ibidem.
Pecockes fleshe is hote and moiste in the first degree. lxxxii.

Q.

Quinces are wholsome. Fol. xiii.
Quinces rawe hurteth. Ibidem.
Quercula minor, the little Oke, or Germander. l.
Quales vnwholsome. lxxiii.
Quickfiluer, or Mercurie. lxxiiii.

R.

Rawe herbes. ix.
Redde wine corrupteth blood. xi.
Rotten sores helped xxxviii.
Bellises of Jarowe, in the Bishopricke of Durisme. xxxix.
Roida healeth the hedde. lb.
Rose water and white wine, for al hotte causes. lviii.
Riach a Heathen kyng, found first Campher. lxxii.

S.

Sore eares to helpe them. Fol. ii.
Serpigo to helpe it. iii.
Swete breathes Fol. vi.
Stinkyng fleume, viii.
Stoppyng of the liuer. viii.
Sowe Thistle the vertue. x.
Stoppyng of vomites x.
Sickenesse in the lunges. Ibidem

Salt water healeth scabbes. xi.
Sodden bread not wholsome. xiii.
Surfettes of Ale and Beare xiii.
Swellynges to helpe them xiiii.
Sweete Prunes bee laxatiue, but tarte be bindyng xv.
Scabius for scabbes, it taketh the name of the propertie, the right name is Stoebe, or Spora, ther be twoo kindes of them. xvi.
Seede agmented. xviii.
Swete Calamus odoratus. Ibidē
Sir Thomas Rushe knight. xxi.
Sundrie names of Woodbinde, as Periclimenon, because it wind aboute the nexte trees and bushes, that it growe vnto. xxii.
Satyrus is a beaste, hauyng a hed like a manne, and bodie like a Goate, and named Gods of the wooddes, and thei firste founde this herbe of Venus, to stirre vp carnall luste. Ibidem.
Sanicle healeth woundes. xxiiii.
Sanicle is good for horse and keen Folio Ibidem.
Staphis Agria Pedicularis, a seede that will kille Lice in children, and Haukes. xxxi.
Solanum, Nightshade, or the slepynge Dwale. Ibidem.
Swallowe dūge will make blind, example of Tobias xxxiiii
Sheperdes purse, to stoppe blood. Folio. xxxv.
Sticados good for the splen. ibidē
Scaldyng and burnyng helped, 38.
Stitchewort will heale the stone, and heale woundes. xxxix.
Sauen of twoo kindes. Ibidem.
Sene helpeth the hedde, with all the sences. xl.
Sir Richard Alie. his pocion, Mathiolus vseth the same in Dioscoridem. Ibidem.
Saincte James worte, called Fellon

An index of the booke of Simples.

lon wede.	fol. xl.
Spatula will kill Lice.	Ibidem.
Swete Botris.	xliii.
Safron haue many vertues.	xlvi.
Sunderie kindes of Spurge, but yet very perillous, the greate Spurge and the seconde excepted, for thei be good.	xlviii.
Shifte water oftentymes, when Atriplex is sodden.	l.
Sauerie the vertue.	li.
Swete Muske is pleasaunt.	lviii.
Swete thynges be good for mankinde, but yet abused of youthfull wantons, it is not to be suffred in them.	lix.
Swete Gloues, their profite.	ibid.
Scepters for kinges, and the Heathen Idols of Ebenus.	Ibidem
Sagapen, or Serapinum, a goodly gumme.	lxiii.
Sagapen will helpe the Lunges, and splene.	lxiiii.
Scamonie is perilous, except it be first prepared.	lxv.
Suber the Corke, will stop bloode and flixe	lxvi.
Sinamon.	lxviii.
Sebesten will helpe struma.	lxx.
Sanders doe coole the hedde, and reconcile sleape, and helpeth the Goute.	lxxi.
Suger of the Cane.	lxxii.
Spicknarde of Spain. helpeth the braine.	Ibidem
Sondrie opinions of Campher.	ib.
Sulpher, or Brimstone.	lxxiii.
Sonderie kindes of Roses, all of greate vertue	Ibidem
Smigma, or Sope.	lxxiiii.
Sope will kill tetters.	Ibidem.
Spodium stop blood.	lxxv.
Salt, what it is in vertue.	Ibidē.
Salte haue vertue to warme and drie.	Ibidem.
Salt not good for leane persones.	
Sir Jhō Delauall, a good knight. Folio.	lxxv.
Sal Gemmæ.	Ibidem.
Sal armoniac.	Ibidem.
Sal amoniac doe clense the skin.	lxxvi.
Salt of Inde.	Ibidem.
Sal Niter, or Peter, for gun pouder.	ib.
Spuma nitri or Barach.	Ibidem.
Salt of Mari mortuum, where as Sodome was.	Ibidem.
Spuma maris.	Ibidem.
Spuma maris do make clene the teth.	ib.
Spunge of the sea.	Ibidem.
Spunge good for woundes.	ibidē.
Spunges newe are good, but olde are euill.	Ibidem
Spunge stones dooe breake the stone in the raines.	Ibidem.
Saphirus resist poison.	lxxvii.
Swines blood	lxxix.
Swine of Inde haue hornes.	ibi.
Swannes fleshe, cholorick.	lxxxii.
Swannes syng.	Ibidem.
Soche meate, soche coplexion.	ibi.
Sea fishe wholsomer, then that of the freshe water.	lxxxiii.
Shell fishes.	Ibidem.
Sundrie kindes of Chese.	lxxxv.
Stones of Oxe bladder.	lxxxvii.
Scorpion breake the stone.	lxxxix.
Snaile helpe ache	Ibidem.

T.

The Arabians call that Nill, whiche wee name Viscum, or Misseltowe.	Fol. i.
The splenaticke loue	Ibidem
To increase heere.	iii.
To cure Serpigo.	Ibidem.
To clense the face.	Ibidem.
The propertie of a good huswife.	4
The king of Bees, & his armie.	ibi.
The iuce of Sage, helpeth consepcion. An example.	b.
To stoppe bloode runnyng at the mouthe how.	Ibidem.

r.ii.   To

An index of the booke of Simples.

To kille the Canker, and quenche Robin goodfelowes feuer. Fol. v.
To clense the stomacke. vi.
To breake the stone. Ibidem.
To washe feete. Ibidem.
Twoo kindes of Fenell. Ibidem.
To helpe a moiste reume. viii.
To helpe the sight. Ibidem.
To helpe the kynges euill. ibidem
To make fatte. Ibidem.
To kill wormes. Ibidem.
To gargarise the hedde ix.
To helpe the iyes. Ibidem.
To prouoke vrine Ibidem.
To clense Leprosie. Ibidem.
To increase milke. x.
To abate the luste. Ibidem.
To kill wormes. Ibidem.
To helpe the Collike Ibidem.
To make swete breathe. Ibidem.
The hedde Ibidem.
To loose the bellie Ibidem.
To helpe the splene. Ibidem.
The goodly vertues of common water xii.
The cause why Nilus doe flow. ib.
The cause of Barnacles. Ibidem.
The cause of Christall. Ibidem.
The effectes of the Bathes, at the toune of Bathe Ibidem.
The dedde sea. Ibidem.
The meane baked bread ye best. xiii
The operacion of Peares. Ibidē.
The operacion of Aples xiiii.
The operacion of Peaches. ibide.
The operacion of Quinces. ibidē.
The operacion of Cheries. ibidem
To comfort digestion xv.
Twoo kindes of Aloes. Ibidem.
To helpe watrie iyes. Ibidem.
To clense choller and fleume. ibi.
To comfort the harte xvi.
The propertie of Uinegar. xvii.
To helpe the Goute. Ibidem.
Theophrastus of Setwall. ibidem
To helpe the splene. Ibidem.

Tyme can not be called again. 18.
To waste winde in the body, ibid.
To digest cold herbes Ibidem
The brain comforted Ibidem
To nese xix.
The belle woodbinde, *Smylax*. Ibidē.
The vertue of Smalage, Louage, Alexander, Percelie, is to open places, whiche stoppeth vrine, and winde. xxiii.
The vertues of Perselies. Ibidem
To heale a bruse, or a fall xxv.
To heale Ringwormes, and Tetters, xxvi.
To moue sweate Ibidem.
The vertue of Lint oile xxvii.
The miserie of vnthriftes semeth pleasaunte, but shame and pain is the ende. xxviii.
The innocente sometyme dieth in the iyes of men, miserable. Ibi.
The consideracion of Hempe in Phisicke. Ibidem.
To helpe the Lunges. Ibidem.
The bread and drinke of the poore, bee the life of the needie: and he that take it awaie from them, is as a murderer. Ibidem.
The old Romaines wer more humble then the newe Romaines, and late Popes, in kepyng names of base titles Ibidem.
The tyme of Cicero. Ibidem.
The beste Pease potage. xxx.
Tares Ibide
Triticum, Wheate, or our bread. ibidē.
To feede on Bran, maketh a man leane, but flower bryngeth fatnesse Ibidem.
The very Diuines and Dunsmen, did neuer agree generally. xxxi.
The sunderie kyndes and natures of wheate. Ibidem.
To kil wormes with Lupines. ib.
Three kindes of Henbane. xxxii.
The white Henbane is vsed in medicene.

An index of the booke of Simples.

dicene. fol.xxxii.
The moste colde herbe, and a poyson. Ibidem.
The death of Socrates was with wine, & the iuce of Humlock. ib.
To helpe hym, whiche haue drunk Humlocke Ibidem.
Twoo kindes of Triple grasse. 33.
Triple grasse hath many vertues, and excelleth againt poison. ib.
To heale woundes and sores. xxxv
Tormentill doe growe, and diminishe with the Wine. xxxvi.
Turmentill kepe shepe from the rotte. Ibidem.
To make the vrine swete. xxxviii.
To clense the Morphewe. xli.
To kill Lice Ibidem.
To heale woundes Ibidem
To gather Iuie gum xlii.
To drawe teeth without pain. ib.
To kill brode wormes, in the chest or bellie Ibidem
The dedde Nettle Ibidem
To helpe the flixe Ibidem.
To helpe the guttes xliii.
To stop the termes of women. ibi.
This place proueth not, that Mandrake will helpe conception, but Mandrake will clense the Matrix, or caste forthe the ded child from the same, then it will kille the liuyng seede. xliiii.
The vertues of Mandrake, is to make one to slepe. Ibidem.
To poyson Wolues and Foxes. xlv
The beste Safron of this worlde, where it is xlvi.
The sea Thistle, called *Eringus*, whiche is so called, because if the roote bee sodden, and conserued with Honie and Cloues, it will preserue nature, or lift hym vp, whiche is decaied, it maie come of *erigo, gis, erexi*, to lift vp, or repaire folio. Ibidem.

The Boze or carle Thistle, called *Chamelion*. fol.xlvii.
The Thistle healeth the pestilence folio. Ibidem.
To vomite. Ibidem.
To purge Choller. xlviii.
Tithimalus Charatias, or *Lathyris* is good in medicene, to purge Melancholi Choller, and Fleume. Ibidem.
The greateste threasoure of this worlde, is a quiet minde. xlix.
Thei, whiche call *Rumex* with the golden Sande Mercurie, dooe greatly erre. Ibidem.
The Kynges euill. Ibidem.
To dye the heere. l.
To clense the stomacke, Ibidem.
The oile of Calamintes, do warm the bodie, and is good againste the Sciatica. li.
To heale sores with *Brionia*. lii.
To clense the face with *Brionia*. ibid.
To cause vrin to passe plentifully. 55
The difference betwene Rubarbe, and Rapontike. lvii.
The crueltie of the Barbarians, is to burne the Spice trees and plantes. Ibidem.
To comfort the spirites. lviii.
The beaste, whiche giueth Muske is like a Goate: that which bringeth ziuet, is like a Catte. lix.
The blaunchyng of Muske. ibide.
Twoo Witches in Suffolke, charmed with Ebenie Beades. lx.
The pore of Fraunce. Ibidem
Three kindes of *Guaiacum*, but the white is moste excellent. Ibide.
The consideracion of *Guaiacum*. ibid
Three moste notable and beste instrumentes of the comon welth the Diuine, the Lawer, and the Phisicion. lxi.
The moste excellent and beste maner, to seeth *Guaiacum* in composicions, with other Simples, to

r.iii. clense

An index of the booke of Simples.

cleanse the Pore, from all the members of the bodie. Fol.lxii.
The diate for the Pore, shortlie declared. Ibidem.
Tartar, made of wine Lies. Ibidem.
Terra Sigillata stoppeth blood. Ibidem.
Thus called Frankensence, or Olibanum. Fol.lxiii.
To clense Galbanum. Ibidem.
To help ye prickyng of sinewes. ib.
Three glewes, ye is of beastes skinnes of Fish, and of Corne. lxiiii.
Terebinthus, or Terebintin, hath great vertue to heale. Ibidem.
The vertue of Terebintine. lxv.
The euill crafte of subtile Apothicaries, doe moche harme. ibidē.
To know good Diacridon. Ibidē.
To seme young, how to doe it. ibi.
To purge tender persones. ibidem
To clense sore iyen. Ibidem.
The Quarce, or Oke tree, wil stop the bloodie flire, or blood, so wil the Barke, Akorns, or Leaues, with the cuppes. lxvi.
The Beeche tree with his fruicte, will stoppe flires. Ibidem.
To stoppe the flire, called *Dysenteria*, and *Tenasmus* with Mirtes. ibidē.
To kill wormes in the belie, with Coloquintida. Ibidem.
To help the teeth, with Coloquintida. Ibidem.
Turpit, whiche purgeth flegme. 67
Tamarinds, or *Tamardactylos* Ibidem.
To helpe Emeroides. Ibidem.
Tamariscus is a little tree, like Quickbene Ibidem.
Tamarix doe helpe the splen. Ibidem
Tamarix against the flire. Ibidem.
The vertue of the pistace nuts. ib.
To helpe broken bones. lxix.
To helpe the splen Ibidem
To kille Lice Ibidem.
To resolue. lxx.
To couer a bone with flesshe. lxxi.

Three kindes of Sanders. Fo.lxxi
The greate vertue of Manna, for mankinde Ibidem.
To cause slepe lxxii.
To stop the whites, and runnyng of the raines. Ibidem.
To clense scabbes lxxiii.
The Rose, a friende to the braine, and iyen. Ibidem.
The best Roses be in Italie. ibidē.
To drye Salt Fol.lxxv.
The flowyng of salt at Nilus. ibi.
To clense sore iyen. lxxvi.
To stoppe blood. Ibidem.
The Magarite or Pearle, good in Cordials lxxvii.
The Magnit stone. lxxviii.
Cripes. lxxix.
The Winter Dere, better then the Sommer. lxxx.
The lunges of the Dere. Ibidem.
The pouder of the Hare, for the stone Ibidem.
The Urchin, or hedghog. Ibidem.
The Weesell, good against the fallyng sickenesse, and *Struma, Anginæ*, or swellyng of the throate. lxxxi
The Fore. Ibidem.
To helpe baldnesse. Ibidem.
The Barnacle of Scotlande, neuer laie Egges, but are bredde onelie of the Ocean Sea: reade *Gesnerus de Auibus lib. iij.* lxxxii.
Three thynges considered in Fishe Folio. lxxxiii.
Tallowe of male beast, are hotter then the female. lxxxvi.
To preserue fatte. lxxxvii.
The prouidence of God. xc.
Trouble hath so hindred me, that I am constrained, presentlie to staie in this little worke. Ibidē

V.

Uiolettes be great coolers, and to colde for the harte. Fol.vi.
Uomites

An index of the booke of Simples.

Vomites strain the bodie. xvii.
Valerian maketh salues of great goodnesse. xxxiii.
Vrtica the Netle. Fol. xxxvii.
Viola Lutea the yellowe Violette, the walle Gillowflower. Fol. xlviii
Very gentlemen, springeth not by extorcion, but by true seruyng their princes, and liuing of their owne, hurtyng not their poore neighbours, preferryng the fauour of the countrey, before lucre, whiche is their chief threasure. Fol. liii.
Virgill. Ibidem.
Vngula Caballina, Horshoue. Fol. liiii.
Vnguentum Egipsiacum. Fol. lxxiiii.

W.

Wormewood hath many vertues. Folio ii.
Welshemennes drinke. Fol. iiii.
Where plentie of Onions dooe growe. Fol. vi.
Woundes from corrupcion. viii.
White wine. Fol. xi.
Wine is an enemie to children. ib.
Wine moderatly vsed, comforteth. Folio Ibidem.
What kinde of water is best. ibidē.
White Poppie is the beste. xxv.
When Venice first began. xxix.
Wheate wil degenerat out of kind that is, from Wheate to Dar-nell. Fol. xxxi.
Walworte maketh medicene for the Goute, and paines in the iointes. Fol. liiii.
When Ebenus came first to Rome Folio. lix.
What euill haue happened, thorowe the abusyng of Guaicum emong the Imperikes. Fol. lxi.
Walnuttes against poison, as Mithridatus reporteth. Fol. lxvii.
Why hogges are diseased. lxxix.
William Hilton, letted William Bullein to finishe his booke of healthfull medicenes. lxxxiiii.
Whate the vertue thereof. lxxxv.
Wine, Oile, and Breade, Gods giftes. Fol. xc.

X.

XXX. Leaues of Azarabaccha doe serue in infusion, but other wayes three, fowere, or fiue, dooe suffice. Fol. i.

Y.

Yellowe and Purple fingers. fo. l.
Yearth wormes. Fol. xc.

FINIS.

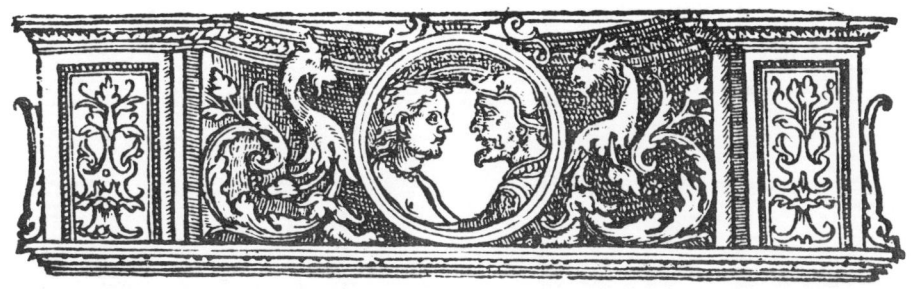

¶Here after insueth a little

Dialogue, betwene twoo men, the one called Sorenes, and the other Chyrurgi: Concernyng Apostumacions, and woundes, their causes, and also their cures, gathered by *VVillyam Bulleine*, the Aucthour, and collectour of all these Dialogues, conteined within this booke. Verie profitable to euery reder, and true obseruer of them. And first beginneth the Sore man to speake, as foloweth.

¶ *A little Dialogue*, betwene **Fol.ij.**
Sorenes, and Chyrurgi.

Sorenes.

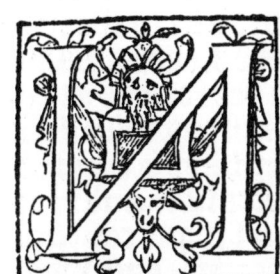

NOw our old frendes haue doen, all their long talke verie profitable to eche other: and also to as many as haue heard them. I trust we shall spend the time to the like effecte, with no lesse profite, then *Marcellus* and *Hillarius*, whiche had comforte, in sekyng foorthe the swete flowers, of sundrie shapes in the fielde, to their no small delite, all this laste Sommer. But now the horie stormie darcke Winter weather approcheth neare, as *Parsius* saieth: Admouit iam bruma foco te basse Sabino. Bassus colde Winter, doe drawe the winde to the fire, in the Mountaine called *Sabinus*, saieth he. Colde weather draweth nere, *Flora* is fled, *Borias* perseth, and causeth all beastes to tremble, bereuyng theim of their pleasaunt Sommer shroudes, vnder the swete leaues of greene trees. The yearth is newe couered with white Snowes, harde crakyng Ice, and horie Frostes. Birdes dooe quiuer and quake, lurkyng in the holes of Rockes, and old barnes, for their relief. The beastes with slender emptie bellies, and cold trebling carkasses, doe cluster in flockes, or shroude theim selues vnder the naked bushes, with their faces from the fierse windes. These shorte daies, and long nightes, causeth bothe man and beastes, to drawe together in warme places, and close houses. Nowe the poor Bees, if thei laboured well in Sommer, thei haue their close swete delites in warme Heues in Winter. Soche doe nature giue prouidence to sundrie creatures, to fore see daungers to come, as hunger, cold storme. Furdermore, God and Nature, haue from the beginning, taught bothe man and beast, not onely to releue thē selues in health, but in the tyme of sicknes and sorenes: eche of theim are taught, how to corrette, stoppe, and purge soche humours, as doe offende nature.

Thus man artificially, and beastes naturally, haue a wonderfull prouidence, whereby the glorie of our Lorde and God dooe appere, of no small maiestie, and deuine power: whiche prepared his insensible creatures, Herbe, Grasse, stone. &c. for his sensible creatures. As Man, Beaste, Fishe, Foule, Serpentes. &c. And one of thē, to be bothe meate and medicen, for an other, his name be praised therefore. Amen.

Sabinus a famous Mountain in Italy
Flora a Goddes of Flowers, a harlot of Rome.
Borias the Northeast winde.

Chirurgj.

SObeit my good brother, you haue reuerently spoken, of the deuine prouidence. I perceiue you did heare and marke well, what ende our good friende *Hillarius* made, praisyng God with the holie Prophete Dauid. Psal.ciii.

Sorenes.

YE forsothe, although I be sore in bodie, yet I trust to begin with good comfort, with a pleasant *Comodi*, and not to ende in a fearefull *Tragedie*. For I haue heard saie in the writing of the holie Euangell, whiche reporteth from the mouthe of God, saiyng:

Tragedy begun euer euill and ende the same.

A Dialogue

Firste seke Gods kyngdome. saiyng: before all thinges seke the kyngdome of God, and then shall al thinges be giuen vnto you. If all thinges shalbe giuen vnto thē, whiche praieth vnto God, then shall cōfort be giuen to the carefull: breade to the hungrie, libertie to the thrall. And finally, healthe to the sicke and sore. &c. As example, Christ gaue healthe vnto the Lepors, Lame, Blinde. &c. Euen so I truste, beyng a sore bodie, to bee releued at the mightie handes of God, or through hym, by his cunnyng ministers, emong whom you are one, whiche haue dooen many happie cures, as I haue harde. Well, saie furder, wee haue presente occasion, and tyme conueniente giuen vnto vs bothe: you to warne, you labour continually, and I again for health, paciently to suffer and learne some wholsome doctrine, for my reliefe. For if the bilders of houses, wherein our bodies bee shrouded, be not to be forborne: moche lesse the repairers of the bodies of men, wherein the soule remaineth, can be spared, when either wounde, sore, botche, or soche like assaulteth our mortall mancion of the bodie. To conclude with you I will, followyng all this shorte Winters daie, in the warme house, to demaunde questions, as well as I can: for my health and learnyng.

Chyrurgj.

Saie on your mynde a Gods blessyng.

Sorenes.

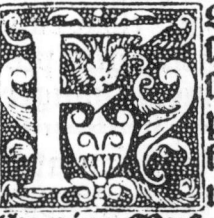

Ignoraunce.

Curtasie.

For that I neuer did drinke vpon the swete flud, or well spryng of Philosophie, in any tēder yeres: neither haue slepte vnder the noble mountaine, and swete twoo topped hille, called *Pernasus*. Furder, I did neuer slumber, or forgotte my self, through golden slepes vpon *Helycon*, that noble high hille and pleasaunt place: where sometyme the nine Muses, gaue forthe their Sacred giftes. But rather I haue drunke and bibbed, vpon the cold seuerus fludde, of the pale water called *Perenne*: and washed my self in the darcke streames, of the forgetfull hellishe broke *Latha*, in cleane forgetfulnes. Therefore to saie the truthe of my self, my sore bodie, and doltishe braine, can receiue but smalle health and comfort, except it shall please thee, sentlie to heare me: For curtesie is a goodly schole maistres, and comfortable are swete Cordials, and wholsome salues: and bitter woordes are bityng corosiue, to feble myndes.

Chyrurgj.

Soft Chirurgians make foule sores. You saie the truth. Euen so, soft *Chyrurgians* maketh foule sores swete woordes are pleasaunt to women, and young childrē: but plaine true tales, ought to be emong men of knowlege, without curious circumstaunce, or Rhethoricall colours. Therefore, go to your matter, the daie is cold and shorte, the tyme passeth spedely awaie, and can neuer come again.

Sorenes.

Forsoth

betwene Sores and Chyrurgi. Fol.ij.

FOrsothe that is moste certain: therefore let vs spende the tyme well. For my parte, I would knowe howe to heale my sores, whiche you doe see here present, before and behinde.

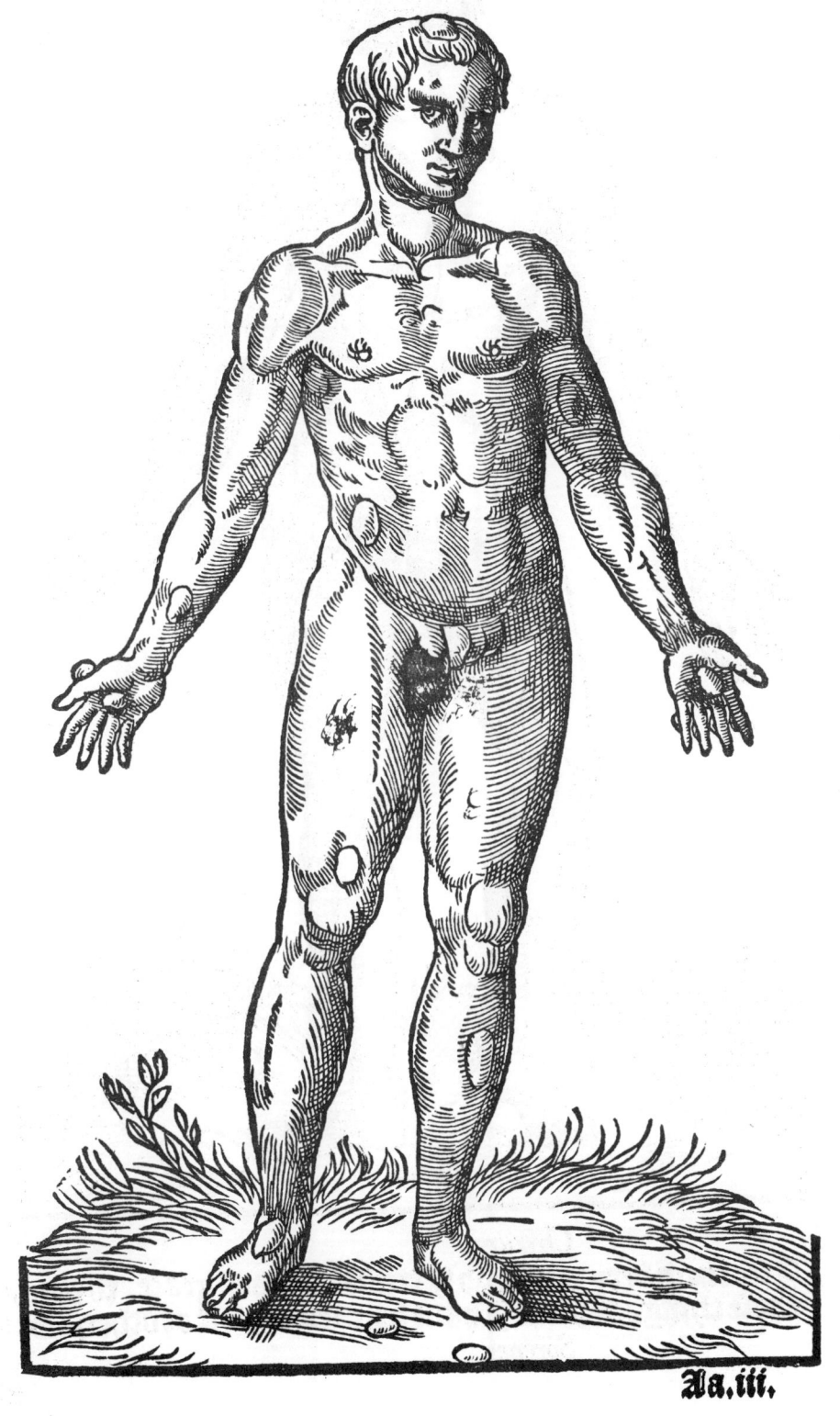

Aa.iii.

A Dialogue

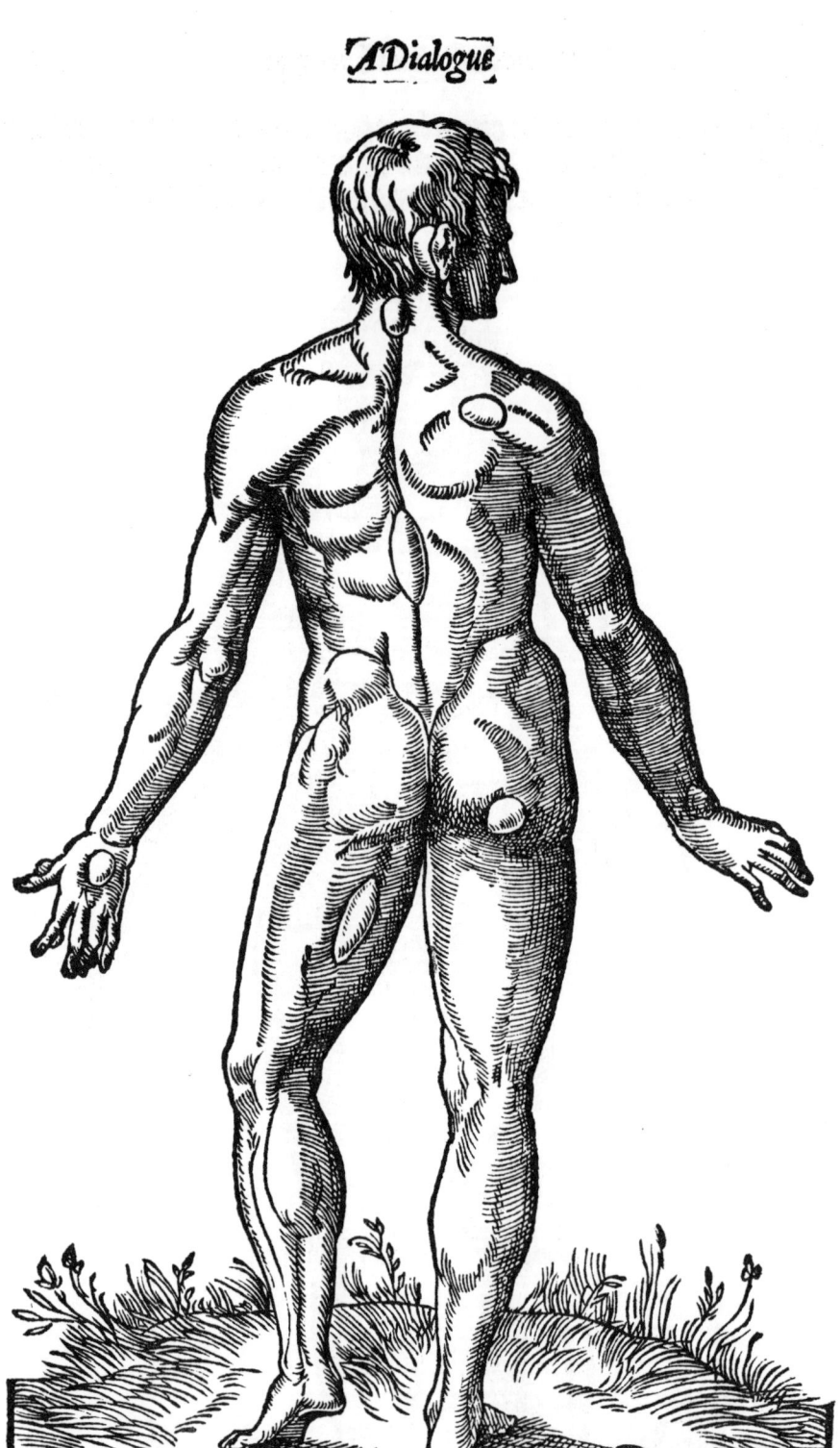

Chyrurgi.

I see them very well, and I truste by Gods grace, to teache you those things, whiche I haue learned my self of others, for cure.

Sorenes.

What

betwene Sores and Chyrurgj. Fol.iiij.

What men of credite, bothe olde and newe, haue written of this moste worthie Arte, of the hande crafte of *Chyrurgj*, or meanes thereunto, shewe me some of their names, for to incorage me to loue this saied arte.

Chyrurgj.

I Shall call to minde, and note with penne, a nomber of worthie men, bothe olde and newe: Heathen and Christians, straungers, and Englishemen, although a great nomber, whom I knowe not in this realme, whiche be worthie persones, and cunnyng men, profitable to our common wealthe. As the moste worthie Fraternitie, of the *Chyrurgians*, of the moste auncient and famous citee of London: wheras, through learned Lectours, and the Secrete Anothomies, by, and through the learned Doctor M. Ihō Kaius: reueilyng vnto this fraternitie, the hidden iuelles, and precious threasours of *C. L. Galenus*, shewyng hym self to be the seconde Linacar, whose steppes he foloweth. — Doctor Kaius.

Who shal forget the most worthy doctor Williā Turner, whose learned actes, I leaue to the wittie commendaciōs, and immortall praise of *Conradus Gesnerus*. Yet his boke of Herbes, will alwaies grow grene, and neuer wither, as longe as *Dioscorides* is had in minde, emong vs mortall wightes. The noble estate of knightes, emong the Englishe, or Bruteshe nacion, whiche of them did euer in race, giue a trippe, out runne, or wanne the victorie of sir Thomas Eliot knight: whiche haue planted soche fruitfull trees, that his graftes dooe growe, in eche place in this our common wealthe, and his Castle of Health, can not decaie. — Doctor Turner. Sir Thomas Eliot Knight.

Thomas Faire Doctor of Phisike, is not dedde, but is transformed and chaunged, into a newe nature immortall: he haue lefte a peece of darke yearth behinde him, and is gone ouer Lethas fludde, forgetting this worlde: and with pleasure spendeth the tyme, emong the heauenly Muses, vnder the twoo topped hill of *Pernasus* hill. Full well he knew *Plini*, whiche taught the goodnes of cleane creatures, and also the pestiferous venome of dedly Melancholie Serpentes, and their present remedie, by the vertues of herbes of sondrie kyndes. — Thomas Faire doctor

Doctor Androwe Borde, wrote also well of Phisicke, to profite the common wealth withall. This man declared, how he was in a greate citee, where he did see three hellishe Tragidies: the one was *Nullus ordo*, the seconde was, *Stridor dentium*, the thirde was, *Horror inhabitans*, and yet this Borde was a birde of this neste or cage, called Rome, whereof he maketh this reporte. I will not forgette Maister Thomas *Paguinellus*, or Pannell, whiche haue plaied the good seruaunte, to the common wealthe, in translatyng good bookes of Phisicke. — Doctor Androw Borde did see at Rome, no order, gnashyng of treth, dwellyng in wretchednesse. Thomas Pannell.

Doctor William Kunyngham haue well trauailed, like a good soldiour, against the ignoraunt enemie: setting forthe the commendaciō praise, and profite of Astronomie, Cosmographie, and Geographe. &c. How well was he seen in tongues, learned in Artes and in Scien- — Doctor William Kuningham.

Ja.iiii. ses,

A Dialogue

ſes, naturall and morall. A father in Phiſicke, whoſe learnyng gaue lybertie to the ignoraunte, with his *whetſtone of witte, Caſtell of knowlege*: and finally, giuyng place to ſlidyng nature, died hymſelf in bondage or priſon. By whiche death he was deliuered and made free, and yet liueth in the happie lande, emong the Lauriat learned, his name was Doctor Recorde, with many other, whiche I muſt giue place to tyme. For the vertues bee not vnknowen in Phiſicke, and *Chyrurgi*, although I name thē not. Yet if you doe further delite, without diſdain to knowe the names of them, whiche haue been excellent in the worthie arte of *Chyrurgi*, Phiſicke. &t. I will declare their names in order, as I haue noted and knowen. As followyng hereafter by letters.

Doctor Recorde.

Achilles.
Aeſulapius.
Aetius.
Agregator.
Aguſtinus Doct.Medic.
Albucaſis Mahumitan.
Alexander Aphradencis.
Alexander Benedictus Veronencis.
Alfonſius Seruius Nepolitanus.
Amatus Luſitanus.
Antonius Fuminellus.
Ariſtotiles Philoſ.Prince.
Arcagathus Peloponenſis.
Auicena lib.iiij.Fen.vj.
Arnoldus de Noua Comen.
Aurelius Cornelius Celſus.
Albertus Magnus.

B.

Bartholomej de proprietatibus rerum.
Bartholmej Montognani.
Bartleus Doc.Medi.
Bunus Doct.Medi.Cant.
Butts Doct.Medi.

C.

C.Plinius ſecundus.
Caſſius Iatroſophiſta.
Chyronem.
C.L.Galenus.

Conradus Geſnerus.
Conſtantius Cataplaſmatis.
Carrus Doct.Medic.
Clemens Doct.Medi.
Caduellus Medicus Doct.Oxo.
Chamerus Doct.Medic.

D.

Damocrates.
Damoxine.
Diocles.

E.

Eucharius.
Euelpiſtus.
Euonimus.
Edwardus Medicus Doc.Cant.
Edmundus Chyrurgus Ebor.

G.

Gariopontj.
Gorgias.
Genus Medic.Doct.Oxo.
Guido Caliacus.
Gulehemus Placentius.
Gulihelmus Turnerus Med.Doc.Cant.
Guilhelmus Variguanj.
Gulihelmus Kunynghamus Med.Doct.
Galus Chyrurg.Lon.

H.

Hactherus medicus Doct.Canta.

Hely-

Helyodorus.
Heraclides Larentius.
Heraclius.
Hera Cappedocis.
Hyeron.
Hieronimus Brunſ.
Hieronimus Cardanus.
Hyppocrates Coy. Princ. Medicorum.
Hugo.
Huycus Medic. Doct.

I.
Iacobus Hollerus.
Iacobus Ruffius.
Iohannes Kayus Medic. Doct. Cant.
Iohannes Almanner.
Iohannes Bauery.
Iohannes Barnardus.
Iohanes Frerus Doct. Medic. Cant.
Iohannes Manerdus.
Iohannes Tagaulius.
Iohannes Vigo Genuenſis.
Iohannes Porterus Norwic.
Hillius. id eſt Albanus Mōtanus doc. me.

L.
Lucas Euangel. Medic:
Lynakerus Docter Medic.
Lamfrancus Mediolanenſis.
Leonardus Bareapalia.
Leonardus Fucchius.
Ludouicus Bonaciolus.
Ludouicus Cælius.
Langtonus Doct. Medic. Canta.
Lurkinus Doct. Medic. Cant.

M.
Machaon.
Mantias.
Martianus Corinbekus Docto. Medic.

Marianus Chyrurgus.
Meges Chyrurgus.
Michaelis Angelus Blodus.
Maſterus Doct. Medic.
Montanus.

N.
Nicolaus Maſſa.
Nicolaus Myrepſi.
Nicolaus Pol.

O.
Oribaſius.
Otho Brumfelſius.

P.
Podalyrius.
Paulus Ægineta.
Petrus Andrias Matthiolus.
Petrus Tolenus.
Philopenus.
Podalirius.

Q.
Querenus.

R.
Raſis tractatus.
Rogerus.
Rolandus Cappellatus.
Robartus Balthropus Chyrurgus.

S.
Sebaſtianus Aquilanj.
Socrate Chyrurgus.
Soranus.
Saſtratus.
Symon Ludfordus Doct. Medic. Oxo.

T.
Tertius Damianus.
Theodorus Epiſt.
Theodorus Priſſianus.
Theophraſtus Peraſelpus.
Thomas Eliotus eques Angl.

Thomas

A Dialogue

Thomas Philologus Rauen.   *Vidus Vidius Florent.*
Thomas Colphus Pharmacopolus Ang.   *VVendius Medic. Doct. Can.*
Tryphon.   *Vickarius Chyrurgus Lon.*

V.

And thus I dooe ende of the names of many menne, besides no small nomber of thē, whiche haue, and doe professe this worthie Arte, bothe of Phisicke, and *Chyrurgj*, to the greate profite of eche common wealth.

Sorenes.

Why doe you rather call Surgerie an Arte, then a Science, whiche I take it to be.

Chyrurgj.

what is called *Chirurgia*

Because it taketh the name of a Greke Nowne, called *Chir*, an hande in Englishe, and *ergon* ministerie, and although bothe together called *Chirurgia* or hande misterie, should be rather hande craft, and not a science: and this is my probacion of this diffinicion. For there bee twoo kindes of *Chyrurgj*, the first is *Theorica*, whiche is the mother schoolemistres, nourishe, and learner of this profitable Arte, without the whiche the workers thereof, haue but one iye, and seeth this Arte

Two kindes of *Chirurgia*

but through a darke paire of spectacles. The seconde and laste part, is called *Practica*, whiche is to put in vse, that whiche *Theorica* haue learned hym, although *Practica* bee very aunciente, and to some men fortunate, for healyng is the singuler gifte of God, as the Apostle saieth. Yet the former called *Theorica*, is reckoned a science, how beit vnprofitably, and by tyme vsurped. Also the laste named *Practica*, I meane not as the common people doe terme euery trifeler, or light doer, to be a practicioner. But rather he is a practicioner, that is able to seperate the qualities of ointementes, and to deserne perfectly of Herbes, Gummes, stones, trees, fruites. &c. And to compounde simples togither, through knowlege, iudgement, and quicke inuencion. For compounded ointmentes maketh plasters, and aleieth Cerotes, accordyng as it is seen in the worthy workes of *Nicolaus Valarius Cordus, Leonardus Fuchius. &c.* And when the bodies of their pacientes bee sore or sicke, then the practicioner must minister, and the medicen must take his effect, with nature & God to giue the health, through his good instrument, whom the auncient learned men doe terme, the artificiall *Chyrurgian*, to whom greate reuerence was giuen, & wer in greate estimacion somtyme, but now not very moche.

Sorenes.

What is then the cause, that so many *Chyrurgians* now a daies, bee despised, and liue so basely, and are coumpted the abiectes of the common people: if the *Chyrurgians* should so bee honoured, as thou saiest thei should be, beyng repairers of decaied men?

Chyrurgj.

Repairers,

betwene Sores and Chyrurgj. Fol. vj.

Repairers? No, rather destroiers, marrars, and mangelers, of the bodies of menne, women, and children: and these men, lacketh not onely learnyng, and knowlege, but also witte, and honestie, through whose wickednes the auncient practicioners, and sober dooers in *Chyrurgj*, bee greatly abused emong the common people: as commonly we see the good men are despised, through the light behauiour of the wicked. For vnder the name of *Chyrurgy*, many young men, liues in the Sentuarie of idelnes, forsakyng their owne handie crafte: and many craftie varlettes, committing sonderie crimes, eftsones thei doe flee into straunge countries, wandering vp and doune. And what bee their shiftes? Mary, to buy some grosse stuffe, with a boxe of salue, and cases of tooles, to set foorthe their slender market withall: For Dogge leaches and Tinkers shall haue worke in euery village. Then fall thei to Palmestrie, and telling of fortunes, daily deceiuing the simple: like vnto the swarmes of the vacabounde Egypcians, and some that call them selues Iewes, whose iyes were so sharpe as Lynx, for thei se all thinges, and some of them talketh of *Nicromancia*, deluding and mocking the people with their knackes, straunge lookes, prickes, domifiyng, and figuring, with soche like fantasies: fainyng that thei haue familiers and glasses, whereby thei maie finde thinges that be lost, and besides theim an infinite nomber of olde toltishe Witches, with blessynges for the faire, and coniuryng of cattell: And that is the cause, that so moche idlenesse and infidelitie is practised, in this euill estate. Of lande leapers, and many simple inhabitours, worse then the subtell Limentours, and begging Freers, whiche deceiued many thorow Ipocrisie: and more hurtfull then the craftie Pardoners, whiche preached remission of sinnes, in euery Parishe Churche, with Belles and Pardones from Rome. These be worse then vacabound beggers, robbing the people, and more hurtfull then priuate murderers, in killyng men, for lacke of knowlege: and in warres often tymes, the good souldiour is caste awaie soner, through the villanie of soche *Chyrurgians*, then by the weapon, and hand of thenemie. And this is a lamentable and a moste pitifull case, and hurtfull to the common wealth: but for asmoche as mankinde, beeyng the principall creature of almightie God, the Angelles excepted, whiche dooe daily beholde the presence of his maiestie. Yet this mankinde, through daiely casualties and misse happes, eftsones is hurte with faules, brused with stripes, pricked with Spere or Dagger, wounded with weapon, burnt with fire, bitten with mad Dogges, whereby his bodie standeth in daily daunger, and perill of death. Therfore poore brother *Sorenes*, like as I doe here discouer, these rabelmente of *Minaruas* seruauntes, whiche liues onely by thefte, yet God forfende, but in the absence of the learned *Chyrurgian*, but that the wholsome medicenes, prepared of good people, and charitable neighbours, should bee greatly preferred, to helpe in soche cases, when tyme, place, and daunger dooe require, or els a greate nomber

should

An ignorant Surgian, is a man slear.

Chirurgie is becomome a Sentuarie.

Of vacabond Chirurgians worse then theues. Lynx can see beste of any creature, and his vrin will tourne into a stone. Plini.

The soldiour is hurte more by an euill Surgiã then by his enemies weapon, often it is so proued.

The miseris of man, whē he is hurte in bodie.

Many good medicens are made of the plain people, to help in the absence of the Chyrurgian.

A Dialogue

Dogge Leaches.

should bee caste awaie, for lacke of helpe. Whereas many for lacke of witte and wealthe, of these Dogge leaches, whiche neuer knewe letter of booke, behaue them selues daiely as foloweth, with their consorted fellowes, as I haue written in plain grosse wordes folowyng.

> Some men in miserie, straunge shiftes will make,
> Spendyng tyme vainly, and labour forsake:
> To liue like lurchers, what force thei of shame,
> Prefarring knauishe knackes, before a good name
> In countenaunces haute, and netnesse of clothes,
> Roystyng like ruffians, thundryng forthe othes:
> Furderers of fraies, with long Dager and Sworde:
> Sowyng of discencion, at eche mannes borde.
> Cariers of newes, proclaimers of lies:
> Liuers by Lecherie, blood succour and spies.

The discripcion of an vnthrift, or a villain of nature striuyng against grace and vertue, vnprofitable for a common wealth.

> Braineleße as brute beastes, and Furies felle:
> Like Plutoes whelpes, trained vp from helle.
> Murcia dʋe teache them, no labour to vse:
> But slouthfull to liue, and vertue refuse.
> Lauernia, theues goddes, all daies of their liues:
> Arme them with horned thumbes, and fine sharpe kniues.
> In Churche, Plaie, and Market, thei hunte for the purse:
> And preache ofte on Pillorie, their eares are the worse.
> Their thumbes be blaunched, with a T. from the fire:
> Soche worke as thei vse, so paied is their hire.
> Dame Penia with palenesse, that Ladie of neede:
> Bryng men into miserie, and euill for to speede.
> Then are thei make shiftes, disceiuers of other:
> Small forsyng to robbe, frende, father, or brother.
> To eche winde that blowe, the thefe set his saile:
> As careleße as the Foxe, whiche waggeth his taile.
> Not forsyng who see hym, in runnyng to his borough:
> Though houndes hym hunteth, all the couerte through.
> When he haue moste curses, then fareth he beste:
> When spent is his spoile, he taketh his rest.
> Then eftsones he searche holtes, felles: woddes, and fennes:
> For rauenyng of Lambes, and stealyng of Hennes:
> Thus lurketh wilie Rainard, without any care:
> But thende of his progresse, is the gallowe and snare.

Soche

betwene Sorenes and Chyrurgj. Fol.vij.

Soche Foxly feates are vsed, emong a greate nomber
To the pubilke weale, moche losse and comber.
More hurtlesse then fatte Monkes, and Friers of deceipt:
Whiche liued in Idolatrie, but had plentie af meate.
To giue to the poore, that had hunger and neede:
But the Ruffen will robbe, meate, money, and wede.
And vnder long cloke lurketh, with tucke and sharpe knife:
For goldes sake the giltlesse, to reaue them of life.
Thus hurtyng the innocent, that trauell with truthe
To suffre soche villaines, it is a greate ruthe.
No more then Thistell, whiche choketh the Corne:
Greate pitie if it please God, soche wretches were borne.
Their parentes doe fantasie them, like relikes and hallowes:
And will neuer corect them, till thei climbe the gallowes.
To no learnyng nor arte, thei train them vp in youth:
But in idlenesse and picking, with tales of vntrouth.
In horehuntyng, beastlinesse, and bellie ioie of life.
In backbityng, baudrie, defilyng maide, and wife.
Yet parentes your tender braunches, easely you maie twiste,
But when it haue greate strength, you can not when you liste.
Then in striuyng for victorie, it is no greate wonder:
Olde boughes will not bende, but first cracke a sunder.
Yet instructe your children so, while youthfull daies doe laste:
That thei maie serue the common wealth, when you are gone and past.
Then shall thei be no brokers, to vsurers handes:
Whereby many oft doe lose their gooddes and landes.
Neither to be pettie Foggers, in cases of the Lawe:
To make mountaines of Molhilles, and trees of a strawe.
Or oppressours of poore men, with wrightes in their bagges
Clothe themselues like Princes, when other lurke in ragges.
Then shall thei not be Perisites, in tyme of prosperitie:
But succour the helplesse, in the stormes of aduersitie.
Neither shall the ignoraunte, counterfeite Chyrurgy:
Semyng to the simple nomber, thei are seen in Astronomie.
With flattryng wordes, and trim tales, glosinges thei can tell:
As though in naturall Philosophie, thei were seen full well.
With retrogradacion, and Lorde of the assendent:
Plasters, oiles, pouders salues, and matter defendent.

Euill parentes, what frutes thei bryng forthe, and to what ende thei come.

For counterfeit Chirurgians.

Bb.j. In

A Dialogue

In semyng to be skilfull,in euery euill maladie:
Whether it be moiste,colde,burnyng hotte and drie.
Yet neither rede Tegaltius,Marianus,Guido,nor Galen·
Olde Hyppocrates,Dioscorides,Rasis,nor Auicen.
Lattine nor Englishe,little or none,doe thei rede:
Small is their knowlege,moche lesse is their spede.
Yet lacke thei no Brimstone,Quicksiluer,or Litarge:
Oiles grosse and lothsome,to beare out the charge.
Thei haue Palmestrie and Charmes,at eche wightes desire:
Good store of blessinges,for tothache and sainct Antonies fire
If young babes through Feuers,with colde be shaken.
Then thei saie an euill spirite,the childe haue taken.
A bad Angell of the aire,an Elfe,or a witche:
When in deede deare frende,thereby fewe soche.
To molest the faithfull,to bryng them to confusion:
But to the infidell and faithlesse,it is Sathans delusion.
Wrought by his instrumentes,loiterers and liers:
Worse then the valeaunt beggers,and mendicant Friers.
Murderers of mankinde,in knowyng of no arte:
Banishe them from Chyrurgj,commende them to the Carte.
To the flaile and the rake,the trace and the togge:
To the dong forke and mattocke,to the shephoke and the dog
To the Naule and the Lingell,the Bristell and the Shoe:
What should the Shomaker,with the Chirurgiās workes doe
For it is the noblest worke,wrought by cunnyng hande:
Excellyng all other artes,in eche citee and lande.
If Princes be wounded,when noble men are sore:

The vertue of Chirurgy.

The Chyrurgen them helpeth,of Chyrurgians what more?
When bones are broken,and members displaced:
When the fetters of the face,with weapon be disgrased.
When blood is shedde,in cuttyng of the vaines:
The Chyrurgian alone,helpeth hym from paines.
Repaireth mankinde,and giueth hym reste:
So of all knowlege,Chyrurgj is moste beste.
For no treasure or arte,can helpe the wounded man:
When the Chyrurgian,by his cunnyng onely can.
Now let this rime passe,God sende vs of his grace:

Aske

betwene Sorenes and Chyrurgj. Fol. vij.

Aske an other question, I will aunswere to that place.

Sorenes.

GOD giue me grace, to beware of soche fellowes, as you haue spoken of before, whiche are an euill compainie, and that I might learne what a very *Chyrurgian* should bee, whiche in your conclusion, you haue commended, and what thynges he should doe in his office.

Chyrurgj.

HE must begin first in youth with good learning, & exercise in this noble art, he also must be clenly, nimble handed, sharpe sighted, prignant witted, bolde spirited, clenly apparailed, pitefull harted, but not womenly affeccionated: to wepe or trimble, whē he seeth broken bones, or bloodie woundes, neither muste he geue place to the crie of his sore paciente, for softe *Chyrurgians* maketh fowle sores. Of the other side, he maie not plaie the partes of a Butcher to cutte, rende, or teare, the bodie of manne kynde: for all though it be fraile, sore, and weake, yet it is the pleasure of God, to cal it his temple, his instrumēt and dwelyng place, and the Philosopher dooe call it *Orbiculus*, that is a little worlde. Therefore seing euery craftes man doe take greate care, bothe daie and night in his vocacion, to helpe and amende dedde thinges, whiche bee insencible, as Shippes, houses, walles, bridges, and an infinite numbre of thinges, whiche mankynde dooeth make, and when it is old, doe renue it, and preserue it from ruyng, and vtter destruccion, although it be not perdurable: Should not therfore mankynde hymself, for his rewarde, bee diligently cured, amended, and renued, when either through falle, wounde, or stripe he is decaied, and that with wisedome and diligence, for when a house is fallen doune the Carpentar maie builde it vp again. But when mankinde departeth, desolueth, and dieth he cannot be reuiued again, by the policie or cunnyng of mankinde, because one mankinde, can not make an other but rather through arte, when thei be decaied, helpe to amende them, through the worke of nature, and the ministracion of the Phisicion: for *Claudius Galen* saieth, that *Natura est operatrix, Medicus vero eius minister*. That is, nature is the worker, the Phisicion is but her minister. Therefore the *Chyrurgicall* Phisicion, is natures seruaunt.

Eight thinges or propertie of a good Chyrurgian.

The Chirurgian is the beste hande craft in the worlde.

Job. 14.

The Chirurgian, is natures seruaunt.

Sorenes.

What then doe nature worke, in *Chyrurgj*?

Chyrurgj.

NAture woorketh three maner of waies, by the reason that conuenente instrumentes and meanes, are applied in the tyme of nede, to helpe here. For firste she deuideth the thinges that are conteined, or vnnaturally knit together. Secondly, she vniteth, knit-

Nature worketh three waies to help her self.

Bb.ii. teth

A Dialogue

The stre[n]gth of nature. teth, and ioineth together, the seperated partes. Thirdly, she expulseth, purgeth, and clenseth, superfluous matter, that doeth abounde, or offende nature.

Sorenes.

Then it should appere, that nature nedes no *Chyrurgi*

Chyrurgj.

Nature must be relieued by sondrie meanes in the time of daunger. Yes, Nature in the tyme of *Sorenes*, can no more be without the *Chirurgian*, then the Smithe can be without his hammer, or the Tailer without his Sheres: and as I haue saied before, although you seem to be forgetfull, yet let the *Chirurgian* be diligent, if he loue to be clothed with honestie, to liue vertuously, and to do thinges artificially, and not to giue *quid, pro quo*, Chalke for Chese, or Dirte for Drinke: for if thei so do, if it springeth of ingoraunce, then thei are worthy to be punished, and after to be reformed. But if thei bee menne of knowlege, and thus abbuse their pacientes, thei are worthy to be punished, as malicious murtherers: but here I stoppe and laie a strawe, I will meddell with no matters of the Lawe, I am no Iudge, although it bee good and the chief regiment, of our common wealth, yet I haue receiued as smalle profite by lawers, and vnquiet men, as wounded men get perfite healthe, by ignoraunte *Chirurgians*, or quiete men leade happie liues with angree wiues, for whom there is no remeadie, but pacience perforce, *quod Socrates*, to *Santippa.*

Sorenes.

Is your name *Chyrurgj*? We thinke by your talke, you haue a domesticall grief, how helpe ye your self, when your feuer taketh you, you beare out the matter as well as you can.

Chirurgj.

If I be diseased of any soche feauer, I do not intende to seke counsell at your handes, neither of *Hipocrites*, nor *Galen*. &c. But onely of *Diogines*, whiche loued to be alone. *Socrates* was taught pacience, but to conclude, no manne knoweth the grief of a straight shooe, but the wearer therof, but for asmuche as many handes make light worke, and many shoulders passe small of greate burdens, I care the lesser, hauing so many parteners. The remedy is this, when stormes be paste, faire weather come at laste.

Sorenes.

Well, well, seke a salue for that sore, I can no skill of your disease, God wote, moche lesse to help mine owne grief, I praie thee therefore helpe vs bothe, yet by your leaue although you bee called *Chyrurgj*, or *Sanitas*, yet I dooe consider, that there is no continuall sanite of bodie, or perfecte quietnesse of mynde, duryng this life of mortalle menne. For if a manne would discende doune
into

into his owne conscience, and see himself with in, he shall easely perceiue, the woordes written of sainct Job the .xviii. Chapiter, in his moste lamentable and pitefull booke: saieth he, a man that is borne of a woman, liueth but a shorte tyme, and is filled full of miserie, and commeth vp, and falleth awaie like a flower, and in the ende passeth awaie like a shadowe, and neuer continue in one estate. For truly we daiely see, aduersitie followeth prosperite, bondage after libertie, pouertie, after riches, sicknes, after healthe, beside an infinite nomber of the passions, and afflictions of the minde. As zeale, strife, gelousie, loue, ioye, care. &c. And as the wise manne saieth, *Omnia tempus habent*, all thinges haue their tyme. And God hath geuen afflicion to the children of men, to be exercised in theim, emong whom, I for my synnes am plagued with this kinde of maladie, as thou seest me haue: I beseche God of his mercie, sende me healthe, and to as many as are sore.

Man is but miserable, & yet is quickly gone.

Chyrurgj.

Thou haste spoken wisely, for al thing is in vain, where God doeth not put to his helping hande, and by his Prophete he saieth, call vpon me in the tyme of trouble, and I will helpe thee make thee whole, and deliuer thee. Behold, how many Lepers, sicke of palsies, blooddie flixes, blindnesse, desenesse, possessed of euill spirites: yea, and death it self, all these haue God helped restored, and made perfecte, for there is *Tempus occidendi*, and *Tempus sanandi* with God, for he is euer occupied, either in punishing the wicked, or conforting of his elected.

Psalm. 50.

Matth. 11.

Ecclc. 3.

Sorenes:

Would GOD, there were soche miracles now a daies, as was then. It were a greate comfort to an infinite number of suche as I am, neither should it be painfull, nor costly, for Christ coueiteth no money, although *Simon magus* delited in nothing els.

Christ is no couetous.

Chyrurgj:

Sorenes, Sorenes? Thou saiest not well, for it is rather a tempting of God, then a beleuing in God, to looke or wishe for miracles, for faithfull men nedes none. And I trust thou art faithfull, therfore thou nedest no miracle, but rather consider this, Christ healed the bodies of Sicke menne, twoo maner of waies, the one by vertue of his heauenlie worde, whereby we be taught that he is God. The seconde he healed somtime with claie, with spitte. &c. Wherein we be learned, and he also haue learned vs, in the tyme of our sorenes, prudentlie to vse Goddes instrumentes and meanes, yea, not with claie or spitte, yet with presious herbes, fruites, gummes. &c. For God hath ordeined theim onelie to helpe his people, to this ende, that his people might serue him. Tobias healed his fathers iyes, with the gaule of a fische, an Angell prepared the medicen. Ezechias the kyng in the time of his

A faithfull man beleueth without miracle, for faith is not seen, but miracles are seen.

Two maner of healyngs.

A Dialogue.

Esaie, 38.
4. Regum, 20

Pestilence, was healed with a cluster of figges. The greate Prophete Esaie, gaue him this medicen. Eliseus did cleanse through the vertue of a swete tree, the foule stinkyng waters, Christ in the Gospell, commaundeth the Apostles to carie oile with them, to heale the sicke. S.

Luke,

Luke the holy Euangeliste was a Phisicion, and some of the antiquites of his Phisicke, remaine vnto this daie. It is saied also that holie Esdras made a goodlie medicene, when the people were in captiuitie in Babilon, to clense them from their malancholie, and heauinesse of minde, whiche medicene is called after his name vnto this daie: these and soche like examples *Sorenes*, should moue thee to vse these meanes to helpe thee.

Sorenes.

I hartely thanke you, I shall by Gods grace, obserue your saiynges, and vse Gods instrumentes reuerentlie, by whose meanes we poore menne be healed. And somtyme the riche infidels, still tourmented with sores. &c.

Chyrurgj.

Men doe vse pretie termes for foule sores and call them by one name, when thei are an other.

Euen so be riche also for sicknes, as we doe daiely see, doe not perticulerlie dwell in poore men, but rather generally in al although the kindes of sicknes be variable, and the complexions diuers, and the causes many, and euery sicknes, and sorenes, haue his proper name, although men, either through ignoraunce, shame of crafte doe abuse their names, although the effect doe stille remaine, as in clenlie termes by your lisence, thei will call it nothing els, but a sausie flemed face, redde or high coloured, when many times in deede, it is not onely so, but the verie Leprosie with all. It is nothing saie thei, but breaking out, or paines of the body, weakenesse of limmes, or a grene sicknes, through the obstruccion of the liuer. &c. with soche nicke names, whose very sure name is, the buttens of Napelles, *Gallicus morbus* comonlie called the frenche poxe.

Sorenes.

Ether to yet stande I in doubt, although I be pained, how to name truly my desease I can not, although of it self it be definable, felte of me, and seen to vs bothe, and knowen onely to thee, what thinke you it is, I praie you tell me.

Chyrurgj.

It is none other then apostumacion, as it doeth planlie appere to me.

Sorenes.

Then I praie you, giue me a difinission, and a deuision, of an apostumacion.

Chyrurgj.

Apostuma-

Apostumacion is a verie euill disease, compounded of. iii kindes of maledies, gathered, and growing together in one quantitie, firste of an euill complexion: Secondly a naughtie composicion, and thirdlie, the continuaunce of time. These three maketh an apostumacion, or swelling within or without the body, notwithstādyng, as *Galen* saieth, not all kinde of swellynges make apostumacions, but soche onely as anoieth the bodie, and the roote thereof is the corrupcion of the fower temperamentes, when thei bee altered, and chaunged into Fleume, Blood, Choller, and Melancholy, through them the shape of a member, is altered, when it is chaunged from his naturall forme, into any straunge, or deformed figure. Also the breache of continuaunce, is caused through insicions, corrosians, breaking, or stretchyng, as *Galen* saith, in the seconde *de arte Medendi*, neuer the lesse, the chief cause is through stretchyng, whereby the partes of the bodie bee seuered one from an other, and this is my conclusion of this diffinition.

Apostumaciō is compounded of thre sondrie euils.

Breache of continuaunce is when the whole partes ar cutte, broken, &c.

Sorenes.

How many kindes of apostumations be there?

Chyrurgj.

There be twoo, the one is hotte, and the other colde, for euery apostumacion is hote or cold, touching their humour, but accidentallie: thei bee diuerfly hotte, as *Galen* saieth, the hote haue their proper signes, to be knowen by, euen so hath the cold, whereby he is perceiued. Apostumations, wherin is boiling and burning, with continuall heate, is iudged to come of blood, or Chollericke humour, euen so iudge them of Melancholie, or fleume, when thei seme to bee colde, pale, deddishe, or partelie not felte, and thus thou shalt perceiue their kindes, and although thei be named a like, yet thei differ one from an other in cure, as thei do in complexion. Moreouer, the apostumacion of blood, hath greate swellyng and heate, ouer all the body, and is seldom seen without some feauer, and the colour is a dimme darke red, also hardnes, if you presse it with your finger, because so moche matter, is gathered grosselie in the place. The pulses will beate very sore, the matter being ouer laden, will kepe doune the artorie, and therfore nature attempting to rase and lifte vp the same, will cause great beatyng in the veines, wherfore the more artories be kept doun, the greater is the labour, and beatyng of the pulses, after whiche, sometyme soloweth soche dollour and pain, that all the partes of the body come to destruccion, as often times in hotte euell complexions, where euill matter is heaped togither in the apostumaciō. That in fine, replexion and tencion, of all the course of the veines doe come, for all the veines in the saied apostumacion, by the meanes of the aboundance of blood, will swell and become great, although before, thei were right, straite,

Thre kindes of Apostumacions, hotte and cold.

How to knowe Apostumacion.

The aboundance of blood in the Apostumacion.

Bb. iiii. cleane:

A Dialogue.

cleane: yea, and some as small as heeres, and these bee the apostumacions of blood.

Sorenes.

What saiest thou then, of them that be Chollerike?

Chyrurgj.

The crueltie of the Chollorike apostumacion, but the bloodie apostumacion is gentler.

APostumacions Chollerike, bee gentiller as touchyng their swelling, but thei doe excell more in pain, and be farre crueller, because of sharpenesse, and bityng of humour, with bitternes, and drinesse of Choller, whereas bloodie apostumacions, although thei doe swell through moistnesse, yet thesame humidite or moistnesse, causith the sore to be more gentler, and of lesser pain then the Chollerike, for thei be twoo contraries, as *Aristotle* saith in his booke of generacion, and corrupcion, *Ignis qui est in vltimo continentis, non est in fine, ebullitionis,*

Of cōtraries of elimentes.

and in an other place, he saieth, *Elementa omnia adinuicem contrarietatem habent,* and that is well saied, for heate is an extreme contrarie to colde, so is moistenesse to drinesse, and more paine in the one apostumacion, then in the other.

Sorenes.

What be apostimacons in quantitie, whiche of theim be greateste, and whiche of theim bee leaste, I would faine knowe, good *Chyrurgj*?

Chyrurgj.

The quantitie of the apostumaciōs.

AS touching their quantites, knowe you that the Chollerike, is lesse then any other, by the reason of his drinesse, and heate, whiche restraineth extencion, but the accidence of the paine, is moste cruell and sharpe, and these be destriyng qualities in this quantite, what time thei are come, to the extreme degre of heate, but apostumacions, depending of cold humours, soche wil bryng their own proper signes, beatyng of the artories, notwithstādyng thei be not comperable to the beating of a Chollerike, or a bloodie apostumacion but more duller, colder, paler. &c. You must allso note, that apostumaciōs that spryng of blood, or choller, be diuersly termed by sundrie names,

Sondrie names of apostumacions, but in effecte are but apostumacions.

as botches, shingelles, fellones, pusshes, vncomes, sainct Anthonies fire, bleanes, bladders, or blisters, crustes, carbūcles, pestilent sores. &c. euen so on the other side, apostumacions, of Fleume or Melancholie, haue ioined vnto them these names, as vndimies, knottes, woundes, Carnelles, wrates, Cankars, Esthachelles, with soche like euilles of mortificacion, in their beginnyng, and bee all called apostumacions, but when thei be growen to a ripenes, and doe breake forthe, then call theim vlcers, speciallie if the matter procede, to the breache of continuaunce. Also apostumacions are sores compounded, and standeth

Sores compounded.

not in one humour a lone, yet often times we saie simplie, that euery one of theim, spryngeth of one humour, as of heate, colde, moiste,

O_j

or drie, of whom, in deede thei doe take their names, as *Aristotle* iudgeth in his Naturalles, as where blood is excessiue, it is called a *Bubo*, or a Sanguine boche, and where as Choller doeth abounde, it is called a Chollerike maladie. And so of the Flegmatike, and Melancholie the like, accordyng to their natures.

Sorenes.

Hitherto I haue heard, but onelie the diffinictons, of the names, or natures of impostumacions, but me thinke to talke of the cures, were more profitable, for onelie vnto that ende, doe I moue these questions vnto you.

Chyrurgi.

I will speake somwhat of their cuers, but or I enter any further in this matter: I thinke it rather necessarie, to speake a little of thinges that be comen, and would bee prudently obserued in their cures, for asmoche as euery apostumacion, dependeth of some cause, and maie not well be cured, except, cause, signe, iudgment of the same with effectes, be perfectly knowen. Therefore seyng there is nothing bolder then blinde bayarde, which falleth ofte in the mire, nor none so hurtfull to the health of mankinde, as ignoraunt *Chyrurgians*, settyng the carte before the horse, and the rootes of the trees vpward, and shoteth at the marke like blinde men, somtyme hittyng by chaunce, more then by knowlege, these thinges considered *Sorenes*. Thinke therfore no time loste, to heare me speake of the causes of apostumacons, for there by the soner, thei maie be healed, therefore I will speake a little more of the causes.

Blinde Bayarde is bolde

Sorenes.

Why? Be there any more causes of apostumacons, where of should thei rise? I praie you shortly shewe me.

Chyrurgi.

Yes: Saieth he, whiche is the Prince of all Phisicke called *Hippocrates*, there bee three kinde of causes, where of apostumacions doe rise, the first is the *Primatiue*, the seconde the *Antecedent*, the thirde the *Coniunctiue*. The *Primatiues*, where meladies happen by misfortune to the bodie, from the outwarde partes, as insision, breakyng, smityng, fallyng, vlceracon of the handes and feete, or any other part, wherof insueth apostumacon. For whē great dolour, that is caused in any part, sone after it foloweth, that ye part anoied crieth vpon nature for helpe, (for suche is his goodnes and prouidence) sendyng out of hande some succour, to the impouerished, and sore partes. But it chaunceth ofte tymes, that this succour, or nourishemente, resteth there or some where by the waie, in ye bacant and weake partes, and so groweth it at length to an apostumacion, in case the vertue degestiue, or expulsiue be not able to maister, and dispache it. The *Antecedent* is diuerslly named, and by diuers termes, as replecionall, humoral com-

Three causes the Primatiue, the Antecedente, and the Coniunctiue, whiche belong to apostumacion.

complexionall, and composicionall, it is called replecctionall, whē the humours increase beyonde their due measure. And albeeit all these haue respect to the qualitie of humours, yet for all that, when all the humours growe beyond measure, it is termed replerionall, humorall, is whē one humour a lone, groweth to apostumacion, as the shingles cometh of pure choller: and an hot botche of pure and laudable blood. Also thei call it complerionall, if the saied humours bee distempered from their first state or qualites, I saie from their first qualities, as if

Composicion Replexion, Complexion, what thei are

their forme in a body wer limited, within the quantitie of. ii. inches, & then if thei had gotten thē iii. inches more, then thereof would spring diuers diseases, taking their names of the qualities, ȳ haue dominion and preheminence of thē. It will be named compositionall, where one humour excedeth the rest, in degree of his qualitie, giuē him of nature in compocicion, and hereof it commeth to passe, that the whole bodie compounded, goeth to ruine, through feuers, and other kinde of maladies. Wherefore no man maie dought, that the complexcion should bee holden for a cause *Antecedent*. Some number dolour with the same causes, whereunto maie be added weakenes of a member, as watrishnesse, and windines. &c. Also a cause *Coniuncte*, is nothing els but the *Antecedent*, when it cometh to a place vlcerated, or well nighe vlceratyng. Here maie not wee passe ouer this with silence, that any apostumacion as touchyng rippyng, or to speake plainer, rottyng, and breedyng of matter, hath propertie fower tymes appropriate to it, that is to wete beginnyng, augmentyng, state, and fall. The beginnyng is, when the

Fower notes in an apostumaciō; beginning, augmētyng, state, & declinyng.

causes *Coniunct*, begin presently to appere. Augmentyng is knowen in that it largeth, and groweth to bignes, and the accidētes increase the matter gathered and heaped together, without further increasyng, sheweth planlie the state. Finally, the fall is knowen (if it bee well loked on) by a certaine softnes, and faintyng in the place. And these tymes muste bee as well obserued, I thinke, as the self maladies: for *Auicenna* with expresse wordes, giueth this admoniciton, saiyng: it is not possible thou shhuldest cure a disease, if thou knowe not, what the disease is. We thinke he dooeth inferre, and conclude, where the tymes be vnknowen, the cure also will be vnknowen, for why: In as moche as the tyme in apostumacion is diuers, the disease is diuers, and the cure will be diuers.

Sorenes.

ALthough you seme to speake somwhat obscurely, and darkly, yet by often tymes readyng, I truste to gette some more knowlege, for it is said of a very wise man. *Omnes homines naturaliter scire dederat*. And I also beyng a man, am desirous of knowlege to helpe my self without the whiche I am the worst kind of beast, and moste vnprofitable vpon the yearth, but hether vnto, you haue spoken, but of the beginnyng of apostumacions, as semeth to me, but how be thei ended and finished, I praie you let me knowe the waie?

Chyrurgj.

Chyrurgj.

GALEN the beste that euer was, and the greatest learned next to *Hyppocrates*, and one to whom chief credēce must bee giuen as vnto a prudent Ship maister, whiche through connyng wisely, doe set his course in the raging seases, defending his Shippe from rocke, storme and tempeste, to the ende, to a riue at the porte, and ende of his trauel so doeth *Galen*, like a worthie maister, defende his pacientes from the shippe wrakes, bothe of sorenes, and sicknes, and saieth if apostumacions tourne not backe againe, then thei doe ende by insensible resolucion, or els by rotting out, and thei be ended fower maner of waies firste by resolucion, as is aforesaid, whiche is vnbindyng, remouyng, or vndoyng of the matter, secondely, to conuerte, change, and tourne the apostumacion into a thyng, called matter, or waire. The thirde is by rotting. The fowerth, is putrifaccion, and of this speaketh *Auicen*, whiche is one of the chief princes of Philicions, in thende of his chapiter, concernyng a hotte apostumacion, and in this cure there is two thinges principallie to bee obserued. The one is, whether the thing be yet a doyng, the other is, whether it be full doen, or ended, I mean by doyng, that is, wether the matter be yet runnyng, or fletyng to the place of apostumacion, and by the thing that is doen, that is, whether the matter be paste, and come already in to the place of apostumacion or not, and note also, that in all soche cures, you maie not prolong, or abuse the time, but diligently go about your busines, for a little loste tyme: put the pacient to great pain, & the *Chyrurgian* to great dishonestie.

Of resoluriō.

Sorenes.

THerefore I praie you, so spende no more tyme any lenger in definitions, names, causes, and signes, of apostumacions, but rather I praie you, begin the maner of their proper cures, and helpes, for els hether vnto, all is but a labourinth, and a croked waie vnto me?

Chyrurgj.

WEll: If you will nedes take vpō you, to minister in your beginnyng, you must reparie repercussiues, which will greatly comfort the sore member, for *Auicen* saieth in his first booke, the fowerth doctrine, that a strong member actiuelie, doe caste from him his superfluous humoure, vnto the weake passiue or sufferyng members, and pulles it backe againe, and eftesones doe powre it foorthe againe, to the greate hurt of the weake parte, where by the weake members is often tymes choked, and strangled with the strength of the humour, whereby the whole bodie is ruined, and finally brought to destrucciō, therfore, to the intente that the weake part be not vtterlie destroied, ouerladen, or choked, with soche superfluous humour, you must, to auoide

the

A Dialogue.

the daunger, make restraint with repercussiues, and medicenes defendent. And this shalt thou dooe, applie, cold, and bindyng receiptes, as *Galen* sheweth in the third of the art, saing: *Repeblemus a paciente particula si infrigidemus & stiptica apponamus, &c.* We shall put of frō the sicke parte, if we coole, and applie binding thinges. &c.

Sorenes.

Doe repercussiues helpe then in this case generally?

Chyrurgj.

Of repercussiue, whē thei are good.

NO. But for asmoche, as this place offereth occasion, to speak of repercussiues, whiche I dooe laude: euen so I shall haue occasion to shewe, where repercussiues ought to bee abhorred and fledde, with no lesse care, then Shipmen doe the rockes in the sea. For it is no lesse pleasure to the *Chyrurgian*, to obtain their purpose, and finishe their cure, then it is ioie vnto the Mariners, luckely to arriue in their owne porte, or restyng place. Therefore *Sorenes*, to the ende that we maie eschue Shipwrackes, and daungerous places, let vs a little inlarge our course, and call to remembraunce, the wise wordes, of that learned man, and famous clarke (maister Jhon Vigo) of Genua, whiche wrote a learned booke, vnto Julius the seconde, wherein he saieth, that apostumacions in vncleane bodies, doe vtterly refuse repercussiues, except thei be firste clensed by purgacions, for moche matter can not awaie with repercussion. In case we should fal sodainly to the cure before purgyng, then should wee greatly erre, for in driuyng it backward, we rather should couche it vp, in the place so

Foule bodies refuseth repercussiues, therefore thei must be clensed.

faste, that it could not be remoued, whereby occasion should bee giuen of euill acsidence. And furthermore, if this come to passe, as God forebedde it should: then would it plainly emport, or threate putrifaccion or corrupcion of the member. Secondly, the emunctorie or cleansyng places, will not desire any repercussiue. Thirdly, take heede how you vse repercussiues, when the matter is fattie and clammie. For *Galen* saieth in the third booke of the Arte, *Corpus existens plenum repercussionem non amittet.* Fowerthly, thinke it no matter of deliberacion, concernyng repercussion, when the cause is venemous, cruell, or furious: but bee occupied wholy, in prouokyng of it forthe, for if you driue it backward, after mine opinion, saith *Tegaltius*, then doe you range farre from the high waie, for this is the cause, why ye shall arre, and not doe well in your cure. Firste, ye shall shutte and close vp the matter, within your senture, whiche of necessitie, ought to be despersed abroade, in the whole circuite, and thereof will followe, by the meanes of the malice, venim and poison assembled together, and so takyng their force in one place will practise no small inconuenience or mischief, against the natural bertues: you shall therefore, firste vse repercussiues, if the matter bee pressed, stopped, thruste, or shutte vp together in one place, doe this, for feare of deformyng of the member, where the sore is, whiche sone will ensue, if it come to putrifaccion in that place. Sixtly, if nature cause

What peril is in the applicacion of a repercussiue, although in some case it is moste beste.

any

betwene Sorenes and Chyrurgj. Fol.xiij.

any apostumacion, by the reason of crises, that is of iudgement, *Hoc est Iudicium,* to auoide, expulse, or put out matter superfluous, in this case, thinke there willbe no meanes founde, to put it backe, without great daunger, and hurte to nature.

Sorenes.

Why? would it hinder anye thing in this case, to apply a repercussiue, or medicene, to driue it backe: shewe me some reason why it should not be: Or what hurte would come thereof, if it were doen?

Chyrurgj.

Mary, this euill might eftesones ensue, for if it bee put backe, or retourned in againe, nature will then inuente, and finde out some other by pathe, from the vnclene, to the clene places, and were not this a greate hurte to nature? yes suerly, it wer no small ieoperdie, therefore we must in soche cases, make euacuasion of the matter, putting a helpyng hande to nature in her crises, as *Gallen* saieth vpon this: *Aphorismus quorum crisis fit, haud facta est, &t.* For the cure of all these causes, you muste vse mollifications, and softenyng medicenes.

what hurte ensueth of a repercussiue.

Sorenes.

Yet againe, I put this question, why you doe vse repercussiues at any tyme?

Chyrurgj.

We vse repercussiues, that we maie apply them, to the intent that the matter yet fletyng, be kept of, and not that, whiche is alredy flowing, be come stubburne, against vs in our workyng, and therefore, doyng accordyng to our rules, we shall order and applie repercussiues in the beginnyng, and augmentyng of apostumacions, for why, the matter at that tyme, is chiefly flowyng to and fro, and *Galen* writeth in the thirde of his arte, that besselles refreshed with binding medicens, put of moche matter from them, how beit this ought to be doen successiuelie, by little and little, because the fluxe of the matter, is with a continuance, and when it is come where it should be, then must it be resolued, and not driuen backe.

what goodnesse cometh of a repercussiue.

Sorenes.

I praie thee gentle *Chyrurgj,* take in hande the cure of apostumacions.

Chyrurgj.

The prince of the Philosophers, *Aristotle* saieth, contraries be, and pertaineth to one science, and doubtlesse, the cures of apostumacions differ not, but in distaunce of more and lesse, for this cause, must I wrastle earnestelie, that the knowlege

Cc.i. of

A Dialogue

of natures, and simples escape you not, for why, the more ye shall excell herein, the better shall you forme your medicenes, for the pacientes behoue, who haue ioined them selues to our companie, now to obtaine this pourpose, ye shall aduisedlie looke, wether the apostumacions fall in a body full of humours, or voide of the same. If it happen in an emptie body: ye shall reken it some cause prematiue, whose cure must be in drawing forthe from the matter, with resolutiues, or softening medicenes, you shall resolue, if you apply, cold and binding thinges together with hot and moist: with cold you must restrain, and kepe it of, if any parte of choller were approching, by reason of dolour, and with bindyng, you shal comfort the member, as I said before, accordyng to the sentence of *Gallen*: that hoote thinges, cause the relentyng of the matter, finally, vse moistening of the same, that the pores harden not, nor be coagulated or stopped, and this spedely muste be doen at the beginnyng, afterward if it take not place, as I haue saied. What haue you to saie, in any other matter?

> *Consider whither apostumacions chaūce in bodies replete with humors or emptie,*

Sorenes.

Shewe me some wholsome medicenne, for apostumacions, I praie you.

Chyrurgj.

> *A good medicene for an apostumaciō.*

I Shall compounde this medicen, for an exemple. ℞. Iuse of Housleke, and Lettice, ana. ʒ.i. oile of Roses, and Camamell ana. ʒ.s.ß. oile Mirtes. ʒ.x. Egges in nomber. ii. Swyng all these with the yolkes and whites, vnto soche tyme, as thei be well incorporated, and then applie it in linnen. Either thus. ℞. Bole Armoniacke, Acasia, añ. ʒ.i. oile of Roses, Mirte, Camamell. añ. ʒ.i.ß. Beane meale. Ɔ.i. duste of Mirtelles, and of Cipers nuttes. ʒ.ß. with a little Waxe, all whiche muste be incorporated at the fire, and applied to the sore place. Furder, for the resoluyng, of an hotte apostumacion, of what cause so euer that it come of: ye shall applie this, which the learned haue greatly commended, & in very deede, I euer founde it, as thei haue said, thorder of it was thus. ℞. Heddes of white Lillies ʒ.v. rootes of the Marrishe Mallowes. li.i. Camamell, Millelotte. ana. M.ß. and a handfull of Bran, sethe all these in water till thei be throughly sodden, and then strain, and presse them, as the Coke doe commonly grated bread, when he maketh his potage, putting it into a clene pan, vnto the which, ye shal put oile of Roses, of Camamill, of Dil, & of lillies ana. ʒ.ii. of the marie of Calues, or Cowes legges, and of Capōs grese ana, ʒ.i. of white Waxe. ʒ.ß. of the softe aples, rosted in hotte embers, if thei maie bee gotten. ʒ.iii.ß. Let all these bee melted together, with that, whiche was searsed at a soft fire, and bee boiled, by the space of halfe an hower, wrought alwaies, that it be diligently stirred all the while, and this will bee a Cerote, whereby ye shall gette profite, and commendacions. Now if the apostumacions, will not bee ruled, and giue place to a resolutiue: for so it fareth oftentimes with them, then prepare molificatiues, or softenyng medicenes, whiche maie be made

> *A more excellent waie to helpe an apostumacion.*

twoo

betwene Sorenes and Chyrurgj. Fol.xiiij.

twoo waies, with Embrocacions, or plasters.

Sorenes.

I praie you tell me, whiche is the beste waie or meanes, to make an Embrocacion?

Chyrurgj.

AN Embrocacion, is made after this maner. ℞. Of a decoccion of Mallowes, Violettes, Barlie, Quince seede, Lettice leaues. ℔.ß. of Barlie meale. ℥.ii. oile of Violettes, and Roses. ana. ℥.i.ß. of Butter. ℥.i. and then seethe theim all together, till thei bee like a brothe, puttyng thereto, at the ende fower yolkes of Egges, and the maner of applying, is with peeces of clothe, dipped in the foresaied decoccion, beyng actually hotte, whiche must be often chaunged, one after an other, by the space of one thirde part of an hower: This will alaie and abate the paine, and cause resolucion, drawing forthe the matter into the skin. Soche decoctions maie be also made, of a Wethers hed, or other fleshe, so that the brothe bee fatte, howbeit, this shall bee, accordyng to thine intente, whether you meane the rippyng, or the resoluyng of it, immediatly after the imbrocacion, let this or the like plaster followe. ℞ Of leaues, of Mallowes, Violettes, and Lettise, ana. ℳ.i. and afterwarde thei shall be sodden, braied, and searsed, make an harde plaster thereof at the fire, with Barlie meale, puttyng thereto ℥.ii.ß. of oile of Violettes, and. ℥.ß. of Butter, this doen, take it of the fire, and then incorporate the yolkes of three Egges, and so applie it to the sore. Now, if he be lothe to take so moche paine, and thinke plasteryng sufficiente, appoincte the pacientes frendes to vse this. ℞. of crummes of breade. ℔.i.ß. let it bee steped in a decoction of Mallowes, Violettes, and Lettes, or in a brothe of Veale, or Mutton: it maie bee doen to with Ewes, or Goates milke, hotte from the dugges. Finally, let it be pressed, and stamped, and drawen rounde in a morter, and then soften it with oile of Violetes, and Roses, ana. ℥.i.ß. and of Butter. ℥.i with a ℈.i.ß. of Saffron. After lette the whole be thicked, at the fire a little, and then put the yolkes of twoo Egges to it: or els take the leaues of Mallowes, and Violettes, or euery of theim, one handfull, and so boile and stampe theim togither, with Bores grease, and vse these hardely. For one of these I assure you, shall ripe a Chollerike apostumacion, whiche thyng ye shall perceiue, by the softnesse in felyng, and by easyng of the paine, as *Auicen* saieth *Cum videris lenitatem quandam & sedationem doloris, tunc scias quod sit in via ad maturationē.* When thou seest a certain softnes, and laiyng of pain, thē thou maiest know, it is in the waie of rippyng, now when the place is readie to bee launced, aboue all thynges, see the inscision, and the openyng be made a longest, with the liyng of the heeres, and sinewes, for why, nothyng will be doen more better, to cause a Cicatrice.

Of an Embroche.

A Cicatrice.

Sorenes.

A Dialogue.

Sorenes.

This is verie well saied: Now I praie you tell me, how you make an Insiscion?

Chyrurgj.

Insiscion how to make it.

AN Insiscion muste be made in the lowest parte, so that the matter maie the better auoide: in especially, if any humour doe vse to fall to that parte, from whens issues would moste naturally fall from. Oft we conducte thē, by their conuenient regions, as saith deuine *Hyppocrates*, & thinsisciō must be made, as it liketh the learned, after a half or croked moon, except the place be sinews, for if it be so, then must it be made a longest, with the course of them. For why, if I would opē it ouertwhart, I might cutte some sinewe a sunder in workyng: Immediatly vpon the inscission, the place muste bee couered with Linte, dipped and wette in the white of an Egge: Neuerthelesse, before ye so doe, ye shall fill the hole of the apostumacion with a tente, made of the same moisted linte, to the intent the matter gushe not out, all at ones, whiche thing, if it were suffred, and the apostumacion greate, the vertue naturall, will bee moche assembled thereby. Whereas wee ought moste warely to saue thesame, that it be sufficiente to feede the place, and worke rightly. For as *Mesue*, followyng the minde of *Galen*, saieth, it is nature, who woorketh health: the Phisicion is but her seruaunte. This also muste bee well remembred, and had in consideracion, in a place apostumated, whether the apostumacion, fall in a fleshie or sinewie place. For when there doe rise a knot in a sinewie place, their loke to be opened, before thei bee full ripen: leaste any sinewe should rotte, by meanes of corrupcion, but in the other, by reason of the freshenesse thereof, we maie abide the perfite riping, sith we bee moued by no inconuenience, to open it before tyme: whiche thyng is not permitted in the other, without some good cause. Now when ye haue well filled, and couered the inscission, let it a lone, and meddle no more with it, for the space of .xxiiii. howers, and when that tyme is expired, ye shall visite the apostumacion, with a digestiue, made of yolkes of Egges, and Teribinth, in continuing thesame, ii. or thre tymes, vntil you se more or lesse, according as necessitie in digestion shall shewe you. At the ende ye maie finishe the cure, with an abstersiue, mingled of Barlie meale, Terebinthen, and rosed Honie. But if it shalbe hollowe (as it is often seen) we giue you this abstersiue in that behalfe. ℞. Of Rosed Honie strained .ʒ.i.ß. of clere Terebintine ʒ.ii. of the iuice of Smallage.ʒ.ß. lette theim boile, till the iuice bee wasted, afterwarde, whiles it is yet warme, put thereto. ii.ʒ.ß. of Barlie flower, and mingle theim together, whiche ye maie kepe, till nede shall require, for the cure.

Consider to open a member, before the sinewe doue rotte.

A digestiue.
An abstersiue.

Sorenes.

What if proude fleshe, dedde or rotten putrified fleshe, chaunce to be in the sore, or apostumacion, what remedie then?

Chyrurgj.

betwene Sorenes and Chyrurgj. Fol.xv.

Chyrurgj.

IN deede often times, there groweth dedde fleshe in soche places, I haue therefore here to saie, how the same must be displaced and remoued, certainly my self did euer vse in remouing of superfluous, and fistered fleshe, the mixt ointmentes, whiche was compounded of *Vnguentum apostolorum*, and *Egyptiacum* of like porcions, and if the parte had been verie sensible, I vsed the pouder, whiche the olde aunctent *Chyrurgians* did vse, to remoue suche fleshe ouer and vpon, that ye shall applie this ointement, whiche the olde anscient *Chyrurgians* had in vse. It is discribed after this maner. ℞. Oile of Roses, of Camamell, ana. ʒ.iii. of fatte Weathers. ʒ.iiii. of fatte Calfes. ʒ.iii. of the mary of a Cowes huckell bone. ʒ. ii. of Letherge of gold, and siluer, ass. ʒ.i.ß. of Ceruse ʒ.ß. of Vermilon. ʒ.iii. of Terebentine. ʒ.iiii. of new Waxe. ʒ.ii. mingle all these togither accordyng to the arte. And let them boile first at a softe fire, encreasing and fortefiyng the same, after a season, and so boile, and sterre it with all, and so doe it, till it get a verie blacke hugh and thus haue you an ointmente to spreade on the sore, like a Cerote. But I sawe one thing comyng to remembraunce, that maie not well be forgotten, by reason of the fearfulnes, of a certaine fainte harted manne, dwelling hereby, now this white liuered ladde, that I speake of, was excedynglie tormented with an impostumation, whiche needed openyng, howbeit, he could abide any thing, rather then the openyng thereof, with an instrument, when I perceiue the importunitie of the man, and the necessitie of the worke, I rotted the apostumation with a potentiall cauterie, whiche was made after this sorte. I tooke a cuppe full of the beste Sope lye, that first distilled furth from the stepefatte, men terme it the mother lye, and caste it into a brasen cauldron, with a dragme of ramain vetriole, whiche I caused to boile, till al the lye was cleane waisted, and then gathered I the some, and frothe, whiche remained therof for my purpose, and truely this is so effectually in writyng, that it semeth to worke sodenlie the acte, and seeyng the woorke began to receiue profite, when as the colour of the place began to bee darke and blacke. This is to bee vsed in the tyme, when the pacient is very feble. But or euer it was aplied, I meane the Cauterie, the hole apostumacion was couerd with a peece of leather, lest that the Cauterie should pearse or hurte some other place, then that whiche I did intende to meddle with all. And furder, that a hole bee made in the middes of the same leather: and furder, to anoint the leather, with some ointment, and in the same hole, to applie the said cauterie. And then with an other pece of leather, to couer the hole, and so let it stande by the space of one hower and a halfe, close couered, and then remoue the Cauterie, and then apparell the place with a plaster as followeth. ℞. Leaues of Mallowes and Violettes, ana, one handfull, let them bee boiled and stamped, puttyng thereunto. ʒ.ii. of Bar-

Cc.iii. rowes

rowes greale, of Butter. ʒ.ſs. of Leauen. ʒ. iii. and. Ə. i. of Saffron, mingle all togither, and plaster wise, laie it to the place, for this will remoue an harde crust, and delaie the pain. Now when the crust shalbe remoued, the vlcer must be cured, as it was afore declared. Hetherto haue we talked of apostumacions, chauncing in clene bodies. Now be cause there goeth one by, by whō I maie quickly certifie my frende of my trauell. I praie you beare with me, for a while, and with all spede possible, when I haue doen, I will I retourne to you again. For I intende to finishe our communicacion, and speake of the apostumaciōs, which hurteth bodies, that be replete of humours, foule & painfull. &c.

Sorenes.

Somtyme an apostumacion, is placed in a grosse foule bodie, full of humours: in soche a case, what is then to be doen, maister *Chyrurgian*, I praie you?

Chyrurgj.

<small>Fower intencions, and six vnnaturall thynges to be obserued.</small>

Then aboue all thinges, my deare frende, you must doe your diligence, to labour and trauell: more then you did in my primatiue cause. And for the cure thereof, it is verie necessarie, that you set fower intencions, diligently before your iyen, and sixe thynges not naturall.

Sorenes.

Whiche are thei, I praie you hartely tell me?

Chyrurgj.

<small>Fiue notable good thynges to be obserued in healyng.</small>

First, that you order your pacientes life, accordingly: and to bryng the humour to iuste equalitie.

Secondlie, to purge the euill humours: whiche doe maintaine the apostumacions hurte, or offence.

Thirdlie, to remoue the cause, coniuncte or knitte to the same thynges, accordyngly.

Fowerthlie, to correct & amende euill accidentes, if any be in place.

Fiuethlie, thinges not naturall, as aire, meate and drinke, sleping and waking, reste, euacuacion, repletion, and accidentes of the minde, as ire, care. &c. All these muste bee ruled with diligence, accordyng to the ebbing and flowyng of the matter: whether the cure doe seme easie or harde, to that ende, that with spedie worke maie be made with wisedome, and the cure quickly finished. Also, that the bellie maie be relaxed, and losed of that humour, whiche doe moste abound. Furder, that the apostumacion bee woorkmanly launced. And here must you <small>No local medicen applied before the bodie be purged</small> chiefly obserue, that no local medicen be applied, before the whole bodie be clensed, and well purged of that humour, whiche doe moste offence to nature. For in so doyng, mischief wil insue to the pacient, and reproche to the *Chyrurgian*: whiche maie rather be coumpted a murderer, then a man helper in soche cases, whereof I haue spoken in the repercussiue

cussiue. &c. So note, that I giue you warning, to obserue diligentlie to losyng of the bellie, in all these causes. And furder, kepe of the matter with repercussiues, as example.

R̃. Oile of Roses, Bole Armoniacke, the three Sanders, with the white and the yolke of an Egge, or els with this. Take Mallowe leaues, Violet leaues, ana. M.i. Wormewood, redde Roses, ana. M.ſs. Barlie meale. ʒ.i. Lintill meale. ʒ.i.ſs. Oile of Chamamell, seethe soche thinges, as ought to be sodden, and let them bee strained, then mingle them together, making a soft plaster at the fire, accordyng to the art. This is a medicene of that greate learned man *Auicen*, his owne inuension, for resolucion, and comfortyng the member: as it maie verie easely bee perceiued, if you marke well the receiptes. Now if these bee founde sufficient, feare not to practise, discomfort not at all. But perhaps you shall finde some matter, verie slimie or tough, to stronge for this, in soche case. Doe thus. Take the leaues of Mallowes, and Violettes, ana. M.i. rootes of white Lillies. ʒ.ii. rootes of Marche Mallowes. ʒ.iii. boile all together, stampe and strain them with a stronge strainer, or Colander, into a Kettle, wherunto put Butter freshe. ʒ.ii. Swines grease ʒ.i.ſs. sethe them, and make a plaster in a stone morter Or els doe thus. Take rootes of white Lillies. ʒ.iii. rootes of March Mallowes. ʒ.ii. and rootes of Garden Mallowes, and rootes of Violettes, ana. M.ſs. sethe them soft, stampe them, and strain them, wherunto put Capons grease. ʒ.i. freshe Butter. ʒ.ii. Barowe grease. ʒ.i.ſs sower Leauen. ʒ.iii. Barlie meale, as moche as shall suffice. Ͽ.i. of Saffron, and make thereof with the former decoction, a conueniente plaster, applie it to the sore place, accordingly.

A goodly repercussiue.

Auicens medicene.

An excellent plaster to asswage paine in a sore.

Sorenes.

What is then to be doen, after this businesse, I praie you maister *Chyrurgian*?

Chyrurgj.

When you be come to this poinct, doe your feate hardely, with lance in hand, trimble not: discomfort not your self, neither your paciente, but open thapostumacion. Somwhat in the forme of a newe Moone croked, and when that is doen, vse the maner of digestion, and abstarcion in maner as I haue saied. But as concernyng the makyng sounde, and the skinnyng, vse the medicen, whiche is compounded of Vermilion. ʒ.i. oile of Roses and Mirtes, ana. ʒ.i.ſs. This is of good effecte, in causyng of a seratrice, cutte or scarre, if the place be annointed with water of Planten, Rose water, Honie of Roses, and a little Allume, it shall bee verie comfortable, with a softe Sponge, to moiste the place: and thus haue the old aunciēt men, euer vsed emong their miserable pacientes. Then there is an other intencion, whiche is verie good: whiche is to amende euill accidence, whiche comber, moleste, and vexe apostumacions often tymes. For if the paciente bee

How to make incisiō.

How to drie humors that doe abounde.

Cc.iiii. long

A Dialogue

longe vexed with soche euill accedence, the vertue naturall will then decaie, and be quickly ouerthrowen: wherof will followe incontinently greate daunger, and moche hinderaunce to the cure of the same, that in fine, it shalbe scant curable: which accidentes be these twoo, the one is called extreme dolour or paine. The other is darcknesse and dedly blacke complexion, of the same place, these twoo bee nere hande desperate cures, and moste daungerous to be helped, in all apostumacions: but commonly these accidentes, are found onely, to be the cause of euill *Chyrurgians* necligences.

Dolour and darkenesse of complexion.

Sorenes.

What moueth the *Chyrurgian* thus to doe? I praie you tell me.

Chyrurgj.

When the matter in the apostumacion, was alreadie ripe, and flittyng, and after the same should quickly haue been expulsed, or auoided by inuisible transpiracion, whiche is one of the forces, or benefites of nature. Then the ignoraunt *Chyrurgian*, ministereth foorthe with repercussiues, which draue backwarde, and pressed the water so faste in the place, that these accidentes did ensue of necessitie. Wherefore I shall exhorte thee, my dere frende, seyng thou arte minded, to enter into the worthie ministerie of this worke: whiche is not onely profitable to thy self, but also beneficiall to the common wealth. That you doe vse repercussiues, namely in the painfull places, that maie be the occasion of riping of the matter, for feare that you repente you, for when matter is ones placed, then neede wee not but to open the pores, whiche thyng euery manne maie doe verie easely, if he doe resorte to the repercussiues, afore described.

What harme insueth of an euill Chirurgian.

Sorenes.

Sir, if in case these accedentes, whereof you haue spoken, be in this daungerous perill, it should seme then, either to be in the falte of the *Chyrurgian*, or els in the malice of the humour, what is then to be dooen?

Chyrurgj.

You shall make a plaster, with these medicenes followyng, whiche the greate learned men theim selues, haue vsed vnto their pacientes. ℞. of hulled Beanes, or Beane that is without the bran. ʒ.i. of Malowe leaues. M.ii. Sethe theim in lye, till thei bee well sodden, and afterward, let thē be stamped, and incorporated with meale of Linte, or Flaxe. ʒ.iii. of Lupine meale. ʒ.ii. and forme therof a plaster, with Goates grese, for this openeth the pores, auoide the matter by transperacion, and comforteth also the member, but if the place after a daie or two: when the applicacion of the plaster, fall more and more to blacknes: it shall bee necessarie to goe further, euen to scarefiyng and incision of the place, accordyng as it maie suffer. Certainlie, these

A good emplaster.

these are soche accidence, that will not so easly be displaced, as I haue talked of, but require moste prudent and circumspect deligence, of the Phisicions. Therefore, who so will come vnto this arte, should dwell no small while, with a learned *Chyrurgiō*, to this ende, that he maie both learne his saiynges and doynges, and obserue thesame, and haue thē euer in minde, that he maie euer bee able to trauise the aire, with his owne proper winges, whithout the helpe of others. And not bee as a blinde guide, neither apte to leade, nor tracte the waie hymself, accordyng to profite, arte and knowlege. For in so doyng, he shalbe like vnto an vnconnyng Shipe maister, whiche bringeth his shippe to ruin, rockes, or wracke, so shall he finishe his course with shame, and his paciente with death. Therefore, when the place is scarified, lette it bee doune bothe quiclie and sodenlie: then laie vpon thesame skarificacion baie Salte. After this be doen, then applie this folowyng, in good order.

what the Chirurgian must doe.

Example.

℞. Of Bane meale, and of Orobus. ana. ʒ. vi. of Lupine meale ʒ. iiii. And boile them in Oxemell, vnto soche tyme as thei shalbe plaster thicke, and after applie them to the place. Or els or plaster it with Beanes, and Lupines, boiled in Barberie lye, and afterward strained and stamped in a Morter. Now perchaunce, ye see euill and corrupte fleshe in the place, ye shall nede no further councell in that behalf. But incontinente anointe the place with *Vnguentū Egyptiacum*, whiche muste bee made after the minde of *Auicen*.

Vnguentum Egiptiacuun of Auicen.

℞. Vert degrece, Roche Alume, Honie, Viniger, an̄. ǯ. ß. that is, as moche as will suffice, sethe them vntill thei come in a red colour, and with this ointment you shall exasperate, and sharpe the place, by the space of twoo or three daies, notwithstanding, if you shall neede, you maie iterate, or often applie the same, vntill the same come to an escharous crust or scabbe, and make separation, whiche must not be roted vp by any instrument, but rather maie bee renued, with one of the mollificatiues, specially young Hogges greace, as it is aforesaid, and when this is fallen of, thesame vlcer muste bee cured, as all other vlcers are, which I shall giue you furder vnderstanding hereafter. Now you doe perceiue, how putrifaction owght and must be handeled, but in the meane while, foresee with wisedome, that this euill be preuented, and auoide thesame, for when a cure is not well handeled, or is cast awaie, then it is to late, to call again yesterdaie. Praier or wepyng in this case, will scant preuaile in the *Chyrurgians* behalfe. Now consequently, after I haue spoken of the asswaging, or mitagating of the dolor, and paine of apostumacion, whiche oppresseth nature, as the prince of Philosophie, called *Aristotle*, affirmeth, saiyng: dolour and paine, be the euilles that dooe dissolue, and vtterly destroie, the humaine nature of mankind. Wherfore it semeth necessarie, that in due order some wholsome waie be taken, to helpe this daungerous matter, and to auoide the dolour.

To abate dedde fleshe.

A Chirurgiš muste haue prouidence to foresee his cure.

Sorenes.

what

A Dialogue.

What is beste to auoide the dolour?

Chyrurgj.

Nothing truelie, but artificiallie to altere, and chaunge an euill complexion, so that it come not by stopping of the matter, or by the breache of continuaunce, or corosion. For then soche grief would aske other succours. For whereas dolour is fallen, it doe plainly appere, a sodaine alteracion of complexion in that parte, as *Galen* affirmeth.

To alter complexion in a sore.

Therfore, if you will make any alteration in nature, inuent some apte proper medicene, for the same purpose: as example. Take Oile of Roses. ʒ.ii. the yolke and whites of.ii. Egges newe laied, beate them all together, and aplie them to the place, then the next daie folowing in the mornyng, aplie this in place or stede of the former. Take crummes of white bread, sodden in Goates, or Shepes milke, or els breade sodden in the brothe of a Chicken, or els you maie take a wethers hed sodden fro the bones, whiche you must presse through a cotten clothe, from the same sodden fleshe, saue halfe a pinte of the decoction, vnto whiche decoction, then put to the same Honie of Roses, and oile of Camamell, ana. ʒ.i. ß. wich yolkes of newe laied Egges. All these muste bee beaten together and recocted, or sodden againe vpon a softe fire vntill soche tyme as it bee somwhat stiffe, when this is dooen, aplie it warme to the dolours pained place, accordingly.

Sorenes.

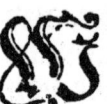
Choise of medicen is good.

What if this medicens preuaile not, what shall I doe then good maister *Chyrurgian*, for I haue hard saie, that one medicen worketh not health in euery complexion, but choise is good.

Chyrurgj.

Then you shall vse this, whiche followeth. For often tymes extreme dolour, and paines of verie necessitie, shall require molificacions, without daunger, wherein there maie bee put soche coolyng thinges, as will not hinder mollificaciō, thus Prince *Auicen* sheweth in his chapiter *de flegmone* therefore doe thus.

Take Mallowes, violettes. ana. ℈.i. seethe them, and braie them, and put in them. ʒ.ii. of Barlie meale, of oile of Roses. ʒ.iiii. and eftsones sethe them againe vntill thei bee in the forme of plaster thicke, whiche in case serue not yet the purpose, note this other.

Take of Fenicreke, meale Line seedes, of flowers of Camamell, of Henne fatte, melted, of Rosed oile. ana. ʒ.iii. Lette all these, the oiles and fattes onely excepted: bee mingled and sodden together, with the decoction of Mallowes, and violettes, vnto soche tyme, as thei bee thickned, to make a plaster. This doen, warme the oile and fatte, and and incorporate the same, with a little oile of Camamill, and of Dill, and so make it to a plaster. This will open the pores, and harde pressed matter, whiche causeth the paine. Now if it be in the augmentyng of a maladie, in this case, ye shall make it after this forme.

Take oile of Roses, and of Camomill, ana. ʒ.i.ß, the yokes of twoo Egges. ʒ.ß. of Barlie meale or more, whiche ye shall shake well together, and so laie it to the place. This suppose I sufficiente, for the appeasyng of dolour: If not, you of your owne hedde, by these maie inuent new, and other confections, to the behofe of your pacientes, and your owne contencion. Sith I haue dispatched this, I will retourne to an hardeined apostumacion, whiche truely, might haue been omitted well inough, the matter beyng so manifeste and plaine.

Neuerthelesse, I will resite here, what the learned haue used in this case, because I would not maime my communicaciō. Certainly this inuencion shall minister diuers fetches and causes, wherin men maie emploie their wittes. Howbeit (accordyng as *Mesue* writeth *De lassitudine post purgationem*) wee will conuerte our intent, to the cause of hardnesse, to the intent we maie cutte it of. For as he saieth, this is the right waie in cures, and the foresight in woorkyng. Wherefore, if it appere that the place tende to hardnes, or euer it come to that poinct, and be fixed it maie be redressed thus. Take ten fatte Figges, of rootes of Marishe Mallowes, smally chopped. ʒ.bi. Seethe theim well, and then braie theim with. ʒ.ii. of Barrowe grece: puttyng thereto a little Saffron, where with couer the place, whiche ye would soften. And ye shall not faile of the purpose. But if it were so, that the praie escaped your wittes, or miste your fingers, you maie be sure to intrappe it with this. *A softenyng emplaster.*

Take of Terebintin medled, and well incorporated with Butter, & this doubtles shall serue your purpose. But or euer it bee applied, the place must be prepared and often made moist, for ripyng of the matter, with blood warme water. Now when it cometh to rottyng, open the place with a potenciall Cauterie, or with some other fetche or meane forseyng alwaie, that it bee doen, accordyng to the rules aboue mencioned. In fine, when it is opened, procede in the cure, as in other. *A potenciall Cauterie.*

These be the thinges, whiche I had this daie to saie, which though thei be not so finelie uttered, ne liuelie declared, as happelie ye looked for: ye shall beare with my simplicitie, in that behalf, for I neuer bestowed labour in Oratre (as I thinke ye perceiue right well) to attain unto eloquence. And so, where I am simple and plain my self, I haue handeled soche thinges, as I had to saie, with semblable simplicitie & plaines, whiche if it like you, also I shall right gladly recite unto you after thesame order and maner: soche thynges, as we haue to utter of woundes. Now, if I haue stombled or missed any where, I praie you correcte it, so if it be worthie of correction. And on the other side, if any thing praise worthie, be come to light, offer and ascribe that to the liuyng God (as I saied in the beginnyng of our cōmunicacion.) That we maie in our self, uerefie the saiyng of the Poet. *Ab Ioue principium, nam sunt Iouis omnia plena.* Of God take thinges their beginnyng, for by hym is all replenished, whose name bee blessed for euer. *Amen.* *Of God beginnyng and endyng of all thinges.*

Sorenes.

I

A Dialogue

YOU haue handeled your self, verie eloquentlie and freshelie inough to daie, also you haue giuen vs cuppes of knowlege, able to quenche the thrust of better men then we are. And I assure you, no man maie greatly wonder at it, seyng we are enuironed on euery side, with soche gentle humanitie, and brotherly loue of eche others. Wherfore, we praie vnto God, that for this your gift, he will prospere you and your cures, and longe preserue you in healthe, to the behoue of your countrie, and frendes. For you haue quenched our thrust, aboue expectacion, with worthie communicacion and medicins. But to giue you warnyng, I praie you haste hether to morowe, with as greate and quicke spede, as ye can passe, after ye haue visited your cures, to the intent ye maie paie vs your promise at full, not without many thankes. Now therfore, sith the of your parte time moueth you, to attende your cures, departe in good time, and remember vs. For we sore people, minde to repaire hether againe to morowe, to heare you although the weather be verie cold.

Chyrurgj.

GO ye on in the name of God, I doubt not, but that I am yours, and all theirs, whiche bee either sicke, or sore, to helpe them, to my power.

Sorenes.

Mannes secrete prouidence.

IT befalleth often times, if any good or euill hang ouer mennes heddes: the deuine minde of man, hath an inglyng, and a smattering thereof, or euer it come to effect, whiche thing is verefied in our self this daie. For where we feared losse of tyme, we haue bainly spent all the daie, in lokyng hether and thether for you maister *Chyrurgion*. And al this together, is doen for you, wherefore to saie truth, we charged you with the matter, and spake liberally of you. Now therefore, if ye recompence it not with diligence, wee will laie all the burthen, in your necke, because we haue taried so long for you this daie.

Chyrurgj.

DOe you herein, as you thinke good. For I am all together yours, and would that you al were helped: specially, because ye begin plainly, to shewe your grieues. And this will I dooe gladlie, omittyng the definicion, in as moche, it liketh you so well: notwithstanding, that all anciēt authours in writing of matters, thought it best to begin at the definiciō. But yet thei, as I thinke, were of that minde and opinion: where the matter was straunge and darke, and where it could not bee well perceiued, but the diffinicion gaue some light to it. And of a truth, so ought thei to doe, where cloudie darknesse and crabbishe knottes, requireth light and openyng by the diffinicion, whiche thing as I trust, shall not happen in my plain wordes. For I intende to speake of woundes, whiche to all men, be as plain as a packe staffe.

Of wonndes For it is giuen men of nature, warely to auoide all noiaunce, and as moche it feareth them also to be hurte, I saie that woundes be manifest

fest to all menne. And if it were otherwise with theim, I might well inough beginne my communicacion, at this diffinicion of woundes. For it were easely saied, that a wounde is a breache of conttnuaunce, newlie made, in an harde or soft parte of the bodie, being without putrifaction and corrupcion. Now therfore, sith there appereth no commoditie curatiue, to rise thereof, I thinke it beste to passe it with silēce notwithstandyng, if you be desirous of it, the saiyng, whiche is rehersed, maie serue the purpose. And now to begin the matter plainly, I suppose I maie laie the foundacion beste, in the deuision of woundes

The diffinicion of a wounde.

Sorenes.

You haue rightlie iudged. But sir, my desire is, that ye will begin, wheras I maie heare one long profitable tale, of the whole matter, and I will occupie myne eare, and kepe silence.

Chyrurgj.

I was mynded thesame my self also.

Sorenes.

Well, go on then, and speake to the purpose, without interruptyng of your talke : vnlesse where necessitie shall cause you to pause, or breath your self, good maister *Chyrurgian*.

Chyrurgj.

I Heard, my friendes and brethren saie, that there were twoo kinde of woundes, whiche dooe no lesse differ in name, then in their cures. The one menne call a simple wounde, the other double or compounded. The simple is, where no substaunce is loste, and is ensounded and cured, with one intencion alone. And of this, wee shall make no further a doe, because of the facilitie thereof. For why? Coblers, Carters, and women bee able to cure soche woundes. Now that whiche is properly called a compounded wounde, is where some substaunce is loste: and necessarily requireth, diuers intēcions in the cure as thus. To vnite that, whiche was seperated, to restore that was loste, and to displace an appostumacion, if it be concurraunt with the same. But here note, that emonges woundes, some be vncurable, and some curable. Therfore we will shewe you, what woundes we holden for mortall, and vncurable. And it is not inconueniente, to begin at the harte, as the chief forte, and principall pece of the bodie.

Twoo kinds of woundes, the one simple, and the other double, or compound.

Then we saie, that euery wounde, anoiyng and perishyng the substaunce of the hart, it is dedly and vncurable. For why? As *Auicen* saith the harte, during the naturall life, maie not suffre any breache of continuaunce. And therefore, to knit vp moche in one knot, soche woundes as giue let and impechemente to the vertue, whiche is necessarie to life, take mankinde awaie, without remeadie. As woundes in the substaunce of the brain: of the winde pipe: of the wesande: of the lunges: of the liuer: of the gaule, of the midriffe, of the mawe: of the splen

what wounde be mortall.

A Dialogue.

Partes most daungerous to be hurte. of the small guttes, of the kidneis and bladder: and generally, al soche woundes, whiche perce through the bulke, and inward partes, be verie daungerous. Because the inwarde partes bee altered, by mouyng of the aire, from out forthe, and the spirites bee offended within, and the vertue naturall, which mainteineth life, is destroied. And the reason why, is that, when these partes be wounded, thei be moste hardly helped, by reason of their continuall mouyng and labouryng. And when this maie not be made whole, thei be not able, ne sufficiente to doe their offices, requisite to nature.

woundes in the muskles. Now must we speake somewhat of woundes, that happen in muskelles, and lacertes. For thei maie bee thought as daungerous, as the foresaid. For as in the one, be manifest tokens of death: so in the other be prognosticable signes, for men enflamed with high and deuine forsight.

Example. For a wounde in a muskell, doeth moche like a woode Snake, whiche lieth awaite for menne out of their waie, lurkyng vnder their grene flowers, where he putteth theim that go by, in doubt or hassard of their life. Therefore my frendes, let vs reason somwhat of them also, that thei leade vs not forthe with vaine hope, and oppresse vs emōges other, as carelesse and idle heddes. Wherefore wee suppose, that woundes chauncyng, three fingers aboue and beneath, the heddes of the muskelles or lacertes, nigh vnto the iointes, be excedyng daungerous:

Of conuulcion mortall. and that prickyng of sinewes, doe often cause conuulsions, by reason of the greate fealyng and felowshippe, that thei haue with the braine. Wherein the saiyng of *Hyppocrates* appereth true, who saith, that a spasme or conuulsion, chauncyng vpon a wound, is mortall for the moste parte. Wherefore, the woundes in soche parte, must be handled warelie, and with aduised deliberaciō. For why, thei will to notablie hinder the *Chyrurgian* his estimacion, if he prognosticate warelie of the same, to them that stande by: whiche thing trulie had, befallen to my self, when I promised a man his life, had not I been admonished of by maister *Rasis*, who secretly and wittely, vnknowen to all the family, pluckte me by the elbowe, and warned me, with these, or like wordes in effecte. And then the pacientes strengthe was agreable to healthe, and no appostumacion risen: but he slepte as he ailed nothyng at all. Consider with thy self, saieth he, as thou doest lightlie alwaie, the signes, which induce conuulsion in woundes. Where as there appereth no swelling in the sore, in good faithe, I conceiue an euill opinion, in the pacientes life, whiche I haue gotten me, with long obseruacion.

A goodly note to be obserued when death is at hande. For the matter, whiche should come forthe, to the pained place, is supped vp of the sinewes. Wherefore, I see a conuulsion euen at hande, for if the matter, though it were little (for in moche it fareth a like) had issued & gathered to the place, it would giue me occasion to thinke well of him. For it should signifie, that the matter did relinquishe the sinewes, and drawe outward.

Now in asmoche as it remaineth, as a slepe within, surely I thinke euill of it: and truely, it was maruailouslie saied of hym. For, or euer the

the fiueth daie came, the man gaue vp the breath, by reason of a spasme or crāpe, whereat I was greatly abashed, reseruyng the signes in memorie, & minde hereafter, as I also aduise you to doe. Yea, & if there be any other els, worthie of obseruacion, marke the vain also diligentlie that it maie stande you for stede, when nede shall require. For this wil require a vigilant iye of the *Chyrurgian*. Wherfore, I appeale here to your secrete hartes, and bid you beware, that ye disgrace not your self thorowe rashenes, but be ripe in prognosticacions, and circūspecte in obseruing of the times, of your workinges bothe for one helpe & others.

Now all other woundes, these onelie excepted, whiche I haue recited, no doubt be curable. And as for the helpe of these curables, there are twoo principall found, the one by the first intencion, the other by the second. The latter is, where deuided partes are ioyned totogether, through a porcion of an other kinde of matter. As for an ensample. Bones are ioyned together, with a certaine harde matter, moche like a bone, but not a bone, whiche is moche like to a Plasarte. The other, when partes are ioyned together, with their like in kinde, as fleshe with fleshe. And these waies, we muste nedes haue before our iyes, to the intente we minister not any thing in woundes, whiche we might afterwarde repent. Wherefore, to auoide these euils I iudge it beste, to begin with soche thinges, as maie bee vsed generally, in all kinde of woundes to helpe mankinde.

Sorenes.

For Gods sake shewe me the beste maner of woundes.

Chyrurgj.

When ye haue determined, to take any soche wounde in hand: incontinent remember to obserue these thinges, that is to saie, an order of the life, locall medicenes, and amendement of euill accidentes. The firste, ye shall obtain by due administracion of the sixe thynges, called not naturall. If the *Chyrurgian* bee ignoraunt therein, the Phisicians maie rule the matter. For it belongeth to them, to giue an order of liuyng, to bryng humours to a qualitie, to trie out inwarde causes, of variable ebbyng and flowyng. And finally, to giue iuste redresse of the same, whiche thyng for the moste parte, *Chyrurgians* laboure not to attain to, because the matter is so secretlie hid, as it wer emonges stones, but onely by meanes of couetousnes, and gredie desire of *Chyrurgians*. For when thei haue gotten onely a little taste, without all excercise, vnder their maister, whiche thyng is mother to Arte, as *Aristotle* saieth. Thei take money hungerlie, thei seke in hande, & rent their skin with their teeth, makyng no consciēce at the matter at all. Now as touchyng the seconde, in applyyng of locall medicenes: ye shall not plaie, make or marre, ne go at all aduenture, as ye sought blindfeled. But perswade your self earnestlie, that you made Argus, to bee your companion in the matter. For in case ye misse but a little, or negligen

What the Chirurgian must obserue.

A Dialogue.

who so dooe graunt to one absurditie, many one wil eftsones followe.

tlſe omit any neceſſarie thyng in the cure, ye ſhall firſt bryng your ſelf in a pecke of troubles, and after will enſue many inconueniences, as ſaieth *Ariſtotle*, graunte one abſurditie, and many inconueniences will folowe. Wherefore, leaſt this doe chaunce, it is good that ye looke narrowlie on the matter, with aduiſed circumſpection. Now therefore, when ye ſtande before the wounded, firſte ponder with your ſelf, how the wound was giuen, of what ſort it is, and how large a gaſhe?

A ſmall wounde.

For be the wounde ſmall, and in a fleſhie parte, without loſing of ſubſtaunce, it maie be cured onely with couenable bindyng. But if it bee greate and depe, firſt ſtaunche the blood, if any be, with ſome medicen coueniēt, as I ſhall declare hereafter, in the place of bledyng & vlcers, whereunto I referre at this preſente. For there I entende to giue medicens, and meanes for that purpoſe. When the bloode is ſtanched, ye ſhall ſewe the wound, with a fine threde, well twiſted and waxed, betwene your fingers. But or I ſpeake of ſewyng, I will recite certain cauſes, where ſewing is daungerous, & therefore forbidden as vnprofitable. And then will I to my purpoſe again in order for your ſake.

Sorenes.

I praie you ſhewe me that order?

Chyrurgj.

You ſhall firſt remember, that woūdes made, with any long and round weapē, as an arrowe or dart: muſt not for a fewe daies, be cured by the firſt intencion, notwithſtandyng thei be cured, partly by the firſt. Some doe ſaie thei be not cured, by the firſt, for why? We kepe thē open, leaſt the matter be impreſoned here. For if it were ſo, woundes might incurre extreme dolour, by reaſon of alliance, with coordes & ſinewes. And therfore we ſaie plainly,

Example.

thei ought not to be ſhut vp in the firſt daies. For my ſelf ſawe this in a valiaūt capitain, at Barwicke, who had a wound in the necke. And a certain Phiſicion tooke the man in hand, & willing to haſte the helpyng of the wounde, whiche ought to haue been kept open, but he cloſed it vp with a ſeame: whereupon, the pacient fell into extreme pain and as it wer, into a continuall conuulſion, inſomoche, that if a cun-

Pate Hardie the Scotte, a good Chirurgian.

ning *Chyrurgian*, called Pate Hardie, a Skot, had not put to his hand the ſoner, he had borne his owne meſſage to the ded. But to our purpoſe, wher I ſaid, notwithſtanding, thei be cured by the firſt intenciō: this is vnderſtanded, that ther is no loſt ſubſtaunce, newly produced in thē

Of the firſte and ſeconde intencion.

For if there were, the cured ſhould be after the ſeconde entencion. And where any ſubſtaunce is loſte, & ought newly be produced, ſewing ſhal be right ſtraunge & vntoward. For why, it can not otherwiſe be well cured, but by the ſecond. For nature ſeketh euer reſtitucion of the loſt parte, with no leſſe carefulneſſe, then the mother her onely loſt ſonne. Wherfore, if we minde to reſtore that, we maie not ſowe vp the woūd, or it be recouered. If the wounde be deepe, and greatlie altered, by the

receipt

receipte of the aire, thinke of no sewyng. For matter is now secretlie **Matter doe couet digestiō**
caused, by reason of the aire, whiche crieth out for digestion, and ab-
stercion. And if the impericke, whom ye knowe of, had thus handeled
the matter, the honeste man ye wote of, had been yet a liue. For when **His name was Iuc, of Swasa in Cambrige Shire.**
he had taken a large gasshe in his legge, and long had left it opē to the
aire, thinkyng to be notablie well cured: caused an *Chyrurgian* to be sente
for, whiche immediatlie in all the haste (a Gods name) seweth vp the
wounde. What will ye more? Immediatlie after the sewyng, importable dolours did arise, and on the thirde daie, the legge was so seastred
that in the.vii. the man would nedes take his *vltimum vale*, and saie farewell to the liuyng. Now if the imperike had first vsed digestion with
abstercion, and then sewyng of the wounde, perchaunce the matter
had not growen, to that extremitie of death. And in case the wounde, **A wounde of a bruse.**
bee by meanes of a bruse, then attempte not to sewe it. For without
doubt, ye shall shortly perceiue, that ye laboured in vaine.

Whereof *Galen* giueth vs a warning worde, saiyng: that it koloweth
of necessitie, that a bruse should putrifie, and tourne to corrupcion. I
adde, and vnderstande it, if it be an extreme bruse. For in a meane, it taketh no place. Therefore, if it be sewed, the seame will sone be corrupted. As we sawe our self, a lustie young man, who came to see a Bull
baityng, in Parisse Garden, and fallen before thesame, I wote not
how, the Bulle gaue hym in the thigh a rente, with the hornes. Now **It is peril-lous to sewe a wound, cō-myng of the bitɩng, or ren-dyng of some beaste.**
when a *Chyrurgian* had taken hym in hande, incontinente he sewed the
wounde, whiche putrified right sone. And certainlie, but if maister
Backter had helped it, I thinke assuredly, the man had died of it. Furder we saie, that sewing is not good in a wounde, caused by bityng of
some beast. For a bitten place, is hollowe & abated, or otherwise, somwhat sauoureth of the nature of a bruse. Howbeit, we leaue this case
to the good *Chyrurgians* iudgemente. For partes seuered by bityng, maie
well be ioyned with a threde, in some cases. Sewing is to no purpose,
where a wounde vncouereth a bone broken, or whole, for it will not
haue adoe with ensoundyng through sewyng: excepte the discouered
be first cladde, and the seconde vnited togither again naturally.

Also a wound in a muscolous place, specially ouerthwart the mus- **Of woundes of the muscles**
kell, vtterlie refuseth sewyng, as *Auicen* saieth, in the chapiter of bindyng of woundes in Lacertes and Muskelles. Or be it a Lacert, whiche is rente in latitude, it is not drawen together, but rather some
thing is put betwene, least the skinne growe together. &c. Wherfore
he would the wounde wente at large, whiles the cure is after the seconde intencion. Thesame doe sinewie places desire also, for if thei be
sewed, the lippes will growe to one, and the sinewes vnder couerte,
wil caste rumetike matter, and shortly cause apostumacion, so that ye
shalbe driuen, whether ye wil or no, to louse the seame, or make a new
insicion. Therfore to auoide this inconuenience, we shall suffre soche
woundes, to run at large for a ceason: and so ye shall haue them, more **A question moued in Chyrurgi.**
tractable in handlyng. How bee it, here is a tedious disputacion mo-
Dd.iii. ued,

A Dialogue

ued, whether a cutte sinewe should be sewed, or not. For there bee sondrie opinions, and aucthorities of the learned, of the one side, and of the other. And verelie, if I should dispute the matter, I would maintaine bothe the opinions, although at this present, I assente with maister Jhon de Vigo, not for that I haue sworne, to saie as he saith, but because his wordes, seme moste consonaunt to reason.

Of sinewes.

And to *Auicen*, where he saieth, if the sinewes be broken in latitude, then it is necessarie to sewe the wounde: and if it bee not sewed, the wound will not growe together. Howbeit, I will omit the prosecuciō of this question: sith it is not necessarie vnto this treatise. But yet by the waie, marke well the saiyng of *Auicen*, where he cōmaundeth to sew the wounde of necessitie. Certes, I, after *Marianus* would let it go open. But he meaneth of a large wounde, whiche would cause greate deformitie, if it be vnsewed. And likewise, if it bee sewed, beyng a greate distaunce betwene stitche and stitche. And on the otherside, where I said, I would suffre it to be louse, I meaned of a small wound, whiche experience shall teache you to be true. Moreouer, many dolorous and apostumated woundes, will none of sewyng, whiche, what for the facilitie, and manifeste apparance, needeth no further declaracion. For the cause is open to theim, that will diligentlie consider the matter. These be the causes, where we vse not to sewe woundes, and bee worthie put vp in memorie. Now will I returne, frō whence I digressed.

How to sewe a wound, and how not.

Now these cases excepted, sewe the wound, with a well twisted thred, drawen through Ware, as we said before, alwaies remembred that ye leaue some place open, in the lowest part, where matter maie haue issue forth. Whē ye haue so doen, ye must applie this medicen, whiche is mingled of the white of an Egge, and a little Oile of Roses. This is doen, because the paciente should not greatlie bee troubled, at the remouyng. For oftime is caused so greate paine, namelie in hearie places, that the pacient semeth to be crampet, or rackt with conuulcion. And let this remain. xxiiii. howers in the wounde, if ye feare any bledyng. And when this tyme is expired, visite your pacient again, with a gladsome countenaunce, and whiles ye be merely talkyng with him take of all the coueryng, and then enbaulme it, with a degestiue of yolkes of Egges, and cleare Terebintine, laied in a clothe. But if the wounde be in the hedde, or any place of moche felyng, take oile of Roses, in stede of Terebintine, wherewith procede in the cure, til mattre be caused in the place. And when that is doen, set the digestiue a part. For if ye procede further, it were but to put putrifaction, to putrifaction. Neuertheles, the brinkes of the wounde, must be oiled with Rosed omphacine, that is Oile of Water Lillies. After ye haue so visited the wounde, ye shall spred this defensiue, one hande breade from it.

The Chirurgian muste looke pleasauntly vpon his pacient.

A defensiue.

Take of Rosed oile. ʒ. ii. ß. of all the Sanders ana. ʒ. ii. of Bole Armoniacke. ʒ. ii. ß. the white of an Egge, and a little Vineger, if the wounde bee distaunte from a sinewie place, if not, wine of Pomegranettes, in stede of Vineger. All whiche, cause to be drawen in a morter
that

betwene Sorenes and Chyrurgj. Fol.xxij.

that it be at hande, when nede shall require. When ye haue thus proceded fower or fiue daies, then muste you giue ouer the digestiue, and vse a mundificacion, whiche is thus mingled. Take of Rosed Honie, ʒ.ij. of Terebintine, ʒ.iij. let thē seeth a little, puttyng thereto .i.ß. of Barlie meale, with Ɔ.i. of Saffron. All whiche must be incorporated at the fire, & vsed the space of .viij. daies, or there about, as is expedient. And as for the sounding, vse the ointment, that I described in apostumacions, wherewith I ensounde or make whole, almoste all kinde of breaches, as our frende can witnesse, whiche (because he would haue the certaintie) would nede be present, when we cured a sore manne of apostumacion vnder tharme hole, whiche *Albenzoar Rasis* reconed for vncurable. If any fattishe fleshe grewe, at the inclosyng thereof, ye shall remoue it with *Vnguentum Mixtum*, mingled of *Vnguentum Egiptiacum*, and *Vnguentum Apostolorum*, of eche like quantitie, or els take this pouder, whiche my self did moche vse. Take of *Citrine Mirabolanes* ʒ.ß, of *Terra Sigillata* ʒ. of burnt roch Alume. ʒ.ij. let them bee stamped small, and the pouder for a corosiue, wherewith ye shall get the victorie and triumphe, ouer the maladie.

Sorenes.

Thus haue ye spoken, of a simple deepe fleshie wounde: now I praie your, procede to the double wounde, and the cure therof.

Chyrurgj.

Restitucion is made, with a matter of an other kinde, as in bones and sinewes. How bee it, some aucthours affirme, that broken and displaced bones in young children, bee vnited againe, with matter of thesame kinde. For why, members, whiche Phisicians call sparmatticall, beyng ones loosed, will not be ioyned again, with *Poros sarcoides*, whiche is of an other kinde. Now therefore, here haue wee to declare, how this meanes maie bee obtained, in a double wounde, of the elbowe or hande. For of all woundes, thei bee moste harde and daungerous, and specially of the hande: for the multitude of sinewes and cordes, and otherwise, scarcitie of nutratiue humours. Therefore let vs take in hande, euen as it were now newly come to our cure.

Now then my friende, when ye bee called to any soche chaunce: remember ye looke seriously, that no shiuer nor gobet of bone be lefte in the wounde, whiche might sharpen and anger, the vertue naturall, through some dolour and prickyng. As it hath chaunced in a famous worthy gentleman and souldiour, called Capitain Rede, whose arme was broken at Lith, in warre, *Anno.* 1559. and many bones remained, to his hurte for a tyme. For if these accidentes a rise, thei shewe an apostumacion at hand: theffect and coming wherof, we ought by al meanes, waies, and policies to imbarre, lest it crepe to the wounded place. And ye shal obtain this, if ye obserue this order, which I wil giue you. First clense the woundes of al sheuers of bones, and then if any bones be fully cut of, place thē in their rowmes, as orderlie as ye can. When

Capitain W. Reede of the holie Ilande

To clense the wounde, and drawe for the broken bones

A Dialogue

ye haue so doen, haue a table at hande, well couched and couered with soft lint, that the hande or member maie be placed to rest theron. And forthwith sewe vp the wounde, in case it be large. For a small wound as we said before, must be left open, to the intente rumeticke matters maie haue free libertie and issue, to come forthe. But take heede in sewyng, that ye pricke no sinewe, and that passage be left in the lowest parte, for sanious matter, whiche shall growe, or be caused there. Whē the woūd is sewed, and the hand laied on the table, then must you apparell thesame with fine linte, dipped in the whites of Egges: and so leaue it gentlie enrolled, for the space of xxiiii. howers, giuing the pacient a conuenient regiment of life in diate according to his nature.

Sorenes.

What shall we doe then, when this is doen, as you haue commaunded, in this moste goodlie wholsome order.

Chyrurgj.

AS sone as that tyme shalbe expired, retourne againe to the pacient, taking a Barbour with you, to make a conuenient blood lettyng, on the other contrary parte: and this is doen, that the matter readie to cause apostumaciō, fall not to the place, which is impouerished, by meanes of the wound. And the bain must be opened for bledyng the second daie, for sauyng of good blood. For if the bain were opened the first daie, then good blood might be drawen, aswell as euill. Now when ye haue dooen, with the bloud lettyng, open the wounde, and applie these medicenes, for the cure thereof, as followe in order. ℞. of moste cleare Terebintine ʒ. ii. of oile Hypericon ʒ. iii. mingle thē at the fire, powre them warme into the wounde. For if it bee applied colde, inconuenience might ensue thereof, as *Hyppocrates* saieth: cold is an enemie to the sinewes, teeth, bones, braine, and nuke of the necke, but heate is profitable and frendly. Therefore it is right conuenient, that in all your woorkes, aboute double woundes, ye eschewe medicenes, whiche shalbe actually colde, and see ye kepe the member warme, as a woman deliuered of her burthen. Moreouer, in the brinkes & circuite of the wound, ye shal apply peces of cloth, throughly weated in Rosed oile, wherin Ingletwitches, or yearth Wormes haue been sodden. For this will comfort the part, and also cause euaporacions of humours, if any should approche. Again, anoint this defensiue about the cubite or elbowe, to defende the wounde from fletyng matters. For this doe thus. ℞. oile of Roses, and of Mirtille oile, ana. ʒ. i. ß. of *Bole Armoniacke, Terra sigillata*, Dragons blood, ana. ʒ. i. ß. of all the Saunders. ana. ʒ. i. ß. of white Waxe. ꝗ. ß. and let it be made to a softe defensiue, in maner of a liniment. And when ye haue thus proceded in the cure, 6. or 7. daies, or more, as vnto the tyme the sinewes caste some rumaticke matter, & then it shall be tyme to goe to abstersiue, or dryyng. The firste, whereof is thus made. Take of Terebintine. ʒ. i. ß. and of Siruppe of Roses

When to lette blood on the contrary side of the bodie.

Cold is an euill enemie to the sinewes.

Abstersiue to clense & drie.

betwene Sorenes and Chyrurgj.   Fol.xxiij.

ſes.ʒ.i.ſeeth theim a little, and whiles thei bee seethyng, put thereto ʒ̄.ſſ. of Barlie meale, and of Sarcocoll, and Frankincence, ana.ʒ.ſſ. of Saffron.Ɔ.ſſ. and ſtire theim well, till thei bee incorporated, and mingled together. This is a gentle abſterſiue, without bityng or nipping whiche is neceſſarie in ſoche woundes.   *A good abſterſiue.*

ʒ̄.ſſ. is as moche to ſaie, as will ſuffiſe

Sorenes.

All this ſhall I gladly dooe to my ſelf and others, but a Gods name, what ſhall I then take in hande, to procede any furder?

Chyrurgj.

YE ſhall miniſter this ointmente, as the learned *Chyrurgians* did order it, whiche is.℞. Of Calues & Cowes fat ℔.ſſ. of oile of Roſes of Roſel an̄.ʒ.ſſ. of letharge of ſiluer ʒ.iii.ſſ of freſh odorāt Wine Ɔ.i. of Ingletwiches or yerth wormes ʒ.ii. of Honie,S. Jhō wort,Madder,and flowers of roſe Marie, an. ℈.ſſ. Let all theſe be boiled together, the Terebintine and Letharge onely excepted: vntill ſoche tyme, as the Wine be waiſted,and then ſtraine the foreſaied coction,and boile it in a newe together with the Litarge, till it haue gotten a verie blacke colour,and laſtlie put the ſaied Terebintine to it, with. ʒ̄.ſſ. of white Waxe. And ſo this will be a ſoft ointment, moſte conuenient for woūdyng of ſinewes. And this kinde of miniſtracion, muſt bee continued, vnto the tyme of ſealing and enſounding: for whiche purpoſe,ye maie vſe this decoction folowyng, or that, whiche was diſcriued before, in apoſtumacions. But ye ſhall finde this decoction folowyng better, becauſe it doeth enſounde and comforte the member withall: and therefore ye maie boldlie vſe it in this place.   *A good ointmente for woundes.*

Take of Roſes,Mirtelles,Wormewood,flowers of Pomegranetes ana. ℈.i. ten Cipres Nuttes, and boile theim in redde Wine, vnto the waſtyng of the thirde parte, whiche vſe, and applie with a Spunge well preſſed,for the repaire of the member. And this was myne order, my frende, whiche in good faith,gat me bothe honeſtie & profite. This I ſuppoſe ſufficient,as far as it appertaineth to the helpe of a double wounde. Now is it tyme,to come to the accidens, wherof we mencioned a little before: whiche thynge, yet neuertheleſſe, I would haue omitted,had I not perceiued,that ye were ſo deſirous of it,and doubtleſſe,not without good cauſe. For why, the greateſt parte and feate of curyng of woundes or vlcers (whereof by Gods helpe,we ſhall reaſon to morowe) ſtandeth in the remouyng of the euill accidentes. And therefore,leaſt I ſhould be ſeen to defraude you, of your deſire, I will ones venter my ſelf for your ſakes, vnder this burthen,heuie though it bee. Verelie I can not but moche maruell, how it ſhould bee,that our nature is ſubiecte to ſo many chaunces, and ſo greate ieopardies: when I conſider the accidentes, in ſewyng woundes, whiche when thei be fallen,thei bryng not onelie the ſlender witted and learned,   *To ende a double woūd and begin accidence.*

Nature ſubiect to many calamities.

A Dialogue

ned, but trouble wittie and farre castyng men also. What thinke you the common sorte of *Chyrurgians* will doe: when thei see learned to seke, to be vncertain, and to run fro medicene, to medicene, thinke ye not, but thei will make light of the matter: if thei see a manne, to bee tormented of paine, burste with apostumacion, bexed with euill complexions, to burne in feuers, to be rackte with crapes, to haue Apoplexes, yea, & to be distracte of their wittes to: Therefore least we be reckened of their nomber, and charged with the crime of vnmercifulnes. Lette vs endeuour our selues, to the vttermoste of our possibilitie, that wee maister euery of thē with many medicens, when thei befal. For if thei be not well handeled, Thei will robbe vs of our honest name, healthe and profite, and all the paciente of their liues, whiche is their chief iewell. Wherefore, we muste bestere vs in the matter diligentlie, when nature is extremelie vexte with dolour: & waie with our selues, whether it come of the breache of continuaunce, or dryyng of the wounde, or els by reason of gatheryng of some humerall matter. And if it come by breache of continuaunce, or dryyng of the wounde, then shall a mollificatiue be beste, for the openyng thereof. But if it come by heaping of humerall matter, then dryyng medicenes shall be beste againste the pain, without any respect of tyme, whiche be mingled of oiles, meale and other dryyng simples. These thynges well considered, firste if the wound be pained, through lacke of digestiō, it maie be eased with this.

whē the Chirurgiā is put to shame.

Take of softe bread sodden, ℥. Goates milke. ʒ. vi. of oile of Roses, and Camamell, ana. ʒ. ii. and yolkes of three Egges, all whiche dooe mingle together in a potte, the yolkes reserued, and boile it, till the oiles be well dronken vp of the bread, and then take it from the fire, and mingle the yolkes withall. Thus shall you haue, if ye boile it accordyngly, an harde plaster, to be applied warme to the place.

Sorenes.

But what if this your medicen, serueth not to the purpose, haue ye no more plentie of medicenes then in store?

Chyrurg.

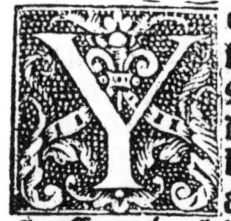Es forsothe, that I haue a medicen of greate vertue folowyng. Take a quarter of a pinte, of the decoction of Mallowes, and Violets, or Mutton brothe of the weader, or els of any beast, that menne vse to eate, and lette bread be well steped therewith, and afterward boile it, as it was saied before. But remember to putte a little Saffron in this, as it maie in the former also, if it please the *Chyrurgian*. But if it come of heaping of matter, vse these medicens that followe.

Take of small grounde branne, ℥. iii. of Barlie and Beane meale ana. ʒ. ii. of Camamell, Melilote, and Wormewood, finelie shorne, an ℥. ß. of odorant wine, three cupfulles, boilyng theim at the fire, with sufficiente Sape, and in the end put thereto oile of Camamell, and of Roses, ana. ʒ. ii. ß. oile of Dill. ʒ. ß. with a little Saffron. And make hereof

hereof a soft plaster, after the maner of a Cerote. I warrant you, with these ye shall asswage the dolour, whiche for the moste parte draweth matter to the place, as a cuppyng glasse, namelie if it bee colde. And if it come of heate, then altre the hotte receiptes, accordyng to the necessitie. And when the dolour is ones appeased, ye shall easelie win the Bulwarke, as touchyng the reste of the cure. Now ye shall represse apostumacion, if ye applie the defensiue aboue described, when ye haue let the paciente bleede, with a diuersiue blood lettyng, a clister goyng before. But if there appere swarte rednesse aboute the wounde, the cause is in an euill complexion, for correctyng whereof, ye maie vse these receiptes. Take oile of Roses. ℥. iii. & mingle the same with the yolkes and whites of twoo Egges, whiche applie, beyng well shaken together in linnen. Or thus. Take. ℥. ii. of *Vnguentum Rosatum*, oile of Roses ℥. i. and put them in a Leaden morter: castyng thereto of iuice of Lettise. ℥. i. ß. of Letharge. ℥. ß. of *Terra Sigellata*. ℥. i. and drawe this, till it bee as a fine leniment, wherby ye shall fully remoue, and correct the euill complexion. But if the pacient shall be vexed with any feuer, conuulcion, palsie, alienacion of minde, swonyng, or soche like, by reason of mouyng of the humours: take a Phisicion to you, and he will amend these accidentes. For if I should now order Sirups, and Pocions (albeit that I entend also at more leisure, to speake more of them in that place, but now) I might seme to put my sithe, in an other manes corn for why, here we talke not of Phisicke, but of *Chyrurgi*, whiche is somewhat contented with Ointmentes, Fomentacions, Plasters, and Leniamentes. This is the money, whiche I had to coigne this daie, to the intente I might bee able to paie you, without farder suite in the Lawe. For ye bound me so straightlie, with an obligacion of an othe. Albeit in this case, euery honeste man will willynglie kepe touche, to discharge his credence to his power.

To correcte a swart woūd.

Sorenes.

O, how rightlie iudge you? But now gentle *Chyrurgi*, in as moche as you haue yelded vs the vse of this daie, let vs depart for the tyme. Howbeit, let vs repaire hether again, I praie you to morowe, to the intent the reste, if any be, maie be paied: and so we receiue the whole some in assuraunce, wherof ye haue giuē vs sore people this earnest penie. And in the meane time, we Sore and Lame, giue thankes to the liuyng God, for his deare benefites, which of his mercie, he haue plentifullie bestowed vpon vs, to releue vs with his giftes, and by his meanes, that wee haue learned, to helpe and heale our selues, when we are lame and sore, whereby we maie be profitable to our comon wealth, I therefore desire you, when you be at leasure, to treate somewhat of vlcers.

God giueth healthe.

Chyrurgi.

Now

A Dialogue.

What an vl=
cer is.

NOw an vlcer is, a breach of continuaunce, with putrifaction and rottennesse, caused in processe of tyme. And their breedyng or ingendering, commonlie (as *Auicen* taketh) is of vlcerated breakynges foorthe of pusshes, and of woundes euill handled. Wherefore woundes (as our chieftaine and graunde maister, affirmeth in the firste treatise of vlcers) as sone as their due tyme of digestion, and abstercio is expired. And yet neuerthelesse, remaine foule and full of corrupcion must be called vlcers properlie, and not woundes: wherof it is a consequent, that euery breache of continuaunce, whiche voideth matter, or virulencie, shall vndoubtedly be called an vlcer. Whereof some bee fathered of an hotte, and some of a colde humour. The vlcers, whiche be founde with rednesse, and itchyng in the edges, come of the hotte: the other, whiche bee without greate rednesse and itche, and haue also wide rootes, are fedde and nourished of colde. Againe, emong vlcers, some bee of small importaunce, and some bee right daungerous. All bee daungerous, whiche breede no *Sanius* matter, when the tyme is to breede: or when some apostumacion is concurrant, whiche shalbe hidden secretlie, without euident cause. For if the apostumacion vanishe, by reason of some medicen, hauyng power to worke that effect, it wer no matter, but if it banishe without cause, and lye secretly a lurkyng: Certes, it importeth no good, but euill, as spasmes, destractions and alienacion of minde. Howbeeit there bee also vlcers, as *Auicen* saieth, whiche properly, and as it were of their nature, produce their effectes now and then, as vlcers of the backe, of sinewes, of the knees, of the hanche, and all soche as haue great aliaunce with the Nuke, wherof some bee tractable, & some repine vtterly against *Chirurgi*, in their cure.

All sores voi=
ding virulent
matter are
called vlcers.

Vlcers bee
harde to cure
that followe
a sickenesse.

All kinde of vlcers be moste harde of cure, whiche succede any sickenesse, and ende thesame, by the waie of euacuacion: for nature vseth to vnburden her self, at that place, from thensforthe, of her euill and vnprofitable superfluities. Likewise bodies, whiche bee accidentall, moistie, or drie, will not easly be cured of their vlcers: as women with childe, and folke sicke of the dropsie: whiche is the caused in the one, through abundaunce of accidentall moisture. In the other, by reason of retained superfluities. Again, drie and ethicall members, maie not easely be ensounded, for wante of good blood: We see the like effecte in olde selie bodies (whiche, what for lacke of digestion of their meates, their naturall heate beyng almoste extinguished, and what for lacke of good blood) bee continually eaten vp of vlcers. Ofte tyme an euill complexion, is cause why, an vlcer is not healed and ensounded. Wherfore in especiall, haue the complexion in consideracion, and neuer rest till ye haue corrected thesame. For why, otherwise the nourishement, which crepeth thether, will be turned into an euil matter, when it is not ruled and maistred of nature. For what is an euill matter els, but corrupted nutriment, whiche nature could not order, ne was able to conuert into the seconde humidities. And to thintent ye maie achiue

this

betwene Sorenes and Chyrurgj. Fol.xxv.

this well, ye shall bestowe a little laboure, to knowe the natures of simples, and signes of complexions, whiche ye maie learne of Galen, in his booke, *de arte medendi*. And spende not your tyme, in trifles and woordes, that passe with the winde, neither in croked and distorted argumentes. For what good shall you dooe to your pacientes, when thei crie for your helpe, when ye haue made a greate sorte of subtill argumentes. Whether there maie be a newtralitie, or meane betwene sicknes and health, in any bodie. Again, sith we se that thei, whiche haue made mencion in their bookes, bee all at square, and none whole of other. Why dooe we embrace soche losyng of time, therefore I will aduise you, to followe with all diligence, Maister Ihon *Tagaltius*, whiche groundedlie and pithelie in his doynges, seketh out fruitfull matters, omittyng trifles.

Galen.

Chirurgians doe not agree

On the otherside, the vlcers, whiche maie bee easelie cured, are tho that chaunce in bodies of good complexions, and bee nourished with good blood, without affluence of many superfluities. Emongest whiche some abide in their newlie caused continuaunce, and some fall to discontinuaunce again. The vlcers whiche fall again to discontinuaunce, bee (as *Auicen* teacheth) where fleshe is caused and generated or euer the mundificacion to bee complete. For in as moche as vncleane superfluites, bee there secretlie hidden, it followeth of necissitie, that the continuaunce be loosed and broken vp again. And for this cause, soche breaches of continuaunce and sores, bee rekened for fistulaies, with the learned Phisicians.

Vlcers in good complexions, ar sone cured.

Further note here, that there bee fiue kindes of vlcers in generall, an vlcer virulent, filthie, caute, rotten and corrosiue. But me thinketh it is meete firste, or euer we meddle with the cure of these generalles, that we recite the accidentes of vlcers, whiche cumber and hinder vs, in the cure: And when we haue so doen, then shal we recite, and treate of their cures. For in case we corecte not the accidentes, whiche make moste for the knowlege *quod quid est rei*, as *Aristotle* saieth in his bookes *De Anima*, we shall neuer winne the victorie of the vlcers, though we striue right stoutly in the cause, because the accidentes holde of the sore, and be of parte against the cure.

Fiue kindes of Vlcers.

Now the accidentes, whiche happen in vlcers, be these, bledyng, superfluous fleshe, euill in sauour, lippes, dolour, apostumacion, hardenes, corrupted bones, swellyng vaines, and roundnesse, and euery of these require properlie a cure, by them self, whiche if it be denaied thē, when thei call for it, or we shalbe conuented before a Iudge, to giue euery manne his owne, or the debt not paied: there maie be no confederacion in amitie with men. Therefore least we be troubled in the law or charged of tirannie, let vs see how we can discharge our handes, of these accidentes, and first of bledyng.

Accidence in vlceres, their names.

Every fluxe of blood, deare brother Sorenes, commonly proceade from a primitiue. For the antecedente, wee will omitte at this present, least happelie, whiles we passe ouer our owne, and rushe rashely

The fluxe of blood proceadyng of a primitiue.

Ee.i. into

into other mennes dooes, might anon be thruste foth by the hedde, for theues. Therefore, to auoide this dishonestie, we will onely speake of bleding, comming of a cause priminet. Now therefore amorofage or bleding, cometh of a late diuision of the continuaunce: or by reason of putrifaction of the same. In woundes wee finde sweting of blood, from a vaine, and somtime wellyng and fletyng of blood, by little and little. A vaine sweateth blood, when he is berefte of his proper couering. Wherefore in this case, we iudge it necessarie, that the Phisicion haste to repaire with gentle medicene, that, whiche was wasted with cruell weapon. This is doen by couenable sewyng of the wounde, but in case the besselles be broken, and the blood run at libertie: it is to bee considered, whether the blood run gentlie, or els spring and amounte fierslie in his streme. If it flete mildlie, then it is plain, that it cometh of vaines, and is somwhat grosse, and dimmishe redde: but if it mount on height, be redd, fomyng and clere, it is an arterie. But as touching the cure: these thinges muste firste bee considered, whether the whole vaine be cutte, obserue the order, whiche shall be declared anon. Next consider, whether the wounde be depe, or superficiall. If it be superficiall, applie incarnatiues to it, whiche shall be soche as followe.

Distillyng of blood from the vaines.

Of woundes depe, and not depe.

Take Sarcocoll, Mirrhe, Aloes Epatike, Dragons blood, Mastike ana. as ye shall thinke conueniente. For so of euery of theim, maie bee ordered by your self, accordyng to the pacientes complexion. And with this ye shall withstande this kinde of bledyng, whiche is wonte to comber men verie moche. Afterwarde, when this medicene is caste into the wounde, ye shall rolle small quisettes of linte, and weate the same in the whites of Egges, well shaken and beaten with duste of Bole Armoniacke, and laie theim orderlie in the wounde. These also must be couered with a linnen clothe, well weate in the same white of Egges, and afterwardes bee bounde, obseruyng alwaie, that the bindyng be handsomely doen, that it cause no dolour. But if the wounde be depe, ye shall consider with diligent heede, whether the gappe maie be sufficientlie stopped, if it bee deepely stitched, and if reason allowe, that ye shall not in any wise omitte the sewyng: that doen, immediatly lette followe a linnen clothe, infused in the same whites of Egges, and duste aforesaied. If ye see that sewyng will not serue, followe the order, whiche I my self folowed, and had euer good successe, as my pacientes can tell and witnesse them selues.

Reperassiues

And first ye shall washe the wounde, with red or binding wine, and that for twoo causes. The one is to comforte the place: the other to washe of the blood, that none maie hinder the sight, to see where the medicene ought to be applied. Againe, that no blood be lefte, to cause corrupcion. For ye shall shortlie after, fele with your instrumēt, what watrishe and filthie sauour it will cause, if ye let any remaine. Now, whē ye are at poinct with these matters, a newe labour and care will handfaste you, that ye shall not bee idle. Then ye shall lute the gappe, or mouthe of the vaines, whiche spout out blood with this medicen.

To stoppe a bleding vain.

℞.

betwene Sorenes and Chyrurgj.   Fol.xxvi.

℟. The dust or pouder of Galles, Beane meale, and Mill dust, an̄. ℈.ii. Jhon Uigos pouder called *Precipitatū.* ℨ.i. and mingle them with sufficient white of an Egge, and applie it to the gappe of the vain, as I said. Now if it shall come of putrefaction, laie all incarnatiues apart, and set your minde to the seperacion thereof: whiche ye shall doe with *Vnguentum Egiptiacum*, if the putrifaction be but small, and betwene two partes of the fleshe. And *Egiptiacum* muste bee made, after the descripcion of *Auicen*, euē at home, Uertgrece, Roche Alome, in quantitie partes a like if it be deper then so, then applie the Trochistes, which I will describe in the ende of the boke: whiche will remoue the rotten fleshe, from the good, without greate pain. But this can no manne rightly minister, except he haue seen it ministered before: therfore if ye set your mindes to attain to this, chose some expert *Chyrurgian* for the purpose, whiche cā distinct these thinges in practise. And in good faith, if trouble did not withdrawe me frō practising, I would shewe you this poinct my self.

<small>when to incarnate, and when to seperate a sore.</small>

On the other side, when the vaine is but partlie opened, incontinent ye muste remember these twoo poinctes, to wete, that the vaine must sullie be cutte of, or bee bounden and knitte. The one poincte we call incision of a vaine, thother bindyng of a vaine. Incision is made and vsed, where the thinges before mencioned, did not serue, as some where thei doe not in deede. And this is practised for this purpose, because the endes of the vain beyng cutte of, should runne backe, and be hid within the fleshe, and so bee couered, whereof will insue stoppyng of the vaine. Howbeit, this maie not bee practised indifferentlie in all baines, but onelie when thei appere small. For when thei bee greate and grosse, then shall you vse one other fetche, not moche vnlike the former. Marke then, before ye make the incision, whether if a smalle drawyng of the fleshe bee made, it were possible to knitte the vaine in the vpper part, whiche thing were moche tolorable in this worke. If that maie not be, cutte of the vaine with an hot Iron, or instrument, made fit to that, or to ẏ like purpose. But take heede, that ye make not thincision to depe, lest ye cut the arterie, which accōpaineth the vain: for there bee fewe baines, whiche haue not arteries associated with thē. Now one cunning man when he was called to one, who had bled twoo daies, and many right skilfull in the matter, had been in a peck of troubles, aboute staunchyng of the bloode. Perceiuyng by questionyng with theim, that were present, that thei had omitted nothyng, that men commonly vse in soche cases, least he should seme a Dorre, emongest labouring Bees. And again, least he should haue failed them who had saied moche vpon his hed, vsed this feate, wherwith he procured hym self profite, and his paciētes sauetie, though men despaired of his life. For some of them that were present, remembred the saiyng of *Auicen*, who saieth, that euill accidentes, are wont to folowe bleding as conuulsions, through emptines, iskyng procedyng of dryng of the villes of the stomacke, and alienacion of minde, with other sinthoms whiche in this case, are argumentes and signes of colde death. For these bee the accidentes that followe bledyng, and when thei appere,

<small>Of incision of small vaines.</small>

<small>Depe incision hurteth the arters.</small>

<small>Euill accidētes followe bledyng.</small>

Ee.ii.   thei

A Dialogue.

Signes of death.

thei signifie death to be at hande, but to my purpose. He perced the lip of the wounde, in the vpper part, euen vnto the cutte vaine, and lefte thesame vntouched of the nedle, on the one parte: then conueighed he his nedle vnderneth the vaine, to the other parte, and perced againe

A good practise.

the lippe, from the lower to the vpper part, in soche wise that he altered the vain, knittyng the endes of the thzede together, and fastyng it to the lippes of the wounde, and thus deliuered he the paciente, euen from deathes doore, and present daunger. But I saie my frendes, one thyng moze, remember that aboute all your wozkes, of staunchyng of bloud (when ye haue filled the wounde with quisettes) laie some pece of clothe vpon thesame, well weate in water, and Rosed Vineger, so that the pece maie compasse the whole member, where the bleding is.

To staunche blood.

Now with soche feates and ingines, shall you triumphe ouer all vnbzidled bloodflowynges, with moche praise, and erecte vp wozthy monumentes of your actes. We haue now, as it maie be thought, spoken inough and inough of bleding: wherfoze least the tyme faile vs, beyng so swiftlie measured, by the first moueable, Let vs now take the cures of vlcers in hand, where we shall bzidle the rest of the accidētes, belongyng to vlcers. For if we would treat properly, of euery of thē, it should be a long matter, and displeasaunt. For why? thesame thinges should nedes be iterated, and repeated again, and yet again in diuerse cures.

Sorenes.

But yet my bzother, me thinketh it were not superfluous, in our cōmunicacion, if you did shoztly declare, oz euer you entred this matter, whereof vlceres take their name in especiall, sithen we haue founde in wzityng, that thei are here and there named, of their causes, as of a matter that went befoze, oz els of their accidentes, by reason of their causes.

Chyrurgi.

Sanguine, Cholorike, Apostumacions.

Thei be named sanguine, cholorike, flegmatike, & melancholike, accordyng as any of these humours, shall excessiuely abounde in them. Or their accidentes, thei call theim harde, cauie, fistulous, rotten, cancrous, corrosiue, dolorous, apostumated, euill lipped, and so forthe, as any accident shall comber the vlcere. Howbeeit the true cause, whereof vlcers take their names, essense and beyng, be but twoo euen, the antecedent, and coniunct: the antecedent, is, where is corrupcion with an excessiue qualitie of euill humours, procedyng of an inordinate regimente of life: hauyng power to frete, viciate, and

Antecedent & Coniuncte.

corrupte the partes of the bodies. The cause coniuncte, is nothyng els but a malicious complexion, caused of woundes breakyng forthe, and opened pusches, namely when thei bee euill handeled of *Chyrurgians* and Phisicians, as wee see daiely in our time, can also deuide vlceres otherwise. For some be plaine, some depe, and of thesame some harde, some softe: Again some standyng, some runnyng oz crepyng. And likewise, some of them be corrosiue, some putrified: but because soche definicions, make better for the dullyng of the witte, then quickenyng.

I

betwene Sorenes and Chyrurgj. Fol.xxvij.

I purpose not to make any speciall mencion of theim in the cures. Ye maie note, that oft tyme, thei be tourned after some propertie or qualitie of the matter, or sanies, whiche shalbe in them. For our Doctors and chief Phisicians saie, there bee fower kindes of matter, or *Sanies*, whiche the Latines thus terme, and cannot well bee Englished *Sanies, Pus, Virus, Sordities*, whereof thei surname them, with like diriued termes. And accordyng to these nomber and termes, I minde to speake of vlcers here consequently in their order. But first of a sanius vlcer.

> Sanies is matter commyng of corrupted blood, or els putrifaction, and somtyme it is taken for poison.

And thus shall we doe, if God so will, when we haue said somwhat of sanies. For in as moche, as we entende to speake of a sanious vlcer, it is reason that we knowe first, what sanies is, whereof it springeth and who be his causes. And by the reason of this, we shal easely know the correction of vlcers, which thing (as we take it) consisteth in knowlege of the causes: rectificacion of complexions, and comfortyng of members. Now sanies is nothyng els, but corrupted foode or nourishemente which natur was not able to digest, neither tourne into the seconde humours, whiche thei call, glewe, dewe, and the humour vnnamed, sanies is caused and generated, when nutritiue matter, compyng or all redie come to a member, maie not be conuerted, into the nature of the member, by reason of the weakenesse of thesame, or superfluities of other members approchyng together. For, as *Galen* writeth, the strong members doe oppresse the weake, and put of their superfluities to them, whiche be tourned into sanies, or virulencie. Wherefore, when we purpose to cure any weake member, wee muste endeuour our self, with all possibilitie, to strengthen it with some medicene confortatiue, that it maie put of straunge superfluities. And verely bindyng medicenes, beyng of soche heate, as shall not exceade the naturall heate of the weake part, shall comfort greatly, as *Galen* saieth in the third *De arte medendi*. Thesame effecte haue defensiues: also if thei be likewise qualified. And after what sort this must be doen, the nature of Simples it self, will informe you. Therefore, bestowe some labour, in the searche of simples, to the intent ye maie fetche theim redily, as it were from a store house, and not seeke at all aduenture, by chaunce medly, as thei grope for a pinne in the darke. The like mischief is committed in administracions of ointmentes, whiche be hotte, or moistie of complexion, and bothe the qualities dooe, promote a sore to putrefaction. For heate and moisture, if heate rewle not thesame, then thei are causes at first dashe, to cause putrefaction. As *Aristotle* Prince of Philosophers affirmeth: therefore, who so euer purposeth, to exercise *Chyrurgi*, must labour with all industrie, to knowe the nature of ointmentes, at his fingers ende. I speake not of the names of ointmentes, as the imperickes, and some of our men doe, whiche professe *Chyrurgi*, as sone as thei can name & recite *Vnguentum Basilicum, Nigrum, Aureum, Apostolorum, Egiptiacum, Rosarum, Album, Camphoratum, Lythargicum, Rosarum, Ceracinum. &c.* whereof thei bragge, and spreade a Pecockes taile againste the simple. But I meane the qualities of ointmentes, whiche must be diuers, in diuers maladies, accor-

> Strong members doe oppresse the weake.

> Chirurgians muste knowe Simples.

Ee.iii. dyng

A Dialogue

dyng to our entencion curatiue, in the maladie. For sometyme we cõforte, somtyme we moiste, some where we drie, as also oftentimes we coole, or heate. Therefore, it is not to be marueiled, that soche venterlynges and younglinges, stomble so ofte at a Strawe. For why, these men be vtterly loste in their bookes, and will not from them one finger breadth, whereof springeth many errours, specially when thei vnderstande not, whiche one learned man recordes, consideryng, spared not to trie out in the matter, in his Aphorismes, saiyng, to worke after bokes, without perfite knowlege, and fine witte, is a right comberous thing. Wherefore I exhorte you, moste dere brethren, that you

Fooles with bookes, bee worse then vnlearned practicioners

order your medicenes, accordyng to the complexion of the member, and your intencion in the cure. And if it be possible, make your medicenes your self, and trust not so moche the Apothecaries, leaste ye be deceiued with the blessed termes, I will not saie cursed, intituled *quid pro quo*, because he is dedde, who made it. For as menne haue diuers phisiognomies, diuers qualities and quantities, with soundrie complexiõs giuen them partly by influences, and partly by tractes, and diuers regions, so haue the simples: also as greate variaunce, emongest theim

Varietie of Simples.

self, in as moche as thei bee of sondrie shapes, places, and countrees, from whens thei acquire proper natures, qualities and powers in workyng. Wherefore *Auicen* crieth out in the Chanon of vlcers, saiyng:

Auicen.

Medicamen quidem vnum, secundum quedam corpora facit nasci carnem secundum quedam est corrosiuum: whiche is thus moche to saie: One medicen in diuers bodies, hath diuers effectes and operacions. In one, by reason of the propertie of the bodie, it causeth flesshe to growe: thesame in some other is waistyng, and right abstersiue, specially, if the bodie be soft and fine. Wherefore this is inferred, that ointementes should bee made, accordyng as the complexion of the member shall require. And this sentence toucheth

C. Celsus.

the fine speached *Cornelius Celsus*, our dearlyng, saiyng: *Ignorari non oportet quod non omnibus egris eadem auxilia conferunt:* Wherefore, be you wise and circumspecte in your confections, leaste it bee your chaunce, to fall into the Noddies had I wiste. Now as touchyng the Judgemente of *Sanies*, that *Sanies* shall be called good, as *Auicen* saieth, whiche is white, smothe, and like in euery part: whiche sentence he borowed of *Hyppocrates*, the diuine Phisicion, in his boke of Prognosticacions, where he saith, *Ea putredo laudatur &c.* White *Sanies* is praised, whiche is like ouer all, egall in the vtter face, and not ill fauoured, the contrary is moste euill. Now if ye will knowe why *Sanies* should haue these properties, rede *Auicen* in the capiter, concernyng the iudgemente of *Sanies*, where ye finde euen your fill, of causes shewed of the saied propertie, whiche ye maie seeke at his handes, and not now at myne, for it would drawe vs farder from our purpose. Ye maie also haue respect to *Galen*, vpon the first of the Prognosticacions: where ye shall rede certaine diuine thinges, for the perfite attainmẽt of this matter. Ye haue now sufficient what *Sanies* is, wherof

Sanious matter.

it cometh and of what sort it is. Now we wil ioyne hereunto, the cure of a Sanious vlcer.

Sorenes.

betwene Sorenes and Chyrurgj. Fol. xxviij.

Sorenes.

Speake now of vlcers, I praie you, that I and my sore brethren, maie perceiue them plainly.

Chyrurgj.

Wherefore, for your better vnderstandyng, ye shall note, that there bee twoo sortes of vlcers: whereof some bee simple, and some be compounde. I meane not, that thei bee simple absolutely, but simple, after some maner of simplicitie. For why, their beyng is of an euill complexion, breache of continuaunce, and somtyme of composicion, also with a concourse of euill qualities. But I saie, thei be simple, so farfoorthe as thei bee opposite to vlcers, where accidentes bee founde, lettyng the true ensoundyng of vlcers. For here we call them compounde, whiche haue soche accidentes. wherfore, when I name a famous vlcer, as we recken the matter, ye shall vnderstande it, of that whiche is fully voide and clere of the saied accidentes, notwithstandyng it be tangled, with some doublenes and composicion. Therefore we will speake first of a simple vlcere, whiche is in the plain: and then of a simple depreste, or hollowed, whiche dooen, we shall in like maner and order treate of the compounded, from whiche kind, the almightie and mercifull God, preserue vs all.

Two sondrie sortes of Vlcers.

And firste we note, that all vlcers in that and as farfoorthe as thei be vlcers, require dryng in their cure: whereof there be twoo kindes, the one hotte, and the other colde. Againe, some be with mordicacion and bityng, and some without. All be bityng, whiche in a certain degree of heate, be drie of complexion, whiche is because heate is yoked, and felowshipped with drought, as *Aristotle* moste learnedly first taught as ye maie reade in his bookes of Generacion, and Corrupcion. And he saieth thus, concernyng the mixture of elementes: If the coldnesse of the yearth, were chaunged to heate, it might no longer bee named yearth, but fire. He saieth farder, if the drought of thesame, wer chaunged to moisture, it should lose the name of yearth, and be called water Whereof it followeth, that thinges so dried, in case thei be found with like qualities: thei will not onely waste and gnawe, but also burne, when thei be applied. And this doe the qualities of the fire, and Mercurie Sublimated apartlie shewe. Neuerthelesse, the one shall bee so moche the lesse of mordicacion or fretyng, as his qualities shall more be oppressed in it, then in the other. And therefore, bee you somewhat the wiser, in chusyng of your simples, least ye take one for an other. Now to the intent ye maie the rather, eschue this foule errour, I will giue you the difference of exiccatiues, or dryng Simples, whiche wee vse in vlcers. For by the knowlege of theim, ye shall sone come to the cure of vlcers. These exiccatiues bee colde: The three kindes of Saunders, Mirabolanes, *Terra Sigillata*, Dragons bloode, Bole Armoniacke, Tutia, Camphire, Ceruse, Letharge, Vermilion, Sinaper, redde Corall, Gum Arabicke: these be hotte, and without bityng or gnawing,

Vlcers hotte colde, and bityng.

Aristotle a good note of Elementes.

Of exiccatiues.

Ee.iiii. Aloes

A Dialogue

Aloes epatike, Mirrhe, Sarcocol, vnholed Galles, &c. Hotte with bityng and mordicacion, vertgrece. Alome. &c. Of these ye maie make medicenes to the purpose, for all kinde of vlcers, so ye knowe perfitely the propertie and workyng of them: ye shall knowe, whether the vlcer be hot or no, by his edges. For if he be reddish in the edges, it declareth heate: as also, if the fleshe be remisse redde, and hotte in felyng, whiche maie be rectified with *Vnguentum Albion*, made after this maner.

To knowe whether vlcers be hotte or colde.

R. Oile of Roses. ʒ. vi. Weathers fatte. ʒ. iiii. Marow of the huclebones of Kine. ʒ. ii. white waxe. ʒ. i. ß. Cerusse. ʒ. iii. ß. Camphorie. ʒ. iii. makyng it to an ointmente, accordyng to the arte, whiche ye shall applie vpon the vlcers, when ye haue firste caste in this pouder, in the sore. R. Of all the Mirabolanes, of *Terra sigillata*, of redde Corall. ana. ʒ. i of Cerusse. ʒ. ii. of roche Alome brent. ʒ. i. of Creuishe shelles. ʒ. i. stape all these together, as small as sande, whiche couer, as I saied with the ointment aboue described. But if the fleshe bee so moche ouergrowen, that the lippes doe appere vpon it, ye shall vse *Vnguentum Apostolorum* for the correction thereof, obseruyng alwaie warely, that the vlcer be not inflamed again. For some complexions be so tender and soft that thei will be altered, almoste at the name thereof, as I sawe my self in a citezein of London: whose name I omit, because he hath been vnkind to our Arte. When I perceiued any soche complexion as he was, I ordered my rectificatiue, with soche cantele, that it should bothe comforte and rectifie. After this sorte. R. Of oile Rosed. ʒ. iiii. of oile Mirtine ʒ. i. ß. of Beane flower. ʒ. iii. of pouder of Roses, Mirtils, and Cipresse Nuttes, ana. ʒ. ii. of *Acatia*. ʒ. ii. of Bole Armoniacke, of *Terra Sigillata*, ana. ʒ. i. of newe waxe. ʒ. ß. and so make thereof a defensiue, betwene hard and softe. And this at twoo applicacions, with *Vnguentum Apostolorum* will rectifie the member, and make the vlcer redie to a Cicatrice. Thus cured Ihon Backter, the learned *Chyrurgian*, soche vlceres in a monethe, where other, whom ye knowe, had theim in hande a yere and more. Now when the fleshe is suppressed, and ye purpose to skinne the vlcer, it is moste expediente, ye vse this Lotion. R. Of good clere wine, one cuppe full, of redde Roses. M. ß. of Rosed Honie strained. ʒ. ß. of roche Alome. ʒ. iii. and as moche Saffron, as shalbe able to colour the wine and sethe all these together, till the Alome be melted, and then moiste the vlcere with this liquere, beyng luke warme: And maintain it, as sone as it maie be, drie the vlcere again, with a fine linnen cloth, that none of the liquer remain there. For it will cause matter and corrupcion, as it befell vnder his handes, who is myne sworne enemie. For whiles he laboured to skinne the sore, as I did, euen with the same medicene, he caused holownes in an vlcere. Now when ye haue so moisted the vlcere, as is saied, laie yet a little cotten in the vlcere, that the moisture, in case any remain, be fully dried vp. Appliyng vpon the same this ointment, whiche is verie effectuall in workyng of a *Cicatrice*.

Vnguentum Album.

To make the skin whole.

Howe to make a Cicatrice.

R. Of oile of Roses and Mirte, ana. ʒ. i. ß. of Vermilonde. ʒ. ii. and sethe them together, till thei gette a verie blacke hugh, and so shall ye finishe

betwene Sorenes and Chyrurgj.   Fol.xxix.

finishe the cure. Lo, here haue you the cure of a sanious plain vlcere: Now will wee to the hollowe, whereof ye shall receiue, large giftes and rewardes, if ye handle your self well, in the reformacion of humours, that fall to the place. Ye knowe that sharpe humours, will properly frete, and consume the fleshe newly growen, and let the growyng of thesame, wherewith the holownes of the vlcere, should bee filled and restored. For the reformacion hereof, shall followe three intencions. The first must be to order the life, with couenable regiment. The seconde to keepe of matter, whiche approcheth thether. And the third, to cause newe fleshe to growe, with the skinnyng of it. The first is had by orderyng of the sore thynges, called not naturall, and chiefly with diete, whiche must be wholly bente, to the contrary of the humours and qualities, whiche feede the sore. The repulse of humours maie be wrought twoo waies: or with competent purgacion, or with some vnctious and cataplasmes, whiche comforte, and put of, as will the defensiue aboue ordered. Fleshe is caused to growe twoo waies, by lettyng of the contraries, and by applyyng of dustes and ointmentes, beyng of like qualities. The duste must bee made, by minglyng of the exiccatiues, aboue rehersed, whiche ye must indolate, accordyng to your nede. But if ye delite more in ointmentes, ye maie make that, after this maner.

Three sonorie intencions.
Of regiment.
Of matter.
Of growing.

℞. Of the clerest Terebintine. ʒ.ii. of Hony rosed and strained. ʒ.i.ß of Plantain water. ʒ.iii. let them sethe, till the water bee wasted, and put thereto of Barlie and Beane meale, ana. ʒ.ii. of Frankencense. ʒ.i with a little Saffron. And so this will be an incarnatiue, with some sturring, whiche ye must couer with *Vnguentum Album*, aboue described. Besides this, the defensiue there ordered, must bee nointed aboute in the circuite, that it bee not inflamed to heate againe. Now if the fleshe grewe to faste, it will be suppressed with *Vnguentum Apostolorum*, applied ones or twise, or more if nede require. And when that is come to equalitie with the edges, then finish your cure, as it was said aboue, in a plain vlcere. There be other feates and engines, whiche can not be written but are left to *Chyrurgians* estimacions. For somewhile one qualitie, somwhiles an other, frouneth or flattereth, and muste bee ruled now hether, now thether, as a Shepe emongest Wolues. Of whiche poincte complaineth *Auicen*, in the entraunce of his worke, saiyng: The tradicion of Phisicke, containeth lesse, then is necessarie for the Phisicion. For the ouerplus, whiche is lefte to their iudgement and estimacion, maie not be expressed, and put in writyng. Wherefore, to the intent ye maie gette this iudgement in thynges, left to estimacion, ye must not lothe, nor be high in the insteppe, to see other experte mennes worke. For there by, with diligent aduertence, ye shal assuredly gather iudgemente, and bee ascertained in your inuencions. Now for asmoche, as we haue giuen you the taste, in a hotte sanious vlcer, wee will ventre (I hope luckelie) the cure of the colde, obseruyng the same maner and order, whiche we vsed tofore in the hotte vlcere.

An incarnatiue.

To abate proude fleshe.

Auicen.

Now

A Dialogue

Colde vlcer.

Now, when a sanious colde vlcere, cometh to our handes (whiche thyng maie easely be perceiued by the iye: for the flesshe will bee semie white, or wanne, notwithstandyng, that sometyme dimme paienesse cometh to an vlcere, through blood, runnyng with cholere. It is also perceiued with feelyng of the hande) now then when soche vlcers, I saie, come to your handes, ye shall not departe in any poinct from the order, whiche before was discribed. Neuerthelesse, we saie for certain, that their remedies as farre differ one from the other, as the vlcers in heate and colde. And here wee will begin with the defensiue, whiche offereth it self, firste in the cure, where our composicion was thus.

A defensiue.

℞. Of oile of Camomell, and Mirte, ana. ℥.ii. pouder of Camomel and Melilot, ana. ℥.ii. pouder of redde Roses, Mirtelles, and Cipresse nuttes, ana. ℥.i.ß. of Barlie and Beane meale. ℥.ii. of newe Waxe. q.ß. and so make the defensiue, betwene hard and soft, wherwith anointe the circute of the vlcere. This dooen, begin the cure with this pouder, castyng it into the vlcere. ℞. Of Aloes, Mirrhe, Sarcocol, ana. ℥.ß. of Frankensence. ℥.ii. of Dragons blood, and flowers of Pomegranetes, ana. ℥.iii. of Saffron. Ɔ.i. and make a pouder of all these, coueryng it afterward with this ointment followyng.

℞. Of oile of Roses. ℥.ii. of oile of Camomel, and Mirte, ana. ℥.iii. of Weathers fatte. ℥.iiii. of Henne greace. ℥.i. of marowe of the Cowe and Harte, ana. ℥.i.ß. of Letharge. ℥.ii. of Ceruse. i. seethe theim, till thei bee blacke, and then putte thereto of cleare Terebintine. ℥.i.ß. of Shippe Pitche. ℥.i. of newe Waxe. ℥.ii. and let theim seeth a little againe: and when ye haue taken theim of the fire, stire theim still, vnto soche tyme, as it be congeled and frame, otherwise, the minerals will fall to the bottome in a residence. This ointmente is *Vnguentum Basilicum*, after our descripcion and entent. Now in case the flesshe appere foggie and fattishe, then *Vnguentum Apostolorum*, shalbe necessarie to drie it. For that without question, will bryng it to equalitie of ensoundyng. And then ye maie finishe your cure, and skinne the same with the lotion aboue ordered.

A sanatiue.

A good foundacion.

Now in as moche, as we bee at poincte with the simples: or right and congruente, we muste laie a fundacion for the compounde, so that we maie like worke men, builde in the humaine bodie, or repaire ruinous and decaied places, and proppe vp soche as are like to fall. Wherfore, ones againe remember the accidentes, before mencioned, to the intent we maie bee able to redresse, and amende theim one by one. For where this maie not be obtained, we shall to our reproche, be kept frō the true ensoundyng of the vlcere. And therefore we purpose, to prosecute the emendement of them, in their order accordyngly. Now when a compounded vlcere is offered vs, lette vs looke what accidentes bee concurraunt, hinderyng the ensounding. For if many maladies or accidentes, were founde in it, we must begin at that, whiche doeth moste comber the vlcere, as *Auicen* saieth, if wee will cure a maladie, where diuers accidentes be concurrant: we muste begin at that, whiche hath

In healing a compounde vlcer, marke the accidents concurrant.

one

one of these three properties *Una earum est q̄ alia sanari non potest antequam ipsa sanetur vt aposteme. &c.* The one is, where the accidente is soche, that if it bee not first cured, the vlcere maie not be cured, as apostumacion ioined with and vlcere. For in this case saieth he, we followe the cure of the apostumacion, vnto soche time as the malice of the complexion be displaced, and then we followe the cure of the principall. Wherefore, to followe and obserue the Canons, accordingly: we shall order principally our intencions, so that wee firste take in hande the accidente, whiche shall chieflie comber and moleste the paciente and vs in the cure. And the first of these intencions shalbe, to order the pacientes life conueniently. Nexte to purge the faultie humour, accordyng to the exigence thereof. Thirdlie, to amende the maliciousnesse of the qualitie, in the vlcere. This last shalbe deuided yet again, accordyng to the disposiciō of the vlcere, requiryng diuers intencions. Now as touchyng the order of life, you maie by your owne iudgement consider, what is to bee doen therein: partlie by his regimente before tyme, and partly in his sickenesse tyme, tournyng his diete to the conttarie qualitie. Is thus. If he vsed a colde regiment before, vse hym to hotte, so if drie, moistie. but dooe it moderatlie, and by little and little. For nature can not awaie with sodaine chaunges: Howbeit this is not seen lightly in humours, without long vse of contraries in foodes. We shall knowe to purge the humours, by the shewyng of the sicke water, in twoo pointes, that is, by the colour and substaunce: whereunto is added the residence, with his qualities, moche or little. And by the significacion of these well considered, wee maie trie out all the sickes complexion.

For if the vrine shall be thicke in substaunce, and redde in colour: it meaneth, that bloud ruleth the manne. If it be thinne of substaunce, and red of colour: doubt not, but cholere hath the preheminence. But if it be thicke in substaunce, and white of colour, then fleume hath the maistrie: as if the substaunce be thinne, and colour white, melancholie. Now of, and by the residence, ye shall perceiue the tyme to giue pocions, and purgacions: for when that beginneth to appere, it sheweth digestion of the humours to be purged. But there be also refractions of colours, and eleuacions, and depressions of residences, whiche signifie, or the denominaciō and seruice, of the naturall heate, and wastyng of the radicall moisture: whiche thynges, now are not to be prosecuted, because this matter partaine to a Phisicion, whereof if God giue me life, I purpose to treate at conueniente laisure: now let this be sufficiēt for the cure of an vlcer. If ye will knowe how an humour shalbe purged, reade *Leonard Futchius* whiche teacheth to purge, accordyng to the faulte of the humour. Other haue at hand, maister *Vygos* boke of *Chirurgj,* where ye shall finde, euen to the full, how to purge an humour. For if I would distemper pocions, make morselles, and mingle pilles, I should be troublesome vnto you, or ye might hit me in the teeth with the prouerbe: ye sette the Carte before the horsse. For my communicacion should bee vnsauerie, as it fareth with a geste, whiche regarde

First handle thaccidence in a cure, and note three thynges.

Regiment of life.

Of vrine considered, in euery sicke or sore man.

Of radicall moisture.

gard not delicate iuncates, being filled before. And therefore, leauing these thinges to you as knowen, I will to the emendyng, of the maliciousnesse of an vlcere, when we applie coole to the hotte, and hotte to the colde. Likewise, if the vlcere be moistie, applyyng drie: if drie, applyyng moistie medicenes. We shall refraine his malice by digestion, mundificacion, corrosion, insicion, and also burnyng and mollifiyng, as it shall please the woorkeman. But when, and how, these meanes shalbe put in vre, that shall we shewe, when we goe aboute to displace the accidentes of vlcers. All whiche thynges we doe orderly, omitting the former matters, for a tyme, because trouble hath preuented me.

Applie contraries.

We haue entreated before, sufficiently of bleding, coming of a cause primatiue, from whens ye must fetche hether, soche thynges as there were spoken. For it were superfluous, to speake more of the matter in this place. Wherfore, being at poinct with that accident, I will make forth to the rest, and speake no more of this. The like would I do with superfluous fleshe, if I had rehersed the cause of it, when we speake of a sanious vlcere. The cause of superfluous fleshe, is to moche moisture and vncleane mundificacion, as *Auicen* thinketh, in the Chapiter of vlceres, saiyng: In some vlcers groweth superfluous fleshe, and in some it groweth not. And the vlceres where it groweth, be thei in the whiche, how moche haste is made, in the repaire of fleshe, before complete mundificacion. Wherefore take you hede, that ye procede not to farre, in moisting of the fleshe. And as for remedies, the matter is plain. for ȳ we knowe the cause: but remēber that ye quicken or delate, in drought and corrosion, the medicen, accordyng as the matter shall require, and as the fleshe shall be more or lesse, swelled vp with foggie fat. We haue seen that this kinde of maladies, hath not felte, nor forsed of other remedies, and hath required an actually cauterie. If this happen vnder your handes, if easie remedies profite not (of whiche sorte bee *Vnguentum Apostolorum, Egiptiacum*, take a corosiue pouder, and brent Alome) feare not to drie it with an hotte iron also. And if ye shall so doe, and a blisterous crust be risen: ye maie displace it, as we shewed before in our treatise of apostumacions, and then retourne to the cure again.

The cause of superfluous fleshe.

If harde and discouered lippes, bee founde in an vlcere, lettyng the ensoundyng, set all your cure, vpon the displasyng of that euill: omittyng no tyme or hower. For if we doe the contrary, we shall in the hast labour in baine, and afterwarde bee compelled, to giue ouer the purpose, and take that in hande at latter cast. Therefore to spend no time in baine, begin with the sheryng or cuttyng of, of the lippes. Ye shall cut them of by little and little, without causyng of greate dolour, if ye applie this pouder, here beneath ordered. For *Auicen* saieth, we should neuer cause dolour in an vlcere, vnlesse we bee constrained to it of necessitie, whiche is, where gentle medicenes serue not, he did not this without foresight. For he was well ware, as a forecastyng man, that there would come after hym, whiche would be more likely, to subuert mankinde, then to preserue: whiche would boast them selues of that,

Auicens prouidence.

that

that thei would no rules of Phisicke in their workes: but will folowe rather the frantike and pestilent saiyng, of a certain counterfaites of our tyme, whiche haue this in their mouthes, and haue brough it to a common prouerbe to, saiyng: that a wounde will brede wormes, vnder a gentill Phisicions hande. As though ignoraunte, and bocherlie crueltie of the Phisicion, should bee cause of healthe. I speake of the crueltie, whiche blinde boosardes doe vse, with all counterfeite boldnesse, and coloured diligence, in euery little felon, to the intente, thei maie thereby winne the name of learned, and expert *Chyrurgians*: and not a whit of necessary sharpnesse, whereunto we be induced, bothe by the rules, and autenticall counsaill, of learned Philicions, and swete perswasions of Poetes. For this saieth the fine witted, and eloquent Naso, *Immedicabile vulnus, est recidendum. &c.* Where the wounde is vncurable, saith he, it must be shorne of, that the holle be not infected withall. Againe, Iuuenall with his satiricall tricke, one Grape draweth an other, only by reason of their aspecte, as one Measelled Hogge, measelleth the whole herde. Virgill also is with vs at our elbowe, saiyng: *Culpam ferro compestite. &c.* Appease, saieth he, the fault out of hande, with the sworde, or euer the cursed infeccion, go farther emong the people. Wherefore, whē ye shall chaunce in soche cures, do that, whiche shal appartain to the preseruacion of the pacient, without all white liuered womālike feblenes. And if ye so bolde your self, and worke accordingly, the matter well considered, ye shall not be called vnmilde and cruell, but prouident and mecifull: notwithstandyng the blustering blames of your aduersaries, because ye haue saued, and not destroied your paciente. For doubtlesse, many sores will not be mended, without the knife, as Cankers, and others, as *Cornelius Celsus* sheweth in his bookes, of hande woorkyng. We haue now runne out of our race, occasioned by blinde *Chyrurgians*, howbeeit, wee haue founde nothyng to moche: their desertes well considered. For who could bee so pacient to heare theim, and would not waxe hote in the cause, namely, beyng exasperated daie by daie, of soche men. For thei can not se the good, liue in quiete by them but thei lye in awaite for them, with all indeuoured mischief. Well, I relinquishe this, leaste I should seme, to bee delited in reprehension of men, where my minde is farre distaunte, from that pathe of writyng. Wherfore, let thē go plaie them: we will repaire to our pouder, which ye shal put on the euill fauoured lippes of woundes or sores, which is this. ℞. Of Citrine, Mirabolaines. ʒ.ß. of red Corall. ʒ.ß. of vnholed Galles. ʒ.i. of Dragons blood, of *Terra sigillata*, and Cerusse, ana. ʒ.ii. Wert degrece. ʒ.ii. of Roche Alome brente. ʒ.i. Sarcocoll, Mirrhe, Frankencense, Mastike, ana. ʒ.i.ß. mingle them all, and pouder them finely as Alcocoll, vpon the whiche, ye shall applie *Vnguentum Basilicum*, after the descripcion in the cure of a colde vlcere. And thus must you procede, vntill the accident be remoued, whiche doen, prosecute the cure, as is aboue prescribed. And in case the pouder, by reason of his weakenes, spede not well the matter, ye maie go to stronger medicenes. Whereof

Soft Chirurgians make foule sores, yet Butcherly mangless, marreth all together.

Ouid: a good note.
Example.

Good counsaill.

How bolde the Chirurgian should be in cure.
C. Celsus.

A good pouder.

A Dialogue

this is the firste. ℞. Of oile of Roses. ʒ.iii. weathers fatte. ʒ.ii. marrowe of the huccle bone of a Cowe. ʒ.i. water wherin sublimatū hath been melted. ʒ.i. seeth theim softly together, vnto the tyme the water be wasted: and then put therto. ʒ.i. of Ceruse, and seeth them againe a little, when it is taken from the fire, ye must stirre it, till it be thicke. This muste bee spreade on a pece of a clothe, and laied on the sore: and peraduenture, ye shall dispatch the matter with this: If not, take this in hande: and without doubt, ye shall winne the castell. But yet be ye hereof warned before hand, that it be not applied in any sinuie place, leaste while ye seke freedome, ye fall into bondage. As it befell in my friend, when he would bicker with the like vlcere, in a womans foote where he could neuer winne the matter, though he lefte no stone vntourned. Neuerthelesse, if ye bee constrained thereto, by any necessitie, or euer ye applie this, ye shall first vse an vniuersall purgacion, of the whole bodie, and also a comfortatiue to the Nuke, that in case there arise any Pestilente fumes, ready to cause a conuulsion, or Spasme: And when ye haue so dooen, procede foorthe to the locall medicenes, whiche maie be thus. Whiche is moste excellent good.

To remoue an escharus scab or cruste.

℞. Ceruse, Vermilion, Sublimatum, ana. ʒ.iii. mingle them, and and pouder theim finely: wherof ye shall sprinckle, so moche in the vlcere, as is able (if I maie so speake) salt the parte, whiche shalbe remoued: and incontinent, couer it with this plaster, whiche shall make for the appeasyng of dolour, and remouing of the escharous crust. ℞. leaues of Mallowes, Violettes, and Lettise. ana. ℳ.i. seeth theim together in Mutton brothe of the weather, and afterwardes stampe thē puttyng thereto. li.ß. of Barlie meale, of oile of Roses complete. ʒ.ii. of Butter. ʒ.iii. and the yolkes of three Egges: with whiche plaister ye must procede till the crust be taken of, and then ye maie prosecute the cure with digestiues, abstersiues, and incarnatiues, as ye were informed afore. If ye woorke after this sorte, and with these remedies, accordyng as thei haue been declared: ye shall winne your Spurres, in soche cures, and great frendship. Now in asmoche, as we be well trained in this, let vs come nerer the accident of dolorous pain, to se how we can ridde our handes of that also. For why, this is now and then so extreme, cruell and sharpe, that it doeth not onelie exclude the cure of vlcers, but vtterly interdite and suspende almoste, all the vertues, as well naturall as animall, and spirituall. Wherefore of verie right we must put our helpyng hande to this also.

Example

For as moche then, as dolour is as it were a cuppyng glasse, in drawyng matter vnto the place, the writers haue vsed moche diligence, in appeasyng of it, consideryng the accidentes. whiche maie insue therevpon, as ouerthrowe of the vertue naturall, failyng of spirites, and contractions of sinewes. All whiche accidentes are perilous, & to be doubted in all maladies. Wherefore, to the intent men maie eschue this by a rule: thei learne men knowlege, in their publicated workes.

that

that it proceadeth of twoo causes, that is: of the breache of continuaunce, and alteracion of qualities. As *Galen* saieth, dolours where as thei be, declare breache of continuaunce, or sodain alteracion of qualities: the continuaunce maie be broken fower waies, by insicion, corrosion, breakyng and stretchyng, as in apostumacion. Alteracion is by heate and cold, moisture, drought, and other. Note, what diligence thei tooke, to finde the causes of dolour. Now if dolour arise, by meanes of insicion, as in woundes: the first waie to appease it, is to sewe it, and next to anoint hote oile Omphacine, in the edges and circuite of the wounde. And this must be doen, not ones or twise, but continually, till it be appeased in a greate part. If it come to corrosion, which accident, properly pertaineth to an ulcere: it must be remoued also, if we entende to cure the ulcere. But here note, that there bee twoo causes of the matter, a proper, and a dependyng: the proper cause is, a certaine malignitie, or shreudnesse in the fleshe, whiche our men call, *proprietas occulta*, the secrete propertie. The cause dependyng is nought els, but euill humours, whiche frete and eate out the fleshe, when thei come to the coniuncte, as doeth cholere, mixte with salte flegme. And certainly, this latter shall neede of euacuacion with *Cassia, Manna, Diacatholicon*, and other like purgatiues. But as for the former, it shall be ruled after an other order, euen by comfortyng of the edges of the ulcere, with defensiues, able to cherishe and fede, the complexion of the fleshe and with the strong pouder, *Precipitatus*, caste in the ulcere, whose descripcion ye shall finde, at the ende of the treatises. If it come by breakyng it is eased by settyng of the bones, and competent bindyng, and situacion of the member. For albeit, the breache bee neuer so well restored, and set in place: there will be yet discontinuaunce, if it be untowardly set to reste. And as for the settyng of bones, ye shall learne at other mennes handes: for their bookes are replenished, with preceptes and rules for the purpose, specially *Galen. &c.*

But if alteracion come of extension, or stretchyng, as it is in apostumacions, mollificatiue medicenes shall be best, to prepare the matter to come foorthe: And *Auicen* sendeth us to soche appeacementes, saiyng, the vehemencie also of dolour, causeth us of necessitie, to use mollificatiues, or softenyng medicenes. But of trouthe my friende, if it grewe through alteracion of the substaunce, the matter muste bee redressed by the contrary qualities. For ensample. If an ulcere be distempered with heate (whiche is perceiued by rednesse in the circuite) it is redressed by a cold ointment. And if the substaunce be fallen to cold, *Unguentum Rasum*, or some like will qualifie the matter sone. If it be engedered with drought, moisture then will pacifie all the grief. Again, if it be disquieted with to moche moisture, drought of an ointment, plaster or dust, wil dispatche it. To be short, if we worke after this maner, we shall discomfite al maner of dolours, caused through excesse of one qualitie, aboue an other. Thus shall we with proper medicens, succor the humain life of mankind, specially when we attain to the cause of the

maladie,

Breache of continuaunce or hurtyng of the whole member.

Alteracion, what it is.

Of dolour.

Two causes of matter.

Alteracion of extension.

When to use contraries in healyng.

maladie, neither shall begge remedies, as doe these Dogleches, which would bee called practicians, a Gods name, and wote not what practise is. For thei dooe as the children dooe in their plaies, whiche when thei liste to haue some sporte, appoincte some marke, and standyng a little of blindfilde, wherle them self about ones or twise on their foot and then gesse to the marke, at all aduenture, in whiche gropyng, thei are founde at laste, when thei thinke theim self sure of it, ferther of, then thei were, where thei stoode at first. Euen so fareth it with these gropyng practicians: for why, thei be not able to distincte, neither tymes of sickenesse, neither knowe the causes of theim, or properties of ointmentes, as he who bare men in hande, with grauitie of woordes, that he was a practician: and when one demaunded, what qualitie *Vnguentum Rosarum* had, he aunswered with greate deliberacion, a Gods name, hotte, ye Marie sir ꝙ the other, a worthie aunswere for soche a practician. Wherefore I exhorte you, to cast awaie all sluggardie, and negligence, that ye maie attain to the knowlege, as well of Simples as of cōpoundes, and stomble not at matters, as thei doe. Ye haue, the causes and cure of dolour: now we will goe to an apostumacion, as the order requireth.

Example.

Now, as touchyng apostumacion, concurrant with vlceres, what should I saie, sithen wee haue largely saied in the matter, when wee spake of apostumacions. But yet to helpe theim, that bee intangled herein: we will talke a little more of it, and put somewhat to the enlargyng of our medicenes, declared before. Then when an vlcere is thus entangled: ye muste vse the remedies, appoincted properly for apostumacions. But in case thei shall not suffice, vse this, wherein ye shall finde soche profite, that for certain, ye shall maruaill not a little at it. But first consider, whether the vlcere be vexed, with an hotte or colde apostumacion. For at that diuersitie, will followe diuersitie of makyng of the medicen. If it be hotte, applie this. ℞ Leaues of Mallowes and Violettes, ana. ℳ.i. of hulled Beanes. ℔.ii. seeth theim all together, vntill the Beanes be soft, whiche doen, stampe theim: and if it be requisite, to put any oile to the same, put a little Rosed Omphacine, and afterwarde spred it on a clothe, and laie it to the apostumacion, for this will apease and resolue. But if the apostumacion be cold ye shall take the same plaster again, howbeit ye shall search, and make it otherwise. ℞. Of Mallowe leaues. ℳ.ii. hulled Beanes. ℔. ii. of Barbors lye. ℥.ß. and seeth them well, after stampe them, and applie it to the place. Certainly, this will woorke moste aptly, for our purpose. But note here, I praie you, that this plaster maie be rectified in our workyng, accordyng as the lye shall be milde or sharpe. Thus haue ye inough, for the displayng of this accident, if ye remember these thinges, with the other aboue. Wherefore we will now talke, of hardnesse of vlceres.

Apostumaciō concurrante with an vlcer

Hotte and cold apostumacions.

Hardnes of an vlcere.

Euery good Phisition, my friende, willyng to cure his pacient rightly, will appoincte himself, twoo principall intentions, that is, is, to preserue and to cure. The firste searcheth for the causes, the other imagineth waies to displace theffect thereof. Therfore to the intent we maye be able to remoue this cause, and withstande the effect, let vs se how many causes hardnes hath. When I was giuen to rede *Chyrurgi*, and delited in the antique bookes, I fell by chaunce vpon *Galens* frist booke, *De simplici medicamentorū*, where I noted him, to put thre causes of hardenes. For it chaunseth, saieth he, of to moche drought of congeling of matter, or els of fulnesse and replexion. If it come of drought, moisture will ease it. And this must be done with ointmētes, plasters, and imbrocations, after the mynde of *Auicen*. Imbrocations bee made with hote water, and Mutton brothe of the Weather. Plaistres maie be of all thinges, as ye hard before. Now the ointmentes be of *Muscilages* and sometyme of *Triapharmacon* as *Myrepsi* thinketh. Howbeit, I suppose *Myrepsi* vsed it in hardenes, caused of frisyng, and not in drought. For I neuer sawe *Tripharmacon* cause moisture, but in hardenes of congelaciōs or frisyng, it serueth well, if it be made with Vinerger, whiche notably cutteth clammy and viscous humours. If it come of fulnes(as it is seen in apostumations) euacuations helpeth the matter: as *Hyppocrates* saieth, sickenes whiche come of replexion or fulnesse, bee cured by euacuation. Now if ye minde to resolue it, let it firste be softened with some mollificatiue, and it will the better banishe and transpire, the pores being opened with the mollificatiue. And if it fall to hardenes againe, ripe it againe with the same medicine as *Auicen* writeth in the cure of apostumations, and then let it be resolued. As for the makyng of these softening medicens, ye must retourne to the treatis of apostumations, wher ye shal finde a special plaster made of Melilote, Sapa or newe wine and lye, and an other of the decoction of Beanes Mallowe leaues, &c. But as for the thirde kinde of hardenesse, partaineth nothing to an vlcere, and for an ende, if the hardenes will not be amēded by these meanes, frete it with some corrosiue, accordyng to the maner as it was prescribed in the correction, of hard lippes in an vlcere.

Now as concernyng corrosie, or gnawing in an vlcere, wee would treate to the full thereof, if we had not medled with the matter, whē we wer about the appesing of dolour, namely, for that that accident is muche more combrous then any of the other. But yet in as muche as we haue there giuen no remedies, we will here haue the matter a little while in consideration againe. Wee suppose then that corrosion is termed of that, that it with his sharpenesse, biting, and fretyng, resolueth, wasteth, and drieth vp the moistnes of the member, after which resolution, the substance of the fleshe is minished, and so falleth to vlceration. Wherefore, accordyng to our determination, there bee twoo causes of this, the proper, and depending. And as for the proper cause, it is, as wee saied before, a certaine malignitie, or filthinesse in the fleshe, whiche Phisicians call the secrete proportie. And for the displacyng of this, ye muste consider the proportie of the member, and then temper and correct it, with defensiues, linimentes, and ointmentes,

ff.iii. made

made, accordyng to your intention, as is that, which I made, respecting bothe complection, and purpose in the maladie, or euill.

A good liniment. ℞. Oile of Roses, Mirte, and Violet, ana. ʒ.i.ß. Bole Irmoniacke, *Terra sigillata*, and Dragons blood ana ʒ.ii. *Acasia.* ʒ.iii. pouder of Roses, Mirtilles, and Cipresse Nuttes ana. ʒ.i.ß. white waxe. ʒ.ß. make here of a linimente, accordyng to the arte, and an ointe the vlcere and his circuite with the same. In case the hinderaunce come of euill fleshe, sprinkle this pouder on it, and ye shall dispatch the malignitie. ℞. Of Citrine, Mirobolanes, of *Terra Sigillata*, of Cerusse, ana. ʒ.iii. of prepared

A consumer of dedde flesh. Tutia. ʒ.i.ß. of Dragons blood. ʒ.ii. of brent Alome. ʒ.ii. mingle them and let it be a fine pouder, to be caste in the vlcere. Whiche ye shall couer with the same liniment, sprede in a clothe: or couer it with *Vnguentum album*, or *Vnguentum de Minio*. The cause dependyng, we take it to bee the antecedent, euen a Cholerike humour, mixt with salt flegme, whiche

Antecedent coniunct. gnaweth the fleshe, when it commeth to the coniuncte, or place. Now for the cure of this, we order twoo intentions, the one to kepe of humours yet fletyng, the other to disconfite thē, whiche be alredie flowyng. The firste maie be doen with *Cassiafistula, Diacatholicon, Manna,* or any like purgatiue. And administracion of the duste and liniment, whiche we ordered now, will accompliche the other. Howbeit, applie this ointment folowing vpon the pouder.

℞. Oile of Mirt, Roses, and Violettes, aū. ʒ.ii. Weathers fat. ʒ.iii. Goates grease. ʒ.i.ß. Iusse of Coleworts. ʒ.iii. seeth theim together till the iuise be dried, and then put therto. ʒ.iiii. of Vermilion. ʒ.iii. of

To make a Cicatrice. Cerusse, and. ʒ.ii. of Letharge, and plaie them againe, till thei become very blacke, stirryng them still, that the Mineralles fall not to the botome, and burne. This doen, put yet thereto. ʒ.i. of Terebintine. ʒ.vi. of newe waxe, and make it to an ointment, betwene hard and soft, in likenes of a Cerote. And this will bring the sore to a cicatrice, and fill your hande full of money for your labour.

Now rottennes and putrefaction foloweth, whose description, I will rehearse, to the intent ye maie thereby be assured of the maladie.

Of putrifaction, or rottennesse. Putrefaction is when the dewe breathing of the spirite, is inhibited and letted in a member, by whom the complection should be maintained and defended. And when this is corrupted, or els letted in his due passage, the moisture of that part is not ruled, and so doeth the parte putrifie and rotte, as *Aristotle* saieth. *iiij. Metheo.* Moisture and heate not ruling the same, is cause of corrupcion at the first meting. But to saie truthe, me thinketh it hath three causes in all. The firste corrupteth the vitall spirite, with holdyng his due breathyng and passage, as doe stuperfactiues or dedde thinges, as Opium, and to coole, repercussiues, thinges lettyng passe, bee grosse, thicke, and clammie humours, whiche by their multitude, thickenes and toughnes, stoppe the priuie spiracles and breathyng pores: but as touchyng thynges that inhibite, thei be causes primitiue. As brusyng, smityng and bindyng to straite. Al these mortifie a member, inhibityng, his spirite and specially

cially bindyng, whiche I sawe befall in a man of muche honestie, liyng in the Hospitall of Saincte Bartholomewes. He was pained of a pushe betwene his tooes, and when one, whom ye knowe, had opened it, there gushed foorthe so moche blood, that the *Chyrurgian* thought it beste, to binde the member, with a right straite bonde, wherevpon the patiente died the nexte date. Wherefore it is expedient, that ye beware ye fall not into suche leude ouer sightes, whereby ye should get the name of Bocherlie manquellers, as he did, not without his desert. Marke here also that, that whiche corrupteth, maie twoo waies bee considered. Firste, as it appereth, the waie to putrefaction, nexte putrefaction alredie caused. If ye consider it, in the first respect, make your recourse to the contrary causes: accordyng to the saiyng of *Hyppocrates*, sickenes caused of replection, be dispatched by euacuacion, whiche doen, the effecte is at a poinct, as *Aristotle* saieth. Remoue the cause and the effecte is remoued. But if ye take on putrifaction the seconde waie, ye must putte on the twoo iyes, whiche *Galen* ascribeth to a good Phisicion. Whereof the right shall beholde the cause, and lefte the effecte, whiche is the putrifaction. The right shall vse contraries to the least applied Ointmentes and plaisters, to repaire the putrefaction, whiche shall be these. ℞. Of Vertdegrece, of roche Alome, and of Honie like partes, with a little Vineger, and haue it to the fire, till the colour alter, from grene to redde, whiche vse, spreadyng this ouer it.

Take of Beane meale, of Barlie and Lupine Meale, ana. li.ß. of Barbours lye. ʒ.ß. and seeth theim vnto soche tyme, as thei bee well mingled together like a paste, whiche must be spred on a pece of cloth. But note, if the rottennesse be so ferre paste, that it will not be displaced, with *Vnguentum Egiptiacum*, of equall partes, ye maie vse this, which vndoubtedly dispatche it. Take of Honie. ʒ.tii. of roche Alome and Vertdegrece. ana. ʒ.ii. of sublimatum. ʒ.iii. incorporate them all together at the fire, till thei be sufficiently sodden, and laie it to the rotten place and then the plaster appointed before. And if there be caused an esthara, remoue it with digestiues, made of Terebintine, and yolkes of Egges, or with Butter. It maie also bee remoued with a plaster, whiche was giuen for apostumacion, opened with a potenciall cauterie: whē this is remoued, the vlcere shall be cured, as bee woundes. Now ye se what is to be doen in putrifaction, or filthie sores.

Sorenes.

What saie you of corrupted bones?

Chyrurgj.

Ow to come to a corrupted bone, the signes of it muste be noted, that ye maie knowe, whether it bee so or not. For it hath proper signes, to be knowen by, as well inwardly, as outwardly. The outward signes bee dulle, and loose fleshe as *Auicen* saieth, in the Chapter *De ventositate spine*. The signes inwardly maie not bee seen with

ff.iiii.   the

the iye, but be founde with the searcher. For if a man searche it well, he shall not onely finde it secretly frete, but also minished and abated in substaunce. Wherefore, if we finde this faulte, and minde to amende it, we shall aboue all thinges, obserue twoo poinctes, one partaineth to the cure, the other to eschue reproche and infamie. We shall auoide infamie, if we refuse to meddle, with the heddes of greate bones and ioinctes. For if we would woorke in soche places, we shall be endaungered of conuulsions, or some euill accidente, by reason of the the fellowship and colligance, whiche thei haue with greate sinewes heddes, of cordes and muscles: whereby we might be utterly disgraced and shamed, as *Auicen* there declareth largely. And as for the cure (these causes eschewed) maie be obtained, specially if the fault be in the middes of the arme or legge, bones and reedes, with conuenient medicenes. There bee also certain kindes of instrumentes, whiche thei calle *Trapanes* and *Raspatories*, very mete for repairing of alterated and corrupted bones. Againe, *Vuguentum Egiptiacum*, made after *Auicens* descripcion, shall bee good, howbeit, ye shall make better spede, if ye use an actuall cauterie, that is, if ye burne it with an hotte iron. Verely my self, when I chaused in soche bones, did euer use actuall cauteries: because thei comfort and rectifie the weake member. Whereof there be two kindes in especiall, the first hath this shape, A. and the parte is plaine, whiche is applied to the bone .C. the other is figured .R. Now in cauterizyng and burnyng, I use this diligence, to eschue inconuenience. I prepared an other instrument, like a finger of a Gloue, with an hole in the middes, through whiche I put my cauterie, to saue the fleshe from burnyng, this used I in plain bones. The seconde was poincted, whiche I used in holes, and hollowe places. There maie bee inuented yet, many other formes of instrumentes, for cauterisyng of bones, accordyng as the worke and place shall require.

Now as touchyng the causes of bones corrupted, thei bee the accident and primitiue: of whiche twoo, the antecedent is the worse. For why, the antecedent will fester the bone, or euer the fleshe bee corrupted, for by reason of the cause primitiue, corrupt and fretyng humors will flete to the bone, and frete it. whiche *Auicen* termeth *Ventositas spine*. Now how this maie bee knowen and cured, ye shall learne of hym, whiche writeth a speciall treatise of it. For wee minde not to meddle with it, because it would drawe us farre from our purpose, by reason of the nomber of intencions. The primitiue cause is, what soeuer befalleth from outforthe, as brusyng, incision, alteracion of the aire (I meane not of alteracion of the aire it self, but of alteracion cause in the bone by the aire) and the use of some ointmentes. And therefore, consider you, whether it come of a wound, or apostumaciō, and so by dilegent calculacion, shal ye come to the cause of the corrupciō. If it procede of apostumacion, corrupt humours be the cause. If it come of a wounde then applicacions of ointmentes, or occursaunce of thaire haue doen it. And if it come of a wounde, then consider again, whether any hole bone

margin notes: A good obseruacion. Auicen. These figures are in the ende. Alteracion of the aire.

betwene Sorenes and Chyrurgj.   Fol.xxxv.

bone were cutte of, or any bone miniched, or els any part. Again, there is no difference, whether a bone were taken out violently, or expelled of nature. For *Auicen* saieth, a fistula maie be feared, where nature expelleth it. Wherefore, if ye couite to knowe, all these particular causes and obseruacions: peruse *Auicen* in that Chapiter, where ye shall finde all thynges, to your full contentacion. This is saied, concernyng corrupted bones. Now in as moche, as our tyme is so shorte by appoinctment, let vs go forthe to the rest of our communicacion. Iuicen.

Sorenes.
I praie you, what is the cause of Varices, and swellyng?

Chyrurgj.
Varices bee swellyng baines in the legges, filled with Melancholike blood. And this is brede diuersly: by stoppyng of the splene, wekenesse of the liuer, to muche feedyng on meates, that increase Melancholie, long standyng and waityng, before men, werines of foote gate, and finally bearing of greate burdens, as it is euidente in them that vse it. And this maladie is verie hard to be redressed, and requireth many intentions and obseruacions in the cure. The first is to order the life conueniently. The .ii. to purge the humour. The third is, to applie conuenable local medicens. Now the regement shalbe to abstain fro meates, whiche brede Melancholie. As Beefe of the oxe Bugle, and Cowe. All salt meates, Pulse, Colewortes, water birdes, Salte Cheese and grosse wine, with other like. The matter is purged with bloodlettyng digestiues and potions. Ye shall taste the blood of *Basilca*, or liuer baine, making a large gashe and hole, that the grosse melancholike blood, maie passe and come foorthe. And it will be the better, and more auaileable a greate deale, if the patient bee exercised by goyng, or some other waie before, so that the humours bee well mingled together. After the bloudlettyng, these sirupes muste followe, sirupe of *Epithimi*, and of Fumiterre, and then a purgation of pilles *De fumo terre*, or Cappers. All which ye shall your self better indosate, accordyng to the patientes state, then I here make farther mention therof. This is spoken in respecte of the accidente, whiche if ye minde to cure well, applie it to the principall intention in the cure. Now as touching the localles, and matter coniunct: when ye wil cure swelling baines, first vse an vniuersall purgation, of the whole body, and then come to the particulare intentions, whiche comprehende three considerations. The first putteth of fleting matter, the second remoueth that whiche is fleten. The thirde comforteth the baines, straineth theim together and resolueth congeled blood. Ye shall kepe of fleting matter with defensiues, applied vnder the knee, whiche maye be soche.

℞. Bole Armoniacke, and claie, ana. ʒ. iii. Dragons blood. ʒ. i. *Terra sigillata*. ʒ. iii. make them in fine pouder, and incorporate theim, with the white of twoo Egges: with. ʒ. of oile of Mirtine, and place it vnder

Of swellynges the cause.

Melancholike meates.

Firste to the whole, then to the particulare.

A defensiue vnder the kne

A Dialogue

How to bind a member. der the knee, bindyng it with a rolle indifferently faste. I saie indifferently fast, because to straite bindyng, wil mortifie the member (whiche were worse then the former euill) neither to slacke. For that is not able to presse the vaines together, neither inhibite the descente, of the Melancholike blood to the place. Therefore lette the bonde be indifferente, so that the blood bee repressed, and the member not mortified.

To open a vain, to purge grosse blood. When ye haue so dooen, ye shall the daie followyng, smite the vaine, whiche appereth aboue the holones of the foote: makyng a large hole that grosse blood haue his passage and milke, or presse doune the blood with your handes, beginning beneath the defensiue, till a great part of the blood of the vaines be auoided. But note, that ye must bathe all the legge with hotte water, before ye presse doun the blood. When the blood is emptied out, stop the vain, & couer the whole legge with this plaister. R. Of Camomell, Melilote, and Wormewoode. ana. ℈. vi. of Mirtilles and red Roses. añ. ℈. iii. of Cipresse nuttes. xx. of *Acatia*. ʒ. iii.

A plaster for the legge, to resolue. of Branne. ℈. iiii. of Beane meale, and of Lupine meale añ. li. ß. braie that is to bee braied, and seeth theim in newe white wine, and Barbours lye, wherein these thynges were sodden before, Tamariske, Moline, Smallage, and rootes of Capers, and plaie all together, till it be like paste: after this, put a little Vinegar to it, that it maie the better cut the humours, & so inroll the whole legge therewith. This plaister (if a man consider it well) hath power to drie, to cōfort, to resolue, and to cutte thinne clammie matter, whiche be necessarie pointes, in this troublesome accident. What will ye more? If ye doe thus, ye shall dispatche and rid your handes of it with honestie. But in case the defensiue so drie, and cause dolour, ye muste chaunge the plaister, and commaunde the paciente, to kepe his legge higher then his bodie, alwaie in his bedde, that blood descende not doune again. For this poincte is necessarie, if he will be cured of the maladie: accordyng to the populer prouerbe, *Gamba al & lesto braso al petto*, whiche willeth the hande to bee kepte at bosome, and the legge in the bedde. And when the pacient is some-

Purge a sore man, after he is amended, for feare of dropsie, &c. what amended, purge hym againe: for otherwise, it were to be doubted, least he fell to an Idropsie, Pthisicke, Phrensie, and dottyng. For the matter, whiche was wont to descende, would be withholden: and in this case his propertie is to rise, and cause soche accidentes, as *Hyppocrates* saieth, to cure olde and antique emeroides, if one bee not lefte open, putteth the pacient in perill, of an Idropsie, Pthisike, and destruction of minde. And in an other place he saieth, of men that be destracted. I fansie is loosed, at the risyng of the swellyng vaines. Wherefore, if a fransie be dispatched, at the prouocacion of them: it is consequent, that the stoppe of theim, will bee cause of the same. Wherefore,

A conclusion *Aristotle* hath this generall rule, in his boke of places. If the presence of a thyng be good, the absence of the same is euill. Therefore, to eschue this euill, we must purge the paciente ones euery moneth, with some purgatiue, which will euacuate the Melancholike humour. There be yet other thynges obserued, as by bindyng, and cuttyng of of vaines,

whiche

betwene Sorenes and Chyrurgj. Fol.xxxvj.

whiche, what for Bocherly crueltie, and otherwise daunger of the pacient, I passe them ouer, sith I neuer practized them, nor neuer intend to doe, the cures beyng so perillous, and full of daungers.

Sorenes.

What saie you of a rounde vlcere? Good sir *Chyrurgion.*

Chyrurgj.

Sir, as touchyng roundnes in an vlcere, we nede not to saie any thyng at all. For ye haue sufficiently laboured the demonstratiue scienses, and haue, as I vnderstande right well profited in them. For ye can erecte triangles, cutte lines, diuide circles, yea, and square theim also, if it were nede: albeit to this daie, the true squaryng of a circle, hath not been inuented. But to the purpose. If ye will deuide the roundnes of an vlcere, by the Diameter, with an hotte Iron, or other instrumente, ye shall deuide the compassyng of villes, and small heres well inough, whiche is one of the greatest lettes, in the ensoundyng of an vlcere. And so shall you withstande the circuicion, whiche dooen, ye maie prosecute the cure of the cutte, burnyng, or otherwise workyng, to your pleasure. Now for that we haue ridde your handes, of these troublesome accidentes: wee will retourne to the cure, of the capitall vlceres, whereof we made mencion before. Whereof the virulent is firste. *Geometrical measures in Chirurgi.*

Good Phisicions haue euer vsed to trie out firste, the cause of maladies, and to cutte them of, whiche dooen, the disease would easely bee displaced. And in good faithe, this semeth to bee the verie pathwaie, to artificiall curing. Wherfore we also, because we would not swarue from the right waie, of our aunciente maisters, will firste declare the cause of a virulente vlcere, and then order the intencion in the cure. The cause then of a virulente vlcere, is Cholerike humours, whiche become sharpe, by reason of salte flegme, mixte with Cholere, and after thei gette virulencie, by adustiō and burning. For virulenci, is not otherwise bredde, as saieth *Auicen*, but of the subtelnesse of hotte watrie humours, whiche originally procede of euill gouernaunce, and order of life. Therefore, we will first appoinct the intencions, whiche muste be observed in their cure. Thei be fiue. The firste ordereth the life, the seconde purgeth the humour, the third kepeth the fluxe of humours. The fowerth drieth them, that be alredie fletyng. The fiueth ensoundeth the vlcere, and comforteth the member. In the first, we must forbid all sharpe, pontike, salted, and hotte thinges, whiche shall be able to alter the blood to heate and adustion, as Ginger, Peper, Cinamon, and giue hym Cheken brothe, Lettise and Borage, as all other thynges, that moderateth the blood, whereof Cheken brothe is thought beste. For it reduceth humours to equalitie, conserueth complexions, and refresheth the vertue. All this is spoken for ensample, that ye take occasion by this, to chuse and refuse thinges conuenient, and disconuenient. *The cause of Sorenes, is first, not considered. Vlcere virulent, how it growe. Fiue good intencions.*

A Dialogue

ueniet. Ye shall purge the matter, if ye giue purgaciõs, that is, thinges that drawe cholere, as *Electuarium de succo Rosarum, Electuarium solutiuum, Diaphinicon*, or some other like in operacion. The fluxe of humours is prohibited, if wee applie this defensiue, in the circuite of the vlcere, fower fingers lesse or more for the same. The defensiue is thus receipted.

A very good defensiue.

Take Bole Armoniacke, and Dragons blood, an̄. ʒ.ß. Beane meale ʒ.i. pouder of Roses and Mirtilles, ana. ʒ.iii. oile of Mirt. ʒ.iiii. iuice of Housleke. ʒ.i. Weathers fatte. ʒ.ß. with a little Waxe: seeth the oile and fatte, with the iuice, till the iuice bee wasted, and then putte to the remnaunt, makyng it to an ointment, after the arte, and order it, as it was now saied. And as for the dryng of humours, vse the dryng simples: howbeit, there must bee diuersitie in compoundyng of theim, accordyng to the natures and complexions, whereof one maie be thus.

Take asshes of Dill, of burnte Leade, and of *Terra Sigillata*, ana. ʒ.i. Letharge of siluer, flowers of Pomegranettes, and vnholed Galles. ʒ.i.ß of Creuis shelles, or house Snailes burnt, of Ceruse, ana. ʒ.ii. of roche Alome burnte. Ɔ.i. mingle theim all together, and pouder it finelie, whiche vse for dryng. And if this profite not, vse the redde pouder, called *Precepitas*, doubtles this will rectifie the vlcer, and digest it. And here note by the waie, that digestion is not causyng of mattre (as some vnlearnedlie holdeth opinion) but it is proporcionating of humours, to the naturall heate, so that nature is animated, to expulse theim, define it thus. Digestion is an ingrossyng of thinne humours, and thinnyng of thicke thynges, with some preparance, to the expullyng. And for this purpose, wee compounde hotte digestiues, in colde maladies, and colde in hotte. Finallie, we ensounde with *Vnguentum de Murio, Triapharmacon, Vnguentum Camphoratum, et de Cerussa*: Or spredde the defensiue aforesaied, in the vlcere. This also that followeth is verie good.

Digestion causeth not matter, but it is the proporcionatyng of the humour.

Take oile of Mirte. ʒ.ii. of Rosed Omphacine. ʒ.i. of Weathers fat ʒ.ii. of Vermilion. ʒ.ß. of Ceruse. ʒ.i. seeth them till thei be blacke, puttyng thereto at the ende. ʒ.ß. of newe Waxe. And after it is taken of the fire, incorporate it with. ʒ.iii. of Camphere, and. ʒ.ii. of prepared Tutie, and so will it be an ointment, like a Cerote. And this will comfort the member, amende the complexion, and bryng the vlcer to skinning. Now for skinning of it, wasshe it with Alome water, which was prescribed before, in skinnyng of vlceres: But one thyng I warne you of, if ye see that the vlcere be enlarged, with these dryng medicens, ye must laie them apart, and vse easier medicens. The signe of to moche dryng, or abstersion by ointmentes will be this. The sore will be like an apostumated sore, and the paciente shall feele paine, nippyng, and bityng, as *Auicen* saieth. Wherefore I will ye forget in nowise, this token and signe, because it will be moche for your aduauntage.

A signe of ouermoche dryng a sore member.

Sorenes.

I praie you saie some thyng, of filthie vlceres?

Chirurgj.

I

IT is euident to see, what glottonous & rauenyng kinde of liuyng we vse, by the alteracion of our blood: whiche is not onely altered to heate, and adustion, but also to foule rottennes. In good faith, reason would we should foresee, that wee fell not to soche excessiue eatyng and drinkyng, whereof might insue, sharpe, filthie, and corrupt humours: whiche cause vlceracion, when thei come thei come to the coniuncte, and afterward feede the vlcere. Well, let them bee their own workemen, and drinke as thei brewe: we wil to our purpose. And first let vs note, what surdities, filthie and corrupt rottennes is. Thei define it, to be a certain white thicke matter, congeled, propense blackenesse, and like lies. This kinde of matter properly, requireth abstercion, and skowryng, as virulencie doeth dryng. More ouer, there bee twoo kindes, a plain and holowe filthie vlcere, whiche require fower intencions: the firste ordereth the life: the seconde pourgeth the humours: the thirde wipeth and scowreth of the filthe: the fowerth partaineth to ensoundyng: ye shall order the life, as in a virulent vlcere, because these twoo differ not, but by the waie of more, or lesse. And therefore, the diet shall respect, specially the qualitie, whiche we there respected in the order. Likewise must the purgatiue be, as there was saied. And the filthe shalbe showred awaie, with these medicenes followyng. ℞. Of rosed Honie strained. ʒ.ii. of clere Terebintine. ʒ.iii. plaie them together, till thei bee well mingled, and then put a. ꝙ.ß. of Barlie flower, and a little Saffron to it. And it will bee a good mundificatiue, for the purpose. But if this shall not serue, let this followe.

Take of clere Terebintine. ʒ.iii. of rosed Honie strained. ʒ.ii. of the iuice of Smallage. ʒ.ß. seeth theim to the wastyng of the iuice, then putte. ꝙ.ß. of Barlie meale to it. ʒ.ß. of Frankensence ʒ.i. of Sarcocol, and a little Saffron, and let it be a soft abstersiue, that maie bee laied in the vlcere, with tentes: And if ye bee sette besides the stoole in this then, make this. ℞. of cleare Terebitine, of Rosed Honie strained ana. ʒ.iii. Iuice of Planten. ʒ.ii. iuice of Dogges toungue. ʒ.i.ß. of Sarcocoll, Frankensence, Mirrhe and Aloes Epatike, ana. ʒ.i. plaie all together, till halfe the iuice bee wasted, but stirre it continually, leaste it burne. After this, let it bee strained, and applied in the vlcere, whether it be plaine or hollowe. But if the praie shall yet escape your nettes, make this, wherewith doubtlesse ye haue your purpose.

Take of Barbours lye. ʒ.iiii. of redde pouder *Præcipitatus*. ʒ.i.ß. of Rosed Honie strained. ʒ.ii. mingle theim well together, and doubtles ye shall scower and drie the vlcere, with this abstersiue. For where as there be but twoo moistures, bred in an vlcere, as *Galen* writeth: whereof the one requireth abstersion, the other dryng. Bothe are respected and considered in this medicene, as it maie easely appere, if a manne consider the simples well. Now ye shall incarnate the sore with ointmentes, that contrary the straunge qualitie of the vlcere: as with hot if the vlcere be colde, and with cold, if it be hotte. For what is ensoun-

Sidenotes:
- Glotonie is no small enemie to nature
- Of filthie matter, what it is.
- Fower intēcions, in two kindes of vlceres.
- A good persite mundificacion.
- To skower and drie all vlcers, plaine or hollowe.
- Contraries when to vse them.

A Dialogue

dyng of discontinued partes, but to rectifie the qualitie, whiche shorteth and hindereth the vertue nutritiue, and to qualifie the complexcion of the member. For if ye dooe thus, nature beyng fortified, will of her self cause fleshe to growe, as it appereth not onely in man, but also in brute beastes. And therefore, I compounde no other ointmentes in this case, then wer ordered before, in the cures of hote and cold vlcers, whither ye maie resort, when ye shall nede. Thus moche haue I said, of the plain filthie vlcere. Now wil we to the holowe and cauie vlcer.

Nature nurisheth her self.

Why should men maruaile, if men of olde tyme, came to the knowlege of Natures sicknesse and causes: for asmoche as thei wer taught, euen by the leding of nature, which thei of that tyme, more diligently obserued then we doe: And therefore, thei came to meruailous greate knowlege, whiche we in these daies, attaine not vnto, because we obserue not in like case. I saie this, in consideracion of a Mouldewarpes moinyng vnder grounde: whiche gaue me occasion to obseruacions, in a cauie vlcere. For because I was presente, where a Gardener stopped the mouthe of the yearth, or hole, where afterwardes (because the cause was not remoued) seuen Moldwarpes came out by sondrie tymes. Truely I noted it, thinkyng it worthie of consideracion in the cure, wherefore, when we be minded, to handle this cure, in his right kinde, we muste trie out the cause, whiche wee seke by humours, accidentes, and qualities of the matter. And therefore, when ye minde the cure of any soche vlcere, consider aduisedly, whether any of the foresaied accidentes by the cause, why the sore refuseth ensoundyng. And if any soche be founde there, and ye thinke that the accidentes, bee the verie lette: retourne then to the correccion of that accidente, whiche hindereth your purpose, and when ye haue amended that, ye shal haue your desire. Now, if the cause be founde in none of theim, then marke the matter, whether it be sanious, virulent, or filthie, and then, accordyng as ye finde it, so resorte to the cure, of the capitalle vlcers, and woorke as is there appoincted, for in so doyng, you shall be assured, to quite your self of it. On thother side, if humours be the cause, whiche is lightly perceiued, by the colours of the fleshe ye muste purge theim: For if it bee ruddie and itchyng, it declareth Cholere. On the other parte, if it bee white, it is a token of flegme, and so of Melancholie, if the colour be dimme and broune. Wherefore, if ye shall alwaie behaue your self thus, in your woorkyng, ye shall not staie, but haue your iye still to the marke, whereat you intende to shoote.

An example of Talpus or Molewarpe.

Amende an euill accidēce and then the cure will prospere.

Here should we speake of a festered vlcere, vnlesse wee had talked of the matter, when we treated of the accidentes of vlcers, where ye shal finde the causes of it, and the cure. Therefore, ye muste make your repaire thither, when nede requireth, and not looke, that I should double it again. Now haue I, my friende, paied my debte, and discharged my bonde, accordyng to my promise: it shall bee your parte, to beare with my trauell, and to take my diligēce in good worthe. And though my stampes bee not so fine, to coigne soche riche money parauenture

betwene Sorenes and Chyrurgj. Fol.xxxviij.

as ye looked for: yet haue I laboured diligentlie, to giue you currante money, whiche I trust to content you. Wherefore thus remaine, that ye be diligent labourers in this, and then within small tyme, ye shall swimme without Corke, and trauerse greate streames, by the aide of these thynges. But if hereafter ye shall looke, to bee holden vp by the chinne (whiche I thinke not) ye must procure, and retaine some other. For I maie not attende vpon you, for businesse that I haue, my deare friende Sorenes.

Sorenes.

TO saie for my self, and my fellowes (whiche I maie, because I knowe their mindes) wee thanke you, as farre as we bee able to saie or thinke, for your faithfull paiemente, brotherly loue, and gentle curtesie. Ye haue so finely coigned all, so orderly laied it foorthe euery some by it self, and so gentelly deliuered it, that wee cannot chose, but allowe it, and highly commende it. But one thing greueth me (I thinke it doeth my fellowes also) that ye leaue vs in the streame to swimme without helpe. Ye knowe right well, gentell *Chyrurgi*, what a nomber of gulphes, bee in the streame of *Chyrurgj*, whiche ye haue not medled withall, it require the helpe of an experte woorkeman. Wherefore, we shall desire you, to graunt vs some aide. Certainly we will repaire to you againe, for other thynges, whiche we will shewe you, at your laisure.

Chyrurgj.

WEll, your desires maie dooe moche with me, howbeeit, I maie not promise at this presente, all your desires or requestes: but of the hedde, I will saie some thyng.

Sorenes.

NArie we praie you, shewe vs the cures of the hedde, when it is wounded, and in perill. For the hed is the prince of members, whose cures are moste harde, and so bid you farewell.

Chyrurgj.

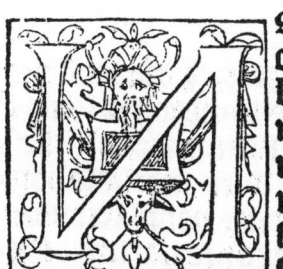NO man, deare Sorenes, that coueiteth to gratifie other, vseth to make light of his frendes requestes, but rather embraceth theim, with all dearenesse of mynde, specially if the thyng truely asked, shall bee righteous and honeste, or bryng the partie, who is required to no hinderaunce. For if those poinctes should appere in any requeste: their peticiōs would seme dishoneste, and worthie of repulse. For why, honestie and righteousnesse, should not please the desired, more then the desirer. Verely, menne should bee farre of, from the waie, if thei thought, that Iustice and honestie, might be acquired, by other mennes losse, and discommoditie. Wherefore, seyng wee consider, that the matter, whiche we coueite to gette all our estimacion (for we desire to

Of honest requeste and friendship.

Gg.ii. here

A Dialogue

here you talke of the maladies, that come of a cause primatiue in the hedde, with their cures) shall be no lesse to you profitable, then to our selues, quiet of conscience.

Sorenes.

WHy should we not boldly require this: namely, sith both of vs, you to declare, and we to hear, be moste at leisure at this presente tyme. We haue also good cause our self in that our conscience dooeth stirre, and encourage vs forth, besides the charitable loue, whiche ye owe emōg our selues, miserably afflicted, in soche causes. Again, if wee did demaunde any thing rashelie, perchaunce euen that, whiche should be pleasaunt to other men, might worthilie be denaied vs. For why, rashnes semeth to import twoo thinges: vnrighteousnes in the demaunder, or els vanitie in the thing demaunded. Yet for as moche as our sute is right iuste and honeste, and you pleasaunte Maister *Chyrurgj*, gentle and free harted to your friendes: let it bee your will and pleasure, to reason with vs, concernyng the matter, to the intente we through your apte and wise communicacion, maie declare so many daungers in the hedde (whereunto these common practisians, rushe out on with all haste, as dooeth Tom a Bedlem, in his naked pro-grace) but redresse thesame, if any soch chaunce, vnder our simple plain handes. For you are the man, as we doe thinke, who is skilfull to cure hurtes in the hedde, and auoide daungers in thesame. And this did we perceiue right well, not onelie at other tymes, but specially in the places, where wounded men are kepte, where ye helped greuous and perilous chaunses in the hedde. Go to then gentle maister, and folowe your friendes desire, whiche be in greate loue with you. And thus do-yng, ye shall doe vs presently greate pleasure, and vnto our posteritie. And albeit, ye can not receiue worthie rewarde, at our handes, for so greate a benefite: yet the almightie God, who doe see no good tourne vn rewarded, nor vice vnpunished, will recompence your paine, and prospere you in your actes and dedes, who euer be praised, for himself and his woorkes. *Amen.*

Chyrurgj.

THE beginnyng of your matter, albeeit, I did well per-ceiue it, yet by meanes the tale was somewhat long, it was almoste fallen out of my remembraunce, whiche I beyng febled, and fallen into decaie, with moche labour of minde, & anguishe that I take for my poore friendes. For accordyng to the debte of our corrupte nature, thei are decessed, and hath giuē vp their soules, to whō the mercifull God, not in respecte of their good deedes, but at the contemplacion of his own bountifull clemencie, graunt endlesse rest and saluaciō with his sainctes and elected. But yet as farre as I can remember, I noted in some, what we are bound to doe, for our frendes and acquaintaunce,

in

in consideracion of our familier conuersacion. Of truthe wee are not ignoraunt, dere frendes, how hard a thing it is for vs, at this present, to satisfie your desire, specially, for as moche as my minde doeth not onely take care, but melteth awaie in floodes of sorowe: for the great affliccion I daily feele. Is it possible, that I should cōtent your desires with like woordes as I vsed, when I talked of woundes, apostumacions, & vlceres: verely, I would I might gratifie you, so that ye should coueite no farther in the matter. But alas, I am rackt and tourmented within my self, when I feele and consider, mine insufficiencie and vntowardnes. But yet, least I should be seen, to tourne my backe, and giue my dearest friendes a repulse or an *vltimum vale* (who bee as myne own iyes) yet I will take the matter, for your sakes vpō me. Neuerthelesse, this would I desire, and obtain at your handes, that none should interrupt me in my tale: but in soche places, where I ende my whole matter. For the time is very short for our matter, whiche we minde to finishe. And certainly, if I thought otherwise, nothyng wer better to me, thā to be questioned with, in euery doubt, which you shal not nede.

Sorenes.

Gentle sir, ye haue moste happely preuented vs. For the matter, whiche wee were appoincted, to gette at your handes, or euer we came hether, by praier or fauour, that haue you offered of your self. Therefore, seyng we are agreed of the matter, set on a Gods name, and luckely make the onsette. For there maie not be greater pleasure to vs, then to heare your woordes, and maner of talke, so that the precious fruite and profite, whiche we looke for in especiall, be preferred, for that is the matter.

Chyrurgj.

I noted, deare Sorenes, and your friendes, that R.R. in his famous worke, vnder whose banner I serued moste and gat all that I haue, at his handes, or not, without his especiall fauour: did fatherlie admonishe his scholers and hearers, that thei should to their possibilitie, trie and searche out, the causes of diseases. Otherwise, thei should attempte, to cure one thing for an other, and giue Chalke for Cheese. And if thei did so, thei should greatly erre in the cure: or rather prouide a beare, to helpe their pacientes to their graue. Wherefore, I haue determined with my self, sith your will is so, that I shall daunger my self in the matter, to recite vnto you the sicknesses, which happen in the hedde, with their causes. And this doe I, to the intente we fall not vnaduisedlie in that, had I wiste, whereof we mencioned before. Thei bee fiue in nomber, that is to saie, apostumacion, vlcere, wounde, bruse, and breakyng. But as touchyng apostumacions, and vlceres without, wee will here make no further a dooe, because wee haue sufficientlie spoken of it before, in our former treatise of woundes: whereunto ye maie repaire at your pleasure. But as for bru-

Chalke for Cheese.

Fiue causes that doe hurt the hedde.

Gg.iii. ses,

ſes, woundes and breakynges, we will laie our foundaciō, as farre as our witte ſhall extende. Ye haue the maladies, wherefore, wee maie procede to the cauſes and cures.

The cauſe of bruſes, what thei are.

And firſte, we will begin at a bruſe or cruſhyng, whoſe cauſes bee falles and ſtrokes, whereof followeth the member, of the continuance broken. And here wee vſe this terme, of the continuaunce, broken, or bruſe: after a large maner, for euery riuyng, or fruſhyng of mannes fleſhe, whiche maie bee twoo waies, that is to ſaie, by meanes of a wounde, and without a wounde. As a bruſe, whiche ſhall be without wounde, maie eaſely be cured, except the bone, whiche is vnder it, bee riuen, the ſkin remainyng whole and ſounde. Whiche hurte, the ſicke hymſelf, will ſhewe to the *Chyrurgian*, by certaine ſignes, as by often ſcratchyng, or touchyng of the place with the nailes, or by ſome other meanes. But if it be ſo, that ye can not be perſwaded, by the pacientes ſhewyng: or if ye be driuen to and fro, and reaſonyng the matter with your ſelf, as in ſoche caſes, mennes mindes bee pluckte, now hether, now thether. Ye muſt conſider the ſmiter, of what ſtrength and force, he might be of, and wherewith the ſtroke was inflicted: as in like maner the place alſo, whether any thing fell on the hed, from an height. For the higher that the place is, and the mightier the ſmiter, ſo moche the greater and worſe muſt the bruſe be deamed. For heauie thynges, fallyng towardes their naturall place, are found of greater force and violence, at the ende of their diſcent and fall, then at the beginnyng, when thei were firſt loſed of their ſtaies. Theſe thinges conſidered, ye ſhall make inciſion vnto the ſcalpe, rulyng the ſame after ſoche ſorte, as ſhall bee declared afterwarde, when wee ſpeake of riuynges of the ſcalpe, with depreſſion of the bone. On the other ſide, ye geſſe by the ſaied ſignes, that the bone remain ſounde and vnbroken, then ſet all your intente, to the cure of the bruſe: whiche ſhall ſtande in a reſolutiue medicene, beyng ſomewhat bindyng withall, if ye feare of putrefaccion. For what ſoeuer is bruſed or fruſhed, muſt nedes putrefie, as *Galen* writeth. But I ſuppoſe, ye are minded to aſke me a queſtiō. How it is, that reſolutiues ſhould bee applied in bruſes, wherein is greate concurſe, and ſhewyng of matter, for aſmoche repercuſſiues ſhould be vſed, as was ſaied, at the beginnyng of ſoche matters. Ye haue well and trimlie doubted at the matter: for this ſhall make moche for the cure of a bruſe, in greate perill, wherof ye ſhall diligently marke, that effuſion of blood, doeth immediatlie folowe vpon a bruſe, becauſe the vaines bee violently cutte of, and the mouthes opened. And the blood whiche ſhall ſo ones be iſſhewed forthe, can neuer returne backe, into the vaines again. Wherefore, ſeyng it is without the beſſelles, it muſt nedes putrefie, & ſo conſequently, corrupt and rotte the fleſhe. For this purpoſe gentle reſolutiues, beyng bindyng thynges withall, muſt bee applied at the beginnyng: where the one reſolueth the blood, and the other being contrary in workyng, cloſeth the vain, that no more commeth foorthe. And hereof appereth the ignorauncie, and ouerſight of

How to finde out a ſtripe, by what tokens.

Of inſicion in the hedde.

Of blood running the chief cauſe and the hurte that do followe the ſame.

theſe

betwene Sorenes and Chyrurgj.　　　　　　　　Fol.xl.

these imperikes, and vagabonde *Chyrurgians*. For thei minister repercussiues, at the beginnyng of euery bruse, without resolutiues: whereof followeth insicion of necessitie, if thei will auoide putrefaccion. And therefore I will giue you the medicen, whiche euer is vsed in soche cases, that ye faule not in the like reprehension and shame.

Take Camomell, Melilotte, branne, ana. ℳ.i. of Beanes, Lupines and Barlie meale, ana. ʒ.ii. of Mirtilles, ℳ.ii. of Cipresse nuttes. ʁb. braie soche thynges as ought to be braied finelie, and then seeth al in newe wine and Barbours lye, vnto the tyme it bee like a Cerote. And at the ende, ye shall put these oiles to the same, that is, of Dille, of Camomell, and of Mirte, ana. ʒ.ii But note, here the oiles must bee vsed, where no putrefaccion is. For in case of putrefaccton, I would vtterly forbid them. Then plaie them again, till the oiles bee well incorporated: and afterward applie it warme. Marke well this medicen. For it were a long matter, and to moche for one daie, to recite to you, how many haue been cured, by the helpe of this medicen alone. But if the bruse be concurraunt with a wounde, or euer ye worke in the matter: ye must diligently consider with your self, whether the rimme or pannicule, whiche from out foorthe, couereth the scalpe, bee cutte or not. And if it be not cutte, the wounde muste be cured, as we shewed in the treatise of woundes, sauyng that the digestiue muste bee made, with Rosed Omphacine, and yolkes of Egges, ouer whiche, ye muste euer applie this medicene, whiche we aboue recited. For it will kepe of putrefaccion, and harde corrupted blood. And after this maner, procede foorthe in the cure, till sanious matter be generated, that doen, laie aparte the digestiue, and applie an abstersiue, in his place. Which maie bee thus. ℞. Of clere Terebintine. ʒ.ii. of Sirupe of Roses. ʒ.i.ß. of Plantane water. ʒ.ß. plaie theim together, till the water bee wasted, and then put therto. ℥.ß. of Barly meale, and a little Saffron as maie be able, to colour the mundificatiue. But take it of the fire, or euer ye put to the meale, and see it bee well stirred, whiles it be well incorporated together. Now, when ye haue thus doen, ye maie vse it, and applie euer the same *Vnguentum Basilicum*, after this descripcion.

Take oile of Roses and Camomell, ana. ʒ.iii. oile of Mirtin. ʒ.i.ß. plaie theim together, till thei acquire theim a blacke hugh, and then put these drugges to them, of cleare Terebintine. ʒ.ii. of Ship pitche ʒ.i. of newe waxe. ʒ.ii.ß. And plaie them again a little, and so take it of the fire, and stirre it cōtinually, till it be thicke. And for asmoche as these woundes, by reason of moche sensibilitie of the parte, bee often tyme vexed, with an *Erisipela*: this place asketh to shewe, howe we withstande that troublesome maladie. And to the entente ye maie so doe, note this, concernyng an *Erisipela*, or Cholorike apostumacion, and put it depely in minde. It is this. An Erisipela maie happē, by reason of boilyng of the humour, or for that that corrupted matter, is retained within. Whiche thing we sawe our self come to passe, by reason of matter, abidyng within, in one worthie capitain. Now this thyng is

Gg.iiii.　　　　　cured

Many men haue been cured by this medicens.

A good abstersiue for the heade.

Vnguentum Basilicum.

Erisipele, is a hotte redde, rounde inflamacion sore, or cholorike boile, with a feuer in the bodie.

A Dialogue

Diseases comyng of fulnes, are helped by emptines.

cured by purgyng of the cause: As *Hyppocrates* saieth *Quecunq; egreditudines ex plenitudine fiunt, euacuatio sanat.* If it bee sharpened and chafed, through heate and boilyng of the Cholerike humour: anointe it with *Vnguentum Rosatum* and lute the wound with the same, as the best learned *Chyrurgiãs* did vse. For if mordicacion or heate bee caused, by meanes of ointementes: it will be pacified through coldnesse, whiche is in the medicene. After ye are at poinct with this, couer the holle wounde with this.

℞. Of Roset Omphacine, and oile Mirtine, ana . ʒ. ii. of *Vnguentum Rosatum.* ʒ. i. of Populion. ʒ. ß. of white Waxe. ʒ. iii. and melte all at the fire: this doen and prepared, infuse a linnen clothe in the same ointement, and see it be all to weated in it, and then take it forthe, and caste it in colde water, that it maie be thicke again. This clothe also muste

Clothes applied to a wounded hed

be applied to the hed, for feare of a noiyng of the place: and be applied where the heare was shauen of. Moreouer, ye shall forme and shape one other clothe, after the same maner, with the saied ointmente, so that ye maie make permutacion, at euen and mornyng, of the clothes But if the panicule or rimme be cutte, and the bone discouered, ye shal neede more diligence and circumspeccion, whiles ye searche, whether the bone be clouen, or riuen in peces. And if neither of these faultes be founde, then is nothing els to bee dooen, otherwise then in woundes, sauyng that this pouder shall bee sprinckled, where the bone was discouered and opened. ℞. Aloes epatike, Sarcocoll, Mirrhe, ana. ʒ. iii.

A pouder for the hedde.

Frankensence. ʒ. i. ß. Flowerdeluce. ʒ. ß. & lette it be in fine pouder, for the saied vse. And as for farther prosecucion of the matter, ye shall do as in the cure of woundes. But in case the bone bee riuen, an other maner of cure will handfast you: whiche will bee farre distaunte, and vnlike the former. And to the intent ye maie be able, to ascertain your self, in soche cliftes and reuynges, ye shall here note the signes and tokens, that followe cliftes and riuynges of a bone.

Signes of broken bones in the hedde.

These thynges bee signes of a broken bone, vomityng, daasyng of iyes, vertige or swinyng, blindnes and fallyng. All whiche muste bee vnderstande, to happen at that presente, when the stroke was giuen. And sometyme an apoplex, a dumpishe priuacion of sense, and a feuer with a behement horrour and colde doe ensue. Now were the pacient taken of a feuer, without colde, there were no greate daunger in the matter, for that accidente cometh oft tyme, of a priuate cause, whiche moueth the accident. And where it is not possible, but the body should bee replete, or bacante of superfluous humours, so it can not bee, but there should insue greate diffrence, at that diuersitie. For if this kind of breakyng, occupie a bacant bodie, the pacient will bee without feuer: but if it fall to a replete bodie, ladē with euill humours, the Phisicians maie thinke the stroke to bee daungerous, and harde of cure.

Dangerous woundes, how to know theim.

For wee haue this lesson of *Auicen*, saiyng: all woundes and vlcers bee daungerous, whiche chaunce vpon superfluities, of a waiwarde and froward bodie. And albeit, it be daungerous, if the pacient bee taken of a feuer, at the beginnyng, yet is the matter more suspecte, if he bee

inflamed

inflamed with feuers, three or fower daies, after the stroke was giue̅: because this should spryng of putrefied bloode, retained within the scalpe vpon the rimmes, whiche thing is knowen by the increasyng of the accidentes. Notwithstandyng, this maie be also, when sanious matter is a generatyng. For why, *Hyppocrates* affirmeth in his Aphoris- mous, that dolours and feuers will happen, more at generatyng of matter, then when it is generated. But this maie easely bee disceue- red: For here the accidentes fall and bee alaied, but there thei bee aug- mented and increased. Therefore, when soche accidentes shall insue vpon a stroke, euen thesame daie, ye maie well iudge, that the breacke or breakyng is complete. Whiche if ye minde to cure rightly, ye shall foorthwith prouide these thynges before your iyes. Firste, when the matter is come to that poincte, that ye must make incision, feare not to cutte the wound, after the maner of a triangle, or one right angle, or els of a crosse, and remoue the fleshe from the bones. When ye haue so doen, fill vp the wounde with small quisettes, well weate before in the whites of Egges. Howbeeit, note and obserue this alwaies, that the quisettes, whiche shall touche the bone, muste bee weate in hotte wine, for feare of alteryng and spottyng of the bone: if thei wer weate in whites of Egges, by reason of the coldnes. For why, *Hyppocrates* saith. *Frigidum inimicum neruis, ossibus, celebro & spinali medullæ, calidum vtile & amicum.* Colde is an enemie to the sinewes, bones, teeth, braine, and the Nuke, or ma- rowe of the backe. But heate is profitable and frendly, and therefore colde must be kepte from the skulle, least we stomble at that blocke by errour. Now this operacion finished, ye shall giue the pacient in com- maundement, to reste hymself: after that maner vntill the nexte mor- nyng, prescribyng him an order, how he shall rule himself, & his diete. His diete shalbe to eate Wheate bread, or tried and boiled Barlie with Almond milke, and drinke boiled Borage water, for the space of fower daies: and after the fowerth daie is paste, giue hym Weaton, for Bar- lie breade, dipped in Cheken brothe, or brothe of Mutton of the Wea- ther, leaste the sicke bee ouermoche weakened, with the slender diatte. Now the nexte daie, retourne to your paciente, and open his wounde gentelly, whiche doen, searche the bone well and warely, with a sear- cher of siluer, whiche must neither be to blunt, to ouer runne the rim- mes, or cliftes, neither so small or fine, that it should enter into them. Ye shall searche it thus. Drawe the searcher to and fro, pretelie vpon the bone: and if it slide plainly without staie, it is a signe the scalpe is saufe and sound. But if it staie, and finde some let, ye maie then think well, that the bone is clouen and cutte. But now, in as moche as we speake of rimmes, and because thei be diuers, this place requireth, to distincte them properly, or euer we medle further in the cure.

Fissures or chinkes, bee caused in the the hedde twoo waies, with a thyng, whiche giueth a blunte stripe, or els with a thyng, whiche cutteth. If it be with a thyng, that giueth a blunte stripe, the thing properly, is called a clifte or a riuyng. And if it bee with a cutte, it is
called

called a chinke or a clifte. And all these varrie in lengthe shortnesse, largenesse, and smalnes thei varrie also otherwise. For euery of them I saie, the chinke and clifte, maie bee with depression of the bone, or without depression. For an instrumente, whiche cutteth, maie cause depression, namely, if it bee thicke or blunte. And albeit, thei agree in the former pointes, yet thei differ in this, that is to saie, the clifte, which is caused by a bruse, is euer thought to be with penetracion, or through goyng and percyng of the bone, where it is not a like alwaie in a cutte or incision. I saie this of mennes scalpes, and not of children. For in children, whiche be within seuen yere of age: we maie be deceiued, as we see by experience. For why, soche sculles will bee infolded, because thei bee not yet hardeined ne strengthed: and moisture also aboundeth in them, whiche propertie is not founde in mennes scalpes that are come to ripe age. For mennes scalpes will riue, and bee cutte through, rather then be infolded, by reason of the hardnes, & drought of the bone. Wherefore, men that are come to hardnesse, are depriued of this, whiche is founde in tender age. And after what sorte, euery of these maie bee cured, we shall declare orderly, when we haue firste premised the intencions, whiche must needes bee obserued, if we intende warelie, to eschue daungers in soche cases. And as sone as we shall be at poinct with this, we shall accomplishe our promise, bothe of a riuyng or clifte, with the depression of the bone.

A clift in the hedde.

A note, betwene a mannes scull and a boies.

Presupposing then the regement of life, these be the chief and principall intencions aboute this cure: that is to wete, to conserue the compleccion of the member, in his proper state, to prohibite apostumacions, and to applie localle medicenes fitte for the purpose. Certes we maie conserue the compleccion, and rectifie it, if it bee decaied, with emplasters, as *Auicen* writeth in the chapiter, of the woundyng of the skinne of the hedde. *Et principium quidem consistit in plastris & erit rectificatio. &c.* The beginnyng standeth in plasters, and so will the rectificacion bee sone had. We shall preuent or put of apostumacions, if we shall worke the thynges, whiche the pacientes strength shallbe able to abide & suffer, as we haue commaundement in thesame place. And doubtles, the disposicion of the bodie, shall awaie with it well inough, if we procede no farther, then till the cause of apostumacion, be intercepted and cut of. These be the causes of an hotte apostumacion, *Siphac*, a gobbetie of a bone, prickyng the vtter rimme, whiche is called *Dura* matter, annoysaunce of tentes, cold approchyng to the rimmes or pannicules, plentie of meate and drinke, and the secrete euill (as thei call it) whiche I vnderstande, to be a certaine malignitie of complexion, and superfluities of frowarde bodies: whiche we shall preuent and cutte of, by purgation and blood lettyng. The pacient shall bee purged, accordyng to the significacion of his vrine. For why, that will shewe the humour, whiche is excessiue in the bodie, as we saied in the cure of vlcers. And as touchyng blood lettyng, it hath, as he saieth, twoo intencions: the one to make euacuacion, and the other to prohibite, or withdrawe.

Auicen.

What thyng doe anoie the brain moste.

Purge the pacient, accordyng to the vrine,

But

But where we treate of blood lettyng, I praie you of good felowship, note this well: for it shall greatlie make for the preseruaciõ, and sauegard of your pacient, which is sore, and for your self also.

Note, derelie beloued, that it maie chaunce, that the sicke come vnder your handes, thesame daie he was wounded, or els after the fowerth. From the first daie vnto the fowerth exquisiuely, you maie vse diuerse blood lettyng, because this is the tyme, when matter causyng apostumacion, vseth to flowe, and turne againe to the place. And this blood letting must be made in the common vaine, called *Mediana*, of the opposite arme. Here ye shall diligentlie marke, and take heede, that ye erre not, in the significacion of this worde *opposite*, as some haue, which were not seen in this woorde at all. For this woorde *opposite*, signifieth contrarietie, as when a thing is placed, ouer againste the contrarie part. Wherefore, the partes of the right side, maie not properly be *opposite* one to an other, within them self, but partes of the right side, to the partes of the lefte. This will appere in the shape of mannes bodie, whiche is erected and figured, after the maner of a quadrant, albeeit, it bee not fully square and shaped, with equalitie of corners, as is a true quadrant or square. Now it is euident, that this quadrangle, in maner is measured, with twoo Diameters, whiche also properlie bee *opposite*. So hauyng respecte to this quadrangle, it shall be an easie matter to see, on whether parte the vaine shal bee opened. And this blood lettyng, as we saied before, is made for twoo purposes, accordyng as the cause requireth, that is to weete, to make euacuacion, or els to diuerte or tourne awaie the blood, to the *opposite* parte. If your entent bee to tourne a side the blood, it muste bee doen in the *opposite* parte. For ensample: When the wonnde is in the lefte side, a vaine of the right side shall be opened, and contrarilie. When the wounde in the right side, a vaine of the lefte, whiche must bee the common. On the other parte, if your purpose be onely to make euacuacion, ye shall worke the feate in the vaine, whiche is moste proper to the parte wounded. As bee the vaines in both handes, called *Cephalicæ*, that is the hedde vaines: whiche will voide matter and blood from the hedde. Wherfore, thei doe amisse and euilly, yea, maliciouslie, to whiche indifferentlie taketh blood, of the one, or other hande at the beginnyng, where the intent should bee to diuerte, and tourne awaie the blood by fleubotomie. For thei make euacuacion, and tourne not awaie the blood, to the contrarie parte, and so consequentlie cause thei the feabled member, to be more feable and decaied in soche wise, that other mẽbers send thither their superfluities, as he saieth. *Quicquid delirant reges plectuntur achiui.* What fault soeuer be committed, emongest the high counsailes, the poor people suffreth for it. For it is certain, that the mẽber is febled, as sone as it is wounded. Wherfore in so doing, thei open the waie to apostumacion whiles thei thinke to preuent and stoppe it, and become occasion of the pacientes death. And thus craftelie woorke the Imperikes and Heathen vagaboundes, coueityng not onelie to slea, and suppe the Christian blood,

but

but vtterrlie to extinguishe the Christian name, if it were possible. Yet a Gods name, we can abide to call theim vnto vs, and intertaine theim with all gentlenesse, where we should not onely forbidde them the arte, but also treade theim vnder our feete, and make theim bonde slaues, as the Turkes doe vs Christian menne, when thei take vs, and vse vs worse then dogges.

 Now, in case the bodie bee full, and replenished with humours, ye shall let your pacient blede againe, in the same place, where ye let him blood before. But if the apostumacion were in the clensyng places, as vnder the arme holes, flankes, and eares, I would in no wise lette my pacient blede, for that maladie: because I finde not, why I should so doe. For an apostumacion maie not a rise, in the emunctorie places, but by euilnes or malignitie, of some principall member, or by reason of the superfluities, of some member adiacen. If the place bee apostumated through matter, expelled from a principall member: Fleubotomie were not to the purpose, because the matter might bee reuoked inward, whiche nature had put foorthe. Neither should it bee well to the purpose also, if the swellyng came of superfluities, of the nexte partes therevnto. For we should putte the matter from the vnnoble and petite member, and burdein againe the principall with it, whereof would ensue greate inconuenienses and daungers. We be also forboden to vse repercussiues, for feare of the like daungers, in the saied emunctorie or runnyng places. (But if I had occasion, in as moche as we liue, and haue a doe with nise, foolishe, and wilfull people, whiche call for thinges to their sauftie, in soche wise, that we must woorke against our rules, to satisfie their lustes: I would open in that case, the *Basilica* or liuer vaine. And it shall make no matter, whether ye open the vaine in the right side, or lefte, so the apostumacion bee in the vpper parte of the bodie: but in case the apostumacion, be in the lower part, blood maie be taken frõ the liuer vaines, in the foote of the *opposite* part, accordyng as ye shall thinke it moste conueniente. Howbeit, it will be surer, and farther from perille, to take blood of the Liuer, in the same parte of the foote. For it were ieopardie, leaste some humiditie, retained in the glandeous fleshe, might by stirryng and angeryng of the matter, cause apostumacions. Well, I haue saied inough, as touchyng blood letting, now wee will to the locall medicenes, whiche shall bee declared in the cure. Wherefore, lette vs come to the cure of a brecke in the scalpe, namely of a clifte, or a riuyng: and firste here marke this figure for blood lettyng, here after this place..

But

Marginalia:
- when to let blood, twoo tymes in one place, & why.
- If an apostumacion bee in the rist of the vpper part of the bodie, thã to blede either lefte arme, or els right is weil.

betwene Sorenes and Chyrurgj. Fol.xliij.

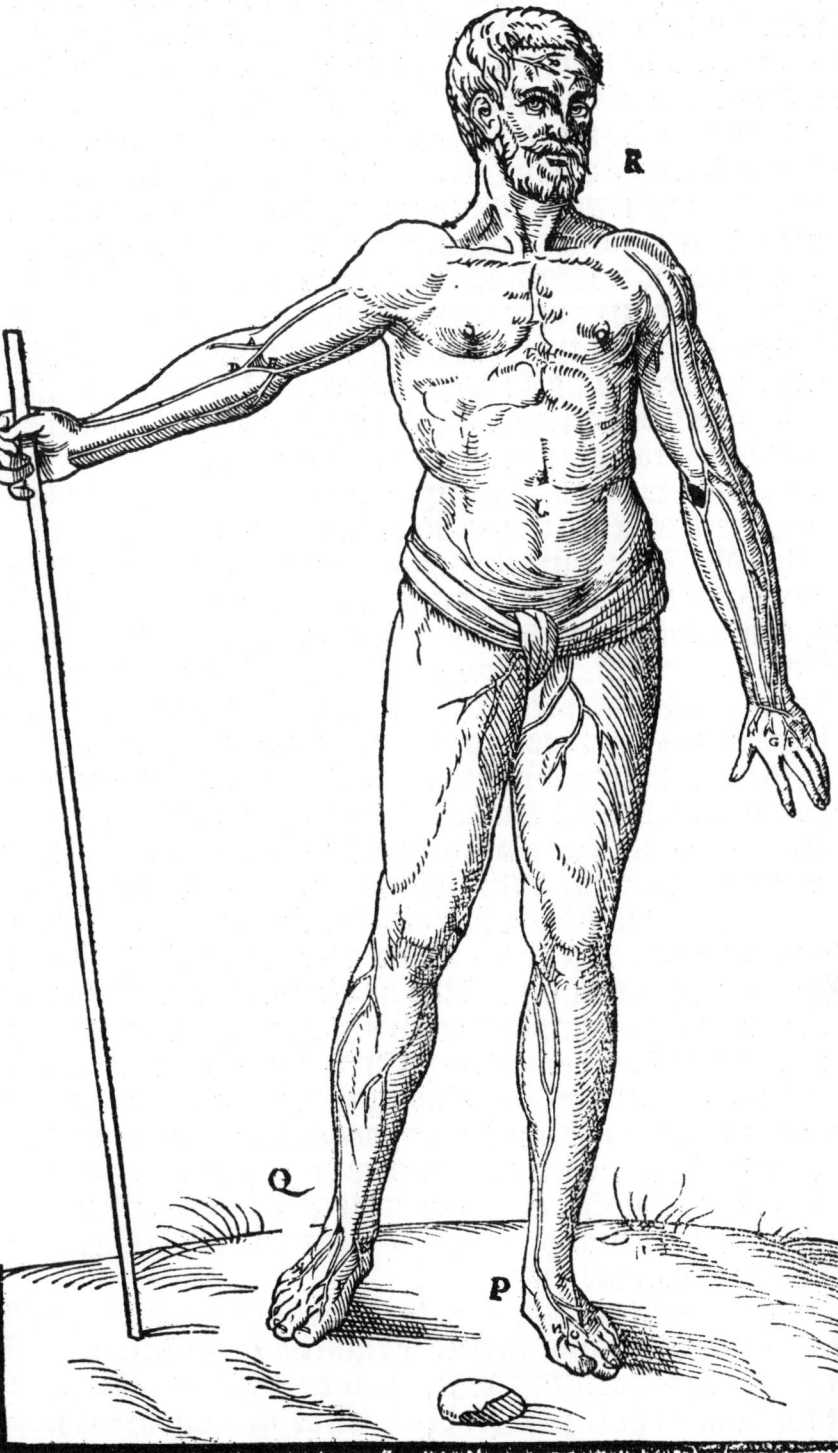

Under the tõg are .iii. vaines, whiche ar good to be opened a=gainst Apople=xia, Anginæ, & stoppyng of the spirites of aspi=racion, and re=spiracio̅, and all the euils of the mouthe, toung, and throate.

K.

The vaine cal=led Sciatica, & cometh from be=neth the knee, dounward, and are .ii. in nom=ber, & are good to be opened in warme water, to help the swel=lyng of the se=crete members and also ye paine called Sciatica

Q

Saphena, co=meth from the holownes vn=der the knee, as Sciatica doeth It is in the in=side of the ancle and is opened for the Splene Matrix. &c.

P.

The vaine of the forhed, to be opened against fransie, Megrē ache in the hed, forgetfulnesse, and sorenesse in the iyes, &c. and this vain spryng from the out=ward throate vaine.

Y.

Vena externa or Cephalica in the arme, is o=pened with a large cutte, not depe, to let forth grosse matter, clense the hed,

from all gre=ues, as falling sicknes, dim=nes of hed, &c

A.

Mediana, whiche is in the middest, it is the chief organe or spryng of the blood, it must bee opened to help the sides Midrife, sto=macke, hotte feuers. &c.

D.

Vena interna, or Basilica, comyng from the harte and liuer, by this vaine is a si=newe like to it, in which is contained the spirite of life, and vnder the same ar migh tie sinewes, therefore it is perilous to o=pen that vain but by greate knowledge, but it help to bee opened a=gainst pleuri=sie, pestilence. &c.

B.

A braunch of Cephalica in the hande.

H.

funius brachij

G.

Saluatella

E.

These three last ar of smal force to open because little blood do cum from thē, but yet to open these small vai=nes in warme water, does helpe Apo=plexia.

But yet or euer we take the cure in hand, I thinke it moche appar=tayning to our duetie, to shewe what waie we minde, to folowe in the cures. For I haue found twoo, after *Auicen*, whereof the one doeth one=ly moiste, and the other onely drie. But to saie trouthe, neither of thē
Hy.i.   liketh

liketh me, by it self a lone. For if I vsed the waie of moistyng, in a bruse, I might well doubt of putrefaccion, because this waie greatly promoteth putrefaccion. For it is doen with oiles, and yolkes of Egges, whiche cause putrefaccion in a brused place. On the other parte, the waie of driyng dooen, with *Aqua vitæ*, and the pouder, whiche *Auicen* describeth in the Chapter, *De incisione cutis*, before alleged, doeth not fullie contente me, though it haue twoo partes: whereof the one defendeth from putrifaccion, but the other parteth not the brused. Therefore, because I would not fall, in either extremitie of onely driyng, or onelie moistyng: I haue gathered a certaine waie of them bothe, consistyng betwene theim bothe. For it shall altogether haue vertue, to drie and to moiste, because, as I iudge, medicenes for the hedde, muste actuallie moiste, and drie potencially. For by the helpe of drought, we preserue the complexion of the bone, and pannicles, whiche be dry of compleccion, as *Galen* writeth. And by moisture, wee procure digestion, if any thing were tourned and brused. All these thinges shall wee obtaine, with Rosed Honie strained, *Aqua vitæ*, and the pouder, whiche wee shall order in the cure. Neither must you maruell at the matter, my friende Sorenes, and your felowes, as did one, whē he heard a man saie, that Honie was moiste in felyng, and driyng in vertue and workyng. Verelie of his corpulencie, if I maie so saie, it moisteth, but as touchyng his qualities & vertue, his operacion is driyng. But it was no wounder, that the young Philosopher, did not perceiue the matter: Alas he had not yet rede ouer bookes of simples, neither the principles of Philosophie. Ladie Ignoraunce caused hym to muse, but not to searche the cause, as did the Philosophers, as *Aristotle* writeth, in his supernaturalles. He would not haue marueiled, if he had rede *Aristotle* concernyng the minglyng of the Elementes: whereby he should haue easely perceiued, that Honie is of the qualities, whereof I reported it to be: by reason of the compleccion in mingling, if it be aduisedly cōsidered, accordyng to his essence and nature. And if there shall be any manne, whiche shall not perceiue throughly, the nature of the Simples, contained in medicenes, yet lette hym assuredly perswade hymself, that I will describe no other waie of cure, then I haue writtē: and haue gote therby, bothe profite and good well spent time, ye haue heard the caurelles and prouisions, whiche I recken necessarie. Now will I orderlie describe you the cure.

Then, when ye finde a clifte, by reason of a bruse, ye shall obserue this order: if ye minde to cure it rightlie, in his kinde. Firste, before all other thynges, consider whether it be with depression, and infoldyng of the bone or not. For if it bee with depression, or infoldyng, all that, whiche is brused, must nedes be taken foorthe: because it would otherwise prouoke, to some apostumaciō. For why, in that case it could not be otherwise, but some gobet of bone, would be vnder the scalpe, prickyng the vtter rimme, or dura matter. And in this case heare thē not, whiche shall counsaill and perswade, to remoue parte of the brused,

and

betwene Sorenes and Chyrurgj. Fol.xliiij.

and to leaue parte. For these men can not remoue the whole cause, in as moche as in euery little parte of the brused bone, maie be some shiuer, whiche by prickyng will come to apostumacion. Therefore to auoide, and eschue the saied cause, let vs take forthe all the brused. But if the clifte be founde, without depressyng of the bone, ye maie not cut out altogether, but onely make an holle in that part, where the matter shall moste easely come foorthe. And to the performaunce of this worke, ye haue three proper instrumentes, the Sawe, the Chesell, and Wimble, emongest which, we haue moste nede of the Wimble, because I finde in it moste commoditie, then in other instrumentes. *Sawe, Chesill, and wimble for the hed*

Firste, it will lightlie make the hole, yea, and that without moche molestyng of the pacient: whiche thyng can not bee doen, without raspatorie. Againe, it will make an hole and euentacion, meete for the passage of matter. Howbeit, there is one great discommoditie, in this instrumente, whiche is, it will lightlie pearce the braine, if it bee not handeled of a right experte woorke manne, in that behalfe. But this chaunseth vnder his handes, who alwaies tourneth the Wimble aboute, after one maner of fashion, where he should vse a trimmelyng kinde of mouyng the Wimble. For if the Wimble passe through, by the rounde mouyng, and so touche the dura matter, it will cutte and rent the same, whiche dooeth lightly happen in a tremblyng mouyng. For if it touched the dura matter, it might well pricke her, but not pearce her through. Wherefore, it would leaue her whole and sounde. *The wimble is beste to perse the hed, to purge forth matter, if it be vsed ducritly*

And therfore, who so would exercise, this feate, ought to haue a light hande, and wittie hedde together, with a sadde iudgement, and not to be taken from emong them, that haue vsed to handle grosse matters, and occupacions: as diggyng or Plowyng, heauyng of timber, and curriyng of horses. For their handes be hardeined with labours, and maie not lightlie feele, when it is through the bone, if thei laie lode on their woorke. And therefore, this woorke muste bee dooen, with moste exquisite diligent, and circumspeccion, leaste we slea men, whiles we labour to preserue them. For this cause, you must giue some attendaunce to theim, whiche handle this woorke manlike: so that ye maie the better, and with more sauegarde, attempte this cure afterward. Now, as sone as the scalpe shalbee holed, ye shall with all spede possible, power in so moche Rosed Honie strained, as shall bee able to couer the rimme of the braine. This hast is made, leaste the aire be entred in, and made alteracion in *Ciphelica*, nexte power *Aqua vitæ* vpon the Honie, till the hole shall be filled, whereunto ye shall caste so moche of the pouder, as maie rise the depth of a kniffes thickenesse, from the rimme. *A wittie hed and a steddie hande, is fitte for a good Chyrurgian.*

Make haste in the cure of the hedde, to defende the aire, whiche will corrupt.

R. Aloes Epatike, Sarcocol, Mirrhe, ana. ʒ.i.ß. Incense. ʒ.i. Dragons blood. ʒ.ß. and Ɔ.ß. of Saffron, mingle theim together, and pouder them finely, for the vse we spake of. All this doe we, to saue the compleccion of the bone, and pannicles, after the minde of *Auicen* and *Galen*, as is alledged before. When ye haue thus dooen, take so moche of a

Hh.ii. Sponge

Sponge, as maie be sufficient to fil the hole: and this is doen for twoo consideracions. The firste is to exclude, the noiaunce of tentes. For a Sponge will giue place to the stretching of the braine, and tentes can not but some whiles cause apostumacion, by reason of the resistaunce and stubbernesse. The other cause is, that the matter be sone drawen forthe, frō the pannicles. For it might alter, if it remained any while, or els be imprisoned, whiche is no rare and straunge thyng, to se daily in the cures, of these light and common practicians. After all this fill the wounde with *Aqua vitæ*, pouder, and linte: applyyng vpon thesame a peece of clothe, anointed with *Vnguentum Basilicum* aboue described, to the intent the medicenes be retained there. And when ye haue accomplished, all these thynges in order, laie this plaister on the hedde shauen.

woorke tenderly in the wounde of the hedde.

Take Camomel, Melilote, ana. ℥. iii. Mirtilles. ℥. ii. Cipresse nuttes. xv. redde Roses, and Wormwood, ana. ℥. i. Beane meale, and Lupine meale, ana. ʒ. iiii. Braie all that ought to bee braied, and seeth them altogether, in newe white wine, and Barbours lye, of like porcions, vnto soche tyme as it shall be like a Cerote. After this, sprede it on a clothe warme, and applie it to the hed. This plaister is vsed for many purposes. Firste, to comforte the hedde, by strengthyng of the complecction, next to defende from colde, and rectifie the aire, whiche is inclosed. This is it that *Auicen* saieth: *Oportet vt vehemens caueatur frigus, etiam in astate, quoniam in eo est timor magnus.* Ye muste beware of vehemente colde, though it were in Sommer, because there is great feare in it. He meaneth that the aire muste bee rectified, namelie, whiche entreth into the hedde, at the openyng of the scalpe. For some will go in, whether ye will or not to fulfill the rome, in as moche as nature, can not suffre any place, to be vacant, or emptie, as the Philosopher dooe write. He meaneth not that the whole aire of the Chamber, ought to bee rectified, as some practicians thinke, and would faine be seen, to be circumspect in the matter. Thirdly, to procure digestion. Fowerthly, to drawe sanious matter, as sone as it is generated, & retained in the Sponge. Fiuethly, to resolue the matter, whiche is wonte to cause apostumacion. For ofte times (as saieth *Galen*, whom *Auicen* citeth) apostumacion soloweth whatsoeuer instrument ye vse, whiche ye shall preuente and eschue, if ye applie the former plaister on the hed. And this maie easely appere, if a man consider diligently, the Simples in the plaisters. Now, thus shall you procede in the cure, vnto soche tyme as the Cicatrice shall be produced: alwaie iteratyng and renewyng, the former medicenes, as often as thei shalbe old, and dismitted. But in asmoche, as the flesh groweth here aboue his place, ye shall represse and kepe it doun, with roche Alome brent, applyyng it alwaie, in the circuite of the superfluous fleshe. But moderate the Alome in small quantitie, that it cause no dolour, by reason of his bityng, and mordicacion. This is the self same maner, whiche hetherbnto haue been vsed in cures, wherewith haue been holpen aboue many hundred persones, in our tyme: but I nede not here make rehearsall of them, sith a manifest thing shal nede

A verie good emplaster for the hedde.

Take heede of colde, in a wounde of the hedde.

There is no place emptie, for aire filleth euery open place.

To corecte proude fleshe.

no witnesses. But I saie, I remember one thing, whiche was almoste forgotten negligētly, and is necessarie to be obserued, about openyng of a scalpe, whiche is this. When ye open the scalpe, in soche cures, and make an hole for the foresaid purposes: be you ware that ye touch not any seame of the scalpe. Thei be fiue in nomber, twoo vncomplet and false, and three true seames. The first is named *Coronal*, of a croune, because the crounes be worne in that place, & it is in the former parte of the hed: the seconde *Lambda* or *Lauda*, whiche is in the hinder part of the hedde. The third true seame, *Sagittal*, like an arrowe, vnder the partyng of the heere, whense one ende toucheth the seame *Coronal*, and the other *Lambda*, in the hinder part: the twoo false seames, be at sides in the regions, or plattes in the temples. Now in case any clifte or chinne, touche either of the twoo, we muste vse moche diligence, and circumspeccion. Note here also, that cliftes and chinnes, maie chaunce in the saied seames: other in length, whiche is, when the clift together with the seame, maketh. iiii. streight angles. Or els in bredth. If it chaunce in length, the bone must needes be bored, & holed on bothe sides of the seame, because the particion of dura matter, maie not bee touched in the woorke. I saie, it must nedes be holed on bothe sides, for as moche as it maie bee, that blood bee fallen from the vaines, in bothe partes, and there bee congeled. For if we would feele, or woorke in the seame where dura matter is bounde and staied (as doe thei, whiche come fro practise to *Chyrurgj*) wee might well feare and doubte, of suffocacion of the braine, because the rimme beyng losed, should presse it doune, and so choke it. And that wee should make no soche losyng of *Cephalica* in the place: we are admonished of *Cornelius Celsus*, in the chapter *De caluariæ curatione* Howbeit, he doeth it in cōsideracion of *Hyppocrates* cōfession, where to the profite of his posteritie: confesseth that he was deceiued, woorkyng in a seame. Wherefore, ye shall not worke in any seame, least ye bee deceiued, as was *Hyppocrates*, prince of Philicians. But if the fissure or *membrana* chaunce in bredth, ye shall make holes in the same, in bothe sides of the seame: alwaies obseruyng this, that neither particion, neither seame be touched at all. When these holes be made, ye shall finishe the *Cura*, accordyng to the order and maner, as was before prescribed. And as for the chinke, ye shall doe in like maner, if ye be assured, that it perce and runne through the scalpe. On the other side, if it go not through that parte of the scalpe: whiche thei call *vitrea tabula*, that is, the Glassie table but onely cometh to the Spongious bone. Ye shall procede to the cure, with *Aqua vitæ*, and the pouder alone, whiche shalbe sufficient. Now if ye liste, ye maie plain and abate the bone, about the riuen place, wherof will folowe soner incarnacion, and causing of the Cicatrice. These be rules, and order in the cures, which are not moche vsed, and yet vsed in harde maladies procedyng of a cause primitiue. Now therefore, haue you that, whiche ye so earnestlie haue required: A gift in myne opinion, as greate as my poore knowlege is able to bryng to passe, worthie for the helpe of mankinde, whiche is in sorenes, but yet keepe these thynges

A Dialogue

thynges long with my self, to the intent I might ones at leaſt, ſo ſone content your mindes. But whether I haue ſo doen, as myne entente was, I am vncertaine. For why, I am become in theſe treactiſes, as one that buildeth his houſe, in the middes of the market ſteede, about the whiche, as touchyng the height, and breadth, the lokers therevpõ ariſe alteracion, and controuerſie, where as the builder thought his worke, of conuenient proporcion. So feare I, leaſt perchaunce my doyng, ſhall ſeme to ſome, abiecte and baſe, and to ſome other, to obſcure or darke. But certes, in aſmoche as I am not able, to pleaſe all ſortes, I thought it beſt, to retain the meane waie in ſpeaking, ſpecially ſith I neuer liked, to flie ouer the toppes of trees: but plainly to go a ſofte paſe, and as it wer with a leadden foote, to thintet, that who ſo liſted to ouer gette me, might the eaſiar attain, without painfull trauell in their iourney. And thus gentle Sorenes: wiſhyng God to ſende thee health, and vs to mete merily again, I make an ende with a Cautery good for thy purpoſe: and a rule to helpe the ſtone.

Sorenes.

But firſt how make you the red pouder, for the parting water?

Chyrurgj.

<small>A goodly water of greate ſtrength, to ſeperate metall good for to coſume rotten fleſhe.</small>

You muſt make it thus. ℞. Of water wherewith Goldſmithes, doe ſeperate golde and ſiluer, whiche is grene, when it haue ſeperated the mettalles: of this take. ʒ. vi. of Quickſiluer. ʒ. iiii. mingle theim together, and put them either into a little ſtone Limbecke, or Still, or els into one of Venice glaſſe, well luted with claie, bothe the hedde of the Still, and the parte wherevpõ it ſtandeth: and alſo the receiuer, where into it droppeth, that none paſſe awaie. Diſtill it on a ſofte fire, in a cloſe furneis. Your partyng water is thus made. ℞. Salte Peter, Alome roche, and Romain Vitriall, ana. li. ii. beate theim together in a Morter, then put it into a double glaſſe, well luted, or ſo ſtopped, that no aire doe tranſpire, or go forthe: this will make a ſinguler good water, drope one gutta or drop vpon the grounde, and you ſhall ſee it boile, as though it were on the fire. Theſe thynges are profitable, to the woorke of *Chyrurgj*, in foule ſores and vlceres: here is good occaſion miniſtered, to ſpeake of the makyng of medicenes. But I refarre that, to the booke of Compoundes, where there are not onely good ſtore of them, but alſo good medicens: no leſſe profitable to *Chyrurgj*, then nedefull to Phiſicke.

Sorenes.

Now how make you Lye, to open, in the maner of a Canterie?

Chyrurgj.

<small>A good Lye for a Cautery</small>

Make it after this faſhion ℞. A pretie rounde tubbe of twoo gallons, with a hole in the bottom, ſtopped, putte into this tubbe, aſhes of the Aſhe tree. Make a hole in the middes, to put in a pottell or more, of vnſlecked Lime, & powre vpon it quickly

quickly hote Lye, as moche as shall couer the Lime, and with al spede couer it with Asshes, that the aire maie be kept in, for twoo daies: the thirde vnstoppe the hole, and let the water distille, from the Lime and Asshes, and keepe this in a close vessell. This will quickly open any parte that is sore, as apustumacions without paine: and if an Egge will not sinke in it, but flete, then it is good Lye, for the purpose.

Sorenes.

Here are good pouders, profitable to your Arte, I praie you learne me some of theim, to clense dedde fleshe: and as for the booke of Compoundes, I will reade that at more leisure.

Chyrurgj.

I will teache you to make a trosse, to clense rotten fleshe, whiche is. ℞. water of Planten. ʒ. vi. Mercurie well sublimated, and made in pouder. ʒ. ß. Seeth theim in a little panne, to the consumyng of the fowerth parte: then let it stand. xii. howers, after knede it with a little Beane meale, and roule theim vp into a trosse. Note also, that you muste mingle so moche vermilion, with the Beane meale, as will colour it: and drie this trosse, in an Ouen, or hotte Sonne. <small>A good pouder for rotten fleshe.</small>

Sorenes.

How make you a potenciall Cauterie?

Chyrurgj.

To make a Cauterie. ℞. Of the strongest Sope Lie, asmoche as will suffise, put it in a brasen Kettle. Put. ʒ. i. ß. Romain vittriall, let all seeth vntill the liquer be consumed, then gather vp the fome, that doe remaine: and kepe this to open apostumacions. For in openyng without pain, this doe excell all other. <small>A potenciall Cauterie.</small>

Sorenes.

But that the tyme is farre spente, and I haue put you to moche paines, els I would haue learned some thing, to haue taken awaie grauell and stone, from the kidneis, raines, and bladder.

Chyrurgj.

At this present, I haue no time coueniēt, to serue that turne at large: it requireth no small trauell. For like as emong all mortall euilles, the stone is the greatest: so the cure is moste cunnyng. Notwithstādyng, I shall by Gods grace intreate, here after at large, the diate, the proper medicenes: cure, and cuttyng of the stone. But yet in the meane time, let the paciēt kepe him warme Eate no salt fishe, or fleshe burnt, rosted meates, harde Chese: or slimie thynges, ingenderers of visos humours, grosse or clammie. Or drinke hotte wines, or eate venison, or any water foule: or be costiffe bellied, or keepe their backe hotte. &c. The signes of the stone are euidente, as paines in the raines, bladder, yarde, loines, &c. with painfull lamen- <small>For the stone a good regimente.</small>

tyng

A Dialogue.

tyng and cryng, stoppyng of the vrine. &c. The causes are many, as of parentes, of euill diatte, with many euill accidentes. The vrine often tymes doe declare, the euilles of those partes, as *Hyppocrates* in the thirde parte of the ix. of his *Aphorismes* affirmeth, saiyng: *Si sanguinem aut pus mingat renum aut vesicæ exulcerationem significat.* To make water, or pisse blood, or els filthy matter: it signifieth Sores and Biles, either in the Raines, or els in the bladder: And assuredly, soche sores and vlcers, come from the stone whiche doe excoriate, frette, cutte, and causeth bothe bloode and matter without vrin, to come forth at the yarde. But somtime pure blood is pissed, of the breakyng of a vaine: and sometyme from women, for the secrete infirmitie, or naturall passion, through clensyng of termes. But grauell in the vrine, betokeneth the stone in the bladder, saieth *Hyppocrates lib. iij. Aphorism. Quibus in vrina velut arenula subsistunt, ijs vesica laborat calculo.* Furdermore, it is skant possible, for old people to be helped, in the raines or bladder, for the stone. Specially in greate glotonous people, as drunkardes with Ale and Bere: or els them, whiche were neuer satisfied with Lecherie in their youth. &c. Howbeeit, to speake a little, for the helpe thereof, twoo thynges must be considered. Firste, the preseruatiue. Secondlie, the curatiue, the preseruatiue, by good diatte, and wholsome regiment of life, as what ye doe eate, the maner of eatyng and drinkyng. The tyme, the place, the qualitie and the quantitie, of the saied meates and drinkes: as meate of light digestion, cleane bread without bran. Not to be to moche hote or cold, neither moche trauell, or sitting still idle, but good exercise. &c. And note, when the stone is in the bladder, then it is harder, then that which is in the raines, & more burnt. Now, if your grauell commeth of heate, or through hotte accidentes, as with hotte wines, labour. &c. Then followe *C. Galens* Syrupe whiche is moste excellent also, in this our age, and is thus made.

R̃. Syrupe of Endiue, of Sorell, of water Lillis, ana. ʒ. v. the waters of Fenel, of Endiue, ana. ʒ. i. mingle them together, and giue the paciente to drinke, Mornyng and Euenyng: and anointe the Raines, with *Galens* colde ointment, whiche is written in the Compoundes.

Sorenes.

But what remedie, when the stone cometh of colde?

Chyrurgj.

GALEN must put to his helpyng hande, whiche willeth, whē soche contraries dooe happen, when nature is so chaunged, from heate into coldnesse, or if it were colde from the beginnyng. Then to helpe with warme thinges, to dissolue, and this was his remeadie. R̃. *Theriace Galeni.* ʒ. i. Sirup of the barkes of the Citri. ʒ. i. warme water, as of *Carduus Benedictus, &c.* ʒ. ii. mingle them together, and giue your paciente, or take it your self ten daies: For it is no light triflyng medicene, but moste effectuall and substaunciall, inuented by *Galen.* And like as in hotte burnyng of the stone, to drinke cleane Whaie, or Butter milke is good, and to eate Purslen. Euen so in the

case

betwene Sorenes and Chyrurgj. Fol.xlvj.

case of coldnes: Hares fleshe, sodden with Capers, and yong Nettles is beste, and a mornynges to eate halfe an vnce of newe drawen *Cassiafistula* mingled with Suger: and to drinke Whaie of Goates milke. Oh that men would forsee, the euilles against nature, as Feuers, Poxe, Lipres Goutes, Stone, Cancers. &c. And take in hand to helpe them, in their firste spring, and then thei would bee sone helped. As example. Fire and water, are good seruauntes, but euill maisters. For if thei get the victory, who can rule thē, the profe is manifest: as it is easie to quench a fire in the beginnyng: but when it haue gotten holde, of the thacke sparres, beames &c. then it is to late. So when bile humour, haue incensed the bloode, vaines. &c. And haue gotten the victorie, rebellyng againste good nature: then it is either to late, or els to harde, to putte them awaie, and bring nature again, to his good estate. Yet it hurteth little the Phisicions, *Chyrurgions*, and Apothicaries, to vtter their knowlege, and also their wares, with promises faire and false, in matters paste cure. For golde hath no corrupcion, although it bee gotten with a corrupted conscience: But to our matter. Take thynges in dewe tyme, for time will neuer be called again, doe what you can. Howbeit while as the bodie is yet liuyng, there is lefte some helpe, to releue, or repaire it againe: and in soche case of grauell, or the stone, what haue euer doen more pleasure, then Clisters, or Enema, ministered beneath at the fundment, nothing truely, cutting excepted. Yet in cuttyng, vnlesse the *Chyrurgian* be verie cunnyng, the pacient will sone crie: *Quare de vuluus eduxisti me?* And although the *Chyrurgian* haue great knowlege, yet one pacient doe skante scape, emong an hundred, happie manne by his dole. On the other side, there be soche bodies, when thei are newlie clensed, and deliuered from grauell, or the stone: eftsone the bodies are soche, that thei haue it againe as painfull, as at the first tyme. And some of those bodies, haue the propertie of the North winde, in dryyng, or turnyng into duste: And other some haue the propertie of Frost, to coagulate, to make colde, and tourne softe thynges into hardnesse, as Ise is. Therefore in soche euilles doe thus. Make a Clister after this maner.

℞. *Milium solis*, or els the berries of Alkakengi. ℥. vi. cleane runnyng water. li. iiii. seeth this vntill the water be halfe cōsumed, then strain it, of this water take a pinte or more, for your Clister, puttyng therevnto the oiles of Dill, Chamomell, and newe Butter, ana. ℥. ii. and a little Salt: thus is your Clister finished and made, minister it warme but not skaldyng. Though this seme a plain Clister, yet it is marueilous good in woorkyng: and clenseth not onelie grauell, but also help the chollicke, and paines in the guttes. When ye haue ministered this then folowyng within three daies, minister this, for it is of great vertue. ℞. Of the decoccion of Mallowes, Parietorie, Colewortes, Holihocke, Smalage, Sitrach, Polipodium, *Cardus benedictus*, Alkakengi sede of eche like quantitie of these. li. i. Oiles of Dill, of Camomell, of Lillies, ana. ℥. i.ss. Butter. ℥. ii. *Hiera simplex*. ℥. i. and a little Salt, mingle all together, and warme put into the Clister bladder, and minister, as is afore

Good potace for the stone.

Menne doe wante prouidence, to forse their owne euilles.

Fire and water bee good seruauntes, but euill maisters.

Cuttyng of the stone, is perilous.

Example.

A goodlie Clister for to help the stone

An other singuler good Clister.

afore saied. If you haue not this choise of oiles, you maie take common oile of Oliues: this Clister is moste excellente good, for the stone and grauell: it haue vertue to open, cleanse, waste, and skower without daunger, perill or hurte. When this is doen spedely, haue this Cataplasme at hande, and warme aplie it to the pained place: whether it bee in the raines, or the lowest part of the bellie, or flankes, let it bee doen often tymes, haue twoo in store, to laie vnto the place warme, one after an other, it is thus made in good order.

A good Cataplasme for the stone.

R. The leaues and stalkes of Pralium, of Mallowes, of Holihock ana. ℥. iii. sodden in the brothe, wherein a weather hedde haue been sodden. Seeth herein also the rootes of Mallowes, well beaten in a morter. ℔.i. the musslege of fenigreke, & flaxe seede, ana. ℔. v. then let it be strained forth strōgly, to this iuice put the oiles of Dill, Chamomell, white Lillis, ana. ʒ. iiii. freshe Butter. ʒ. vi. Honie. ʒ. v. boile al together in a cleane panne, put in branne of Barlie, and meale, temper all with a sticke, vntill it come to the thicknesse of soft paste: sprede it in two seuerall Cataplasmas, and warme applie one of them after after an other, to the dolorous place. And when one is colde, then applie on thother often times, this is of a singuler operacion: with this, that greate learned manne, maister Doctor *Marianus* haue doen moche good, and this I haue also proued many tymes. Then to make the matter perfite, giue your pacient to drinke *Benedicta laxatiue* ʒ. vi. tempered with cleane odoriferous, warme white wine, a quarter of a pinte or more, when this is doen: wrap hym in warme clothes, with hed well couered, and so let him sweate. And this clenseth the raines and bladder, equall with any other: excepte you will hasarde your life, in cuttyng. Furdermore, note a greate secrete, whiche I doe disclose for the sake of mankinde. Let the paciente haue the stilled waters, of Sarifrage, Perietarie, Persilie, *Filipendula*, and Smalege, altogether ana. ʒ. iii. and putte into this water, this precious pouder followyng.

A drinke for the stone.

A mostewor-thie pouder for the stone.

Ɔ.i.ß. or Ɔ. R. Perselie rootes cleane washed and scraped, I meane their rindes, and Percelie seede, ana. ʒ. vi. or more, and. ʒ. viii. of the flowers of *Iringium*, or the sea Thistil, and also *Iringium* rootes, and the rootes of *Cardus Benedictus*. ana. ʒ. ß. Cutte your rootes finelie and thin, and put al together in a close vessell. into the Ouen, vntill thei bee drie, and then make pouder: keepe it close from aire. And when occasion dooe serue, temper your foresaied quantitie into your waters, or els while wine or Chicken brothe, drinke it warme. Also note well this Syruppe for the stone, wherein the pacient maie take euery seconde night warme ʒ. ii. R. Rootes of Holihocke. ʒ. iiii. the leaues of Mallowes, *Filipendula*, and Perietarie, ana ℥. ii. the seede of Perselie, Fenegrece, and flaxe ana. ʒ. i. *Iuiubes* in nomber. xxx. clene scraped Liquoris. ℔. i. the rootes of *Sparagus, Cardus Benedictus, Iringium*, Perselie and Fenill, ana. ʒ. ii. ß. seeth al these in. x. ℔. waight of cleane runnyng, or well water, vnto the third part be wasted: then strain it, & put vnto this decoction ℔. i. ß. of clene white Suger, stirre it, and make your Syruppe, and kepe it in a close double glasse,

A Syruppe for the stone.

glasse. These foresaied thinges are excellent good, to be sodden in clene white wine, puttyng therevnto .li.i. of the white *Guiacum* rased, and put in a vessell of three gallons, made close in the mouthe: and so put into a faire greate hollowe Caldron of water, and so to seeth fower howers, then take it from the fire, and stande vntill it be colde. Then open it, and strain it, and kepe it close, to drinke at all times.

And thus also haue Richard Bullein, a zealous louer in Phisicke: more for the consolacion & help of thafflicted sicke people, beyng poore then for the lucre & gaine, of the money of the welthie and riche. This man I saie, although he professeth comfortable cordialles, and heauenly medicenes for the soule, beyng a deuine: yet he hath good experience of many infirmities and sicknesses, infecting the bodies of man kinde, and haue doen many goodly cures, whiche I doe leaue vnwritten, bothe for the prolixitie of tyme, and also for that no adulacion, flatterie, or any priuate affeccion should appere, or be suspected in him the aucthour hereof, towardes hym the saied Richarde Bulllein, because he is his naturall borne brother: but to the matter, his medicene for the grauel in the raines and stone. And thus he writeth in his pretie woorke, whiche if it please God, shall hereafter come to the profite of the common wealthe, of the Englishe nacion. And this is his compendious order: Saieth he, the greate dolour, flegmon, or vlcere of the raines, by the whiche raines, vrine is conueied into the bladder. &c. or the stone in the bladder: dooe cause greate paines in making of vrine, whiche vrine is often stopped, or els pisseth little stones, with excoriacion, and blood. Where grauell, and ragged stones, commyng of grosse, salte hotte matter, viscuous humours: after long hotte burnyng Feuers, euill diatte, Chese, olde poudered Beefe, Bakon, venison, salte fishe, hotte wine haue been vsed in diatte. The stone is oftener in the bladders of the leane hotte men, whiche haue larger vesselles, then in fat persones hauyng small vesselles, and colde moiste fatte bodies. &c.

Richard Bullein his practise for the stone.

The stone, saith he, after the minde of *Galen*, in the raines is lighter, lesser, softer, and redder, declinyng somewhat into graines, but in the bladder, it is greater, heauier, harder, greuouser, in colour whitishe, or more adusse, and bothe these are daungerous, and skante curable. After one is .xl. yere olde: as saieth *Hyppocrates. Aphoris. Quicunque nephretici sunt non sanantur post quadraginta annos.* Who so haue the passion in the raines, after .xl. yeres, is paste cure: the regiment in the cure is double. The first is, to prohibite the generacion of the stone. The seconde is to displace, or remoue it, when it is growen. The firste intencion haue fiue thynges, not naturallie, directly contrary against the stone. Is aire, grosse, mistie, cloudie. &c. to be fled, for it doeth ingender grosse matter.

Twoo thinges consideredand the stone, for the cure of the same.

Meates and drinkes, as grosse wine, and salte meates, burnt thynges, colde water, whiche will bryng grosse matter, and brede stone.

Labour imoderate, to moche excercise, which ingrosseth the blood.

Solitarinesse, moche studie, no trauell, or lecherie imoderate, whiche are greate enemies to nature.

Greate

A Dialogue.

Greate affliccion of the mynde, watchyng, fastyng, &c.

To helpe these euilles, doe thus, as folowe.

Use meates of light digestion, in due tyme, place, and order.

Moderate labour betwene meales, to helpe digestion, and make the bodie strong: and to beware of listes, wrastlynges. &c. that will hurte the body, beyng vsed imoderatly.

Of all thynges to beware of Idlenesse, the mother of euilles, and nourisher of as many sicknesses to the bodie, as is made through glotonie: and speciall, of to moche copulacion carnall.

Use pleasaunt Musicke, and thynges to delite the spirites: for Melancholi, whiche is colde and drie, is a greate furderer of the stone: and when these are doen, vse these thynges folowyng.

R. Bulleins Siruppe for the stone. ℞. Syruppe of the twoo rootes, Honie of Roses, Syruppe of Vineger simple, Syruppe of Fenell, Syruppe of Sarifrage, ana. ʒ.ſſ. the water of Fenill, of Wormewodde, of Persilie, of Maidenhere, of Alkakengi, ana. ʒ.i. mingle theim, and temper theim warme, and drinke this often times, mornyng and euening, vntill the matter flegmatike bee digested. Then vse this potion, to purge the saied digested matter in this order followyng. ℞. Of the decoccion of the fower greate hot rootes, into whom put these seedes, Percelie, Sarifrage, Anisseedes, Smalage, Fenell, *Asparagus*, ana. ʒ.i. seeth these together, then strain it,

R. Bullein his electuarie for the stone. and put into the same, *Electuari de Cassia, Diacatholiconis*, ana. ʒ. iii. *Diaphæniconis*, ʒ. ii.ſſ. mingle theim in warme drinke, with Honie of Roses, to make it swete, and drinke it warme in the mornyng, within fower daies followyng, swallowe these Pilles followyng, whiche are of greate vertue.

R. Bullein his Pilles for the stone. ℞. Pilles of *Hiera Nicolai*. ʒ.i.ſſ. make fiue pilles in number, rounde, newe and gilted, and take them earely. Drinking the brothe of a Chekin, with .ii. howers followyng. Then applie this implaster warme in to the raines, the daie nexte after your Pilles.

Richard Bullein his emplaster for the stone. ℞. Crummes of twoo manchettes newe baken, and thirtie Figges three yellowe yolkes of Egges, Saffron. ʒ.i. fresshe Butter. ʒ.ii. sweete Rose water. ʒ.vi. let all stande in a morter tenne howers, then beate al with a pestle. Then sprede it vpon a clothe, and verie warme applie it to the raines, renue it stil warme, and applie it to the raines again. Then haue at hande this Clister followyng, to take after the emplaster haue remained, by the space of fiftene howers.

R. Bullein his Clister for the stone. ℞. Oile of Dille ʒ.vi. clene white wine. ʒ.vii. newe fresshe Butter. ʒ.iiii. Capons and Duckes greace, without Salt, *Cassia fistula*, newe drawen from the Cane, ʒ.ſſ. the yolke of one Egge, with a verie little fine white Salte, temper all in a panne, to the order for a Clister, and warme put it into the bladder, and so minister towardes euenyng, and assuredlie, these bee goodlie remeadies for the stone. The whole regimente for the stone, the saied Richard Bullein, shall by Goddes grace, shortly come forthe, to the profite of the common people.

The index betwene Sorenes and Chyrurgj.

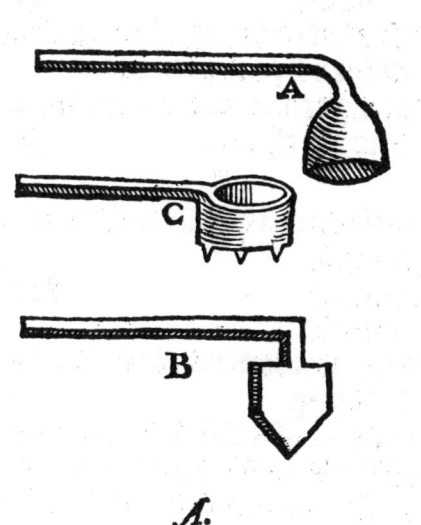

A.

A faithfull man neede no miracle. Fol. ix.
Apostumacion is compounded of thre thynges. xi.
An igno aunte *Chyrurgian*, is a man slear. fol. vi.
A good medicen for an opostumacion. fol. xiii.
A Cicatrice. Ibidem.
A digestion. Idem.
An abstersiue. Idem.
A good repercussiue. xv.
Iuicens medicen. Idem.
An excellent emplaster, to asswage paine Idem.
A verie good emplaster Idem.
A softnyng emplaster xviii.
A wounde for a bruse. xxi.
A good question Idem.
A defensiue verie good Idem.
An abstersiue to clense xxii.
A good ointment for woundes. 23.
A good practise xxvi.
Anticedent, Coniunct, &c. Idem.
A good exiccatiue to drie. xxviii.
Aristotle, a good note for the Elementes. Idem.
An in carnatiue to cause flesh. xxix
A defensiue. Idem.
A sanatiue Idem.
A good foundacion Idem.
Iuicens wise prouidene. xxx.
A good pouder
Alteracion of nature, what it is. folio. xxxii.
Alteracion of extencion. Idem.
A good liniment. xxxiii.
A consideracion of ded flesh. Idem.
Anticedent and Coniuncte, what thei are. Idem.
A verie good obseruacion. xxxiiii.
Alteracion of the aire. Idem.
A defensiue vnder the knee. xxxv.
A conclusion. Idem.
An other good defensiue. xxxvi.
A signe of ouermoche dryyng. ide.
An other good mundificaciō. xxxvii.
A verie good abstersiue for the hed folio. xl.
A good pouder for the hedde. idem.
A diate xli.
A clifte in the brain pan. Idem.
A note, betwene a mannes braine panne and a childes Idem.
A good note for a *Chyrurgian* xlii.
A wittie hedde, and a stedfaste hande for a *Chyrurgian*. Fol. xliiii.
A verie good emplaster for the hed folio. Idem.
A water to consume rotten fleshe. Folio. Idem.
A good Lie for a cauterie. Idem.
A good pouder for rotten flesh. xlvi
A potenciall Cauterie Idem.
A reward for lecherie. Idem.
A Syruppe for the stone. Fo. xlvii.
A good plaster for the stone. Idem.
An excellent pocion for the stone. Folio Idem.
A good Clister for the stone. Idem.

B.
Borias the North East winde. Fol. i.
Blinde Baiarde is boldeste in the Carte. Fol. xi.
Blood proceadyng of a primatiue cause Fol. xxv.

A.i. Breache

The index betwen Sorenes and Chyrrurgj.

Breache of continuaunce. xxxii.

C.

Curtesie. Fol.ii.
Chyrurgerj is a Sentorie for vagabõdes. Fol.vi.
Christ is not couetous xi.
Composicion, Replexion, and Cõplexion. xi.
Consider in what bodies, apostumacions are bred xiii.
Consider to open a member, before it doe rotte. xiiii.
Cauterie potenciall. xvi.
Choise of medicens are very good. Folio xvii.
Capitain William Rede of the holie Ilande. xxii.
Colde is the greatest enemie to the sinewes of all. Idem.
Chyrurgians doe neuer agree. xxv.
Chyrurgians must knowe Simples. 28.
C. Celsus xxviii.
Colde vlcer xxix.
Consider the brine, & so woorke. 03.
Corosiõ bityng or gnawing. xxxiii
Contraries, whẽ to vse thẽ. xxxvii.
Chalke for Chese xxxix.
Clothes applied to a wounded hed folio xl.
Cuttyng of the stone is perilous. folio xlvii.

D.

Doctor Turner. Fol.iiii.
Doctor Kaies Idem.
Doctor Recorde Idem.
Doctor Kuningham Idem.
Doctor Faire Idem.
Doctor Androwe Borde Idem.
Dogge leches, what thei are. Fo.i.
Dolor in complexion xv.
Distillyng of blood from the hed. folio xxv.
Depe cuttes hurteth the arteries. folio. xxvi.
Digestion causeth not matter, but it is the proporcionatyng of the humour Idem.
Diseases comyng of fulnesse, are helped by emptinesse. xl.
Daungerous woundes, how to knowe them. Idem.

E.

Euill parentes, their fruictes. vi.
Example xvii.
Example Fol.xix.
Example xx.
Euill accidentes, followe moche bledyng xxvi.
Example of a Moldwarpe. xxxvii.
Erisipele, is a hotte, redde, rounde inflamacion sore, or Chollerike boile, with a feuer in ẽ body. xl.
Example of blood lettyng. xlii.

F.

Flora a goddes of flowers, or an harlot of Rome Fol.ii.
First seke Gods kyngdome. Idem.
For counterfeit *Chyrurgians* vii.
Eight thynges or properties, of a good *Chyrurgian*. viii.
Fower notes in an apostumacion beginnyng, augmentyng, state, and declinyng. xi.
Foule bodies doe repulse repercusiues except thei be purged. xii.
Fower intencions, and sixe vnnatural thinges to be obserued. xv
Fiue notable thynges to be obserued in healyng. Idem.
Fooles with bokes, be worse then vnlearned practicioners with practise. xxvii.
First handle thaccidence in a cure, and note three thynges. xxx.
Firste to al the whole bodie, & then to the perticuler member. xxxv.
Fiue good intencions xxxvi.
Fower intencions, in twoo kindes of vlcers xxxvii.
Fiue causes that dooe hurte the hed.

The index betwene Sorenes and Chyrurgj.

hedde xxxix.
Fissures or chappes xli.
Fiue semes in the braine pan. xlv.
Fiue kindes of vlcers xlvi.
Fire and water are good seruauntes, but euill maisters. xlvii.

G.

God giueth health Fol. xxiiii.
Galens note xxv.
Greate clarkes are not the wisette men. xxviii.
Geometricall measure in Chirurgi xxxvi.
Glotonie is no small enemie to nature. xxxvii.
Galens Syrup for the stone. xlvi.

H.

How to knowe apostumacion. x.
How to rebate flesshe superfluous. folio xv.
How to make incision. xvi.
How to drie humours that doe abounde xxi.
How to sewe a wounde, and how not. Idem.
How to make a Cicatrice. xxviii.
How bolde the Chirurgian should be in cure xxxi.
Hotte and colde apostumacions. folio xxxii.
Hardnes of an vlcer Idem.
How a pacient died, by euill cure. folio xxxiiii.
Hippocrates order. Idem.
How to binde a member xxxvi.
How to find out a stripe, by what tokens in the hedde xxxix.
How to cutte, to the ende to heale folio xlii.
How cold hurteth Idem.
How to searche a wounde. Idem.
How suffocacion of the brain may come xlv.

I.

Ignoraunce Fol. ii.
Incision, how to make it xiiii.
It is perillous to sewe a wounde, commyng of the bityng, or rending of some beast xxi.
In healyng a compounde vlcere, marke the accidentes concurrant xxix.
Imbrocacion xxxiii.
If an apostumacion, bee in the middest of the vpper parte of the bodie, then to blede either in the lefte arme, or els right is well folio xlii.

K.
L.

Linx can see beste of any creature, and his vrine will tourne into a stone. Plini Fol. vi.

M.

Many good medicens are made of the plaine people, to help in the absence of the Chirurgians. vi.
Manne is but miserable, and yet is quickly gone ix.
Menne doe vse pretie termes, for foule sores, and cal them by one name, whē thei are an other. ix.
Mannes secrete prouidence. xviii.
Matter doe couet digestion xxi.
Melancholie meates xxxv.
Manne is made Geometrically in order xlii.
Make haste in the cure of the hed, to defende the aire, whiche els will corrupt xliiii.
Menne doe wante prouidence, to forsee their owne euilles. xlvii.

N.

Nature worketh three waies to helpe her self Fol. viii.
Nature must be releued by sonderie meanes, in the tyme of daunger Ibidem.
No locall medicen applied, before

Ii.ii. the

The index betwene Sorenes and Chyrurgi.

the bodie be purged   Fol.xv
Nature nourisheth her self, xxxvii.

O.

Of vacabond Chirurgians, worse
    then theues   Fol.vi.
Of contraries of elementes.   x.
Of resolucion   xii.
Of repercussiues, when thei are
    good   Idem.
Of an Embroche   xiiii.
Of God, is the beginnyng and en-
    ding of all thynges.   xviii.
Of woundes   Idem.
Of conuulcion mortall   xix.
Of the first and seconde intencion
    folio   xx.
Of woundes in the muscles.   xxi.
Of sinewes   Idem.
Of woundes depe, & not depe. xxv.
Of incision of small vaines.   xxvi.
Of exiccatiues   xxviii.
Of vrine considered, of euery sicke
    and sore man   xxx.
Of radicall moisture   Idem.
Ouid: a good note   xxxi.
Of dolour.   xxxii.
Of putrifaccion, or rottennesse.
    folio   xxxiii.
Of bones, whiche are corrupted,
    two thinges considered. xxxiiii.
Of swellynges, the cause.   xxxv.
Of filthie matter, what it is.   37.
Of honest requeste and frendship.
    folio   xxxviii.
Of incision of the hedde   xxxix.
Of blood runnyng, the chief cause
    and the hurte that dooe folowe
    the same   Idem.

P.

Partes moste daungerous to bee
    hurte   xix.
Pate Hardie the Scotte, a good
    Chirurgian   xx.
Purge a sore manne, after he is a-
    mended, for feare of dropsie. 35.
Purge the paciente, accordyng to
    the vrine.   xli.
Poore men are corrected, for great
    mennes faultes   xlii.
Preseruatiue, and Curatiue. xlvi.

Q.

R.

Reperassiues   Fol.xxv.
Regiment of life   xxx.
Remoue the cause, and the effecte
    will cease.   xxxiiii.
Richard Bullein, his practise for
    the stone.   xlviii.
Richard Bulleins Syrup for the
    stone   Idem.
Richard Bullein, his Electuarie
    for the stone   Idem.
Richard Bullein his Pilles for the
    stone   Idem.
Richard Bullein his emplaster for
    the stone   Idem.
Richard Bullein his Clister for
    the stone   Idem.

S.

Sabinus, a famous Mountaine in
    Italie.   Fol.ii.
Softt Chirurgians, make foule
    sores   Idem.
Sir Thomas Eliot knight   iiii.
Sondrie names of apostumaciōs,
    but in effect, are but apostuma-
    cions.   x.
Sores compounded   Idem
Signes of death.   xxvi.
Sanguine, Cholorike, apostuma-
    cions.   Idem.
Sanies is matter, commyng of
    corrupted blood, or els putrifac-
    cion, and sometyme it is taken
    for poison.   xxvii.
Strong members, doe oppresse the
    weake   Idem.
Sanious matter.   Idem.
Softe Chirurgians, make foule
    sores, yet Bocherly manglers,
    mar-

marreth all together. Fol. xxxi.
Signes of broken bones in the
hedde. xl.
Sawe, Chesill, and Wimble, for
hed are good instrumētes xliiii.
Sagittalis siue discriminalis xlv.

T.

Tragedie beginne euer euill, and
ende thesame. Fol. ii.
Thomas Phayre Doctor iii.
Thomas Pannell Idem.
Twoo kindes of Chirurgians v.
The souldiour is hurte more by an
euill Chirurgian, then by his e-
nemies weapon, often it is so
proued vi.
The miseries of manne, when he
is hurte in bodie Idem.
The discripcion of an vnthrifte, or
a villain of nature, striuyng a-
gainst grace and vertue, vnpro-
fitable for a common welth. idē
The vertue of Chirurgi. vi.
The Chirurgian is the best hande
crafte in the worlde viii.
The Chirurgian is natures ser-
uaunt. Idem.
The strength of nature Idem.
Twoo maner of healynges. ix.
Twoo kindes of apostumacions,
hotte and colde x.
The aboundaunce of blood, in the
apostumacion Idem.
The crueltie of the Cholericke a-
postumacion, but the bloodie a-
postumacion is gentler Idem.
The quantitie of the apostuma-
cions. Idem.
Three causes, the Primitiue, the
Antecedente, and the Coniunc-
tiue, whiche belong to the apo-
stumacion xi.
To abate dedde flesh xviii.
To alter a complexiō in a sore. idē
The diffinicion of a wounde xix.

Twoo kindes of woundes, the one
simple, and the other double, or
compounde xix.
The Chirurgian must looke plea-
sauntly, vpon his pacient. xxi.
To clense the wounde, and drawe
forthe broken bones xxii.
To ende a double wounde, and be-
gin accidence xxiii.
To correct a swart wounde. xxiiii.
The fluxe of blood, procedyng of a
primitiue cause. xxv.
To stoppe a bledyng vaine. Idem.
To staunche blood xxvi.
Twoo sundrie sortes of vlcers. 28.
To knowe, whether vlcers be hote
or colde Idem.
To make the skin whole Idem.
Three sondrie intencions: of regi-
ment, of matter, of growing. 29
To abate proude fleshe Idem.
The cause of superfluous flesh. xxx
To remoue an escharus scabbe or
cruste. xxxi.
Twoo causes of matter xxxii.
To searche the cause, and displace
the effect xxxiii.
Three causes of hardnesse. Idem.
To make a Cicatrice Idem.
To helpe putrifaccion xxxiiii.
These signes are in the ende. idem
To open a vaine, to purge grosse
blood xxxv.
The cause of Sorenesse is first, not
considered of many. Idem.
To skower and drie all Vlceres,
plain, or hollowe xxxvii.
The cause of bruses, what thei are
Folio xxxix.
To let blood on the contrary part,
why it must be, by reason xlii.
The Wimble is beste, to pearse the
hedde, to purge forthe matter, if
it bee vsed discritly xliiii.
Take hede of colde, in a wounde of
the hedde Idem

ji.iii. There

There is no place emptie, for aire filleth euery open place. xliiii.
To correct proude fleshe. Idem.
Twoo thynges considered in the stone, for the cure of the same. Folio. xlviii.

V.

Vnguentum Egipciacum of Auicen. xvii.
Vlceres bee harde to cure, that followe a sickenesse xxiiii.
Vlcers in good complexions, are sone cured xxv.
Varietie of simples xxvii.
Vlcers hotte, colde, and bityng. 28.
Vnguentum Album Idem.
Vlcer virulent, how it growe. 36.
Vnguentum Basilicum, xl.

W.

What is called Chirurgi v.
What perill is in the applicacion of a repercussiue, although in some case, it is moste best. xii.
What hurte ensueth of a repercussiue, some tyme xiii.
What goodnesse cometh of a repercussiue an other tyme Idem.
What harme ensueth of an euill Chirurgian alwaies xvi.
What the Chirurgian must do. 17.
What woundes bee mortall xix.
Woundes in the muscles. Idem.
What the Chirurgian muste obserue in his cure xx.
Who so dooe graunt to one absurditie, many one wil eftsones folowe the same. Idem.
When to let blood on the contrary side of the bodie, and why. xxii.
When the Chirurgian is putte to shame xxiii.
What an vlcere is xxiiii.
When to incarnate, and when to seperate a sore. xxvi.
When to vse contraries in healyng xxxii.
What thyng doe anoye the braine moste of all. xli.
When to let blood, twoo tymes in one place, and why. xlii.
When to drie, and when to moiste a wounde in the hedde xliii.
Woorke tenderly, in the wound of the hedde xliiii.
Why men doe pisse blood xlvi.
When the stone cometh of cold. idē
Why corrupcion cometh from the yarde Idem.

¶ *The ende of the Dialogue, betwne the*
Sore manne, and the Chyrurgian
By william Bulleyn.
Marche. 1562.

The Anatomie.

IN this place good reader, but that infortunate happe haue preuented me with lettes, els assuredly, I would haue written at legth, the whole large *Anatomie* of the bodie of mankind: but here I do ende, onely with the names of these bones, at this present time, vntill hereafter, if God will suffer me to doe more, I am then yours.

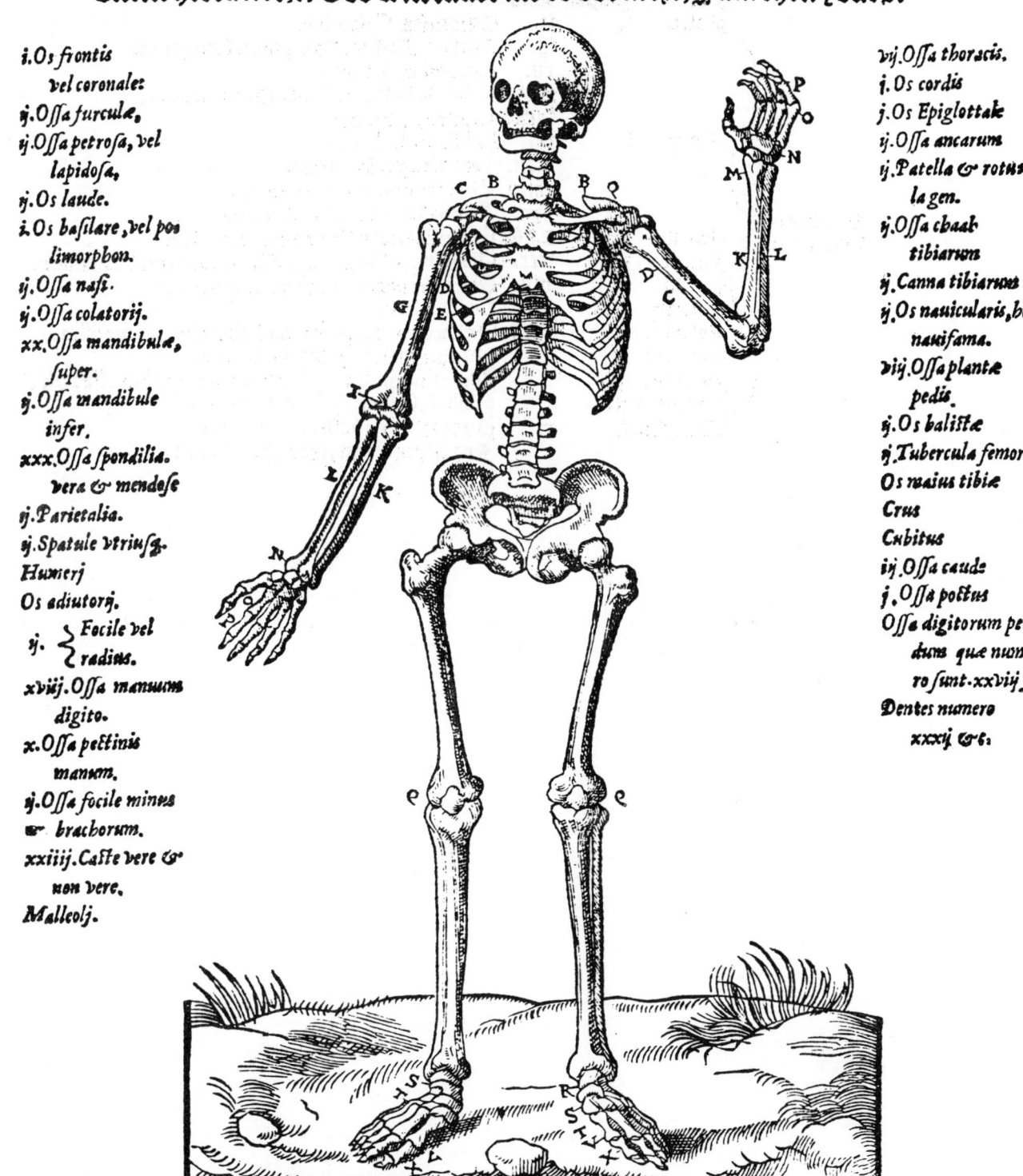

i. Os frontis vel coronale.
ij. Ossa furculæ.
ij. Ossa petrosa, vel lapidosa.
ij. Os laudæ.
i. Os basilare, vel poslimorphon.
ij. Ossa nasi.
ij. Ossa colatorij.
xx. Ossa mandibulæ super.
ij. Ossa mandibulæ infer.
xxx. Ossa spondilia vera & mendose
ij. Parietalia.
ij. Spatulæ vtriusq.
Humerj
Os adiutorij.
ij. { Focile vel radius.
xviij. Ossa manuum digito.
x. Ossa pectinis manum.
ij. Ossa focile minus & brachorum.
xxiiij. Caste vere & non vere.
Malleolj.

vij. Ossa thoracis.
j. Os cordis
j. Os Epiglottæ
ij. Ossa ancarum
ij. Patella & rotula gen.
ij. Ossa chaal tibiarum
ij. Canna tibiarum
j. Os nauicularis, hoc nauisama.
viij. Ossa plantæ pedis.
ij. Os balistæ
ij. Tubercula femoris
Os maius tibiæ
Crus
Cubitus
ij. Ossa caudæ
j. Ossa pectus
Ossa digitorum pedum quæ numero sunt. xxviij.
Dentes numero xxxij & 6.

A tergo & a fronte me finxisti.   Psal. 139.

Whereas through sondrie lettes, and also swifte printyng of these Dialogues, many errours haue been committed, yet by Gods grace, thei shalbe shortly all amended: And in the meane tyme, good reader, beware of these faultes here noted, and take all the reste in the better part, and helpe to amende them in the readyng I praie you.

	Fol.	Page.	Line.	
	Fol. i.	i.	ii.	Calamita. Calamitæ.
			iij.	Amber, Ambre. Camphire. Camphoræ.
			xij.	Amonum. Amomi.
			xiiij.	Cassifistula. Cassiafistula. Peter, Peper.
			laste. Iaunes, Iaundes.
	Fol. ij.	i	xxi.	Indictum Indicum.
			xxiij.	Sarafrage, Sarifrage.
			xxiiij.	Rhapreontion. Rhaponticum
Reade alwaies for			xxx.	Xilobalsanum. Xilobalsamum
	Fol. iij.	i	Laste Benedicta adde therevnto, laxatiuæ
	Fol. v.	i.	xxx.	Diagalinga, Diagalanga. Cardamonium Cardamom
	Fol. vi.	ij.	viij.	Diatreon pepereon. Diatrion pipereon
	Fol. xiij.	ij.	xxix.	Loche Lohoch.
	Fol. xvi.	i.	xviij.	Oxisaccara compositum. Oxisacchara composita
	Fol. xvij.	ij.		Flowerdelise, Flower de luce.
	Fol. xxi.	ij.		Pilule sine quibus noli. Pilulæ sine quibus esse nolo.
	Fol. xxiij. ij.			pilule Asseyeret pilulæ Assaieret.
	Fol. xxvi. i.		xx.	Put forthe de before Acerositatis.
				For Myrabolan, rede Myrobalan.

¶ The booke Fol. j.
of Compoundes.

Sicknes.

How make you Alypta Muschata?

Health.

First take the best gū of Laudanū. ʒ. iii. of Storar or Styrar Calamita. ʒ. ß. of ligne Aloes. ʒ. ii. stacte or the fattest part of Mirrhe. ʒ. i. of Amber. ʒ. camphire. Ɔ. i. ß. of Muske. Ɔ. ß. of Rose. water asmoch as you will. This doeth helpe children, whiche be short winded, and the straightnes of the breast and wombe, whiche cannot kepe their milke, of this we maie make excellent perfumes, whiche noble men be accustomed to vse, it is oftentimes mixed with electuaries.

Sicknes.

How make you your owne Antidotari, **whiche you vse your self?**

Health.

First take of Mirrhe. Ɔ. i. of Opium, whiche is the iuce of blacke Popie. Ɔ. xviii. of Amonum. Ɔ. vi. of Percely Ɔ. xv. of Smalage seede. Ɔ. xii. of Squinantum. Ɔ. ix. Cassifistula. Ɔ. iiii. white Peter. Ɔ. iiii. blacke Peper Ɔ. xv. of the beste Mustarde. Ɔ. xii. Storar. Ɔ. vi. Siler Montan. Ɔ. iiii. of the best Michrydatum Andromachi Ɔ. v. of Honie clarified, as moche as will suffice, and as you iudge meete. The quantitie whiche shall bee receiued at one tyme, of this is. ʒ. ii. Take your Storar with Honie, sprinkell or caste the other on drie, seth your Opium with swete wine, soden to the thirde parte, vntill it shall bee as thicke as Honie. This is good against a quarten Ague, long hedache, the turnyng sicknes, the fallyng euill, ouermoche wakyng, fransines, the pain of the iyes, reumes, tothache, shortnes of winde, sighyng, olde coughes from the lunges: it causeth also the spitell to be thicker, and apt to auoide, taken with Hydromell, whiche is made of Honie and water soden together, and if a man doe spit bloud, then it must be taken with Acetum mulsum, whiche is made of Uinegar and Honie, or els it ought to bee receiued with Uinegar, mixed with water, or with. ʒ. ii. of the iuce of Knotgrasse, or Plantan, howbeit, you must adde or diminishe, accordyng to the strength of the paciente. It is also a present remedie for the stomake, for it consumeth superfluous humors, and causeth a good apetite. It cureth the Hikeope and stopeth vomityng, it moueth a man to auoide winde, bothe from the liuer, stomack, and lower partes. It helpeth paine of the liuer, the yelowe Iaunes, and all diseases of Melancholie, the grief and heauines

The gooblie vertues of Asincritum.

nes of the splene: it ingendreth good couler, it purgeth dounewarde fleume and choler, it doth distribute meate disgested into his partes, it prouoketh vrine, and causeth the grauell in the raines and bladder to auoide, it cureth Illica & collica passio, taken with drinke it moueth a man to the stoole, and cureth inflamacions in shorte time, it doth mitigate the gnawyng and paine in the belly, it doth heale and take away the ouermuche stretchyng forthe of the Matrice, whan it cannot be easelie taken in at the mouthe: then let it be ministred with the iuice of Fenegreke at the fundament, and so it will take away the payne in al the lower partes, it doth cuer all diseases of the matrice, it asswageth the paine of women which labour of childe, it cureth the Mother and drawyng vp of the Matrice and stretching of the same, it stoppeth vnnaturall purgations and purgeth corrupt and superfluous humours it stoppeth fluxes of bloud from the Matrice, if it be taken alone or with olde wine, we may also vse this in the goute of the feete, and in Arthritica passio, whiche is a weakenes in all the ioinctes of superfluous humours Spasmus, called the crampe or contraction of sinewes.

Sicknes.

For as muche as you haue shewed me the vertue of sundrie simples before, now would I gladly learne how to cōpound medicines of sundrie kindes, to helpe me now in the time of sicknesse, and first what is Aromaticum Rosarum and howe should it be made.

Health.

Gabrielis Ioannis Damascen.
Nicholai Myrep.
Leonardus Fuc. De cō. Medican.

First take cleane redde Roses. ʒ. xb. and the best Liqueris scraped. ʒ. vii. Lingni Aloes, Sanders yellow, ana. ʒ. iii. Cinamom ʒ. b. Macis, Cloues, ana. ʒ. ii. ß. Gum Tragaranthi, ana. ʒ. ii. Ɔ. ii. Nutmegges, the greate Cardamom called the graine of Paradise, Galangall. ʒ. i. Spickenarde, Amber grise. Ɔ. ii. an Muscke. Ɔ. i. & cleane white Suger, as much as will suffice, and so dissolue all together in the pure syrup of redde Roses.

Sickenes.

What is this to my helpe beyng Sicke.

Health.

This healeth the weakenes of the Stomacke, and dothe comfort al the principall partes of the bodie, and wyll clense corrupte humors, foule and groce matter remainyng in the breast and stomacke: it also refressheth the braine and comforteth the hearte, and causeth good digestiō, and drieth vp superfluous moister in the goutes. And euen so reporteth Nicholaus Myrepsi, Gabriell, Iohannis Damascenus, and Leonardus Fucchius, men learned and daiely approned to whom we must geue credens as to most worthy teachers.

Sick-

Sicknes.

God is so iust and merciful that he wil nether suffer any vice vnpunished or vertue vnrewarded. Therfore these men haue receiued the fruites of thier owne labours, being good instrumentes to comforte the troubled, and heale the sicke that be aflicted with sūdrie infirmities. Where as an infinite numbre thorough the bestly abusyng them selues, be plaged with their fonde foolish delites as inordinate riotes, banquetes, surfetes, actes venerus, wrath, and other passions which bryngeth them all to my house, except diet with his brother quiete, and merie man meete these companions in the waie, and tourne them backe again, into the plesaunte Paleis of you goodman Health, whiche in all poinctes are contrarie to me poore sicknes, now subiecte to all miseries, as feuers &c. Yet of charitee shewe me some holsome medicine for diuers infirmites.

Health.

I shall shew thee a very excellent medicen against sundrie infirmities, whom Leonardus Fucchius in his cōpounding of medicens doeth greatly commende, and it is thus made. Take of Asarabacca, Balme seede, Henbane seede, ana. ʒ. ii. ß. of Cloues, Mirrhe, Cipres, Opium, ana. ʒ. ii. the iuce of Balme, Cinamom, Folium Indictum, Setwall, Ginger, Coste, Corall, Casiafistula, the Gumme Tragantum, Spike, wilde Fenell, Frankinsence, Euphorbe, Storax Calamita, Cardamonium, Siler, Montan, Mustarde, Saxafrage, Dill, Anisede, ana. ʒ. ii. Ligni Aloes, Rubarbe, Rhapontike, the confeccion called Alipta muschata, the Otters stones, Galinga, Opopanax, the fruite Anacardin, Masticke, Brimstone vnsleked, Pionie, Seholme, Roses, Time, Gladian, Peneriall, bothe rounde and long, Aristologia, Gentian, the outward rinde of mandrage, Germander, Baiberies, yelowe Carottes, ana. Ualarian rotes, long Peper, white Peper, the woode of Balme, called Xylobalsami, Carawaies, Amonium Parselie, Louage, Rewe sede, ana. ʒ. ß. fine Golde, little Perles, smale fishes, called of the Apoticaries Vnguis odoratus, the bone in the hart of the redde Deare, the shauing of Iueri, Calamus Aromaticus, Pelletarie of Spaine, ana. ȝ. xi. of Honie asmoche as you iudge mete.

Fucchius in libr. cōmp. Medicum.

Aurea Alexandrina Nicholaj.

Sickenes.

And what is the vertue of this.

Health.

It helpeth reumes of the hedde, whiche come of colde, the moistnes and runnyng of the iyes, the tothe ache, and hedde ache, if the forehed be therewith anointed, it doeth also cure the fallyng euill, madnes, turnyng sickenes of the hed, and

The booke of Compoundes.

to conclude, all maner of diseases, whiche be aboute the hedde, it healeth also those, whiche be troubled with the cough, or haue superfluitie of humours in the breast, the gnawyng and grippyng of the mouth of the stomack, whiche the Grecians call Dispepsia, and the Latines Appetitus prostratus, whiche is a corrupted appetite, it cureth spittyng of bloud, and the ache in the hippe, or huckelbone of humours, it asswageth also the Collike, and scoureth the reines, it prouoketh a man to pisse, and cureth the strangurian, breaketh the stone congeled, and taketh awaie all diseases in the bellie, it cureth quotidian and tercian Agues, takē with the iuce of stichados, in the beginning of the fittes.

Sickenes.

I doe hartely thanke you. I praie God I maie receiue comforte by your holsome composicion, called Aurea Alexandrine. Now sir, for as moche as I haue red the bare names, bothe of simples and compoundes, euen as menne passyng through Citees, fieldes, wooddes and riuers, smally regardyng their vertues, condicions or properties, euen so haue I doen, but now if it shall please your mastership, that in short questiōs, you shewe me the Compoundyng of Aromaticum Garyophillatum.

Health.

Wherunto are we mortall wightes borne, but one to help the other, the poore to the riche, the wise to learne the ingnorant, the whole to cōfort the sicke. For we whiche now bee in good health, and fele no grief, ones shall decaie, and fall into your miserable estate, and finishyng our tyme in dolour, agonie and paine. And thus I am perswaded, that our liues can not bee prolonged one minute: for the almightie haue set our course and ende, whiche we maie not passe, no more then the Sonne, Moone and the Starres, can goo out of their course and order, whiche thei be placed in. But Medicine easeth, maketh cleane, and comforteth nature, taketh awaie paine, but prolongeth no life, and thus our Diuines saie. But I beyng thy Poticarie, neighbour Sicknes, dwellyng nere thy doore, will teache thee many goodly medicines: and now how thou shouldest make Aromaticū Gariophillatum. Firste take of Cloues. ʒ. vii. Mace, Setwall, Galinga, yelowe Saunders, Crochisdiarodonis, Cinamō, ligni Aloes, Spicknard, long Peper, the great Cardamō ana. ʒ. i. Roses. ʒ. iiii. grated Licores, Gallia muschata, Folium, Indicū, Cubebes, ana. Ɔ. iii. of Amber. ʒ. i. of Muske Ɔ. ſs. of syrup of Pomecitron, as moche as you iudge mete. This comforteth the stomacke and the hart, stoppeth vomityng and the disposicion vnto vomiting, it consumeth also the corrupt humours in the stomack, and doeth nourishe all the principall members it causeth heate, and dissolueth winde.

Sicknes.

How

The booke of Compoundes.   Fol.iij.

How make you Acaciæ?

Health.

Take the plant or brauch of a Bulles or flow tree, with the fruit and laie it in a vessell certaine houres, and so let it stande, then seth it vpon a fire, and straine forthe the licour, the which streined, seth it on the fire againe, vntill it bee thicke, and then kepe it in fine vessels like shelles, and so drie it.

Sicknes.

How make you Auryli.

Health.

Take wheate and beate it lightly, not to small, and put it into a vessell of glasse, and couer it with water, so that the water be aboue it, twoo or three fingers, and so let it stande by the space of a Night: in the Morning presse it doune well, vnto the substaunce, whiche Amilum is made of, doe dissende to the bottome, afterwarde straine it with a Siue, and cast awaie the Bran, whiche swimeth on the water aboue, let the residue, whiche shall make Amilum, stand til it goo doune to the botome of the vessell, and the water swim aboue, then caste forthe the water softly, so that nothing remaine, and drie it with a little Cotten: let this be doen in Somer, and also Sonne dried lest it waxe sower, and so corrupte. Couer the vessell with a fine cloth. that nothyng fall in: If you will make this in Winter, then you must take greate hede, that it be not sower, ye must also prouide, that it bee sone dried, either in the Sonne, or in the wind, or in the fire, and thus you maie make Amilum of Rice.

Sicknes.

How make you Aquæ odorifera, **whiche is swete water.**

Health.

Take of Rose water, li. iiij. Storax Calamita, Beniamen, Cloues ana . ʒ. i. of Muske, Ciuet, Amber Grece, ana . ℈. xx. of Camphire, ʒ. ii. some put vnto this, ʒ. i. of Ligni Aloes, let the be put into a vessell of glasse, couered with a couer, hauyng holes in it, then let them boile in a vessell full of water, as it is in a Balneo Marie, whiche is a glasse or vessel, set within an other greater on the fire: this doen strain them with a fine linen clothe, and so to be reserued in a vessell in the Sonne, by the space of. xv. daies, and then it will proue an odoriferus water moste pleasaunt.

Sicknes.

How make you Benedicta.

Health.

                                    A.iij   First

The booke of Compoundes.

Irst take of the best Turbeth, Suger, ana. ʒ.x. Diagridion. ʒ.v wilde Liles, Roses, ana. ʒ.v. Cloues, Spicknarde, Ginger, Safron, Sarafrage, long Peper, Amonium, Cardamoniū, Smalege sede, Salgem, Galinga, Mace, Carowes, Fenell, Spenage, Kneholme, or Buchers Bromme, Gromell seede ana. ʒ.i. of Honie as much as will suffice. This dooeth cure the wekenes of the iointes, and the cold goute in the feete, it doeth also purge the reines and the blader.

Sicknes.

How make you Balsamum artificiall.

Health.

Irste take Turpentine. ʒ.xii. gumme Elomi. ʒ.v. of Rosen. ʒ. iii. let them be melted together, and when thei be molten, mingell these pouders folowing, of Aristologia longa ʒ.ii. of Dragons bloud. ʒ.iii. make these in greate peces. This medicine dooeth heale bothe newe and olde woundes, and chiefly, those that be aboute the hedde.

Sicknes.

How make you Confectio dulcis de musco.

Health.

Irst take of Safron, the swete roote Doronicke, Setwall, Ligni Aloes, Mace ana. ʒ.ii. white Perles, silke in pouder, Amber, redde Coral, ana. ʒ.ii.ß. the confection, called Gallia Muscata, Spicknarde, Folium Indicum, Cloues, ana. ʒ.i. Ginger, Cubebes, long Peper, ana. ʒ.i.ß, Muske. ʒ.i. Ɔ.ii. make this with Honie not clarified, the fowerth parte of the weight of all the other. This doeth cure the tremblyng of the harte, and all diseases of the of Melancholie, and those men, whiche be heauie without a cause, it remedieth also the diseases about the braine, as the tournyng sicknes, and falling euill, the writhyng or pullyng of the necke, or the mouthe on the one side, and all diseases of the lunges, and shortnes of winde.

Sicknes.

How make you Confectio Hamech.

Health.

Irste take the fower kindes of Mirabolans. ʒ.iiii. Rubarbe ana. ʒ.ii. Agarike, Coloquintida, Polipodi of the Oke ana. ʒ. xviii. Worme woode, Tyme, Sene, ana. ʒ.i. Violettes. ʒ.xv. the flower of harder Tyme. ʒ.ii. Anisede, Roses, Fenell, ana. ʒ.vi. the iuice of Fumitari. li.i. Prunes in nomber. lx. of Raisens, of Coraines the stones taken out. ʒ.vi. powre all these into a vessell of glasse, whiche hath a straight mouthe, and stop the mouthe, by the space of. v. daies, afterward let them boile ones, then strain them, and dissolue into the

strainyng

The booke of Compoundes. Fol.iiij.

straining of Casia fistula. ʒ.iii of the fruit of the wilde Date tree, called Thamarinde.ʒ.v. of Manna or swete dewe ʒ.ii. breake them with your hande, and straine them. Then caste on Suger li.i. of Scammoni.ʒ.i.ß. seth them vntill thei shalbe as thicke as Honie, then caste vppon them, the pouder of all the fiue kindes of Mirabolans, Reubarbe Fumiterie seede ana.ʒ.iii. Anissede, Spicknarde ana.ʒ.i. This cureth all diseases, whiche come of fleume and choler, but chiefly the ryngeworme, scabbes, keper, cankers, and soche others.

Sicknes.

How make you Cerotum Stomachale.

Health.

First take of redde Roses.ʒ.xx. of Worme woode leaues.ʒ.xv. of Masticke.ʒ.xx. Spicknarde.ʒ.x. beate them small, then take of Virgine waxe.ʒ.iiii. oile of Roses.li.i.ß. make your confection there bee some, whiche dooe washe the oile and the waxe, and then resolue them with a gentill fire, and afterwarde mingell them with the other, and so it is iudged better. This doeth mitigate inflamacions, and hote impostumes, whiche be in the stomacke and liuer.

Sicknes.

How make you a confection for the iyes.

Health.

First take of white Leade washed.ʒ.x. of Amile ʒ.iiii. of gumme Arabike, and Trangantum ana.ʒ.ii. of Camphire.ʒ.ß. make these into pouder, and dissolue them in Rose water, afterward make thereof little balles.

Sicknes.

How make you conserue of Buglosse.

Health.

First take of the leaues of Buglosse li.iiii. beate them in a morter of stone, and then caste vpon theim li.iii. of Suger, make your conserue like Opiata, whiche is a thin Electuarie. This comforteth the stomacke, and healeth diseases, whiche come of Melancholie, the sownyng and tremblyng of the harte, it purgeth also Cholere.

Sicknes.

How make you a conserue of Rosemarie?

Health.

First take of the flowers of Rosemarie, li.ß. of suger, li.i.ß. make your conserue. This doeth comfort a moiste braine, and molify hard & stife members, it also purgeth Melancholie and fleume.

A.iiii.   Sicknes

The booke of Compoundes.

Sicknes.

How make you a conserue of Borage or Buglosse.

Health.

First take of the flowers of Borage. ʒ. iiii. Suger. ʒ. xii. make your conserue, accordyng to the arte. This doeth remedie the trembryng of the harte and sownyng, it also purgeth Melancholie, and causeth a man to be merie.

Sicknes.

How make you conserue of Roses.

Health.

First take of Rose leaues. li. i. beate them in a stone morter, and caste vpon theim of Suger. li. iii. make your conserue after the fashion of Opiata. This doeth comfort the stomacke, hart and all the principall partes, it molifieth also those partes, which be hard and purgeth Melancholie.

Sicknes.

How make you a conserue of Violettes.

Health.

First take the flowers of Violettes. li. i. beate them in a morter of stone, and caste vpon theim. lib. i. of Suger, make your conserue accordingly. This dooeth cure inflamacions of Choler, quenche the thirst, and moueth a man to the stoole.

Sicknes.

How make you a conserue of Maiden heere.

Health.

First take of Maiden heere. li. beate them and put Suger vnto them, as in the other. This helpeth the Plurasie, deceases of Melancholie, and red Choler, and the Splen or Milte.

Sicknes.

How make you a conserue of Gladian.

Health.

First take of the rootes of Gladian. li. seth it in water, vntill it be well soden, afterwarde drie it, and searse it through a Siue then set it on the fire againe, and put. lib. iii. of Suger vnto it make this conserue like to the Electuarie Opiata. This remedieth deceases of the braine and senewes, with all soche as come of fleume.

Sicknes.

How make you a conserue of Enulacampana.

Health.

The booke of Compoundes. Fol.v.

Health.

Take of the roote of Enulacampana.li.ii.seeth it well, afterwarde drie it, then searce it through a Siue, and then set on the fire again, and put.li.vi.of Suger vnto it. This doeth comfort the stomacke, and principall partes against fleume, and help the hart.

Sicknes.

How make you a conserue of Cychory, or Succhory?

Health.

First take the Succhory flowers.li.i. beate theim in a morter of stone, and caste vpon theim.li.iii.of Suger. This purgeth Melancholie and Choler.

Sicknes.

How make you conserue of Sorell?

Health.

First take the leaues of Sorell.li.ß. beat it as you did the other, cast vpon them of Suger.li.ß. This helpeth Choloricke persones.

Sicknes.

How make you Conditum Cotoneorum.

Health.

Take as many Quinces as you iudge conuenient, and seth them and take the decoction of them.li.iii.of Suger.li.i. seeth them well, and reserue theim, some Apoticaries put in the whites of Egges, when thei be clarified. I will also teache thee an other waie to make this confeccio̅. Take of the seede or kirnell of Quinces.ʒ.iiii. tempre theim by the space of halfe a daie, with.li.iii.of the iuice of Quinces, then boile them alittle, and straine them, and cast vpon the̅ li.ii.of Suger, afterwarde seeth them well, and kepe them in bores.

I will also teache thee an other waie, to make an other confeccion of the same. Take of Quinces.li.vi. when thei be sodden, put vnto the̅ li.iii.of Suger, and seeth theim well, as you did before, kepe theim in little bores.

Sicknes.

How make you Diagalinga.

Health.

First take of Galinga, ligni Aloes, ana.ʒ.vi.of Cloues, Mace, Louage, ana.ʒ.iii. Ginger, longe Peper, Cinamon, white Peper.ʒ.i.ß.of Calaminte, Mintes, and dried.ana.ʒ.i.of the lesser Cardamoniu̅, Spicknarde, Louage seede, Fenell sede, Anessede, Carowaies ana.ʒ.x.of Calamus Aromaticus.ʒ.i.of the best Suger.ʒ.x.ß. of Honie clarified, asmoche as will suffice. This doeth cure the deceases,

The booke of Compoundes.

ses, that come of winde and belchyng, whiche semeth sharpe in the mouthe like Vineger, it is proued to cause good digestion, & fortefieth the weakenes of the stomacke and liuer beyng colde.

Sicknes.

How make you Diacyminum Nicholai.

Health.

Take of Cummin laied in Vineger, by the space of a daie, and afterward dried ʒ. viii. Ɔ. i. of Cinamom, Cloues ana. ʒ. ii. ß. black Peper, Ginger ana. ʒ. ii. ℈. v. of Galinga, Sauerie, Calamint ana. ʒ. i. Ɔ. ii. Charuill seede, Louage, ana. ʒ. i. ℈. xiii. longe Peper. ʒ. i. Spicknarde, Cardamom, Nutmegges, ana. Ɔ. ii. ß. of Honie asmoche as you iudge conueniente. This helpeth the stomacke and principall partes, whiche be troubled with winde, it causeth good digestion, and bringeth heate to the stomacke, & other principall partes that be cold.

Sicknes.

How make you Diambra of Mesuæ.

Health.

Take of Cinamō, Doronicke, Cloues, Mace, Nutmegges, leaues of Galinga and Spicknarde. ʒ. iii. the greate and lesser Cardamom, ana. ʒ. i. of Ginger, Saunders, ligni Aloes, longe Peper ana. ʒ. ii. of Amber. ʒ. i. of Muske. ʒ. ß. make it with the best Suger, and the water of Roses. This comforteth the braine, harte, stomacke, and all the principall members, it causeth good digestion, and maketh a man merie, and ingendreth heate in the principall partes, it is very comfortable to olde men, and those whiche be cold of nature and complection, to women also, and cureth the deceases of the matrice.

Sicknes.

How make you Dimargariton calidum.

Health.

Take of Cloues, Cinamon, Spicknarde, ligni Aloes, Galinga, Liquores, Crochisti Diarodonis, and little balles of Violettes an. ʒ. i. ß. Nutmegges, Mace, the confectiō of Muske, Setwall, Reubarbe, Storax Calamita ana. ʒ. i. Perles, Ginger, the bone in the harte of the redde Deare, the shauyng of Iuori, Vnguis odoratus. ʒ. ß. Muske, Amber, Cardamon, Louage, Basell seede ana. Ɔ. i. ℈. ii. of Camphire ℈. vi. of Mel Rosatum, asmoche as will suffice. This doeth cure the weakenes of all the bodie, sounyng, and faintyng, bothe of the stomacke, and also of the harte, and comforteth the liuely partes, and those that bee pensiffe and sadde without a cause, it cureth the cough and consumpcion, it doeth also recouer those, whiche be weake with long deceased.

Sicknes.

Sicknes.

How make you Diamargaritum frigidum.

Health.

Take the .iij. kindes of Sauders, the flowers of Roses, and Violettes, the seedes of Melons, Trochisti Diarodon, rawe Silke, made in pouder, ana. ʒ.ij. the bone in the hart of the red Deare, Spodium, Doronike, the roote bothe of red and white Behen, Spicknarde, Safron, ana. Ɔ.ij. shauyng of Juerie, flower gentill Saphire, Jacinte, Emeraude, Sorell, and Endif seede, Ligni Aloes, graie Amber, ana. ʒ.ß. of fine golde. ʒ.j. Camphire. Ɔ.j. of Muske. ℈.ij. mixe thē and make therof a pouder: putting in perles. Ɔ.j. and Currals red and white, ana. Ɔ.j.ß. and white Suger.

Sicknes.

How make you Diathameron of Dates.

Health.

Take of Cloues, Ginger, ana. ʒ.v. ℈.xvj. of Cinamom. ʒ.iij. of the substance of Dates, Galanga, Spicknarde, Setwal, Coste, Pelletarie of Spain, whit and red Coral, the gumme Rhaponticum, Spike, Fruite, Anacardium, Date stones, Balme seede, Anis seede, Ginniper seede, ana. ʒ.j. Ɔ.ij. of fine Golde, the bone of the Hart of the Red Deare, ana. Ɔ.ij.ß. of the shauing of Juerie, of Muske, ana Ɔ.ij. of Amber. Ɔ.j. of Honie Roset asmuch as you iudge best, but few Apoticaries do make this, for it is not greatly vsed, yet some do occupie it verie muche. This will recouer a man from daunger of death vnto life. It also helpeth those that be shorte winded or haue any disease in the winde pipe, or haue the coughe or be in a consumption, it cureth also all diseases of the breast and stomacke, the dropsie & paine in the raines, it bringeth mirth, it maketh a man lustie and fat.

Sicknes.

How make you Diarodon Abbatis.

Health.

Take of white and red Saunders, an. ʒ.ij.ß. of gumme Arabike and Tragantum, Spody. ana. Ɔ.ij. Asarabacca, Masticke, Aniseede, Fenell, Cinamon, Rewbarbe, Basill seede, Berberies, wilde Succhorie seede, Porseline seede, white Popie seede, seedes of Gourdes, Cucumers, Melons, Citorons, ana. Ɔ.ß. Suger candie, Roses, ana. ʒ.j. ʒ.iij. of Camphure. ℈.vij. of Muske, ʒ.j. make this with the sirup of Rose water. This helpeth the yelow ganders, weaknes of the liuer, consumptions, diseases aboute the harte, and those whiche be troubled with the heate aboute the stomacke, longes or the whole bodie, and also those which be recouered, from longe and litle agues.

Sicknes.

The booke of Compoundes.

How make you Diacalamintha.

Health.

First take Calamintes, Peneriall, Hysope, blacke Peper, Siler Montan, Percellte ana. ʒ.ii. Ɔ.ii. of Louage. ʒ.i. Ɔ.i. of Smallege, Aminthine, Dill, Aniseede, Cinamom, Ginger ana. Ɔ.ii. of Honie asmuche as will suffice. This cureth diseases of the stomack whiche come of colde, causeth digestion, and chiefly in olde men, it taketh awaie the cough, whiche doeth come of a colde cause.

Sicknes.

How make you Diatreon Pepereon.

Health.

Take of the Pepers. ʒ.vii.ß. Ginger, Time, Aniseede. ʒ.iii. Spiknerde, ana, Amonium, Cinamom, ana. aure. Casia fistula siler Montan, Enula, Campana dried, ana, aure.ß. make it with Hony clarified. This doth engender heate in the stomacke and bealy, it remoueth all paien of slumatike causes, it purgeth the stomacke of raw humors, and helpeth digestion.

Sicknes.

How make you Dyarreos.

Health.

Take of flowerdelice. ʒ.i. Sugar Candie, Tragantum, ana. ʒ.iii. mingle them and so make them in pouder.

Sicknes.

How make you Diairis Salamonis.

Health.

Take of flowerdelyce. ʒ.i. Peneriall, Hisope, Licores, ana. ʒ.vi the gumme Tragantum, Almondes, Pineaples, Cinamon, Ginger, Peper, ana. ʒ.iii. Figges, Dates, Reasons, of Corans picked, ana. ʒ.iii.ß. of redde Storax. ʒ.iii. of Hony asmuch as will suffice. This is ministred against the Coughe, shortnes of winde, and also restoreth the speche loste.

Sickenes.

How make you Diatragacantha calida.

Health.

Take of Gumme Tragantum Hisope, an. ʒ.iii. Pineaples bothe kindes of Almondes Blaunched, Linseede, ana. ʒ.vi. seede of Fenegreke Cinamon, ana. ʒ.ß. Licores, Ginger, ana. ʒ.ii. make a pouder of these. This is good against the hardnes and straightnes of the breast which cometh of a grose and colde cause.

Sicknes.

The booke of Compoundes. Fol. vij.

Sicknes.

How make you Diatrangacantha Frigida.

Health.

Take of white Tragantum.ʒ.ii.gumme Arabike.ʒ.ii.ʒ.ii. of Jmili.ʒ.ſſ. of Liqueris.ʒ.ii. of Penedis.ʒ.iii. the foure greater colde seedes, pared & picked, ana.ʒ.ii. of Camphere. Ɔ.ſſ. of the sirup of Violets, as muche as will suffice. This doth cure all diseases aboute the lunges, breast, and those whiche be in a consumption, and euell likyng, the Plurasie, Coughe, and those which be hotte and drie the roughnes of the tongue, and the weason, let the pacient hold it in his mouthe, and swalowe it doune, when it is melted.

Sicknes.

How make you Dyamoron.

Health.

Take of the iuce of Mulberies.li.ſſ. the iuce of blacke beries and straberies.li. of Hony.li.ſſ. swete wine sodden to the third part ʒ.iii. make it after this forme. Take your iuce, let it boile with your Hony and sweete wine vppon a softe fier in a vessell of glasse or tinne, vntil it be wel sodden, and to know when it is well sodden you must take a drop of it, and lay it vpon a Marbel stone, and if it will abide vpon the stone, and cleaue like thick Honi, the stone being turned on the one side, then it is well sodden, and this doen strain it and kepe it in a vessell of Tinne. This is very good against sores in the throte, & al kindes of strangling, & paines in the mouthe, to gagaris therwith.

Sicknes.

How make you Dyacodium.

Health.

Take.x.heades of ripe blacke Popie of a meane bignes, cast vpō thē.li.ii.ſſ. of raine water, and if thei be more moiste then drie, then let them lie in the water a day and a night, but if they be drier let them lie longer, after this seeth them vntil two partes of the water be consumed, then straine theim, then put in swete wine.ʒ.iii. good Honie.ʒ.i. then seth it again, and put in Acacia, Hypocistis, Safron, Myrrhe, and the flowers of Pomgranettes, ana.ʒ.iii. and seeth it againe, this helpe Catars, paines in the lunges, and cause slepe.

Sicknes.

How make you Dyaprassium.

Health.

Take of grene Horehounde.ʒ.v.ſſ. Tragantiū, Pine aples, swete Almondes, of a kind of Nuttes called Pistici, the substaunce of Dates, Figges, Raisens of Corans, the stones taken out, ana ʒ.iii.ſſ. Cinamum, Cloues, Nutmegges, Mace, Galinga, ligni Aloes, ℈.i. Spicknarde

Spicknarde, Ginger, Setwall, Lickores, Rhapontike Anacadin, storax Calamita, Galbanum, Turpentine washed, Mastike, Mirrhe Flowerdelice, Aristologia, Rotunda, the roote of Cipres, blacke peper Aniseede, Fenell, Dyll, Smalage seede, Parslie, Sarifrage, ana. ʒ. ii. wilde Lilles, Organne, Wormewoode, Squinantum, Cardimonium, white Peper, Carowaies, Louage, Daylie, ana. ʒ. ii. ß. Peletorie of Spayne, water Mintes, Peneriall, Dittan, Coste, Sauerie, Basill, Pionie, longe Peper, Amonium, Orobus ana. ʒ. i. Ↄ. iii. the woode of Balme, Casia fistula, Corall, chauyng of Iuorie, Balme seede, yelowe Carittes, ana. ʒ. ß. Muske, Amber, the bone in the hearte of the redde Deare, ana. Ↄ. riiii. of hony clarified, as much as you iudge sufficient make it after this sort folowing, put into. li. iii. of Hony, and of grene Horehound, Betony, & yong Pine aples pared, ana. ʒ. v. put also vnto the ʒ iii. of the best old wine, & let them boile together with a soft fier vntill the wyne be consumed, let your Figges be made cleane with in and without, dresse lykewyse your Dates, and let your Reasyngs be picked, and then dresse also your Pine appels, Almondes and the nuttes, Pistaci, drye euery one of them by them selues, afterward beate them in a Morter, and put vnto them Turpentine washed, after this beate all again, and let them be tempered with the same Hony, in the Morter where they were before, and mingle them with the spices whiche we haue spoken of before. This dothe cure the weakenesse of the stomacke, chiefly Reumes, and the braine which is colde, the turnyng sicknes, the eye sight, the winde pipe troubled with grose fleam it doth also mitigate the tothe ache. The iuce. This is ministred in all Fluxes, & chiefly in the bluddy flux, with the decoction of rain water, in the whiche Spidie was sodden in, or with Rose water, it stoppeth also the flux of meate vndigested, which the Phisiciōs cal Lienteria.

Sicknes.

How make you Diapapauer.

Health.

First take of white Popie. ʒ xxv. sweet Almondes blāched, Kirnels of Pineappel, gumme Arabike and Tragantum, the iuce of Liqueris ana. ʒ x. of Amili, ʒ iiii. of Purslen seede, & Lettise seede, kirnels of Quinces, ana. ʒ iii. of Saffron, ʒ i. of Penedis. ʒ iiii. take of the syrup of Popie asmuch as will suffyce. This helpeth those which be in consumption, and those whiche can not sleape.

Sicknes.

How make you Diacurcuma.

Health.

Take of Tragacāth, Safrō of Azarabacca, parsly, yelow Carrits Anisede, smalage sede, ana. ʒ. iiii. Reubarbe, wilde Fenel, Spicknard, ana. ʒ. vi. Cost, Mirtle beries, Casiafistula, Squinantum Balme seede, Mader, the iuce of Wormewoodde, Egremoni, & Balme

ana

ana. ʒ ii. Calamus, Iramaticus, Cinamum, ana. ʒ. i. ſſ. wilde Garlike, Ceterach, the iuce of Liqueres. ʒ. ii. ſſ. the gumme Cragatū. ʒ. i. make it with clarified Hony. This cureth olde diseases, and the euell likyng and deformitie of the body, when the meate beyng receiued doeth not nourishe, that is corrupt in the body: it also healeth the Dropsie, and diseases of the Liuer and the Splene whan thei be harde or indurate, it purgeth the stomacke of corrupt humors cold and windy, it mitigateth payne in the raynes and blader, and prouoketh vryne.

Sicknes.

How make you Diaſatirion.

Health.

Take of the rootes of Satirion whiche be like stones, the garden Parsnipe, the Nuttes called Piſtaci, Pineaple seede, Cloues ana. ʒ. xii. Ginger, Iniſſeede, Rocket, Birdes tongue or Stichworte. ʒ. v. Cinamum, cloue Garlike. ʒ. ii. ſſ. of Muſke, ℈. vii. make it after this forme, put the rootes of Satyrion in so much clarified Honie as will suffice, let also the Parsnipes and Pineaple seede bee well beaten by them selues, and then put thē into the same Hony, and ſtiryng them well, ſuffer them to seeth a certein space, then mingle with them your Pineapels and the nuttes Piſtaci well ſtamped, and when thei haue boiled a littell while, take them from the fier, and put vnto thē the pouders of the ſpices, and at the laſte put in your Muſke with Roſe water. This doth reſtore and fortefie the weakenes of the reines of the blader, it prouoketh vrin, and moueth a man to haue greate deuocion, to praie in Venus temple, or to be Venerus.

marginal note: The two ſtones of Satyrion or Orches, the one will flete, and thother ſinke in water.

Sicknes.

How make you Diaprunes ſolutiue.

Health.

Firſt take a hundred Damſones, and put theym into a Tinne veſſell with ſo much water, that they may be well couered and let them boyle well till they be ſofte, afterward take them from the fyre, and when your water is so colde that it is but luke warme, then take them forthe, and put them into a Syue ouer a great veſſell and chafe your Prunes so long with your handes, that nothynge remaine but ſtones and ſkins. Then put into the water, in the whiche the Damſons were ſodden in before. ʒ. i. ſſ. of Vyolettes, and boyle them, and make a ſyrrupe with. li. ii. of Suger, into the which Sirup put the ſubſtance of the Prunes, let them ſeeth vntill they be thicke, and then put into the same water. ʒ. i. of Caſiafiſtula waſhed, putte therto alſo. ʒ. i. of the fruite Thamarinde, diſſolued and ſtrained into the same water, remember alſo that ye boyle in the same of Prunes ʒ. i. of Vyolettes, ſeeth them well, ſtiryng them continually, and whē they be ſodden, take them from the fyre, and ſprinckle on these pouders folowyng, Saunders, Spodie, Reubarbe, Roſes, Violets, Pur-

The booke of Compoundes.

stine seede, succorie seede, Berberies, the iuce of Licores, the Gumme Tragantum, ana. ʒ. iii. of the foure greater colde seedes, ana. ʒ. i. if ye will make it laxatiue, put vnto euery pounde when it is taken frō the fire. ʒ ß. of Scamonie Diaprunes not losyng this, is ministred in hote and burnyng Agues, and chiefly in Synocha, whiche is a continuall feuer of aboundaunce of bloud, in this Ague it may safely be ministered in the beginnyng, increase, and at all times, and without Diagridion it maie be geuen at all houres of the daie, and with Diagridion, but in the mornyng, and that sircūspectly, because it is very laxatiue.

Sicknes.

How make you Diaphœnicon.

Health.

Take of Dates infused in Uineger three days and three nightes ʒ. vi. ʒ. i. of Penedis, which be litle wrethes of Suger, desolued in the decoction of Barly. ʒ. iii. ʒ. i. of blanched Almones, ʒ. xv. of Turbyth. ʒ. ii. ß. of Scamonie, ʒ. vi. Ginger, longe Peper, the flowers of drie Rue, Cinamum, Mace, ligni Aloes, Aniseede, Fenell seede, yelow Carottes, Galinga, ana. ʒ. ii. beate them well, and make them with clarified Hony. This doth cure mixt Agues of diuers humours the Colicke & paine in the belly, it purgeth all rawe humours of cold.

Sicknes.

How make you Diacartami.

Health.

Take the roote of Tragantum. ʒ ß. the substāce of Quinces. ʒ. i. thickest chifes of Saffron. ʒ. iiii. of white Ginger. ʒ. ii. Diagridion. ʒ. iii. white Turbithe. ʒ. vi. Manna or sweete dewe, Mel Rosatum strayned, ʒ. i. of Suger. ʒ. viii. wylde Lilles. ʒ. iiii. make an electuari, puttyng vnto it asmuch Hony as will suffice. This purgeth choler and fleume.

Sicknes.

How make you Diacorallium magistrale.

Health.

First take of the spices of the confection Diarodon Abbatis, whiche I did speake of before. ʒ. iiii. of both Coralles, litle peeces of Perles, ana. ʒ ß. beate them to fine pouder, and put vnto them of Suger resolued in the water of Roses. ʒ. viii. ß. make them into small peeces. This doth comfort the harte and stomacke, and chiflie those which haue ben longe sicke of colde.

Sicknes.

How make you Diacasiafistula pro xnematibus or Glisters.

Health.

The booke of Compoundes. Fol.ix.

Health.

First take of flowers of violets, the leaues of Malowes, Marcurie and Parietarie, ana. ℥. of wormewod, ℥.ß. take al these grene & yong, make a decoction of these in a sufficiēt quantitie of water, then straine them, and pressyng them with your handes into this strainer, you must dissolue a. li. of Casiafistula ℥. li. of the best Hony or suger. This purgeth and moueth a man to the stole, it is very expedient for tender & delicate parsons, because it is gentle in operaciō.

Sicknes.

How make you Dyasene.

Health.

Take of ligni Aloes, Cloues, Galinga, Witumges folīu nidicii, Mace, Cinamum ana. ʒ.ii. the stone Lazure. ʒ.i. of Sene twise asmuch as of all the other of saffron. ʒ.i. of the shauynge of Iuorie, Spodie, Anacardin, the bone in the hearte of the redde Deare, littell fysshes called Unguis odoratus, ana. ʒ.ii. wylde Lylles. ʒ.i. beries of Myrtes, Gentian, Bayberies, Eleborius, Ynger or Beresoore ana. ʒ.ii. Walnuttes made in pouder, in number. xb. of Amber. ℈.ii. of Hony asmuche as wyll suffice. To heale the Lepzie, some phisicion mingle with these serpentes fleshe. This doth remedie all diseases of Malancholy & madnes, the gnawyng and grypyng about the mouth of the stomacke called Cardiaca passio, it taketh away heuines, quarten Agues, and diseases of the splene.

Sickenes.

How make you decoctio Pectoralis.

Health.

First take of drie Hysop, Maidēhere, Figges, Sebesten, Raisens of Corantes, Barley, Liquores, ana. equall partes, boyle these together in a sufficient quantitie of water, then strain them, & so reserue them. This aswageth all paine about the brest, it cureth also the cough and horsenes, and if Aster be put in, it helpeth the reume.

Sicknes.

How make you Decoctio comunis.

Health.

First take of Prunes, wylde Dates, Raysons or Corans, Violets, Lyquores, Barley, ana, equal partes, boyle them in a sufficient quantitie of water, then straine them, and kepe them. This decoction is muche vsed in hot Agues and other hote diseases, and whan the yere is hote, to temper medicines with all, which be receiued in such hote Agues all times. This decoctiō is chaunged accordyng to the diuersitee of diseases, because some be hotter then other.

B.iii

The booke of Compoundes.

Sicknes.

How make you Electuarium Catholicum.

Health.

First take Sene & Casiafistula newe drawen, Thamarinde, ana. ʒ. vii. Reubarbe, Violets, Polipodie, Aniseede, ana. ʒ. iiii. the foure greater colde seedes, ana. ʒ. i. take. li. i. of Polipodie, and beate it, and seeth it well in water and straine it, then make a syrupe with the beste suger, temper your Casiafistula and your Thanarinde together, and whan the Decoction is almost made, put them into it with the other spices, and so make the electuarie. This is ministred in hote and burning Agues, because it doth molifie, dispers and comfort, it doth also cure diseases of the lyuer, of the Splene.

Sicknes.

How make you Electuarium Rosatum.

Health.

Take of Sugar, the iuce of Roses ana. li. i. ſſ. of the three Saunders ana. ʒ. vi. of Spodie. ʒ. iii. of Diagridion. ʒ. rii. of Champhire. Ɔ. i. temper it after the forme of an Electuarie, with a Syrup made of the same Sugar and Roses. This doeth purge Choler easely, and healeth hote diseases in the ioinctes, the hedde ache, the paine of the iyes, tournyng sicknes, and it hath been proued againste the yelowe Iaunes.

Sicknes.

How make you Electuarium de psyllio.

Health.

Take of the iuce of Buglosse, bothe harde and the wilde, the iuces of Endiue and Smalege, sodden al together and fined, ana li. ii. Aniseede, Sene, ana. ʒ. ſſ. of Maidenhere. Ɔ. i. the iuce of Fumitarie. ʒ. iii. of Asarabacca. ʒ. iii. Spicknarde. ʒ. ii. lette theim lye a daie and a night, then sette theim on the fire, and suffer theim to boile ones, then caste vpon theim. ʒ. iii. of Violettes, of the harder Time. ʒ. ii. boile them ones again, but with a soft fire, then strain them, and when thei be strained, put vnto them. ʒ. iii. of Fliewoꝛte, and let them all stande a daie and a night, but stirre the continually, this doen, presse forthe the slymie sappe of them, and take li. iiii. of it, and put vnto it. li. ſſ. of fine Suger of Scammonie, rosted in an aple. ʒ. iii. ſſ. after this set it on the fire againe, and seeth it alittle, and then put into it of Trochici Dyarodon, Trochistes of Spodie and Trochisti de Rubarbarie ana. ʒ. i. little balles of Barbaries. ʒ. ſſ. then make your Asarabacca into a grosse pouder, that it maie bee the moꝛe laxatiue, you maie put also to these confections, grene Violettes, and drie Damascens. This purgeth yelowe Choler, and healeth the

(margin: Fliewoꝛte is called Psyllion.)

The booke of Compoundes. Fol.x.

the turnyng sicknes of the hed, whiche cometh of a cholorike humor.

Sicknes.

How make you Electuarium inde maioris.

Health.

Take Cinamom, Cloues, Spicknard, Roses, Casiafistula, Mace Cypresse, ana. ʒ.iiii. yelow Saunders. ʒ.ii.ſs. ligni Aloes, Nutmegges, ana. ʒ. ii. Turbith. ʒ. i. of Suger Penedis ana. ʒ.xx. Gallinga, Cardamom, Asarabacca, Mastike ana. ʒ.i.ſs. of Scamonie. ʒ.xii. beate these altogether with the oile of Almondes, then take of the iuce of Quinces, Pōgranetes, the iuce of Smalege, Fenell ana li.ſs. seeth these iuces with clarified Honie, vntill thei bee thicke, and then make the Electuarie with the other spices. This purgeth superfluous humours, and chiefly flegmatike and corrupt humours in the stomacke, in the other principall partes, it dissolueth winde, and cureth those diseases, whiche come thereof, as the paine of the stomacke and the inwarde partes, the Collike and paine in the raines, it doeth also consume corrupte humours in the iointes.

Cardamom is the graine of Paradice.

Sicknes.

How make you Electuarium stomachi, to comfort the breast.

Health.

Take the beries of Mirtes finely beaten. ʒ.xii. of Roses, Spodie Manna, whiche is the flower of Frankensence, of the thre Pepers, of yelowe Saunders, the flowers of the wilde Pomgarnettes, gumme Arabike, ana. ʒ.i.ſs. the kernelles of the Pomgarnets, made in pouder. ʒ.vii. of Corriander steeped in Vineger, and made in pouder. ʒ.iii. Sorell and Plantan seede, of Roses, ana. ʒ.ii. breake thē all well, and rubbe them with your handes, then put theim into Sorel water, and so make your electuarie. This comforteth the stomacke and the inward partes, it stoppeth a laske, whiche cometh of to strong a purgacion, and moueth a man to meate.

Sickenes.

How make you Electuarium de Gemmis.

Health.

Take of white Perles. ʒ.ii. little peces of Saphire, Jacinct, Corneline, Emeraudes, Granettes, ana. ʒ.i.ſs. Setwall, the swete roote Doronike, the rinde of Pomecitron, Mace, Basell seede, ana. ʒ.ii. red Corall, Amber, shauyng of Iuorie, ana. ʒ.ii. rootes bothe of the white and redde Behen, Ginger, long Peper, Spicknard, Folium Indecum, Safron, Cardamom, ana. ʒ.i. of Trochisti Diarodon, ligni Aloes, ana. ʒ.v. Cinamom, Galinga, Zurubeth, whiche is a kinde of Setwall, ana. ʒ.i.ſs. thinne peces of Golde and Siluer, ana

Doronicum a roote whiche growe in Mauritania Ruellius call it Aruabo.

B.iiii.   aur.ſs.

aur. ß. of Muske. ʒ. ß. make your Electuarie with Hony, of Emblici, which is the fourthe kinde of Mirabolans with Roses strained in equall partes asmuch as wil suffice. This healeth colde diseases of the brayne, harte, stomacke, and the Matrice, it is a medecine proued against the tremblyng of the harte, fayntyng and sounyng, the weaknes of the stomacke, pensifenes, solitarines, Kinges and noble men haue vsed this for their comforte, it causeth them to be bolde sprited, the bodie to smell well, and ingender to the face good colour.

Sicknes.

How make you Emplastrum diachilon album.

Health.

Take of Fenegrike, Lynseede, the roote of Holioke, presse oute of all these the slimy sape, and take of it one part, and of Litharge wel beaten, and closed from drosse, one part. ß. of olde and clere oyle. iii. partes, beate the Litharge and the oyle longe, in a morter of stone with an yrone pestel. Then boyle them on the fier softly, stiryng them vntill the Litharge runne together, then take it from the fier, & suffer it to coule, after this take the slimie sape, and boyle it once. Then cast by littell and by littell, the slimy sape of the herbes vpon the Litharge and the Oyle, beatyng them with a pestell, till it be thicke: Ye may put vnto this emplaster, the fine pouder of Flowerdelice, & you may vse for your common Oile, which is salet Oyle, the oyle of Flowerdelice, some mingle with this the slimy sappe of Melilot. This emplaster is very good against impostumes and hardnes of the liuer and splene or stomacke, swellyng aboute the throte, and all hardnes of euery place.

Sicknes.

How make you Emplastrum diachylon magnum.

Health.

Take of Litharge broken and sifted. ʒ. xii. oyles of Flowerdelice Camomile, Dyll, ana. ʒ. viii. of the slimy sape of Lynside, Fenegryke, Holyoke rootes, Figges, Reasons of Corans, and of the fat in the belly of the Seele fishe, the iuce of Flowerdelice, Squilla, and of Hysop, ana. ʒ. xii. ß. of Turpentin. ʒ. iii. the gumme of Pineaple tree, yelow waxe, ana. ʒ. ii. make it after this fashion: beate the Lytharge and the oyles which we did speake of before in a Morter of stone, with a leaden pestel, by the space of halfe an houre, then let them boyle vpon a softe fire, stiryng it continually til it be thicke, then take it from the fyre, and suffer it to coule, afterwarde take the slimy sape with the other, and boyle them vntill they be hard, then take it of and lay it vpon a Marbell stone, and make it in great peeces. This emplaster is stronger in operacion, and better to ripe, and to resolue al hardnes and inflamacions, and is daily vsed of good Chirurgians, for the excellent vertue therof.

Sicknes.

The booke of Compoundes. Fol.xi.

Sicknes.

How make you Emplaſtrum de Mucilaginibus.

Health.

Take you the ſlimie ſape of Holioke ſeede, of Linſeede, of the inner rinde of the Elme tree, of Fenegreke, an̄. ʒ.iiii.ß. of the oile of Camamyle, of Lylles, and of Dill, ana. ʒ.i.ß. of Amoniacum galbanum, Opopanar, Serapinum ana. ʒ.ß. of new waxe. ʒ.xx. of Saffron.ʒ.ii. Turpentine ʒ.ii. make it emplaſter accordyngly. This emplaſter doth molifie all hardnes of apoſtumacions.

Sicknes.

How make you Emplaſtrum ad ſtomachum.

Health.

Take of ligni Aloes, Wormewode, gumme Arabike, Maſtike, Cipers, Coſte, Ginger, ana. ʒ.ß. Calamus Aromaticus of the fineſt, Frankinſence, Aloes, ana. ʒ.iii.ʒ.iii. Cloues, Mace, Cynamum, Spicknard, Nutmigges, the cōtection called Galita Muſchata Squinantum, ana.ʒ.i.ß. mingle all theſe together, with the confection called Miua Aromatica, whiche is made of Quinces, Peares, and ſuche other bindyng thynges, laye all vpon a clothe, and parfume thē with the wood of Aloes. This emplaſter doeth comfort the ſtomacke and liuer, it encreaſeth alſo heate in them and make digeſtion perfite.

Sicknes.

How make you Emplaſtrum de granis lavvri.

Health.

Take of fine Frankenſens, Maſtike, Mirrhe, ana.ʒ.i. of Baiberies.ʒ.ii. of Cipers, Coſte ana.ʒ.ß. clarified Honie, aſmoche as will ſuffice to make it, then ſprede it vpon a clothe, and ſo laie it to the ſore. This is a very excellent plaſter againſt the Dropſie, and wil aſwage all ſwellynges of winde, if you triple the quantitie of Cipers, and put vnto the plaſter alſo a little quantitie of Cowes donge, or Goates dries, it doeth alſo aſſwage all griſes, whiche come of colde winde, and chiefly the paine of the ſtomacke, bealie, raines, matrice, and blader.

Sicknes.

How make you Emplaſtrum de Melilote.

Health.

Take Melilote, and Fenegreke ana.ʒ.bi. the flowers of Camamil Baiberies, the rote of Holioke, Wormewood, ana.ʒ.iii. Smalege ſede, wilde Carrowes, Flowerdelice, Cipers, Spicknard, Caſiafiſtula Annie Aniſſede.ʒ.ii.ß. Margerā.ʒ.iii. Ammoniacum.ʒ.x. Storar, Calata, Bdellū, ana.ʒ.b. Turpentine.ʒ.i.ß.xii. Figges, the fat of a Gaote

Bucke

The booke of Compoundes.

Bucke, Reisons, ana. ʒ.ii.ſſ. Waxe. ʒ. vi. Oile of Mergerum, Oile of Spike, asmoche as will suffice to beate them in. This emplaster doth molifie all hardnes of the stomack, liuer, splene, and al inward parts.

Sicknes.

How make you Emplastrum coronem, a plaster of greate vertue.

Health.

Take of the Pitche, whiche is aboute shippes, pressed or strained of ana. ʒ.ii.ʒ.iii. of Serapinum. ʒ.ii. of Amoniacum, Turpentine, drie Pitche, Safron, ana. ʒ.i.ʒ.iii. of Aloes, Frankensence Mirrhe ana. ʒ.i. Opopanar, Storar Calamita, Galbanum, Mastickes, Alume, Fenegreke, ana. ʒ.iii. of the Dreges, of Storar liquida, which the Apoticaries cal stacte, Bdellum, ana. ʒ.iii. of Litharge. ʒ.i. ſſ, make it after this fashion, beate your Serapinum Galbanum, Opopanar, and Amoniacum a litle, and temper them with wine. Then boyle them vnto the wine be halfe consumed, then set it on the fyre in a vessell of Tinne, and when it shall begin to boyle, put vnto it your Pitche, and stirre it well, vntil it be melted, and whan it is melted put waxe vnto it, and that beyng also melted, put in drie Pitche, whiche is called Collophonia, the Storar beaten small with an hote pestell must be put therto, afterward Mastike, Frankensence, Mirrhe, Bdellium, and some after these put in Turpentine, Alum, Lytharge, and at last of all Fenegreke, when it is sodden, powre it vpon luke warme water, and than incontinently take it foorth again, and presse it with your handes, till all the water be foorthe, this done, make your pouder of Aloes mingled with the oyle of Laurell, vpon a Marbell stone. Then make of all mingled together, baules or great peeces with pouder of Saffron, your hande beynge annointed with the same oyle of Laurell. This emplaster taketh away al pain which is caused in spittyng, the grief of the stomacke which cometh of colde, it doth also dissolue congeled humors in the stomacke, and the hardnes of the splene it helpeth the Dropsie which cometh of coldenesse of the Liuer, & also the coldnesse of the Matrice, if it be layde vpon it, it is excellent.

Sicknes.

How make you Emplastrum Oxycroceum.

Health.

Take you Pitche whiche is aboute shippes, Saffron, Colophonie, of waxe, ana. ʒ.iii. Turpentine, Galbanum, Amoniacum, Mirrhe, Frankinsence, Mastike, ana. ʒ.i.ʒ.iii. make it thus, breake the Galbanum et Amoniacum a litell, then lay it in Wineger, by the space of a night, in the mornyng set them on the fyre, and melte them, and whan they be melted strayne them, and seethe them again, till the thirde parte of the Winiger be consumed, then put in your pith beyng

The booke of Compoundes. Fol.xij.

beyng pressed or strayned before. When as this is melted put in waxe, the which also melted, put in Colophony and Turpentine, and sone after Mastike, Frankinsence and Mirrhe, styrryng it alwaies fro the beginnyng vnto the ende, when it shall be sodden, put in colde water, afterwarde washe it vpon a Marbell, anointed with oile, and make it softe and gentill, then cast vpon it the pouder of Saffron and so make it in greate peeces. This cureth broken bones, and asswageth all griefes in what part soeuer thei be of the body, it doth also mollefie harde impostumes, in any parte of all the body of mankinde.

To cure broken bones.

Sicknes.

How make you Emplastrum de Ianua.

Health.

Take of the iuce of Gilofloures, Plantain, Betony, & Smalage, ana.li.i. of Waxe and Pitche, Rosen, and Turpentine, ana.li.ſs make of these an emplaster, sodden on a soft fire, vntil ẏ iuce be wasted, then put in your Turpentine, but stirre it well, ẏ it burne not.

Sicknes.

How make you Emplaster Gratia dei.

Health.

Take Turpētine.li.ſs. Rosē.li.i. white Waxe.ʒ.iiii. Mastike.ʒ.i. of Veruin, Betoni, Pimpernel, ana.ℳ. beate these herbes, and boile them in strong white wine, vntil the thyrd part be consumed, then straine them and cast awaie the substance of the herbes put vnto the waxe strained, with the iuce Rosen, Mastike, & let them boile styrryng them till thei be thicke, take them of and put in Turpentine, and mingle all together, and make your emplaster, saieth Nicolas.

Sicknes.

How make you Emplastrum contra rupturas.

Health.

First take of Pitche aboute shippes, of Aloes, ana.ʒ. of Litharge of red waxe, Colophonie, Galbanum, Amoniacum, ana.ʒ.i. Misselto of the oke, ʒ.vi. of chalke or plaster, of both Aristologia, Longa, and rotunda, Mirrhe, Frankensence, ana.ʒ.vi. Turpentine.ʒ.ii. of comen erthe wormes, of Oke apples, ʒ.iiii. of Campher, and of Dailie of Bolearmoniake, ana.ʒ.iiii. of the bloud of a man, li.i. make it thus, put the Misselto firste into the water, and suffer it to boyle long in a decoction wherin a Rammes skin was sodden in, and let it seeth by the space of a daye and a night, then take it from the fire, and put vnto it Turpentine, lytharge, Colophonie, Mastyke, the whitest Frankinsence, Mirrhe, Galbanũ, Amoniacum, and sone after Cumferie and Dayses, Chalke or plaster, and Bolearmoniake, after this set it on the fire againe, and put in the bloud

Misselto, is called Uiscũ or Misken, that groweth in Oke, or Thorne.

Bloud of man is to bee had at Barbars, or bloude letters, it muste bee dried in the Ouen.

of

The booke of Compoundes.

of man, and bothe Astrologias, and laste of all Aloes, you must sturre it continually, when it is well sodden, take it from the fyre, you shall know it to be well sodden when it wil not cleaue, nor sticke vnto your fingers, then lay it vpon a Marbell stone, anointed with oyle of Uiolets, and make it softe with workynge and laborynge of it with your handes, after this you must beate it again in a morter, continually by the space of two or three daies, then reserue it.

Sicknes.

How make you Emplastrum pro Matrice.

Health.

First take of the roote of Sinckefoly. li. i. of ligni Aloes, yelowe Saunders, Nutmegges, Berberies, of the flowers of Rosemarie or Roses, ana. ʒ. i. of Cinamum, Cloues, Squinantum, Camomil flowers, ana. ʒ. i. ß. Mastyke, frankinsence, the confection called Alipta muschata, and Gallia muschata, of Storax liquida, which is called also Stacte, an. ʒ. iii. fyne Muske. ʒ. ß. of Waxe. li. i. ß. of pitch about olde shippes. li. iii. make an emplaster.

Sicknes.

How make you Emplastrum Diuinum.

Health.

Take of Galbanum. ʒ. i. ʒ. ii. of Amonyacum. ʒ. iii. ʒ. ii. Opopanax. ʒ. of Litharge. li. i. of newe Waxe. ʒ. viii. of oile Oliue. li. ß. Frankincens. ʒ. i. ʒ. i. of Mirrhe. ʒ. i. ʒ. i. of Uergrece. ʒ. i. of Bdellum. ʒ. ii. of Aristolochia longa. ʒ. i. of Amentis, whiche is a kinde of Chalke. ʒ. iiii. mingle all these together, and make an emplaster.

Sicknes.

How make you Emplastrum de minio.

Health.

Take of the oile of swete Roses. li. i. ß. oile of Mirtelles the ointmente, Populeon, ana. ʒ. iiii. of Hennes grease. ʒ. ii. the Tallowe of an Oxe or a Cowe, ana. li. ß. Swines grease. ʒ. vii. Litharge of golde and siluer, ana. ʒ. iii. ß. of white Leade. ʒ. iiii. of Turpentine. ʒ. x. of Waxe asmoche as will suffice to make your emplaster, accordyng to the arte, somewhat blacke.

Sickenes.

How make you Emplastrum de Cerusa.

Health.

Take of the oile of Roses. li. ii. of white leade. li. iiii. of white wax ʒ. vi. make an emplaster. This is verie pleasaunte emplaster, against

The booke of Compoundes. Fol. xiij.

gainst all sores, whiche come by reason of the heate of the sonne, or by any other hoote cause, againste rubbinges, gallynges, or excuriacions of heate.

Sicknes.

How make you Emplastium Palmen.

Health.

Take Litharge of Golde. li. iii. of oile Oliue, yong swines greace ana. li. i. ß. of grene Coporas ʒ. iiii. buddes or toppes of the Date tree, seeth theim altogether on the fire, and stirre them continually, with a sticke of the same Date tree, and if you cannot haue the buddes or tippes of the Date tree, you maie take the rootes of Redes. This is a verie excellent plaster against woundes, festered with bloud and againste greuous emposthumes, burnynges, brosynges, shotyng, prickyng of humours.

Sicknes.

How make you Emplastrum Tripharmacum.

Health.

Take of oyle Olyfe, li. iiii. of Litharge, of Golde. li. ii. of Vineger. li. ß. make the plaster accordyngly. This emplaster dothe bryng new flesh again in woundes, and doeth heale them.

Sicknes.

How make you Emplastrum desiccatiuum rubrum.

Health.

Take Litharge of Golde. ʒ. iii. Oyle of Roses, oyle of Violettes, ana. li. ß. of waxe. li. xii. the stone called Lapis Calaminaris, of Terra Sigillata, of redde Leade, ana. ʒ. iiii. of Camphur. ʒ. i make the emplaster. This doth drie vp Byles and sores cleansed.

Sicknes.

How make you Hiera picra Galeni.

Health.

First take of Saffron, Spicknarde, the wood of Balme, Casiafistula, Cinamon, Mastiche, ana. ʒ. vi. of Aloes, a hundreth. ʒ, and take of Honie, asmoche as will suffice, beate them, and worke them all in the iuce of Coleworts, wormewood, or wine, that thei maie be so mingled together, as Leuen in Dowe, put vnto them Scamoni that thei maie the better cleaue together, and also purge the bodie of Choler, if you will put Agarike, and the inner parte of Coloquintida then it will purge Fleume, and if the flower of harder Tyme, bee mingled with it, then Melancholie is purged. To make it the more gentil in operacion, and least noisfull to the stomacke, the Poticaries put vnto this composicion, twise so moche Aloes, as of all the other kindes. Your Aloes must be broken and washed, that it maie better goto the botome of the water, and the drosse whiche swimmeth aboue, ought to be cast awaie with the water, and this must be doen twise or thrise, when it is well washed, then it will bee a verie holesome medicen for the stomacke, and nothyng hurtfull to the inwarde partes: after this the other simples and medicines ought to be mingled, and so it shalbe a verie good purgacion for weake stomackes. This purgacion, whiche is made with Aloes, doeth remedy iliaca passio, and consumeth superfluous humours in the stomacke, it doeth amende the palenes of tye face the iye sight, whiche is dimmed with grosse humours frō the stomack, it prouoketh a man indifferently vnto the stoole, woorkyng and purgyng from the Liuer, it doeth hurte those, whiche haue a hote Liuer, but the stomacke thereby is helped, whiche is cold and flegmatike.

Sickenes.

How make you a Julep of Roses.

Health.

FIrste take of Rose water. li. iii. of fine Suger sodden and clarified. li. ii. make your Julep with a soft fire. This quencheth the thirstie in hote Agues, and dooeth asswage the heate, bothe of the liuer, and of the harte, it doeth also resiste corrupcion of humours, and kepeth a man in health.

Sicknes.

How make you Julep of Wiolettes?

Health.

TAke of the water of Wiolet flowers. li. iii. of fine Suger sodden and clarified. li. ii. mingle theim, and seeth theim with a softe fire. This is a pleasaunte remedie in all burnyng Agues, and for those, whiche haue a hote liuer, or harte, it helpeth also those, whiche haue any roughnes in the winde pipe or throte, it helpeth the plurasie, and drie cough.

How make you Loche de Pino.

Health.

TAke of the kirneles of the Pine aples, take. ʒ. xxx. of sweete Almondes, walnuttes made in pouder, the gumme Tragantum, gumme Arabike, Liquores, the iuce of Amilum, Maidenhere, Lillie rootes, ana. ʒ. iii. of Dates. ʒ. xxxv. of bitter Almōdes ʒ. iii. Hony mixed with the iuce of greate Raisens, fine Suger, fresche Butter, and ʒ. iiii. of the best Honie asmoche as will suffice. This doeth heale olde coughes, shortnes of breath, & causeth a man to auoide grosse spittell.

Sick-

The booke of Compoundes. Fol.xiiij.

Sicknes.

How make you Loche de Squilla, or Scilla.

Health.

First take the iuce of Squilla and of clarified Hony, ana. li.ß. seeth it vntill it shalbe thicke. This purgeth grose and toughe fleame congeled in the winde pipe, and causeth it easely to auoide, it cureth also shortnesse of winde, and the payne of the breast and side.

Sicknes.

How make you Loche sanum.

Health.

Take Cynamom, drie Hysope, iuce of Liquoris, ana. ʒ.ß. of Iniubes, Sebesten, ana, in numbre.xxx. Raysons of Coranes, picked Figges, Dates, ana.ʒ.ii. of Fenegrike.ʒ.v. of Maydenhere M.i. of Aniseede, Folium indicum, Flowerdelice, Calamint, Linseede ana.ʒ.iiii.seeth all these in foure pounde of water, till halfe be consumed. Then put into this.li.ii. of Penidis with a confection of Suger, seeth it vntill it be as thicke as Hony, then mingle with this of Pyneaples pared, ʒ.v. of blanched Almondes, Liquoris, the gumme Arabyke of Amili, ana.ʒ.iii. of Flowerdelice.ʒ.ii. labour this confection vntill it shall be thicke and white. This cureth the coughe and hoorsenes of the voyce, whiche cometh of colde and fleugmatike humours whiche be in the breast and lunges.

Sicknes.

How make you Loche de Caulibus.

Health.

First take of redde Colewoorte.li. of Saffron.ʒ.ii. of Suger, Hony, ana. li.ß. make your syrrup.

Sicknes.

How make you Loche de pulmone vulpis.

Health.

Take the Lunges of a Foxe dried, the iuce of Liquores, Mayden heere, Fenell seede, ana. ʒ.iiii. make it with Suger, sodden in water, asmuch as will suffice. Some make it with the iuce of Mirts, and then it is bothe Laxatiue, and also a comforter of the stomacke. This is a plesant remedie in al consumptions and diseases of the stomacke it doth both comfort and clenseth the lunges.

Sicknes.

How make you Methridatum Manardi.

Health.

C.ii. Cake

The booke of Compoundes.

Take the Duckes and Drakes bloud, the bloud of a Goose, & of the herbe Grace called Rue, Fenell, Dil, Nauewes, an. ʒ. iii. ye roote of Gentian, Trifoly, Squinantum, Frankensence, drie Roses, ana. ʒ. iii. white and longe Peper, Coste, Valerian, Anyseede, Cinamom, ana. ʒ. ii. Mirrhe, Spicknarde. ʒ. vi. Turmentill, Asarabacca, Amoniacum, ana. ʒ. iii. Mace, Agarike, ana. ʒ. ii. Balmeseede. Ɔ. i. Flowerdelice, Saffron, Rhaponticum, Mastike, ana. ʒ. i. of Stichades. ʒ. v. make a fine pouder of all these, and put foure times so muche Hony as of the other and mixt them, beate your pouders finely, and seeth them softly.

Sicknes.

How make you Methridatum.

Health.

This is an excellēt Mithridatum, that is of Andromachy, but the beste is made at Bisanz.

First take of Storax Calamita. ʒ. i. Ɔ. i. of cloues, Spyknarde, the wood of Balme, Orobus, Louage, the gumme Tragantū, Mastike, Galbanum, Sandarike, the sweete thorne, Aspalthus, the Otters stones, the gumme of Iuie, Bdellium, Terra sigillata, and Lemmia, Melilote, the gumme of Ladanum, Opopanar, Canonia cum Opium, Brimstone vnsleked, Liquores, Salte Peter, Hipoquistis, Acacia, Roses, Germander, saint Johns worte, Sothernewoodde, Pionie, Hysope, Organie, Enulacampana, Sauin leaues, the leaues of Baye tree, Aristologia Longa, the flowers of harder Time, Worme seede, Rosemarie, Centaurie, Seeholme, the flowers of the wilde Pomegarnet, the inner rinde of the Mertill tree, the flowers of Pomgarnet, Raddish seede, Squilla, Aniseede, Balme seede, Gette, Henebane, Fenell, Comyn, Cardamoniū, Silermontan, white Mustardseede and Parsely seede, Rue, white Popie, Smalage, yelow Carets, Clarie, longe Peper, Basill, Amonium, ana. ʒ. i. Gladium, the common Bure, Swines Nuttes, Capars, Tutsan flowers, the horne of the Redde Deare, ana. Ɔ. ii. of the iuce of Balme, or of Myrte tree, Cynamom, Saffron, Coste, Squinantum, Ginger, Folium indicum, and in the steede of it, Cloues or Spicknarde, Turpentine washed, Myrrhe, Frankinsence, Casiafistula, Agarike, Spica Romana, Rhaponticum, Flowerdelice, Asarabacca, Dittan, horehounde, the inner rinde of Coloquintida, Sticades, Mougwort, Calaminte, Pelletarie of Spayne, grounde Pine, blacke and white Peper, Manna or swete dewe, Cresses, sinkefoly, ana. Ɔ. i. of Bayberies. ℥. vi. ß. of stronge and olde Wine. ʒ. i. of Hony asmuche as will suffice. This doth cure al diseases of the head, whiche come of colde and chiefly Mellancholy, and fearfull person, the faulyng euill, the Mygram, runnynge iyes, and all other diseases of them, the tothe ache, and all griefes and sores of the mouthe & Iawes, if it be layde on the place infected, if any Reume distill from the head, then it must be layde to the Temples, after the fashion of an emplaster, it cureth also the Quincie and Apoplexion, whiche is whan a man can neither feele nor moue, it helpeth also the

Coughe

The booke of Compoundes. Fol.xv.

Coughe, shortnes of winde, spitting of bloud from the lunges, and all inwarde diseases, it cureth also stiffnesse of mēbers, whan the sinewes be so stiffe that the parte can not moue, it also helpeth the Crampe, Conuulsions, Palses, diseases about the Mydref, Raines & the bladder, it breaketh the stone, prouoketh the flowers stopped, and healeth all diseases of the Matrice, it molifieth all hardnesse, and cureth the Goute, and it is a chief remedy for all poysons, and against the byting of a mad dogge, or any other beast, if it be layde to the place or dronke, it cureth also Quarten Agues and Quotidian, also take with it luke warme wine, an hower before the fit cometh.

Sicknes.

How make you Micleta.

Health.

Take of the three first kindes of Mirabolans dressed and made in pouder. ʒ.ii.ß. Commin, Aniseede, Folium indicum, amios, Carowaies. ana. ʒ.ii.ß. Cresses seede. ʒ.ii.ß. Bellericum, the fourth and fift kind of Mirabolās, made in pouder, an. ʒ.ii. infuse al these in vineger a day and a night, afterwarde make theym in pouder, then mingle with them Spody, the flowers of the wilde Pomgranet, Mastike, gumme Arabike, Manna, or sweet Dew, ana. ʒ.ii. stampe them all with the oile of Roses, and temper thē with the syrrup of the Mirtle tree. This cōfection hath been proued against the Emeroides, gnawyng and grippyng of the belly, the bluddie fluxes of the body, and is to be giuen in the Syrup of Planten. ʒ.iiii. in the night.

Sicknes.

How make you Miua simplex seu Aromatica.

Health.

Take a hundred. li. of the iuce of Quinces, put it into a cleane vessell of stone, and let it boyle softly, scumyng of it til it be half consumed, then straine it, and let it stande. iiii. howers, & caste vpon it. lx. li. of olde wine, this done set it on the fier and seeth it vntill it be thicke, some Poticaries make it with these spices which folow, and some without: they take of thē best Cinamum, the lesser cardamom, ana. ʒ.iii. of Cloues. ʒ.ii. of Gynger, Mastyke, ana. ʒ.i.ß. of Saffron. ʒ.ii. of ligni Aloes, Mace, ana. ʒ.ß. stampe all these groselie, except Saffron, and hang them in a clothe, and make them sweet with. ʒ.i. of Muske, and with. ʒ.ii. of the confection called Gallia Muschata, there be also some other Poticaries which make this cōfection with Suger. This confection fortefieth the stomacke, lyuer, and all the principall partes, it causeth good appetite and digestion, it stoppeth also vomityng, and fluxes of the body.

Sicknes.

How make you Mel rosatum.

C.iii. Health

The booke of Compoundes.

Health.

Take of Redde Roses, prepared and dressed, as in the Conserues before, ana. ii. partes, of good Hony. vi. partes, seeth them with a gentill fier accordyngly, some Poticaries put in equall partes, bothe of Hony, and of the iuce of Roses without any leaues, some other put also of the leaue. i. parte and ß. and of the iuce. i. parte. ß. of Hony. iii. partes. This comforteth the stomacke, and doeth digest and purge Fleugmatike humours conteined in the Stomacke, or in the Weynes.

Sickenes.

How make you Mel violatum.

Health.

Take of the Flowers of Wyolets. i. parte, of good Hony. iii. partes, seeth them with a softe fier. This is a singuler good remedie in hotte Agues, because it maketh the body moyste and also laxatiue, it asswageth the drinesse of the stomacke and breast.

Sicknes.

How make you Mel Anthosatum.

Health.

Take of Rosemary flowers. i. parte, of Hony. iii. partes, make it as the other before.

Sicknes.

How make you Manus Christi.

Health.

First take of Suger clarified and melted in the water of Roses li. ß. seeth these two till the water be consumed and the Suger harde, in the ende of your decoctiõ, put in. ʒ. ß. of Perles or precious stones, made in fine pouder, then lay it vpon a Marbell stone anoynted with oyle of Roses or Wyoletes, or Rose water.

Sicknes.

How make you Oximel simplex.

Health.

Take of good Hony. ii. partes, of Wineger. i. parte of well water iii. partes, your Hony and water ought to be sodden together, so that no some be suffered to abide aboue, then put in your vineger, and let it seeth well, vntil your Hony sease somyng. This doth purge grosse and Fleugmatike humours, by makynge of them thinner by dissoluyng them by opening, and breakyng of them, it doth also disgest the mattier which remaineth of longe Agues.

Sick.

The booke of Compoundes.   Fol.xvj.

Sicknes.

How make you Oxymel diureticum.

Health.

Take of the rinde of the roote of Smalage and Fenell, ana. li.s. Parsely, Kneholme, or Buchers broume, Sperage, Smalage seede, Fenegryke seede, ana. ʒ.j. seeth these rootes and seedes into one. li. of water, and one. li. of Vineger, vntill they come to the half and a littell more, then take of Hony asmuch as will suffice, and seeth it well, and make a sirup.

Sicknes.

How make you Oximel Squilliticum.

Health.

Take of clarified Hony. li. iij. of vineger, of Squilla li. ij. seeth it sufficiently. This dissolueth groase, toughe, & fleugmatike humors, it cureth also belchyng which cometh of raw & disgested humours, it healeth also the bladder, exulcerated in mollifiyng of it.

Sicknes.

How make you Oxysaccara simplex.

Health.

Take of Suger. li. j. of the iuce of Pomgranettes. ʒ. viij. of Vinegar. ʒ. iiij. seeth it on the fire, till it come to the forme of syrupe. This is verie good in tercian, quartan, and burnyng Agues. In the springe tyme, it purgeth the choler in the stomacke.

Sicknes.

How make you Oxisaccara compositum.

Health.

Take of Maidenhere, Ceteracke, Hartes tong, Liuerwort, Violettes, Fenell, Sperage, Kneholme, or Buchers broume, Stichworte, ana. li.j. make it after this fashion: laie your herbes and rootes, in the iuce of Pomgarnettes, by the space of three daies, vpon the fowerth daie, boile them a little, and strain them well. Afterward putte vnto theim asmoche Sugar as will suffice, seeth theim till thei shalbe thicke.

Sicknes.

How make you oile of swete Almondes.

Health.

Take Almondes and blanche theim, and take awaie also the inner rinde, then stampe them well, and make them in massie peces in a hote place, by the space of fiue daies, then beate and stampe theim together againe, and then presse theim, so

The booke of Compoundes.

that the oile maie issue forthe, and if you will seeth it againe in a vessell, set within an other, by the space of an houre, and then presse it, it wil runne moche better: you shal haue much plentie of oile, if you fill bagges with Almondes stamped, and then laie them vnder hote ashes or sande, betwene a clothe, and afterward presse theim. This oile mollifieth the roughnes of the throte, the hardnes of the lunges, and of al the inwarde partes, it healeth consumpcions, and encreaseth seede in men, it asswageth the heate of the matrice, and of the priuie partes of a woman, and also heate of the reines, and of the blader, if it bee laied to the place.

Sicknes.

How make you oile of bitter Almondes?

Health.

This oile must be made in al thinges, like vnto the other before. This openeth al obstructiō and apilacions, and causeth winde to auoide, maketh the fleshe smothe and faire, it doeth also take awaie spottes, and deformities in the face, ache in the senewes, and all hardnes.

Sicknes.

How make you oile of Baie?

Health.

First take ripe Baiberies, and stampe theim well in water, and straine theim, when thei bee colde, gather of the fatte, whiche swimmeth aboue, and it shal bee your oile. This oile bringeth heate and molifieth, in so moche that thei, whiche bee troubled with scabbes, ringwormes, or any soche sores, be cured therewith, if thei be anointed, when thei bathe theim, Cholorike persones, and all those, whiche bee suspecte to haue the Lepere, or any parte thereof, must eschue and auoide this oile: it is a singuler remedie against colde complexions, moiste and fleumitike, & those whose iointes be affected with cold, it cureth falling awaie of the heire, taken with the water of saltpeter: this doen, you muste also washe your hedde, with wine and Honie, and with the flower of Fenegrike, howbeit, if your hedde be vexed with any grief of heate, then you must vtterly eschue this oile.

Sicknes.

How make you Oleum Sesaminum.

Health.

First take and washe the little grain Sesanium, from all filth, then sprinkell vpon it a little water with Salte, and rubbe it with your handes, then caste water vpon it againe, till it bee moiste, afterwarde laie it forthe to drie, whiche thing doen, you must take it againe, and drie it better by the fire, so moderately as you can,

and

and after this put it into a bagge of courſe clothe, and rubbe it again with your handes, til the huſke go of, when the huſke is taken of, you muſte then grinde it, and preſſe forthe the oile, as you did in makyng the oile of Almondes, you maie make after this faſhion oile of Lineseede, Popie seede, or Lettice seede, sauyng that your Lineseede, maie not haue the huſke taken awaie. This oile encreaſeth fatnes, and sede in man, it moleſieth the throte, you maie alſo mingle this oile, with many other.

Sicknes.

How make you oile of Spike.

Health.

Firſt take of Spike. ʒ. iii. of wine and water ana. ʒ. ii. ß. oleum Sesaminum. li. ß. seeth theſe in a double veſſell, that is one ſet within an other, with a ſoft fire, by the ſpace of fower houres, and ſtirre it continually. This is a verie good oile, againſte all deceaſes of colde winde, grieues of the ſinewes, ſtomacke, liuer, ſplene, reines, blader, and matrice, the hedde ache, and megrum.

Sicknes

How make you Oleum de Coſto.

Health.

Take of drie Coſte. ʒ. ii. of Caſiaſiſtula. ʒ. i. the bloudes of Copres, of Mergeram. ʒ. biii. of ſwete wine, aſmoche as will ſuffice to laie the ſtuffe in two nightes, take of the oile of Sesaminum, li. iii. seeth it as the oile before. This oile engendreth heate in the ſinewes, and in all partes of the bodie, it openeth obſtructions and opilacions, it fortifieth the ſtomacke and liuer, it kepeth the heere from fauling of, and the hedde from horenes, it cauſeth good colour, and ſauour in all the bodie.

Sicknes.

How make you oile of Rue?

Health.

Take oile Oliue. li. iii. the leafe and iuce of Rue, ana. ʒ. ii. make an oile accordingly. This doeth heale and drie, thereof it is a preſent remedie againſt all diſtillacions and reumes, it aſſwageth griefes of the breaſte, and bringeth heate to colde members.

Sickenes.

How make you the oile of Dill.

Health.

Take of oile Oliſe. li. ii. ʒ. ii. the flowers of Dill. ʒ. ri. laie the flowers of Dill three daies in oile, and seeth theim the fowerth, with a ſoft fire a little, and then take them of, this doen put in

The booke of Compoundes.

to thesame decoction. ʒ. iii. of Dill flowers, and seeth it in thesame, and kepe it. This oile aswageth all greues and aches, it openeth, looseth, and prouoketh a man to sweate, it doeth mitigate the colde, and shakyng in Agues, if the backebone be therewith anointed, it causeth slepe, and cureth the hedde ache.

Sicknes.

How make you oile of Camomill?

Health.

Take of oile Olife. li. iii. of the flowers of Camomile. li. i. make it as the oile of Dill. This doeth mitigate all aches, it stoppeth fluxes of humours, bicause it doeth alose, and not binde, Paulus Aeginetae doeth take. ʒ. ii. of the drie flowers of Camomile, without the whites, and doeth couer the bessell with a linen clothe, so that the aire maie pearse through, and then doeth set it in the Sonne, by the space of fourtie daies, after this the mouthe ought to be well stopped, and so kept, and if you cannot haue grene flowers, you maie take drie, and seth them in a double bessel, that is, one set within an other, howbeit, the oile shalbe of lesse strength and efficacitie. This oile is electuarius to the teeth, anointed by it self, or by some other temperate thyng, doeth open the poores, and causeth the skinne to bee thinne, it cureth long Agues, and all grieues, if the place bee anointed with it, and swete wine.

Sicknes.

How make you oile of Mirtes?

Health.

Take of Salet oile. li. iii. of Mirtes stamped. li. i. of the best wine li. ii. mingle these together, and suffer them to boile, vntill the wine bee consumed, then straine theim, and so reserue it. This oile doeth refrigerate and binde, & therfore it cureth the fluxe, whiche cometh of weakenes of the stomacke, burnynges, pimpelles, kibes and gaulinges, if the place be therewith anointed, it healeth clistes about the fundamente, and the broade piles, the weakenes of the members, it stoppeth also vomityng and sweatyng.

Sicknes.

How make you oile of Flowerdelice?

Health.

Take the rootes of Flowerdelice. ʒ. ii. and of the flowers. ʒ. iiii. and of the decoction of the rootes. li. i. of oile Oliue. li. ii. lette theim boile in a double bessell, vntill the water bee consumed, after this straine theim, and chaunge the rootes, and flowers, and decoction, this ought to be twise, and then strain them, and reserue thē: the Poticaries commonly make it after this fashion, how bee it, you
shall

The booke of Compoundes. Fol.xv.

shall rede in Dioscorides another forme of makyng this Oyle. This Oyle scoureth, purgeth, loseth, openeth, ripeth, and aswageth aches of colde, it ripeth rawe humours in the breast and lunges, it taketh away paine in the ioyntes, and molifieth the hardnes of them, all impostumes and swellynges about the necke, or in any other place, it aswageth payne of the Matrice of colde, the Crampe and payne about the Reynes, and the stenche also of the nose.

Sicknes.

How make you Oyle of Roses.

Health.

First take oyle Olyfe, or the oyle of the graine Sesanium washe them ofte with well water, then take a sufficient quantitie of leaues of younge and redde Roses beten, and couer them with the oyle wherin thei were washed, and stop the mouth of the vessell, & set it in the Sunne by the space of .vii. daies, afterwarde seeth it in a double vessell, by the space of three howers, then chaunge againe the Rose leaues, and take freshe, and set theim in the Sonne other seuen daies, after this seeth them againe, and chaunge theim as you did before, and put vnto theim infusion of Roses, asmoche as of the oile, and stoppe the mouthe of the vessell, and set it in the Sonne, by the space of fourtie daies. This oile (as Mesuae writeth) doeth comfort, lose, open, and aswwage all aches, it is also good against inflacions, and fluxes of humours, therfore beyng droken, it is a present remedie against bloudie fluxe, and all other fluxes. There be twoo kindes of this oile, the one is made of ripe Roses, leaues, and the other of oile Oliue, and Rose leaues: the first kinde doeth molefie, and make the skinne thin, it openeth, and aswwageth all maner of griues: The second kind doeth refrigerate and binde, and therefore it cureth the headache in Agues, or of the heate of the Sonne, it aswwageth burnyng, whiche is engendred of winde, in a full stomacke, and finally it cureth all aches of the hedde, if the place be therewith anointed, it is also a presente remedie against paine in the stomacke, or bowelles, of sharpe humours, if it be mixt with .℥.ii. of Mastike, and with a little quantitie of waxe, it aswwageth all redde inflamacions, if the place be anointed with it.

Sicknes.

How make you oyle of Violettes.

Health.

First take oyle Oliue .li.ii. of younge Violetes stamped .℥.iiii. put them into a glasse, and set them in the sonne by the space of .vii. daies, afterwarde boyle them in a double vessel by the space of three howers, then strein and reserue theim, Paulus Agineta doth call this oyle Iaton and writeth that it is made either of purple Violets, or els of yelow Violets, which many iudge to be Hartesease, he willeth also that the Violets shal stande .x. daies in the sunne

and

and be thrise changed, and the vessell to be so stopped that no ayre may enter in and in the meane time you may put in drie Violets. This asswageth all inflamacions in what parte so euer they be, it molefieth exulcerations and horsenes of the breast or lunges, it mitegateth hot apostumes and the pluracies.

Sicknes.

How make you Oyle of Quinces.

Health.

First take of the Quinces whiche be not fully ripe, and stampe them, and of the iuce of thē, ana, equal partes of the oile of vnripe Oliues, asmuche as will suffice, put it into a glasse, & set it in the sunne by ye space of .xv. daies, then set it in a double glas, which is one vessell set within an other by the space of foure howers, then change your Quinces and the iuce of them once or twise, and make it as you did the other, after this streine it, and reserue it. Dyoscorides doth shew an other and a better way to prepare this oyle. Paulus Ægineta doth call this oyle Melinon, and maketh it after this sorte he doth take of Quinces vnpared. ʒ. iii. of the oyle of vnripe Oliues ʒ. xviii. and dothe set it in the sunne. xl. daies. This oile forteseth the stomacke, the principall members, and the sinewes which be lose and weake, it prohibeteth ouer much sweatyng, it is also a present remedie against all fluxes.

Sicknes.

How make you Oyle of Masticke.

Health.

This Oile is so good, that it is called the seconde, that is fewer better, for the vertue therof

Take of Masticke. ʒ. iii. oyle of Roses. ʒ. xii. of good wine. ʒ. viii seeth it in a double vessell accordyngly. This Oyle, as Mesue writeth is the seconde for his vertue, for it comforteth the stomacke, sinewes, liuer, and ioyntes, it doeth molifie harde apostumes, and aswageth aches.

Sicknes.

How make you Oleum Castario.

Health.

First take. ʒ. i. of the Otters stones, and seeth them in one pond of oyle Oliue, vntill the thyrde parte be consumed, then keepe the oyle in the pouder of the Otters stones.

Sicknes.

How make you Oleum de Euphorbio.

Health.

Take of Euphorbe. ʒ. ß. of oile of Hartesease. ʒ. v. of swete wine as moche, seeth it till the wine bee consumed, and then reserue it. This oile is verie good against cold deceases of the sinewes, the

The booke of Compoundes. Fol.xix.

the ache of them, and of the ioinctes, the paine of the liuer and splene, the hedde and the reume, the vertigo and forgetfull diseases. Galine doeth make this oile Oliue of Euphorbe, accordyng to the pacientes infirmitie, as it dooeth appere in the seconde booke De composicio Medicamentorum.

Sicknes.

How make you Oleum vulpinum.

Health.

Take a whole Foxe, except the bowels, and put hym in a vessell, and powre vpon hym welle water, and salte water. ʒ. xviii. of olde oile. li. iiii. seeth this ouer a softe fire, with. ʒ. iii. of Salte, vntill the water be consumed, then put it into a vessell, and powre to it swete water, wherein the herbes were sodden. li. ii. and Time. ℈. ii. seeth theim againe, till the water be consumed. This oile is a chief remedie againste the paine in the iointes, that is called Arthritica passio, against the goute in the seate, and paine in the raines and backe.

Sicknes.

How make you Oleum de Tartaro.

Health.

Take of the lies of white wine. li. ii. or els asmoche as you iudge beste, make it in pouder, and wrape it in linen clothe, or in towe, then mingle it again with strong white vinegar, afterwarde drie it againe vnder hote ashes, vntill it shall bee verie blacke, then make it in pouder againe, and set it in a vessell in a colde place, and so let it stande by the space of. viii. daies, till it shall be resolued in to oile and runne, and if it will not runne of it self, then presse it with your handes into a glasse. With this oile women doe anointe their faces, to make them smothe and faire, for it cleanseth the face meruelus well with Camphere.

Drie your Tartar in an Ouen.

Sicknes.

How make you Oleum de Scorpione.

Health.

First take twentie Scorpiõs, more or lesse, accordyng to their quantie, putte theim into a vessell of glasse, and powre vpon them. li. ii. of oile of bitter almondes, stoppe the mouth, and set it in the Sonne. xxx. daies, then straine it, and so vse it. This oile is the moste presente remedie, to breake the stone in the reines, or the blader, chiefly if the reines or the necke of the blader, or the places there aboute, bee anointed with it, or els it bee ministred in by the yerde, it is also made with olde oile, and mixed with many other medicines, whiche be good against poison: it is also a present remedie against the pestilence, or stingyng of Scorpions. &c.

You shal haue Scorpions at the Poticaries.

Sicknes.

D.i. How

How make you oile of garden Lilles?

Health.

First take of oyle Oliue. li.i. of flowers of white Lylles. ʒ.iiii. make this oyle, as you did the oyle of Camomill Paulus Aegineta doth shew another way of making of this oyle. This oyle is very good against womens diseases, runnyng sores of the head, the scurfe or any other breakyng forth, if the place be therwith anoynted, it is also good against all diseases, and aches of colde, and inflamacions, also anointed with Saffron, if it be dronken, it wil purge choler but it is noysome to the stomacke.

Sicknes.

How make you Oleum de Papauere.

Health.

First take of the flowers, and greane heads of Poppie stamped, ana. ʒ.iii. of oyle Oliue not ripe. li.i.ʒ.iii. make your oyle accordingly. This oyle aswageth head ache, and causeth a man to sleape whan the cause of waking cometh of heate or vapers assende to the head, if ye temples, nose, eyes, or forehead be therwith anointed.

Sicknes.

How make you Oleum Nimphæatum album.

Health.

Ninuphar is the water lilly, white or yellowe.

Take of oile Oliue not ripe. li.i. of the flowers Ninuphar whan thei be fresh, and stampe. ʒ.iiii. kepe theim in a vessell of glasse and repare it as you did the oyle of Violetes, both for settyng it in the sunne, and for the sething and changing of the flowers and the mixing of the decoction. This oyle hath almost the vertues of the oile Poppie, but because it is not so cold, & doth not so much dulle senses, therfore we mingle with it the Oile of Popie to cause a man slepe the better, it altereth a hot complexion, vnto what part so euer it be laid.

Sickenes.

How make you Oleum Menthæ.

Health.

First take of Mintes leaues, and of the iuce of it. ana. ʒ.iiii. vnripe oyle Olyue. li.iii. put these into a vessell of glasse, and set it in the sunne by the space of. xv. daies, stoppyng the mouth of it, this doen, boile them. iiii. houers, then straine them wel, this being doen, afterward straine it, and so let it be kept. This oile is good for a weake and a colde stomacke, it stoppeth vomityng, and causeth digestion, it moueth a manne to his meate, and mollifieth all hardnes in what parte of the bodie so euer it be.

Sicknes.

The booke of Compoundes. Fol.xx.

How make you Oyle of Wormewood.
Health.

Take the buddes, toppes, and iuce of wormewood, ana. ʒ.iiii. of oyle Oliue. li.iii. you shall make this as you did ye other. This doth comforte and bringe heate to colde members, it fortefieth the stomacke, and causeth good appetite, it openeth obstructions and healeth diseases which come of a coulde cause, it destroieth wormes and doth bring them forth, if it be mixt with oyntmētes and plasters and layd to the place.

Sicknes.

How make you Oleum Lumbrecorum.
Health.

Take of earth wormes. li.i.ß. of oyle Oliue. li.ii. of wine. ʒ.ii. boile them all together, and make an oyle accordingly. This is comfortable to the sinewes vexed of colde, and good for the ach of the ioinctes.

Sicknes.

How make you Oleum de Cherua or alba viola.
Health.

Take flowers of Hartesease. ʒ.xii. of oile oliue. li.ii. the flowers of Hartesease, must be laid. iii. daies in oile seeth them well on the fourth day with a soft fier, this done, put vnto the decoctiō ʒ.iii. of the flowers of Hartesease, then set it in the sunne and reserue it. This oyle openeth, loseth and asswageth paine of the ioinctes and sinewes, breast, reines and bladder.

This sweete herbe growe, vpon walles and in Gardens, it florishe in April and Maie.

Sicknes.

How make you a Pomander.
Health.

Take of Storax Calamita. ʒ.i.ß. of Beniamin. ʒ.ii. of the gumme of Ladanū. ʒ.ß. of Cloues, white Saunders, ana. ʒ.iii. of Roses, Mergeram, ana. ʒ.ii.ß. mingle with these pouders of Muske and Ambergrice, ana. Ɔ.i. make your baule with the infusion of Rose water and Siuet, in a morter somewhat warme.

Sicknes.

How make you Diahyssopus Nicolai, which is greatly commended of Cordus.
Health.

It is a very holsome medicine, and must be thus made as foloweth, take Hysop, Yreos or Flouerdeluce roote, Time, black Peper, ana. ʒ.xxx. Pulsall royal, Sauory, Rue, Commen. ana. ʒ.xx the fruite of Dates, Tragacante, Liqueris, fatte figges, Raisens of

D.ii.　　the

The booke of Compoundes.

the Sunne without stones, Fenel, ana. ʒ.x. Ginger, vncullerid Carowaies, Louage seede, ana. ʒ.v. and Suger, beate your dried thinges in a brasse morter, and your moist thinges in a stone morter, & then temper them together according to arte as Manus Christi or softer, this Dia is good to be eaten for the coldnes of the head, and fasten vp the Uuyla, purge the arters stomack, Lunges Cough, and helpeth Plureces, and this is good for thee, for thou arte much troubled with these euils.

Sicknes.

How make you Diacost, after Mesue.

Health.

You must make it thus, Take swete Cost, Arabicum, or for that Costmary the whitest, the wood of Cassia, Sinamom, ana. ʒ.v the sedes of smalage, of Inissede, and Rubarbe and Squinans ana. ʒ.iii. Azarabacca rootes, Saffron, Aristologiae, Myrrhe, añ. ʒ.ii. & Suger as wil suffise, stampe your dried thinges in a morter, and serse them, and stampe your moyst in a stone morter, and mingle them together, and seeth your Suger with Rose water, put in your receptes in the ende, and make it as harde and as soft as you will, this helpeth Dropses, and stoppinges of the guttes, winde, colde or rawnes, paines of collike.

Sicknes.

How make you Diatrion Sandalon Nicolai.

Health.

Take the three kindes of Sander, white, red and yellowe, of red Rose leaues, fine white Suger, ana. ʒ.iii. Rubarbe, Spodium the Syrup of Liquires, Purslen seede, ana. ʒ.ii. Ɔ.ß. Ǥ.v. Imile gum of Arabike, and of Tragacath, the seedes of Melons, Cucumers Gourdes, Citrons, Succorie, or Endiue, añ. ʒ.i.ß. Camphere. Ɔ.i. and Suger to seeth it in, when the pouders be finely cerced, and the gummes resolued, and so temper them in your panne, hauyng Endiue or Burage water, this is moste holsome against all the sicknes of the liuer, coming of heate aboue nature, and helpeth the yelow Jaunders, and causeth slepe.

Sicknes.

How make you that moste worthie and excellent Cordiall Diamuscum dulce.

Health.

You must vse these simples folowing. Take Saffron, Doronik, Setwall, wood of Aloes, Mace, ana. ʒ.ii. white fine perle, rawe white silke, dried and beaten into pouder, Carabe or Crabfishe, red Corall, Gallia Mulchata, swete Basell, or Balme, the white and the

The booke of Compoundes. Fol.xxj.

the red Bene, or the flowers, Spicknard, Cloues, ana. ʒ.i. white Ginger, Cubebes, longe Peper, ana. ʒ.i. sweete Muske, Ambergrice, ana Ɔ.i.ß. beate this finely in pouder, and with Suger and Rose water, seeth them accordingly into a thicknes, temper it still, and powre it vpon a Marble stone. This is good against the passions of the harte, in swellyng of the stomacke, lacke of slepe, fallyng sicknes, and shortnes of breath, to be eaten mornyng and euening. You maie make an other good Diamuscha Amarum, of a stronger effecte, againste Dropsie, to drie moiste humours, and to clense corrupcion, or putrifaction within the body: if you adde these thinges. Take dried Wormewoode, fine yellow Aloes, Castor which be Beuers stones, & louage sede ana. ʒ.iii.ß.

Sicknes.

How make you pouder of Violets.

Health.

Take of flowers of Violets, li.ß. of Roses, ʒ.iiii. of Cipers, ʒ.ß. of Mergeram, Cloues, ana. ʒ.i. white Saunders, Beniamin, ana. ʒ.iiii. of Storax Calamita. ʒ.i.

Sicknes.

How make you Puluis contra pestem.

Health.

Take of Sinkefolie, Dittan, Tunis, Scabuos, Buglosse roote, ana. ʒ.ß. the kirnels of Pomcitron, Sorell, ana. ʒ.iiii. of Coriander. ʒ.ii. of red Roses, ʒ.i. of Purselin seede. ʒ.ii. the shauinge of Iuerie. ʒ.ii. of white and red Corall, ana. ʒ.i.ß. of Terra Sigillata ʒ.ß. of Bolermoniake. ʒ.ii. mingle them and make a pouder.

Sicknes.

How make you Puluis de Boloarmenio.

Health.

Take of the three Saunders, Galanga, Aloes, Cinamom, redde Corall, red Roses, the seede of Melons, ana. ʒ.ß. the rootes of Tunes and Sinkefolie, ana. ʒ.iii. the shauynge of Iuerie, of Hartes horne, ana. ʒ.ß. of Aniseede, Fenell seede, Ginger ana. ℈. rb. of Sorell seede, of the kirnels of Pomecitrone, Iuniper seede, Cloues, ana. ʒ.ß. of Bolermoniake. ʒ.ii. make a pouder therof.

Sicknes.

How make you puluis contra Lumbricos.

Health.

First take of wormewodde. ʒ.i. of Lupines. ʒ.ß. of Hartes horne made in pouder. ʒ.i.ß. mingle them and make a pouder.

Sicknes.

D.iii. How

The booke of Compoundes.

How make you puluis Bezeardicus.

Health.

<small>Let this bole armoniake be put in a little Vineger, and so dryed.</small>

Take of Bolermoniake.ʒ.ii.of red Roses, of Sorell seede, of the Kirnels, of Pomecitron, of Hartes horne made in pouder, Rue seede, the roote of Doronike, Imber seede, of Southistel or Cardus Benedictus. ana.Ɔ.iiii.of bothe Corals, of ligni Aloes, of rawe silke, nether coloured nor died, but as it cometh from the silke worme of the three Saunders, of Perles, of the bone in the harte of the redde Deare.ana.ʒ.i.of the Emerode.Ɔ ii.of the pouder of Perles, of Sink folie, Dyttan, Tunis, Scabios, Coriander, Terra Sigillata, ana.ʒ.ii of Camphire.Ɔ.ii. of Saffron.Ǵ.xv.of Imber.Ɔ.ii.of Mushe.Ɔ.iiii. and make a pouder, if it be put in the syruppe of Rybes, it is a goodlie cordiall.

Sicknes.

How make you penidias.

Health.

Take of the best Suger.li.i.or.ii.and at the most three, and put it into a vessell of Brasse, beyng couered within with Tinne or els into an earthen vessell, one of brasse is better for this purpose, mete your Suger with such a quantite of sweete water as will couer it, and if your Suger be very good and stronge, mingle with it for euery pounde of it.ʒ.i.of Pony, then sprinkle vpon it oile of sweet Almondes, and if you haue not this Oyle, you may vse some other in the steede of it, set your vessell on a fier of coales without smoke, and seeth it vntill the water be almost consumed, you shall know whether it be sodden inough or no, thus, take a drop of it, & lay it vpon a Marble stone, and touche it with you finger, if it appere like threades, and will cleaue and sticke vnto your finger, then take it from the fier and lay it vpon a Marble stone, and drawe it abroade, after that ye haue mingled it with the Oyle of Sweete Almondes, or of Syzamyn, after this gather it together againe as hot as your handes will suffer, afterwarde drawe it foorth againe with your handes, as sweet Electuaries be drawne, and then sticke a croked naile very hie in the wall, and cast it vpon the croked naile, and so drawe it long till it be white, you must kepe it by the fire, as longe as you doe drawe it, that it maie bee hote, and more gentill to drawe, when you iudge it to bee white enough, then cutte it with sheres in peces, if you make this confecciō rounde, long, or otherwise, then take of white Amilum, breake it and stampe it, and laie it vpon the Marble stone, and then cast vpon it the paste of Penidis, and rolle and cutte it, and so make it in what kinde so euer you will, howbeit, you must make it quickly, lest it ware colde betwene your handes, this doen laie it in a siue, or in some other like thing nye the fire, by the space of an hower, then take it awaie, and reserue it: this is good for the lunges or cough.

Sickenes.

How make you pignolatum?

Health.

This confection is made with Sugar, dissolued in Rose water, and well clarified, and when it is sodden enough, put in Pine-aples pared, and let it stande and coule, till it come to the forme of a harde confection, and then reserue it.

Sicknes.

How make you pilule sine quibus nolj.

Health.

First take of Aloes washed. ʒ. xij. of the fiue kindes of Mirabolans, Reubarbe, Mastike, Roses, Wormewood, Violtes, Sene, Agarike, Dodder, ana. ʒ. temper theim with the iuce of Fenell, into the whiche you shall put. ʒ. vj. of Scamonie well broken, how be it, mingle your Scamonie with the iuce of Fenell, then presse foorthe your iuce with the Scamonie, so moche as will suffice for the concoction, then make your pilles with your handes, anointed with the oile of Violetes, or oile Oliue. These bee presente Pilles to purge Choler, Fleume, and Melancolie, against euill sight, whiche cometh of abundance of humours, against paine of the eares, and of iliaca passio.

Sicknes.

How make you pilule Auræ.

Health.

Take of Aloes, Diacridion, ana. ʒ. b. of Roses, Smalege seede, ana. ʒ. ſs. of Aniseede, Fenell seede, ana. ʒ. i. of Mastike. ʒ. i. of Saffron, of the inner parte of Coloquintida, make your pilles with the infusion of gumme Tragantum. These bee very excellente Pilles to purge the hed, and to amende the iye sight, the winde in the stomacke or bowelles, and thei purge without any paine.

Sicknes.

How make you pilule Cochie.

Health.

First take of the pouder of Hiera picra. ʒ. r. of Coloquintida. ʒ. iij. ℈. i. of Scamonie. ʒ. ii. of Turbith Sticades, ana. ʒ. b. mire it with the syrup of Sticados, and so make your pilles. These doe purge the hedde merueilouslie well, but chiefly of grosse and colde humours, it asswageth the hedde ache and reume.

Sicknes.

How make you pilule de octo rebus.

Health.

The booke of Compoundes.

Ake of Aloes Diacridion, ana, ʒ.ii. of the inner parte of Coloquintida, and of the flowers of harder Time, Agarike, Mastike the thirde kinde of Mirabolans, wormewood, ana.ʒ.i. temper them with the iuce of night shade.

Sicknes.

How make you pilule de Mirabolanis.

Health.

Firste take of the fiue kindes of Mirabolans, Agarike, Diagridion, Coloquintida, Sene, ana. ʒ.ſſ. the flowers of the harder Tyme, Turbithe, Aniſſeede, Fenell, Mastike, the stone Lazure, ana.ʒ.iii. of Aloes.ʒ.i. make these pilles with the iuce of wormewod, and if you mingle a little Ginger with them, your pilles shall bee the better. These pilles be verie good against the ache of the hippe, or huckell bone, the goute and the splene. Thei doe clere the sight, and purge burnt choller.

Sicknes.

How make you pilule Elephaneniæ.

Health.

Firste take of Cinamom, Cubebes, ligni Aloes, Calamus Aromaticus, Mace, Nutmegges, Cardamom, Cloues, Asarabacca Mastike, Squinantum, Spicknarde, the fruite of Balme, ana ʒ.i. of drie Wormewood and Roses, ana. ʒ.v. stampe thē, but not smal, and then put vnto theim.li.xii. of water, seeth theim till twoo partes of the water bee consumed, then rubbe theim with your handes, and strain them, and presse forthe the water, this doen, take of Aloes Succotryne.li.i. wasshe it in a Skillet, or soche like vessell of stone, couered or elles with glasse: you muste wasshe it ofte, and with raine water, then drie it, and cast vpon it.li.ii. of that whiche you did presse forthe before, drie it in the Sonne, then mingle it with your Aloes of Mirrhe, Mastike, ana, ʒ.v. of Saffron.ʒ.iii. beate them well, and caste vpon them the residue of that, whiche was strained, and rubbe theim with your handes, vntill thei be broken: many Poticaries wasshe Aloes, with infusion of Rubarbe. These pilles asswage paine of the stomacke, whiche cometh of fleume, and purgeth the stomacke very wel, the brain and the instrumentes of the sences, from grosse and corrupt humours.

Sicknes.

How make you pilule Aggregatiue.

Health.

Firſt take of the first kind of Mirabolans of Reubarbe, añ.ʒ.iii of the iuce of Egrimonie, and Wormewoode, ana, ʒ.ii. of Diagridion.ʒ.vi. of the thirde kinde of Mirabolans, Agarike, Coloquintida,

The booke of Compoundes. Fol.xxiij.

loquintida, Polipody, ana. ʒ. ii. of the best Turbith, of Iloes, ana. ʒ. vi of Mastike, Roses, Salgem, the flower of harder Tyme, Iniseede, Ginger, ana. ʒ. ſs. of the Electuarie of Roses, as moche as will suffice, to make it thicke. These pilles be verie good against long Agues, and those whiche be vexed with superfluous humours, ache of the hedde, stomacke and Liuer, thei purge corrupte Choler, Melancholie, and Fleume, thei quicken and refreshe the instrumentes, of the senses.

Sicknes.

How make you Pilles of Reubarbe.

Health.

Take of Liquores, iuce of wormewood, Mastike, ana. ʒ. s. of the first kinde of Mirabolās. ʒ. iii. ſs. of Smallage seede, wilde Lillies, Fenel, ana. ʒ. ſs. of Trochisti, Diarodon, ana. ʒ. iii. ſs. of Hetra Picra. ʒ. x. of Reubarbe. ʒ. iii. make them with Fenell water. These pilles cure long Agues, and those, whiche be also engendred of diuers groce and corrupt humours, thei asswage the paine aboute the liuer, and chiefly thei cure the dropsie: some Phisicions vse these in the ende of a mirte tercian, you maie make thē stronger with other simples, as you iudge best for the paciēt, take of these in the morning. ʒ. ii. or. ʒ. i. ſs

<small>Citrine Mirabolans, bee taken for the first kinde.</small>

Sickenes.

How make you pilule de Sarcocolla.

Health.

Take of the gumme Sarcocolla. ʒ. iii. of Turbythe. ʒ. iiii. of Coloquintida. ʒ. i. ſs. of Salgem. ʒ. i. dissolue the Sarcocola in Rose water, and mingle all the other with it, and so make your Pilles, these purge fleume, how be it, few Phisiscions do vse them.

Sicknes.

How make you pilule fœtide maiores.

Health.

First take you of Serapinum, Amoniack, Opopanax, Bdelliū, Coloquintida, wilde Rue, Iloes, the flowers of the harder Time, ana. ʒ. b. of Spurge, Clammony. ʒ. iii. of Cinamum, Spyckenarde, Saffron, the Otters stones, ana. ʒ. i. of Turbythe ʒ. iiii. of Gynger. ʒ. i. ſs. of Euphorbe. ʒ. ii. dissolue your gumme in the iuce of Leekes, and so make your Pylles. These Pilles purge grose humours, and be very good against ache in the ioynctes, and goute in the feete, againste paine in the backe, knees, stomacke, the Colike, white Leaper and Pore.

Sicknes.

How make you pilulæ de Euphorbio.

Health.

Take

The booke of Compoundes.

A good pille for Sciatica.

Ake Euphorbium, Coloquintida, Agarike, Bdellium, Serapin ana. ʒ.ii. of Aloes. ʒ.v. make Pilles, with the iuce of Leekes. These purge fleame, and do also mollifie, they cure the Paulsie, and purge grose humours, which haue course to the ioinctes and sinewes, they cure the ache and paine in the hippe and huckell bone of humours.

Sicknes.

How make you pilule lucis maiores.

Health.

First take of Roses, vyolettes, wormewoodde, Coloquintida, Turbythe, Cubebes, Calamus Aromaticus, Nutmigges, Spicknarde, the flower of harder Tyme, the seede and wodde of Balme, Siler Montanum, Rueseede, Squinantum, Azarabacca, Mastyke, Cloues, Cinamum, Anysseede, Fenell, Smallage, Casiafistula, Saffron, Mace, ana. ʒ.ii. of all the kindes of Mirabolans of Rewbarbe. ʒ.vi. of Aloes, Succotrine asmuche as of them all, make them with the iuce of Fenel. These be present remedy against dimnes of the sight, they purge the instrumentes of the senses, and superfluous humours, they kepe the body stronge and in health.

Sickenes.

How make you Pilule lucis minores.

Health.

Ake of the wodde of Balme and the seede of Balme. ana. ʒ.i. of Selyden. ʒ.v. of Roses, vyoletes, wormewod, Eyebright, ana. ʒ.iii. of Sene, the flowers of harder Time, of all the kyndes of Mirabolans, of Agarike, Coloquintida, Squinans, the stones Lazule and Licius, ana. ʒ.ii. of Aloes, Succotrine, asmuche as of them all, make them with the iuce of Selendine or Fenell. These doe purge Melancholy better than the other.

Sicknes.

How make you pilule de Lapide lazule.

Health.

Ake of the stone Lazule washed. ʒ.v. ȳ flowers of harder Time, of Polipodie, ana. ʒ.viii. of Scamonie, of Salte, ana. ʒ.ii.ß. of Agarike. ʒ.viii. of Cloues, Anisseede of Hiera Picra. ʒ.xv. make them with the iuce of Endif. These be excellent Pilles against longe diseases of Melancholy and burnt choler.

Sicknes.

How make you pilule de Bdellio.
Health.

Take

Take of Bdelliū. ʒ.xii. of Inniseedes. ʒ.iii. of all kindes of Mirabolās, of Amber ana. ʒ.ii.ß. mingle your Bdelliū with the iuce of Leekes, and so make the Pilles. These Pilles haue bene proued against runnyng Emerodes, and the sores of them, and to stoppe the termes menstruall in women.

Sicknes.

How make you pilule de Hermodactylis.

Health.

Take of wilde Lilles, of Aloes, of yelow Mirabolans of Turbith Coloquintida, Bdelium, Serapinum, ana. ʒ.vi. of the Otters stones, of the gumme, Sarcocolla, Euphorbe, Opopanax, wilde, Rue, Smallage, anna. ʒ.iii. of Saffron. ʒ.i.ß. mingle these with the iuce of Colewortes, and make them in Pilles.

Hermodactili bee. ii. kindes, one like a Lilly hauing one rote the other like Saffron, both roote and flower, but greter, but this is called in y Greke Ephemeron.

Sicknes.

How make you pilule Arthiticæ.

Health.

First take of Ephemeron, Turbythe, Agarik, ana. ʒ.iiii. of Casia fistula, Spicknard, Cloues, the wood and seede of Balme, Ginger, Mastike, Fenel, Iniseede, Saxafrage, Sperage, Kneholme or Buchers Brome, Roses, Gromell seede, Salgem. ana. ʒ.ß. of Aloes Succatrini, asmuche as of them all, make them with the iuce of Fenell. These Pilles cure the goute of the ioynt of the feete.

Sicknes.

How make you pilule Stomachicæ.

Health.

Take of Aloes. ʒ.vi. of Masticke, of Roses, ana. ʒ.ii. make theim with the iuce of Nightshade. These purge the stomake and hed. You maie make theim with Mirabolans, Citrine, Aloes, Turbeth ana. ʒ.x. Roses, Spicknarde, Mastike ana. ʒ.ii.ß. Inisedes. ʒ.i.ß. sal Gemme, and Safron ast. ʒ.i. make this with syrup of Wormwood.

Mesues pilles for the stomacke.

Sicknes.

How make you pilule Ante cibum.

Health.

Take of ligni Aloes, Cloues, Folium indicū, Mastyke, the wodde and seede of Balme, Cassia wood, Mace, Nutmegges, Cynamū Cubebes, Saffron, siler Montan, Spicknard, ana. ʒ.ii. of Reubarbe, & Aloes Succatrine, asmuche as of them al, mingle them with sweet wine, and make your Pilles. These Pilles cause good digestion, and distribute meate vndigested, and must be taken before meate.

Sicknes.

How make you Pilles of Agarike, or Agarici.

Health.

Take

The booke of Compoundes.

Take of Agarike, Mastike, ana. ʒ. iii. gardē Lillie rootes, Horehoūd ana. ʒ. ii. of Turbith. ʒ. ß. Hiera picra. ʒ. ii. of Coloquintida, the gumme Sarcocoll, ana. ʒ. ii. of Mirrhe. ʒ. i. make these Pilles with the iuce of Erbes or frutes fined either in the sonne or by the fier and this iuce so fined, is called of the Pothicaries *Rob.* These Pilles purge the stomacke from grose and corrupt humours, and thei bee verie good against shortnes of the wynde, and olde coughes.

Sicknes.

How make you Pilles of Fumiterre.

Health.

Take of the fiue kindes of Mirabolans, ana. ʒ. ß. of Aloes. ʒ. vi. of Scamonie. ʒ. ß. mingle them with the iuce of Fumiterie, & let them stande til thei be drie, then sprincle on againe the iuce of Fumeterie, and suffer them againe to drie, and so do the thirde time then let them stande vntill they be thicke, and then make your pilles.

Sicknes.

How make you pilule Comunis.

Health.

This pille is agaīste the pestilēce, and called Ruffy.

Take of Aloes. ʒ. ii. of Saffrō, Mirrhe, ana. ʒ. i. make them with sweet wine. These Pilles be muche vsed of the Phisicions, if they be taken in sommer, and if you take them in ẏ plage time, then you must put vnto them as much Bolermoneake as of Aloes.

Sicknes.

How make you pilule de Asseyeret.

Health.

First take of Hiera Picra. ʒ. i. of Mastyke, of yelow Mirabolās ana. ʒ. ß. of the best Aloes. ʒ. ii. make your Pilles with the iuce of Stycados. These Pilles be a present remedy agaynst the headache.

Sicknes.

How make you pilule Bichiæ.

Health.

Take of the iuce of Liqueris, Amili, Tragantum, gumme Arabyke, sweet Almōdes, ana. ʒ. i. of Suger. ʒ. iii. make them with the slimie sappe of the seede of Quinces.

Sicknes.

How make you pilule imperiales.

Health.

Take Cinamom, Amonium, Aniseede, Mastike, Cardamom, Ginger, Setwall, Mace, Nutmegges, Cloues, Saffrō, Cubebes, ligni Aloes,

The booke of Compoundes. Fol.xxv.

Aloes, Turbyth, Manna, or sweet dewe, Agarike, Sene cods, Spicknarde, of the fiue kindes of Mirabolans, ana. ℈. i. of Rewbarbe, as muche as of them all, of Aloes as much as of all the other, make them with the sirrup of Roses or Uyolets.

Sicknes.

How make you pilule de Hiera picra.

Health.

Take of the pouders of Hyera picra, simpler. ʒ. i. make them with the conserue of Roses as much as will suffice.

Sicknes.

Some tyme the bodies of menne, women, and children, bee so weake and febell, that thei bee not able to receiue purgacions by Electuaries, Pilles, or Glisters, what easie meanes is then to be founde, to purge the bellie, I praie you tell me.

Health.

There bee diuers meanes to bee founde, as appereth by Nicolaus Myrepsi, whereas he teacheth how to make Suppositores: as for example, here is one of them. ℞. Elleborus the black. ʒ. ii. and good yelowe Aloes. ʒ. i and Mousedounge. ʒ. iii. beate these in pouder, seeth them in Honie, vntill the thicknesse of a suppositorie, then make one or twoo, in the forme of a longe small finger, then put a little fine Cotten vpon the ende thereof, and so put it in the bodie, and this will bring foorthe bothe Choler and Fleume, also here foloweth an other, to pulle doune the swellyng of the bellie, winde in the greate guttes, Chollike, or soche like, take the seede of Rewe, called herbe Grace, or of wilde Rewe, of Agarike, ana. ʒ. iii. Commine well dried, Turpete, ana. ʒ. ß. Dacridium, ʒ. ß. ℈. iiii. beate these fine in pouder accordingly, then put in salt Peter, or comon salte. ℈. iiii. and seth it in Honie, as is aforesaied: Here also doeth folowe the making of an other, to relaxe the bellie, take of ye iuce of Rapes, or Panis Porcinus ʒ. i. and salte of the yearth, or comon salte. ℈. iiii. & Honie as moche as will suffice, as in the maner aforesaied. But if you will purge Choler aduste, fleume, or winde in the bellie, Colocynthidis, called Coloquintida, the inward parte therof, but not the seedes. ʒ. iii. Polipody clene washed. ʒ. iii. Bulles or Ore gaule. ʒ. i. and Honie, as example before. I haue shewed you the waie of purging suppositers, now shall I shew you the maner to make some suppositers to heale Dysenteria, or flux of bloud, coming from the apostumacions bred in the liuer, and sometime a perilous flixe, with rasyng or excoriacion, continuall turmentes, and moste greuous paines in the guttes, with casting out yellow choller, sharpnes of bloud, choller aduste, salte fleume, whiche sicknes haue slaine many men, women, and children, for lacke of helpe.

To make good suppositors laxatiue

Suppositors to help colike

Suppositors to stop fluxis.

E. i. ℞. Opinum

The booke of Compoundes.

℞. Opium, whiche is the iuce of Poppie dried, Mirrhe, Castorium, whiche be the dried stones of Beuer, Safron, Frankinsence, Hypocistidis, ana. ʒ. vi. Styrax. ʒ. iii. and a little wine and Honie accordingly, and so seeth your suppositer to the thicknes, and roule it three finger lenth. In other for the same.

Caster, is Beuers stones.

℞. Opobalsamum, and the fine lockes of Wolle, roule theim together, in the maner of a suppositer, this hath a merueilous workyng, saieth Nicolaus Myrepsy in this case: an other for the same.

℞. Opium, Myrrhe, Safron, Dragones bloud, Bolearmoniake, Lemmy, called Tarra sigillata, Mastike, ana. ʒ. i. the iuce of Planten and of Knotgrasse, and a little Goates milke, asmoche as will suffice, putting in a little of Icacia, or the iuce of Slose, or wilde Plummes, beaten together in a morter, and then seeth it in a little panne, powryng in a fewe droppes of Oile and Winegar, and when it is thicke, roule it in a suppositer: prouided that your saied suppositers bee. ʒ. i. in waight, and those be beste, saieth that learned man Nicolaus Myrepsi, also his counsell is, to make them in length, more then thre fingers. Now shall I shewe you the maner, of an other laxatiue suppositer, and so I will make an ende of theim.

℞. Mercurie and Wormwood, dried and beaten in pouder, the rind of Colocinthida, Igarice, and Hierapicra, ana. ʒ. i. comon salte, or salt Peter. ℈. iii. and Honie as moche as will suffice, and then make your Suppositer.

Sicknes.

Oftentimes chaunceth great perilles emong women, when as either nature is to weake, wherby menstruall termes are stopped, or the childe within the belly dedde, wherbpon women oftentimes doe die, I praie you tell me some spedie remedie, and approued medicene, that will so open the matrixe, whereby the dedde childe maie be cast forthe, to helpe the woman.

Health.

Opophalion is an excellēt Emplaster, to deliuer or bryng forth a dedde childe from the mother.

There is no better medicene, then this folowyng, called Ompophalion. ℞. Rapeseede, Sal Niter, Elleborus, the white and the blacke, Colocinthidis, called Coloquintida, Staphes agre, ana. ʒ. iii. Scamoni. ʒ. ii. the iuce of Elaterii, whiche is a wilde Cucuber, or Cucumeres anguini. ʒ. ii. ß. beate your dried thinges into pouder, and put theim into the Oile of Ireos, and the gaule of an Oxe, or Bull, ana. ʒ. iii. mingled together with the pouder of Carthamus. ʒ. iii also dissolue in your saied oile Amoniac. ʒ. iiii. then stampe bitter Almōdes. li. ß. with your foresaid receiptes, in a stone morter, then spred it vpon a pece of leather, and make a greate broade plaster, and aplie it vpon the bellie of a woman, for soche a case as I haue saied, and it will worke accordinglie.

Sicknes.

How make you Pomatum.

Health.

Take of the fatte of a yonge Kyd. li.i. temper it with the water of Muske Roses, by the space of foure daies, then take fine apples and dresse them and cut them in peeces and larde them with Cloues, then boyle them all together in the same water of Roses, in one vessell of Glasse, set within another vessell, let it boyle on the fier so longe vntill all be white, then washe them with the same water of Muske roses, this done, kepe it in a glasse and if you will haue it to smel better, then you muste put vnto it a littell Ciuet or Muske or of theim bothe, and Amber grice. Gentilwomen doe vse this to make their faces smothe and faier, for it healeth cleftes in the lippes, or in any other place of the handes and face. &c.

Sicknes.

How make you Rosata nouella.

Health.

Take of Roses, Suger, Liqueres, ana. ʒ.i.ʒ.ii. of Cinamom. ʒ.ii ℈.iii. of Cloues, Spicknarde, Gynger, Galinga, Nutmegges, Setwall, Storax, Calamita, Cordaniom, Smalage, ana. ℈.i. ℈.viii. make these in pouder. This pouder stopeth bomityng and castyng of the stomacke, it fortefieth those whiche haue been longe sicke, and letteth ouer much sweatyng.

Sicknes.

How make you Syrupus de acetositatis citri.

Health.

Take of the tarte and sower iuce of Pomecitron. li.xii. seeth it in a vessell of Glasse, on the coales with a soft fier, till the thirde parte be consumed, then straine them, and let it stande til it be cleare, and take of that which is cleare. li.vii. and then power vpon it fined Iulep. li.v. seeth theim vntill it bee thicke, if it bee in Sommer, then let it stande in the Sunne till the water be consumed. This is a present remedy agaynst all diseases whiche come of grose and corrupt humours, against the pestilence and all poysons, it dothe also quenche thirste.

Sicknes.

How make you Sirupus de Acetosæ.

Health.

Take of the iuce of Sorell clarified. li.iii. of Suger clarified. li. ii. make of these your sirup. This sirup is good against colerike persons, and tercian Agues, the burning of the stomacke, and the harte, it is a singuler remedy in plages, and in Agues of corrupte humours.

The booke of Compoundes.

Sicknes.

How make you Syrup de Agresta labrusca, oꝛ vnripe Grapes.

Health.

First make this syꝛup of vnripe grapes, as you did the syꝛup of Pomecitron. This cannot be made but onely in sõmer, because the iuce of the vnripe grape cannot be gotten but at that time.

Sicknes.

How make you syꝛup of Calamintes, oꝛ de Calaminta?

Health.

Take bothe of the Garden and wilde Calamintes, ana. ʒ.ii. of Louage, yelow Carots, Squinantum, ana. ʒ.ʋ. of Raysens of Coꝛans picked. li.ſſ. of Hony. li.ii. and so make it: you must take li.ʋ. of water, to boile your Reasons in theim, then this beyng caste foꝛthe, take asmoche again, and let it seeth till the halfe be consumed, afterward put you Honie vnto it, and make your syꝛuppe accoꝛdingly. This syꝛup is a pꝛesent medicine against all diseases of the splene, and chiefly if it be made hard, it doeth cõfoꝛt those, whiche haue their inwarde and pꝛincipall partes colde, oꝛ be shoꝛte winded, oꝛ haue any cough, foꝛ it doeth purge the stomacke, bꝛeaste, and bowelles merueilous well, of grosse and coꝛrupt humours.

Sickenes.

How make you syꝛuppe De mentæ.

Health.

Take of the iuce of Quinces, and sowꝛe Pomgranettes, cast vpõ these iuces, of dꝛie Mintes. li.i.ſſ. of Rose leaues. ʒ.ii. lette it stande a daie and a night, then set it ouer a softe fire, with Honie and Sugar, vntill the halfe be consumed: mingle with your syꝛup the confection called Gallia Muschata, to make theim pleasaunte. This syꝛuppe is good foꝛ a colde stomacke, it stoppeth vomityng, and the disposicion vnto it: it taketh awaie the hicket, and fluxes and cold, oꝛ winde in the guttes.

Sicknes.

How make you syꝛuppe De abſinthio.

Health.

Take of Woꝛmewoode. li.ſſ. of redde Roses, ana. ʒ.ii. of Spickenard. ʒ.iii. of good olde wine and newe, of the iuce of Quinces ana. li.ii.ſſ. let it stande a daie and a night, in a vessell of stone, then seeth it with a soft fire, till the halfe bee consumed, with. li.ii. of Honie, and then make the syꝛuppe. This is an exellente medicine to foꝛtifie the stomacke, and to cause good appetite, to make strong the bowels & liuer, and chiefly when the diseases cometh of a cold cause, it helpeth also in hote diseases, if it be tempꝛed with colde thinges.

Sick.

The booke of Compoundes. Fol.xxvij.

Sicknes.

How make you syruppe of Fumitarie?

Health.

Take of all the kindes of Mirabolans, ana. ʒ.xx. of the flowers of Borage, Buglosse, and Violettes, of Wormewoode, Dodder ana. ʒ.i. of Liqueres, Roses, ana. ʒ.ß. the flower of garden time Polipodie, ana. ʒ.vii. of Prunes a hundred, of Raisons of Corans piked, ana. li.ß. of the fruite Thamarind, Casiafistula, ana. ʒ.ii. let these boile in. li.x. of water, till it come to. li.iii. make your syruppe with the iuce of Fumitarie, sodden and fined with. li.iii. of Sugar, sething them accordyng to the arte. In this syrup makyng, you must obserue this order, in putting of your simples, bicause some require more time and some lesse, therefore first of all putte in Polipodie, then Prunes, Raisens, Liquores, Wormwood, Roses, Dodder, and Borage flowers, afterwarde Violettes, Mirabolans, flowers of harder Tyme, Casiafistula, Thamarinde, whiche after some Phisicions iudgemēt should not boile, bicause it is verie tender, how bee it, other learned menne thinke it beste, to putte it in the latter ende of the decoction, and so to suffer it to boile ones, that it maie the better be mixed with the other and if a man would contende, that softe and tender simples, dooe lese their moistnes in boilyng, then wee muste answere, that thei lese not their naturall moistnes, but the vnnaturall and accidentall, and you must also obserue this order whiche foloweth, if you will make your syruppe well, when your decoction is made, then clarifie your Suger with welle water, the whiche beyng sodden and clarified, put into it the iuce Fumetarie, when it cometh nie to the fashion of a syruppe. The same decoction must be sodden oftentymes, by little and little, til it shall be well and perfectly sodden, then put in your fruite Thamarinde and Casiafistuly, and so make an ende of your decoction. This syruppe openeth, and taketh awaie all obstruction, bothe of the stomacke, and of the liuer, and fortefieth all the members, it cureth all the sores about the inwarde partes, whiche come of salte, and burnte matter, as the scabbe, leaper, and Frenche Pocke.

An obiection for syruppes.

how to make Syruppes.

Sicknes.

How make you sirupus de Fumoterre simplex.

Health.

First take of the iuce of Fumetarie well fined. li.iiii. of Sugar clarified. li.ii.ß. make a syruppe, this clense the liuer.

Sicknes.

How make you a syruppe of Liqueres?

Health.

E.iii. Take

The booke of Compoundes.

A Medecine very good for the Pleurici.

Take of Lyquoris. ʒ. ii. of Maydenheere. ʒ. i. drie Hysop. ʒ. ſſ. caste vpon these. li. i. of water, & let it stande a day and a night, then seeth it till the halfe be consumed, this done, put these vnto the decoction of Sugar, Hony, Pendice, ana. ʒ. viii. of Rose water ʒ. vii. make of these a syruppe. This is a presente remedy againste the Pleurici, olde coughes, to purge the stomacke and lunges.

Sicknes.

How make you Syrup of Hysop.

Health.

This syrupy excelleth in vertue for the Lunges.

Take of drie Hysop, the roote of Smalage, Fenel, Lyqueris, ana ʒ. x. of barly the huske taken of. ʒ. ſſ. of the seede of Malowes, the gumme Tragantum, the kirnels of Quinces, ana. ʒ. iiii. of Maydenheere. ʒ. vi. of Iuiubes, Sebesten. ana. xxx. of Raisons of Corans, picked. ʒ. xii. of Figges, Dates, ana. x. of white Penidis. li. ii. make a syrup. To this syrup makyng take. li. viii. of water and seethe it vntill it be come to three, then presse it, & let it boyle with Pendice, vntill it come to the forme of a syrup, and in makyng of it you ought to kepe this order for your simples first take Iuiubes Sebest, Raisons Figges, Dates, the roote of Smalage, Fenel, then Barly, Malowseede kirnels of Quinces the gumme Tragantum, Hysop, Maydenheere. This sirup cureth diseases of the stomacke, the coughe, pleurici, shortnesse of winde, and all griefes of the body.

Sicknes.

How make you Sirupus de Marubio.

Health.

A good medicine for olde men to clence Fleume.

First take of greene and younge Horehounde. ʒ. ii. drie Hysope, Maydēheere, ana. ʒ. vi. Liquoris. ʒ. i. of Calaminte, Anisseede the rootes of Smalage and Fenell, ana. ʒ. v. of Malowes seede Fenegrike, Flouredeluce, ana. ʒ. iii. of Lynseede, kirnels of Quinces, ana. ʒ. ii. of Raysons of Corans picked. ʒ. v. Figgs. xv. of Penedice. li. ii. of Hony. li. ii. make of these your syrup, you must take to the makynge of this syrup. li. x. of water whiche shall boyle till the halfe be consumed, because the Hony and Penedice require muche seethyng. This syrup cureth olde coughes, longe diseases of the breast & lunges, shortnes of the winde, and chiefly in olde men, if it come of a fleugmatike humour, grose, corupt and harde to be dissolued.

Sicknes.

How make you Sirup de Epithymo.

Health.

first

The booke of Compoundes.   Fol.xxviij.

First take of harder Time of the garden. ʒ.xx. of the twoo firste kindes of Myrabolans, ana. ʒ.xv. of Dodder, Fumiterre, ana. ʒ.x. of Tyme, Buglose, Calamynte, the fouerth and fifte kinde of Mirabolans, of Liqueris, Polipodie, Agarike, of Stycados, ana. ʒ. vi. of Roses, Fenel, Inysseede, ana. ʒ.ii.ß. of Raysons of Corans. ʒ.iiii of Thamarinde. ʒ.ii.ß. of Sugar. li.iiii. and here you muste putte to the makyng of this. li. x. of water whiche muste bee sodden to three. li. this muste bee kepte, as concernyng the puttyng in of your Simples, fyrst take Polipodie, Agarike, Raysons, Liquores, Fenell, Iniseede, Stycados, Fumiterre, the Roses, Doder, Buglosse, Myrabolans the stones taken out, and the flowers of ye harder Time, dissolue your Thamarinde in one parte of the decoction, and let your Suger boyle with new wine, boyled to the thirde parte, whan your decoction shall be as thicke as Hony, yet seeth it a littell more, and in the ende put in your Thamarinde, and let them boyle once or twise, till they come to the thicknes of a syrup. This is aproued medicen agaynst the French Pockes, Cankers, fallyng of the heere, greate and deepe woundes, lepres, and all diseases of Melancholy and burnte Choler. This doeth purge meruelous well, yf a man take therof a good quantitee, comenly we ought to take from. ʒ.iiii. to. vi.ʒ.

There be. v. kindes of Mirabolans, whose names be, Citrine Cheduli Indu Bellerici Emblici.

To help a common knowen malady bothe in Englande and Fraunce called the pox

Sicknes.

How make you sirupus de Eupatorio.

Health.

Take of the rootes of Smalege, Endiue, ana. ʒ. ii. of Liquores, Squinantum, Dodder, Wormewood, Roses, ana. ʒ.vi. of Maidenheer, Cardus Benedictus the flower, of rootes of Buglosse, Inisede Fenel sede, Agremonie, ana. ʒ. v. of Reubarbe, Mastike, ana. ʒ.iii of Spicknarde, Asarabacca, Folium indicum, seeth them in. li. viii. of water, vntill the thirde parte be consumed, and make a syrup with. li iiii. of Sugar, and with a sufficient quantitee of Smalage and Endiue. This sirup is good in longe Agues, chiefly to fortifie the weakenesse of the liuer and stomacke, it cureth the dropsie, and euill likynge of the body, olde and almost vncurable sores, deliuereth the stomacke from wind and coldnes, it aswageth also the payne of the midref and swellyng therof.

Againſt Dropſie.

Sicknes.

How make you syrup of Sticados.

Health.

Take of the flowers of Sticados. ʒ.xxx. Tyme, Calamint, Organie. ana. ʒ.x. of Iniseede, Pellitarie of Spaine, ana. ʒ.vii. long Peper. ʒ.iii. Gynger. ʒ.ii. of Raysons of Corans. ʒ.iiii. of Suger li.v. put also vnto them these pouders folowyng, Cynamom, Calamꝰ Aromaticus, Saffron, Ginger, blacke Peper, longe Peper, ana. ʒ.i.ß.

E.iiii.   bynde

The booke of Compoundes.

bynde them in a thinne clothe, and hang them in the sirup. This hath ben proued against all colde diseases, of the sinewes, as the Paulsie, faulyng euell, crampe, shaking, writhyng of the necke on the one side, reumes from the head to the breast, and doeth comforte the stomacke and the inwarde partes of the bodie.

Sicknes.

How make you sirupus de Violes, or Violettes?

Health.

Take .li.b. of the infusion of violets, of Sugar clarified .li.iiii. mingle them together, and seeth them with a soft fier, & kepe them. This is a present medecine against hote Agues and heat of the liuer and harte, the plurasie, drie coughes, the roughnes of the windepype and throate.

Sicknes.

How make you syruppe de Papauere simp. or Poppie?

Health.

Take of the heads of white and blacke Popie, ana. lx.z. seeth thē in .li.iiii. of raine water vntill it come to .li.ss. and with .z.iiii. of white Sugar and Penedise make your sirup. This siruppe causeth a man to sleape, and quencheth the thyrst, it stoppeth reumes running to the breast, and doth mitigate the pain. This is not so cold as the compounde Papauer.

Sicknes.

How make you sirupus de Papauere Compositum?

Health.

Take of white and blacke Popie. ana. z.l. of Maidenheere. z.rv. of Sugar. z.v. of Iuiube. rr. of Lettise seede. z.xl. of Malowes seede, of the kirnels of Quinces, ana. z.vi. seeth them in .li.iiii. of water, vntill the halfe be consumed, then make your sirup with. z. viii. of Sugar and Penedise. This compounde sirup hath the same vertue, which the simple hath, but it causeth great colde & aswageth paine better. Mesuas doth iudge it to be good agaynst a drie coughe and a consumption.

Sicknes.

How make you Sirup of Mirtes comp.

Health.

Take .xx. Mirtes, of Saunders white and red, of Manna or swete dewe of heauē, the flouers of wilde Pomgarnets, Barberies, ana. z.rv. of Medlers. z.l. of well water .li.viii. boile thē al to the half then strain them, and put into the strayning, the iuce Pomgarnets & Quinces, ana. z.vi. of Sugar clarified .li.iii. mingle these, and seeth them

The booke of Compoundes.   Fol.xxix.

them vntill they come to the fashion of a syrup.

Sicknes.

How make you Syrup of Myrtes, simp.

Health.

Take of the iuce of Myrtes. li. xii. seethe it in a vessell of glasse with a soft fier vntil the thirde parte be consumed, then strain it and let it stande vntil it be clarified, then take. li. viii. of that which is clarified, and put vnto it. li. v. of Hony, seeth it till it come to the thicknes of a sirup. ʒ. i. if it be sommer set it in the sunne, vntil the water be consumed. This comforteth the stomacke and al the inward partes, and cureth also an olde coughe.

Sicknes.

How make you sirupus Acetosus simplex.

Health.

Take of good white Sugar. li. viii. and putte it into a vessell of stone, and cast vpon it. li. iii. of cleare welle water, seeth it with coales or els with a littell fier, without smoke, alwaies scommyng it, seeth it till it shalbe cleare, and vntill the water be half consumed. Then put vnto it of Uineger of white wine very strong. li. iii. seeth it vntill it be enough. This is a present remedie against all hoat diseases, subtill or grosse matter, prouoketh vrine, quenche Choler, and doeth extenuate and make grosse thinges soft, and clenseth stinkyng matter in the stomacke.

Sickenes.

How make you sirupus Acetosus compositus.

Health.

Take of well water. li. x. put vnto it the rootes of Fenell, Smalage, Endiue, ana. ʒ. iii. of Anysseede, Fenell seede, Smalage seede, ana. ʒ. viii. of Endiue seede. ʒ. ß. seeth them with a softe fier, vntill they come to. li. v. then straine it, and put to the decoction li. iii. of Suger, let it bee carified as before, and mingle with it a sufficiente quantitee of good vineger, accordyng to the forme of the syrup before. This syrup purgeth groase, and fleume it scoureth, and openeth opilacions and obstructions, whiche be aboute the liuer, splene, and reines.

Sicknes.

How make you syrup de succo Endiuiæ, or Endiue simplex.

Health.

Take the iuce of Endiue fined. li. viii. of Suger clarified. li. v. ß. make your syrup, sething. This is a principal medicin to aswage the

The booke of Compoundes.

the heate of the lyuer, the harte, and the other chief partes, and it cure the Pleuresie.

Sicknes.

How make you sirup of Endiue compositus.

Health.

Take the iuce of Endiue and Fliewoꝛte, ana. li. iii. these iuces must be clarified, then take of Roses, Violets, Letels, Boꝛage, Egrimon, ana. ʒ.ß. of Maydenheere, Barly the huske taken of, of the foure great cold seedes. ana. ʒ. i. of sugar, asmuch as wil suffice make the syꝛup, and pouder it with white and red Saunders, Barberies, kirnels of Quinces, ligni Aloes, Cynamon, the rynde of Pomecitrone, ana. Ɔ. i. This aswageth the great heate of the liuer, and hart and of the other principall partes, it is very good foꝛ all hoate complexions, it loseth and openeth all opilacions, and obstruction it doth comfoꝛt weake members which be troubled with heate it dothe also digest cholerike and sharpe matter.

Sicknes.

How make you syꝛup of Suckerie oꝛ Cichoꝛii.

Health.

Take bothe of the garden and wilde Suckery and of bothe Endiues, ana. M. ii. of Goꝛdes, Lyuerwoꝛte, white Endiue, Lettis Sumterre lupius, ana. M. Barley the huske not taken of, Galtakenge, ana. ʒ. iiii. of Liqueris, Maydenheere, Ceteracke, Centwoꝛt Dodder, ana. ʒ. vi. the rootes of Fenell, Smallage and Sperage. ana. ʒ. ii. boyle them in a sufficient quantite of water and strain them and make your syꝛup with good sugar and foꝛ euery pouñde of Sugar take ʒ. iiii. of Reubarbe and. Ɔ. iiii. of Spicknard bounde in a thinne cloth which shalbe often time pꝛessed, till your syꝛup be well sodden: the quantitee that a man shall take at one tyme is. ʒ. iii. with the water wherin the fower common colde seedes were strained.

Sicknes.

How make you syꝛup of Quinces.

Health.

Take of the iuce of tarte Quinces, fined and clarified, partes. x. Sugar, partes. ii. make a syꝛup accoꝛdyng. This stopeth vomityng, quencheth the thirst and doth comfoꝛt the stomacke.

Sicknes.

How make you syꝛuppe of Nenuphar, oꝛ water Lillis.

Health.

First take. li. ii. of the flowers of Nenuphar, and seeth them ones, then pꝛesse them, and put into the iuce pꝛessed. li. ii. of sugar, and seeth it till it come to the foꝛme of a syꝛuppe.

Sicknes.

Sicknes.

How make you syruppe of Barberies?

Health.

First take of the iuce of Barberies fined. li. iii. of Sugar clarified li. iii. make a syruppe accordingly.

Sicknes.

How make you syruppe of tarte Pomgarnettes?

Health.

First take of the iuce of Pomgarnettes. li. ii. ß. of sugar clarified. li. iii. make this syruppe as before. This syrup is good, againste hote Agues of choler and fleume.

Sicknes.

How make you syrupus de Bizantijs?

Health.

First take of the iuce of Endiue and Smalage, ana. li. ii. of Hops, the garden or wilde Borage, and Buglosse, ana. li. i. boile theim ones and then straine and fine them, this doen, take. li. iiii. of the iuce clarified, of fine Sugar. li. ii. ß. seeth it with a gentill fire, vntill it be thicke as syruppe. This is very good againste Agues, whiche come of obstructions and of choler, of fleume, and also the yelowe Jaunders.

Sickenes.

How make you syrupus de infusione Rosarum viridium? Or grene Roses.

Health.

First take of the infusion of yong Roses. li. v. of Sugar. li. iii. mingle theim, and make a syruppe. This is good for the thriste in burnyng Agues, and to assage the heate, it doeth comforte the stomacke, harte, and liuer, beyng troubled with heate, it preserueth the body fro all corrupcion, and from the pestilence, it resisteth poison.

Sicknes.

How make you syrupus de Rosis succis? Or dried Roses.

Health.

First take you of the infusion of drie Roses, and Suger ana. li. ii. mingle them and make a syrup. This doeth comfort the stomacke, and binde meruellous well.

Sicknes.

How make you syrupus de succo Rosarum?

Health.

First

First take the iuce of Roses fined. li. i: ß. of Sugar clarified. li. i. ß. make a syruppe accordingly.

Sicknes.

How make you syrupus de Iuiube?

Health.

Take. ix. Iuiubes of violetes, Malowes seede, ana. z. v. of Maydenheire. z. i. the kirnell of Quinces sede, of white Popie, Mallowes, and Letice. z. i. the gumme Tragantum, ana. z. iii. of Liquores, Barley, the huske taken of, ana. z. viii. seeth them in. li. iiii. of welle water, or els Raine water, vntil the halfe bee consumed, then strain it, and put vnto the iuce strained. li. iii. of sugar clarified, make your Syrup accordingly. This is very good against horesenes of the voice and the cough, the plurasie, and exulcerations of the bladder.

Sicknes.

How make you syrup of Maydenheere comp.

Health.

First take of Maydenheere. M. ii. of Tentworte, Cetorake, ana. M. i. of Iuiubes, Liqueris, ana. z. ii. make a decoction puttyng vnto it. li. iiii. of Sugar, make your sirup, then take of Maidenheere. li. iiii. of Iuiubes. li. iii. Liqueris. z. iii. of sugar. li. vi. and this syrup is iudged to be the better. This purgeth grose humours, loseth and openeth obstructions, scoureth the raines, and clenseth the brest of grose humours.

Sicknes.

How make you Syrup of Maydenheere, simp.

Health.

First take of the decoction of yonge Maydenheere. li. iii. of Suger li. make your syrup.

Sicknes.

How make you an other syrup of the same.

Health.

First take of Liqueris scraped. z. ii. of Maydenheere. z. v. caste vpon them. li. iiii. of well water, and so let them stande a daye and a night, then boile them vntil the halfe and strayne them, and put vnto the decoction. z. viii. of Sugar clarified, Penedice, and Maydenheere, seeth it till it come to the forme of a syrup.

Sicknes.

How make you syrup of Mugworte.

Health.

Take of Mugworte, ℈.ii. of Calamint, Folium indicum, Sauerie, Organy, Time, Quikebeme, Stichados, ana. ℈.i. of Camomill, Melylot, Mergeram, Roses, ana. ʒ.i. of Vngius odoratus Calamus Aromaticus, ana. ʒ.iii. of Spikenarde. ʒ.i. Germander, Moderworte, Gelofflowers, Sothernwodde, ana. ℈.ß. gladyan, Horehounde, Madder leues, Siluer Montan, ana. ʒ.i. Azarabacca, Squinantum, Anisede ana. ʒ.vi. Fenel, Anyp, Smalage, ana. ʒ.vi. boile thē in a sufficiēt quātitee of water according to the art, then put vnto thē asmuche Hony as wil suffice, and make your sirrup. This is a present remedie to prouoke the naturall termes of women beyng stopped.

Sicknes.

How make you Siripus de Limonibus?

Health.

Take of the iuce of Lemondes. li.i.ß. of Sugar clarified. li.iii. make your sirup. This is very good to consume grose and corrupt humours, and wormes, it aswageth heate in Agues, and purgeth raw humours.

Sicknes.

How make you Sirupus de Cetrach.

Health.

Take of Cetrach, Hartestonge, Endiue, Liuerworte, wormewod Sichorie, ana. ℈.ß. of Dodder, Linseede. ʒ.i. the fower commō great seedes, flowers of Borage, Buglosse, Langdebief, añ. ℈.i. Maydenheere, rootes of Fenell, Parsely, Kneeholme or butchers Broume, ana. ℈.i.ß. make your syrup, and cast on these pouders, Folium Indicum, Spicknard, the gumme Lacca, Casiafistula, ana. ʒ.ii. binde these in a thinne clothe, and boile them in the syrup, and reserue it. This doeth comforte the liuer, scoureth the reines, and deliuereth the splene fro all obstructions.

Sicknes.

How make you the syruppe of Buglosse?

Health.

Take of the infusion of the flowers of Buglosse, or Langedebefe, li.iiii. of sugar. li.ii. make a syruppe.

Sicknes.

How make you an other of the same.

Health.

First take of the iuce of Buglosse, fined. li.iiii. of sugar. li.iii. make your syruppe. This syruppe doeth comfort the stomacke, and maketh a man merie, it is also ministred against sounyng and faintyng of the harte, and franfey.

A present syruppe for the stomacke.

F.i. Sicknes

The booke of Compoundes.

Sicknes.

How make you Sapo Moschatus?

Health.

A very swet Baule to clese the skin.

Take white Uenice Sope. li. iiii. cut it into smal peeces, and the pouder of Cloues, Iuncus Odoratus, Spicknard, white Sañders, ana. ʒ. i. ß. the pouder of Beniamen and fine Masticke, & Storax Calamite. añ. ʒ. i. fine Muske. Ǯ. xxx. Amber greece. Ǯ. xxiiii Ciuet. Ǯ. xvi. put these in a morter with sum Rose water, or els sweet compouded water: you may put in Oyle of Been, or els a litle oyle of Almondes or Jenuper: and so make this sweet baule, & washe therw̄.

Sicknes.

How make you Theriaca Galeni?

Health.

Nicholas prepositus do put in white Coporas.

Take of *Trochiscie, Squillini* or *Scillini*. ʒ. iii. of longe Peper. ʒ. ii. of Trochisci, Theriaci, Diacorallion, añ. ʒ. i. of the woode of Balme. Ɔ iii. the iuce of blacke Popie, Agarike, wilde Rapes seede, Cinamom, the iuce of Balme, añ. Ɔ. ii. of Reubarbe, Safron, Spicknarde, Roses, Yreus, Calamus, Coste, Squinantū, Ginger, Casialyng, Storax Calaminte, Mirrhe, Turpentine washed, white Frākinsens, Calamint, Dittō, Sticados, wilde Tyme, rootes of Sinkefolie, Persely, white Peper, añ. Ɔ. ii. Folium Indicum, gum Arabike, Serapin, terra Sygillate, Hipocistis, Spicknarde, Gladium, Germander, Gentiā, wilde Fenell, the seede of Balme, Smalage, Amonium, Fenell, wilde Carowaies, Siler montan, Cresses, Aniseede, S. Jhons herbe, wilde Aspaltum, which is a thing compouded, and made of Jewes, Pitche, Castor, Opopanar, Galbanū, Mummy, Centaurie, Aristologia longa, wilde yelowe Carettes, ana. Ɔ. i. of Honie asmoche as will suffice.

This is a Triacle of an incomperable vertue agaynste poysen, Pestilence, and venime.

This is iudged to be the chief and principall of all medicines, bicause it bringeth quietnes, and doeth cure the greatest diseases, and greues in euery parte of the bodie, as the fallyng sicknes, and insensibilitie, whiche is a disease, when a manne can neither moue, feele, nor vnderstande, it healeth conuulsions, the hedde ache, paine of the stomacke, megram, horsenesse of the voice, and straitnes of the breast, shortnes of winde, and diseases of the winde pipe, spittyng of bloud, yelowe Jaũders, Dropsie, & the diseases of the liuer: Iliaca passio, woundes exulcerated in the bowelles, fransinesse, the stone, it prouoketh the Termes stopped, and deliuereth women of dedde childzen, it cureth lepres, meselles, and olde diseases: It is a present remedie againste colde, and all poisons, stinging of benemous beastes, and here you must vnderstand that the quantitie ought to be changed in ministryng of it, accordyng to the quantite, and qualitie of euery disease, this doeth refreshe also and comforte the sences, harte, braine, liuer, stomacke, and doeth kepe all the bodie safe and pure, from all corrupcion.

Sicknes.

How make you Trifera?

Health.

Health.

Take the iuce of blacke Popie.ʒ.ii.of Cinamom, Cloues, Galinga, Spicknarde, Setwall, Ginger, Coste, Storar Calamita, Calamus Aromaticus, Cipres, Flowerdelice, Wormesede, Gladian, Mandzager, Spicknard, Roses, Peper, Aniseede, Smalage sede Persely, yelowe Carotes, Henbane, Comine, Basell, of Honie asmocn as will suffice. This is a present medicine against all inwarde diseases of women, and against the paine of the stomacke, taken with the decoction of Aniseede and Mastike: It cureth also all diseases of the Matrice, whiche come of colde, taken with wine, wherein Mugwort was sodden, and if you make a rounde thing of silke or wolle, to seen after the fashion of a finger, and anointe it with the oile of a Wesell, or soche other Oile, and put it into the matrice, then it will moue the flowers of women, whiche doe not conceiue. It is also a singuler remedie for children, whiche speake in their slepe, or cannot slepe, if it be taken with wine, wherein Mandzag or Elder hath been sodden: It will also helpe them, if it be taken with womens milke, accordyng to the quantite of the little graine Cicer.

Sicknes.

How make you *Diatrion Sandalon*.

Health.

First take of white, redde, and yelowe Saunders, of Sugar, an. ʒ.ii. some Poticares take Fleworte for sugar, which is thought to bee better. And Galline doeth make this composicion, after this sorte. Take of Reubarbe, Spodie, Liquores, Purselin seede, ana, ʒ.i.ß. of Amile, Gumme Arabicke, Tragantum, of the fower comon greate seedes, white Endiue seede, ana.ʒ.i.ß. of Camphere.Ɔ.i. so put vnto these fower times as many Roses, as of all the other, and of the syrup of Roses, asmoche as will suffice. This doeth cure the paine of the liuer and stomack, and those whiche be in a consumpcion, or haue the yelowe Iaunders.

A goodly dis to coule the liuer.

Sickenes.

How make you *Trochisci Diarhodon abbatis?*

Health.

Take of Roses, ligni Aloes.ʒ.ii.of Mastike.ʒ.i.ß. Wormewoode, Cinamom, Spicknarde, *Cassiælignum*, Squinantum, ana. ʒ.i. make your balles with old wine, & with the decoctiõ of the cõmon rootes, as Smalage, Percelie, Louage. These balles bee verie good againste olde Agues, and those whiche come of diuers causes, against quotidian and all other Agues, by the whiche the beautie and forme is corrupt & this is put into great confections saith Nicholas.

Sicknes.

The booke of Compoundes.

How make you Trochisci de violetes?

Health.

Take of the young flowers of white violetes, ʒ.v. of Amili, ʒ.iii. the seede of white Popie, ʒ.iii. of Reubarbe, Ɔ.v. the seede of Plantein, ʒ.i. of Balme, Ɔ.i. of Rose water, as moche as will suffice, make it after the forme of the balles before, this is not used but when it is mingled with other composicions.

Sicknes.

How make you Trochisci de Squilla?

Health.

First take one bolle Squilla, and bake it well in paste, and caste awaie the outward rinde, beate the substaunce of Squilla in a morter, and put unto it asmoch of the fine flower of Orobus, and temper it with wine and Honie, and if you haue not Orobus at hande, then take asmoche breade, well and finely broken: make your little balles, and drie theim in the Sunne. Some Poticaries take in this confection, one parte of Squilla, and partes, ii, of Barly flower.

Sicknes.

How make you Trochisci Theriaci.

Health.

First take a yong Adder, of the length of a spanne, with redde iyes, a shaking tongue and hornes, like the graine Sesanium, cutte awaie the hed and taile, about three fingers, that which is in the middes must be dressed, the skin taken of, and the inward partes cast awaie, washe it oft in swete water, and seeth it so long, til the fleshe fall from the backe bone, and temper the fleshe and the iuce of it together, putte unto it asmoche of the flower of Orobus, or of breade, make little balles of the weight of ʒ.ß. drie thē in the shadowe. These be not taken, but when thei bee used with other greate conposicions, except it be in curyng the Leper.

Sicknes.

How make you Trochisci Diacorallion?

Health.

Take of redde Corall, Cinamom, Mirrhe, Amonium, Popie ana ʒ.iiii. of Squinantum, Safron, ana. ʒ.ii. of Calamus Aromaticus, the wood of Balme, Casiafistula, Folium indicum, Masticke, wilde Tyme, Valerian, Azarabacca, herbe Robert, ana. ʒ.i. and these beyng first made in pouder, forme your little balles with wine. These are a present remedie to staunche the bloudie flux, it doeth also fortefie the stomacke, and causeth good digestion.

Sicknes.

The booke of Compoundes. Fol.xxxiij.

Sicknes.

How make you Trochisci de Camphiere?

Health.

Take of Rose leues.ʒ.iiii. of Spodie.ʒ.ii. of yelowe Saunders, ʒ.ii.ß. of Safron.ʒ.ii. of Liquoris.ʒ.ii. of ligni Aloes, Cardamom, Amili, Camphire, ana.Ɂ.i. of sugar, of Manna or sweete dewe, ana.ʒ.iii. make your balles with the sappie parte of flewoꝛte, and Rose water. These be very good in hote Agues, and to quench the thirstie and burnyng of redde choler oꝛ bloud: it aswageth the heate of the stomacke, liuer, of all the inward partes, it cureth the yelowe Jaunders, and those whiche are in consumpcion.

Sicknes.

How make you Trochisci de Alchachengi?

Health.

Take of the Beries of Alchachengi, thꝛee of the lower greater colde seedes, ana.ʒ.iii.ß. of Bolermoniacke, gumme Arabike, white Frankinsence, Dꝛagons bloud, white Popie, bitter Almondes, Liquoris, Tragantum, Amili, the kirnelles of Pineaples, ana.ʒ.vi. of Smalage seede, Amber, Henbane, the iuce of blacke Popie, an̄.ʒ.ii. make your balles with the sappie iuce of the beries of Alchachengi. These bee a pꝛesent medicine against exulceracions in the reines, and the blader, and the paine in pissyng.

Sicknes.

How make you Trochisci de Mirrha.

Health.

Take Mirrhe.ʒ.ii. of Lupus.ʒ.v. the leaues of Rue, wilde Mint Peneriall, Comine, Mader, Peietarie of Spaine, Serapin, Opopinax, ana.ʒ.ii. make balles of the waight of.ʒ.ii. of whiche let the pacient take.ʒ.i. on the daie tyme, in the water wherein Juniper seede was sodden. These be so strong a medicine, to purge the termes in women, that it will cause the childe to discende, if thei vse thē oft, the termes shalbe moued very well: also in boryng the crokyng & bowyng of the hamme, oꝛ in cuttyng the vein, whiche lyeth by the ancell, you maie also vse boryng about the thies.

Sicknes.

How make you Trochisci de Musco?

Health.

Take of the wood of Aloes.ʒ.v. of Amber.ʒ.ii. of Muske.ʒ.i. the gumme of Tragantum, with Rose water asmoche as will suffice, to temper theim together, so make your balles. These doe comfoꝛt the stomacke, harte, and liuer, & be vsed with great medicins.

F.iii. Sicknes.

The booke of Compoundes.

Sicknes.

How make you Trochisci de Rubarbaro.

Health.

Take of Reubarbe.ʒ.x.the iuce of Egremony.ʒ.iiii. of Roses.ʒ. iii. of Spicknarde, Aniseede, Madder, Smalage seede, wormewood, Azarabacca. ana.ʒ.i. bitter Almondes.ʒ.iiii. make your balles of the weight of.ʒ.ß. These doo aswage the paine of the liuer, and do deliuer it from obstructions they cure inwarde impostumes, old griefes, the dropsy and yelow iaunders, and restore good couler, to drinke them is a presente remedy, for these whiche bee of euill lykyng or in consumption. Many Phisicions do vse them in hote Agues, and when the body beginneth to fall into consumption.

Sicknes.

How make you Trochisci de Spodio.

Health.

Take the red Roses.ʒ.xii.of Spodie.ʒ.x.of Sorell seede. ʒ. vi. of Purfline seede, of Coreander seede, infused in Vineger and afterwarde dried, the rinde of the Frankensence tree, ana.ʒ.ii. Ampli made in pouder, the flowers of wylde Pomgarnets, Berberies, ana.ʒ.ii. gumme Arabike made in pouder, ana. ʒ. i. make thele with the iuce of vnripe grapes. These bawles taken with the iuce or seedes of Sorell, be very good against Agues of choler, which haue a continuall flux, they aswage the burnyng of the stomacke and liuer and quenche also the thurst and drinesse.

Sicknes.

How make you Trochisci de Abfintnio.

Health.

Take of Roses, Wormewod, Anysseeds, ana.ʒ.ii. of Rewbarbe, the iuce of Egremonie, Azarabacca, Smalage, bitter Almondes, Spicknarde, Mastike, Folium indicum, ana.ʒ.i. make your balles with the iuce of Endiue. These be good in longe Agues, and deliuer the stomacke and liuer from the principall partes, and doo cause good appetite, if they be dronken in longe Agues they profitte very muche.

Sicknes.

How make you Trochisci de Eupitorio.

Health.

Take of Manna or sweet dew, the iuce of Egremonie, ana.ʒ.i.of Roses.ʒ.i.ß.of Spicknard.ʒ.iii.of Reubarbe Azarabacca, Aniseede, ana.ʒ.ii. of Spodie. ʒ.iii.ß. make your balles with the iuce of Egremon. These be necessary against long Agues, and the cold,

and

The booke of Compoundes. Fol.xxxiiij.

and shaking of them, against obstructions of the liuer and splene and inwarde inpostumes, the yelowe Iaunders, and the dropsie, if thei be taken at the beginning.

Sicknes.

How make you Trochisci de terra sigillata.

Health.

Take of Dragons bloud, gum Arabike made in pouder, Ciuet, Rose seede and leaues, Impli made in pouder, Spody, Acatia, Hipoquistis, the stone which doth stanche bloud, the flowers of the wilde Pomgarnet, Bolermanie Terra Sigillata Hempseede, Cokell, Perles, Amber, ana. ʒ. ii. Cragantum, blacke Popie, ana. ʒ. i. ß. Purslane seede made in pouder, Frankensence, Oke apple, Saffron, an ʒ. ii. make your balles with the iuce of Plantaine. These be excellent balles to staunche spittyng of bloud, and chiefly if they be taken with the water of Plantaine: if the forehead be therwith annoynted, they stoppe the secret termes, and to conclude they stoppe any fluxe, if so be that the place be therwith anoynted.

Sicknes.

How make you Trochisci de Ambre.

Health.

First take of Amber. aur. vi. of Hartes horne made in pouder, gumme Arabike, Corall in pouder, Cragantum, Acatia, Hipoquistis, the flowers of wilde Pomgarnetes, Masticke, the gum of Ladanum washed, blacke Popie made in pouder, ana, aur. ß. make these with the slimie iuce of Flewozte.

Sicknes.

How make you Tela Galterij.

Health.

Take of comon sallet Oile. li. i. of Ceruse. ʒ. iiii. of Litarge. ʒ. iii Mirrhe. ʒ. ß. make these like a ceare clothe, whiche is made of waxe. This doeth heale and drie vp sores.

Sicknes.

How make you Vuguentum Apostolicum.

Health.

Take of Turpentine, white waxe and Rosen, take. ʒ. xiiii. Opopanaxe, the pouder of Brasse, ana. ʒ. iii. Amoniacum. ʒ. xii. Aristologia, Rotunda, white Frankinsens, ana. ʒ. vi. Mirrhe, Galbanum, ana. ʒ. iiii. Opopanax, Verdegres, Bdellum. ʒ. vi. of Litarge ʒ. ix. infuce your Bdellum in good Vineger, and so dissolue it, and seth it in Sommer with. li. ii. of osle, in winter in thre. This cureth easely olde fistulas, swellyng, and harde kirnelles, it eateth awaie deade

F.iiii. flesshe

fleshe, and clenseth the wounde.

Sicknes.

How make you Vnguentum Rosarum.

Health.

Take of yong swines greate, as moche as you will, and washe it in hote water. ix. tymes, and as oft in cold, then stampe it with a greate quantite of yong Roses, and let it stande by the space of seuen daies, afterward seeth them with a soft fire, and straine thē, then take again as many Roses, and stampe them with the greace & so let them stande by the space of .vii. daies then caste vpon them one parte of the iuce of roses, and of the oyle of Almonde .vi. partes seeth all together with a soft fier vnto the iuce be consumed, and if you wil put vnto this Vnguentum rosarū a littell quantitee of Opium, then it wyll proue a very excellent medicine to coole heate and to anoynt the back with all.

Sicknes.

How make you Vnguentum basilicum maius.

Health.

Take of white waxe, Rosen, Talow of a Cowe, drie pitche, the Greke pitch, the fat of the belly of the Sele, fine Frankēsence, Mirrhe, ana. ʒ. vi. of liquid or moyst pitche. ʒ. iii. of al the other ana. ʒ. ii. ß. This is a present oyntment against woundes inflamed & woundes in the sinewes, it doth clense them and brynge new fleshe agayne. The learned Surgens, thinke this oyntment not to bee layde to hot sores or woundes, because it is of his nature also hot, & so shall cause greater inflamacions wherfore vse it rather in woundes without all inflamacions of heate.

Sicknes.

How make you Vnguentum aureum.

Health.

First take of yelow waxe. ʒ. vi. good oyle. li. ii. ß. Turpentine. ʒ. ii. Rosen dried, Pitche, ana. ʒ. i. ß. fine Frankensence, Mastike. ana. ʒ. i. Saffron. ʒ. i. make your oyntment. This hath ben proued for to heale bruses and strokes.

Sicknes.

How make you Vnguentum basilicum minus.

Health.

First take of Rosen, Pitche, waxe and oyle as much as wil suffice and make your oyntment.

Sicknes.

How

The booke of Compoundes. Fol.xxxv.

How make you Vnguentum Populeon.

Health.

Take buddes of Poplar tree.li.i.ſs.blacke Popie, Mandrage leaues, the buddes of Bramble, Henbane, Dwale, Stoncrope, lettice, Howſelike, Burre, Vyolettes, Maydenheere, ana.ʒ.iii. of yonge freſhe ſwines greaſe.li.ii. drie all your herbes and boyle them with the greaſe and ſo make your oyntmēt accordingly. This is good to anoynt the temples, pulſes, the palmes of the handes, and the ſooles of the feate in hotte Agues.

Sicknes.

How make you vnguentum Martiaton.

Health.

Firſt take of white waxe.li.ii. of oyle.li. viii. of Roſemarie, of Bay leaues, ana. ʒ. viii. of Rue. ʒ. viii. of Quikebeme. ʒ. vii. of Sauine, watermintes, Sage, Baſell, wilde time, Calaminte, Mougworte, Enula Campana, Geloufflowers, Brankurſine, gooſe greaſe, Peritorie, Pimpirnell, Egremony, Wormewoode, Primeroſe, Borage, younge buddes of Elder, Orpin, Millefolie, Houſleke Germaunder, Centaurie, Strawberie leaues, Sinckefoly, herbe Judaice ana.ʒ.iiii. the roote of Holy oke, Comin, Mirtell, ana. ʒ. iii. of Fenigreke. ʒ. i. ſs. of freſh butter. ʒ. i. ʒ. ii. of Nettels, Violettes, red popie, of the thyrde kinde of Mintes, of Balme, Dockes Maydenhere, Waleͦthiſtle or Cardus Benedictus, Woodebyne, Valerian, herbe Robert, Sorell de Bois, Hartes tongue, Ore iye, Camphere, Storax, Deareſuet, ana. ʒ. ſs. Maſtyke, ẜ fat of a Beare, and of a whelpe, ana. ʒ. i. of Frankenſence. ʒ. ſs. oyle of Spyke. ʒ. ii. let al your herbes be gotten in May, in one or two dayes together, if it may be, ẜ from.iii.of ẜ clocke in the mornyng vntil. xii. thē ſtampe al your herbes together ẜ infuſe them in ſweet wine. vii. daies, on the eight day ſeeth them ouer a ſoft fier, and whan your wine doeth begin to conſume, then put in your Oyle and boyle them al together vntil your herbes begin to conſume then ſtrayne them, and caſte away the herbes, and ſet the iuce ſtrained on the fier againe, and when it boyleth, put in Storax, and ſoone after the butter and the greaſe, the oyle of Spike, Maſtyke, Frankenſence, waxe, and whan the waxe is melted, then take it from the fier, ſturryng it alwaies til it ſhalbe thicke, and then reſerue it. This is a ſinguler oyntment for a colde headache, the paine of the breaſte and ſtomacke, and agaynſt hardnes of the breaſt, the ſplene and the lyuer, it cureth, *Illiaca paſſio*, if the place be anoynted with the oyntment hot it healeth the Paulſie, the ache of the hippe, and the goute in the feet, the frenſie, ſwellinges, hardened kirnels, the crampe, the conuulſiōs and all other aches of colde.

Sicknes.

The booke of Compoundes.

How make you Vnguentum arogon.

Health.

Take Rosemary, Margeră, the roote of wake Robin, or Kucko pzike wild Tyme, Rue, wilde Cucumer rootes, ana. ʒ. iiii. ß. of Bay leaues, Sage, Sauin, ana. ʒ. iii. of Horsemintes, *Laureolæ*, ʒ. ix. of Brionie rootes. ʒ. iii. of Neppe, wilde Cucumer leaues, ana. li. ß. of Mastike, Frankensence, ana. ʒ. viii. of Pelletarie of Spaine, Euphorbe, Ginger, peper, an̄. ʒ. i. oyle of a Wesel. ʒ. ß. *Olei Petcolii*, the greace of a Beare, oyle of Bay, ana. ʒ. iii. of Butter. ʒ. iiii. of salet Oyle, li. v. of waxe, li. i. ʒ. iii. gather your herbes in May, and vse al other thinges, as in the oyntement before, stampe them well and lay them in oyle in a morter by the space of. viii. dayes, and on the eight day set it on the fier vntill the herbes go downe to the bottome, afterwarde straine them, and then set the iuce strained on the fier again, & whan it beginneth to boyle, put in your oyle of Baye, Butter, the Beares greace and waxe, the which beyng melted, put in Mastike, Frankensence, at the last, Ginger, Peper, Pelletarie of Spaine, Euphorbe, and when they be well sodden, then take all of and reserue. This curethe colde aches, annointed after this fashion, take an Eggeshell & warme the oyntment in it at the fier, then anoynt the place, whan the place is anoynted, lay also the shell vnto wherin the oyntmente was warmed. It helpeth the crampe and conuulsions, and whan a man is so stiffe for colde that he can not moue his necke : it is good against ache and paine in the hippe and ioinctes, and against a quarten Ague, if so be the backbone be therwith anoynted before the fitte come.

To cure aches in the ioinctes, comyng of colde,

Sicknes.

How make you Vnguentum Dialthæ.

Health.

First take of Holioke rootes. li. ii. of Linseede, Fenegreke, ana li. i. of Squilla. li. ß. of oile. li. iiii. of waxe. li. i. of Turpentine the gumme of Iuei, Galbanum, ana. ʒ. ii. of Colophonie, Rosen ana. li. ß. washe the rootes well, and beate your Fenegrike, Lineseede, and Squilla altogether, afterwarde put them all into. li. vii. of water, by the space of three daies, and on the fowerth daie, boile them till thei be thicke: then put them softly into a bagge and strain them, puttyng vnto them a little hotte water, to cause the iuce to strain the better, after this take. li. ii. of that iuce, and boile it with oile, vntill the iuce bee consumed: Then put in the waxe, and when it is melted, put in Turpentine, Galbanum, gumme of Iuei, and at last pouder of Rosen, and drie Pitche, when it is thicke, take it from the fire, and make your ointment. This asswageth paine of the stomacke of colde, and the pleurasie, if you anointe the place therewith, it dooeth also bryng heate, molifieth and causeth moistnes.

Sickenes.

How

The booke of Compoundes. Fol.xxxvj.

How make you vnguentum Agrippæ?

Health.

Take of Brionie rootes .li.ii. the rootes of wilde Cucumer and Squilla. ʒ.vi. of Flowerdelice.ʒ.iiii. of Ferne rootes.ʒ.ii. of Walworte, & Seathstell an̄.ʒ.ii. washe the rootes twise or thrise, & beate theim in a morter of Marbel, then put theim into .li.iiii. of oile Oliue, & Masticke.li.ii. by y̆ space of seuē daies, to encrease the better their heate, sauour & efficaci, boile them on the eight daie, vntill the rootes be softe, then straine them, and when thei be strained, set them on the fire again, and when it beginneth to boile, take.ʒ.xv. of white Waxe, and when it is melted, take it from the fire, and make an ointemente of it, when it is colde. This is a presente remedie againste the Dropsie, and all swellynges, in what parte so euer thei bee: it asswageth paine in the sinewes, prouoketh vrine, causeth a man to be laxatiue, and cureth paine in the raines of the backe.

<small>An ointment agaynst the Dropsie and swellyng.</small>

Sicknes.

How make you vnguentum diapompholigos.

Health.

Take oile of Roses.ʒ.x. of white Waxe.ʒ.v. of the iuce of Nightshade beries.ʒ.viii. of white Lead.ʒ.iiii. of comon Lead made in pouder, of Tuthie, a kinde of Leade, an̄.ʒ.s. of Frankinsens, ʒ.i. make those simples in pouder, whiche be fitte to be made in pouder, seeth the iuce of Night shade, with the oile of Roses, vntil the iuce be consumed, then mingle the waxe with the pouders, and beate thē in a morter, and then make your ointement. This drieth *Erypsipelæ* & old stinkyng sores in the legges and thighes.

<small>Erysipelæ is a redde inflamation in y̆ body, with a feuer or horror.</small>

Sickenes.

How make you vnguentum de Enulacampana.

Health.

Take of Enulacampana rootes sodden in Wineger, and afterward well dried.li.i. of swines grease, oile Oliue, ana.ʒ.iii. of newe waxe.ʒ.i. of salte made in pouder.ʒ.ß. of quicke Siluer, and Turpentine washed, ana.ʒ.ii. make this ointmente accordingly.

<small>An oyntment against extreme iche, scabbes, and Pore.</small>

Sicknes.

How make you vnguentum contra Scabiem.

Health.

Take of Swynes greace.ʒ.v. oyle of Baye, Quike siluer sleked, of Waxe washed, of Frankensence made in pouder, ana.ʒ.ii. of salt ʒ.viii. of the iuce of Plantain and Fumiterre, asmuche as you iudge sufficient. Make it after this fashiō, set the iuces with the wax, oyle of Bay and swines greace on the fier, and let them boyle vntill all be melted, then put to Salte, Frankinsence, Mastike, and boyle them

<small>Another for the same.</small>

all

The booke of Compoundes.

all vnto the iuce be consumed. Then take them from the fier, and put vnto them the Quickesiluer flecked, as you did in the other oyntment before and so vse it. This is a very stronge oyntment and therfore you must take diligent hede, least that you touche any principall member with the oyntment, because of your quike siluer you must also mingle a greate quantite of Mastike with it.

Sicknes.

How make you vnguentum propueris scabiosis.

Health.

First take of Turpentine washed. z.iii. of Butter washed. z.ii. of Salte. z.i. of the iuce of Pomecitrones, of the yolkes of. iiii. Egges, of oyle of Roses. z.i. mingle all these together & make an oyntment.

Sicknes.

How make you vnguentum desiccatiuum Rubrum.

Health.

Take the stone called lapis Calaminaris, of terra Sigillata an. z.iiii. Litharge of Golde, white leade, ana. z.iiii. of Camphere z.i. of wax. z.v. oyle of Roses, oyle of Vyolets, ana. z.vi. make the oyntement accordingly. This will drie moste humours.

Sicknes.

How make you vnguentum contra Lumbricos.

Health.

Take of bitter Almondes, and the iuce of Peche leues, and Motherworte, ana. z.ss. of Roses, Lupine flowers, the pouder of Hartes horne, ana. z.i. of Aloes, Succotrini. z.ii. some put vnto these. z.ii. of Orgals. Take a littell quantitie of Vinegar, and as moch Hony as will suffice, this applied to the belie, will kil wormes.

Sicknes.

How make you vnguentum Resumptiuum.

Health.

Take of Swynes greace. z.iiii. of Hennes greace, Gouse greace, and Duckes greace, ana. z.ii. of Hysop. z.ss. oyle of Vyolets, Camomill and Dill, ana. z.ii. of fresh butter. li.i. of white ware, z.vi. of Tragantum, of the slimy sape of the kirnels of Quinces, Linseede, and Holyoke, of Gumme Arabike, ana. z.ss. mingle them together and make an oyntment.

Sicknes.

How make you Vnguentum Album.

Sic.

Health.

Take of Oyle Oliue. li. ii. of fine white Leade. li. i. white Ware, ʒ. vi. some Poticaries put to these. ʒ. ii. of Camphier, make the oyntment accordyng.

Scknes.

How make you *Vnguentum Matritum.*

Health.

First take of Lytharge, of Golde. ʒ. iii. of Salet Oyle. li. ß. of Wineger. ʒ. iii. make the oyntment in a Leadē morter accordinglie: This cooleth and dryeth, and killeth itche.

Sicknes.

How make you *Vnguentum Ægyptiacum.*

Health.

First take of the flowers of Brasse, called Wardegrece, of Hony, ana. riiii. of stronge Wynegar, aur. vii. seeth them vntill they be thicke, and make your oyntment. This is a singuler good ointment against old woundes and Fistulas, whiche stande in nede of clensyng. It doeth also eate away dead flesh and purgeth also from al corruption.

Sicknes.

How make you *Vnguentum Citrinum.*

Health.

Take of Borax whiche is a kynde of Salte Peter. ʒ. ii. of Camphire. ʒ. i. of white Corall. ʒ. ß. of Sea glasse burnt. ʒ. i. of Merbon stones, of the Gumme Tragantū, Imili, Merbull, Cristall of fine Frankinsence and white, of Salte peter, ana. ʒ. iii. of white Marbell. ʒ. ii. of Serpentarie, white Lead. ʒ. vi. make it after this fashion, stampe your Tragantum, and the Marbull stones in a Morter with an Jron pestell, stampe the other alone in the same Morter, and serse them thorough a Siue with a fine clothe, with. li. of fresh swines greace, and Goates greace, and of Hens greace. ʒ. i. These greaces must be put into a Skillet, or some other suche like vessell, the whiche vessell ought to hange ouer the fier, in a cauderne ful of water let the water in the caulderne so boyle that the greace may be melted, by the heate of the water in the cauldern. Whan the greace is melted, strain it through a fine clothe into a dishe, and put vnto it all the pouders, except Camphire and Borax, stirryng it continually, vntill all go together on a lumpe. This done mingle with it twoo Pomecitrones or mo, stirryng it all waies, and whan it beginneth to boile, put in Cāphire and Borax, it must be continually stirred til it be cold, after that it be taken from the fier the which done, make the oyntment. And here

The booke of Compoundes.

here you must note that one pounde of pouder, will requier. li. viii. of greace.

Sicknes.

How make you *Vnguentum Neapolitanum.*

Health.

These ointementes bee good for the buttons of Naples, sores, ache, &c.

First take of Oyle of Camamil, Dyll, Spicknarde and Lilles, ana. ʒ. ii. of Swines greace and the saite of Veale. ana. li. i. of Euphorbe. ʒ. v. of Frankinsence. ʒ. r. Oyle of Bay. ʒ. i. ß. greace of a viper. ʒ. ii. ß. of quicke Frogges, of earth wormes washed in wine ʒ. iii. ß. iuce of Walworte, and Enula Campana rootes, ana. ʒ. ii. of Squinantum, Stichados, and of Motherworte, ana. M. ii. of sweete wine. li. ii. boyle them all together vntill the wine be consumed, then strain them and put vnto the straining, Litharge of gold. li. i. of Turpentine wasshed. ʒ. ii. make this ointment or cearclothe with white Wax, putting vnto it, whan it is almost sodden. ʒ. i. ß. of Stackte, or of the saltest and tendrest parte of Mirrhe, then take it from the fier and stirre it till it be luke warme, after this put vnto it. ʒ. iiii. of Quicke Siluer slecked with your spittell, stiryng it till the Quickesiluer be runne together on a lumpe with other Simples, and so make your oyntment.

Sicknes.

How make you Another. &c.

Health.

Take of Oyle of Spyke. ʒ. i. Olei de Tartari, Oyle of Baye, olei Petrolei, and Swines greace. ʒ. iiii. of Frankinsence. ʒ. ß. of Euphorbe. ʒ. i. ß. the oyntment of Holioke, and of Agrippa. ana ʒ. i. of Quickesiluer. ʒ. iiii. mingle all together & make your oyntmēt.

Sicknes.

How make you *Vnguentum Galeni.*

Health.

A good colde vnguentum.

Take of white Waxe. li. i. oyle of Roses. li. iii. let these be melted all together, and wasshed well and ofte with colde water, vntil they be white, the better that they bee wasshed with a littell Wineger.

Sicknes.

How make you *Vnguentum ad Combustione ignis,* to heale burnyng with fier.

Health.

An ointment for burnyng.

It is an oyntment whiche I haue often times proued to helpe many, whose vertue excelleth in healynge the flesh, whan it is combust or burnt with fier, and it must be thus made. Take of the

the rinde or tender barke of Eldar, & the Pith or corke of ye same Eldar ana. ʒ.ii. boyle it in .iiii. pintes of water vntill half be consumed then strayne it, and put in Oyle of Nuttes. ʒ.iiii. and seeth it softly in a cloase vessell vntill your water be wasted, then put in new cleane clarified Wax. ʒ.ii. mingle them together and so is your oyntmēt made.

Sicknes.

How make you Sugar Roset.

Health.

Take fine Sugar and dissolue it with Rosewater, and seeth it well, then cast it on a Marbell stone, till it be colde and harde, afterwarde cut it in great peeces. Thus you may also make Sugar Violet, and Buglosse.

Sicknes.

I haue been troubled with a blouddy Flixe many a longe daye, with paynfull turmentes in my guttes, and runnynge oute of yellow choler, excoriation, or as I thinke the scrappynge of my guttes, with pouryng out of bloud, my body is cleane wasted, my flesh consumeth, I cannot tell what to doe, I take no rest in my bed, I haue a continuall drinesse, this paine hath brought vnto my minde, an infinet number of cares, and miserable afflixtions of the soule: I haue been with many, I haue sought euery where for helpe, but I haue founde none. I pray thee deare Health bestow vpon me some worthie medicine which may recouer me, and heale me of this sore, and greate Disease?

Here sicknes describeth the flixe with the effectes.

Health.

This assuer your selfe, I haue helped many, and hindered none that haue vsed it, for I my selfe haue oftentimes proued it, euē so do you. Take the iuce of Planten, of Knotgrasse, of Shepperdes purse, of Nightshade, of Ribworte, the water of Roses, ana. ʒ.ii. the whites of three Egges, the seede of Ryse, the dried Flowers of Pomgranets, the rinde of Pomgranets, the wilde white Rose, finely beaten in pouder and searsed, ana. Ɔ.ii. *Acaciæ.* ʒ.i. clarified Oxe tallow ʒ.ii. Goates mylke pinte. ß. seeth al these together, then put in Terra Sigillata fine in pouder. ʒ.i.ß. put these all into your glister bladder, and receaue it luke or more then bloud warme in at your foundamēt, and lie doune vpon your bedde and reste, hauyng the lower partes of your belly warme anoynted with Oyle of Rue, and afterwarde take Wormewod, Southernewod, Rose leaues, Sauery, Puleole, Rosemarie, ana. ℳ. the beries of Myrtels, the pouder of the barke of Pomgranets, ana. ʒ.ii. Wheate Bran. ℳ.ii. seeth all these in rayne water, and white wine, ana. li. iiii. vntill parte be consumed, then with warme clothes be washed, and after apply all these thynges to your Raynes of your backe and belly, then drinke Red wyne, wherin tarte ploūmes

A glister to stop the bloody flixe.

G.ii. haue

The booke of Compoundes.

Bulleyn haue vsed this ofte tymes to his frendes.

haue bene sodden, Planten water, and vnripe Mulberies: and this is myne aduice Sicknes, to make thee whole, for with this I haue helped many withall.

Sicknes.

How make you an Epithema to stoppe the flixe?

Health.

I Shall teach you a very good holsome Epithema, whiche hath helped many a hounderd, make it and proue it as occasion shall moue thee. Take a Linnen bagge a foote square, put therin Red Rose leaues, red Briar leaues, Myrtill beries with the leaues, Polei of like quantitee to fill this bagge accordynge to greatnesse of the body so make this Bagge, but commonly. xii. inches is vsed, let this seeth in Red wine, then applie it to the belly very warme, and make it warme againe, yea. x. or. xii. times, and kepe it to the belly: and somtime there appereth knottes like litle Figges in the nether partes, through the aboundance of humours, in suche cases, with a Sponge washe that place often times with the decoction of the Epithema aforesaied, and drie Mulberies, and Briar bearies whiche bee skant ripe, make them into pouder and burne Hogges heere, and the ashes therof put into this pouder, and. viii. graines of Masticke in pouder, cast or rubbe your sore place therwith. iiii. times a daye, and here after foloweth most excellent for that same purpose. Take gum Arabike, Frankinsence, Masticke, Aloes flaua or yellow, ana. ʒ. ii. Dragons or mans bloud, the stone called Hematist, ana. ʒ. i. ß. the burnte pouder of the cloue of a Crabbe or any shell fishe. ʒ. ß. with twoo hard rosted Egges, this gumme dissolued with a littell Red wine tempered with the rest of these pouders and Egges, make them warme and in a linnen longe bagge applie it to the raynes, and so make it warme betwene. ii. platters vppon the Coales, and giue the sicke Theriaca ʒ. i. mingled with Red wine. ʒ. iiii. warme to drinke at that presente time, and this will stoppe any extreme flux, if you will make a glister to helpe the Colike or winde in the guttes. Take Hysop, Sentaury, ana. ʒ. i. and one good white Coloquintida, seeth it in a cloase bessell in twoo quartes of water vntill halfe be wasted, then straine it, and take a pint or more of this decoction, & put therbnto oyle of Rue. ʒ. i. and warme let it be ministred, if this be somewhat weake to a verye stronge body, adde to this Hony. ʒ. i. Hyera simplex. ʒ. i. and common Salte. ʒ. i. ß.

Epithema to stop fluxis.

A glister for the Collicke.

This did doctor Mansfeld vse to his pacientes at Norwiche, many tymes.

Sicknes.

How make you Collyria which be vsed for sore eyes?

Health.

Collyrium. Sieff.

T Hey be made of twoo kindes, the one liquid or moist called Collyrium, the other drie, made in forme of a Suger loafe, called Sief, but in waight not. ʒ. ß. & of them speaketh *Galen, lib.* 4. *medic. localium*

The booke of Compoundes. Fol.xxxix.

*localium cap.*4. and *Paulus Ægineta in libro septimo. Cap.*16. They bee made of iuces, liquors, sedes, fruites, partes of plants, mettals. &c. But I will thee shew how to make some for the comforte of eyes: and first whan the eyes begin to be sore, hotte, redde, dimme. &c. Take the white of an Egge well beaten, and oftentimes drawne through a strainer with the lyke quantitee of cleane Rose water, & Planten water mingled together, and drop parte of this into your eyes. Another, take Tuthia or Lapis Tuti prepared, and the stone called Calaminari, ana. ℈.iiii. the white of an Egge, Rose water, womans Milke, the decoction of the curnels of Quinces, ana. ℈.iii. mingled together, you may put in fine cleare yellow Aloes. ℈.i. if you will. This Collyria will drie vp watry and gummy matter in the eyes. *Verie good Collors for sore iyes.*

Another to quicken the sight. Take the stone Tuthi or Tuti prepared, Amoniaci, Bras burned or adust, lapis Calaminari, ana. xii. peny waight, Myrrhe, the stone called Hematist, Opium, ana. vi. peny waight, yellow Aloes called Hepatici, Bulles gaule, Galbanū, gum Sagapeni, ana. iiii. peny waight, Salt Armonyake, the iuce of Chelidon, ana. iiii. peny waight, and therbnto Rosewater, and beat it in your Morter, then rowle them in small sharpe peeces, and drie them, kepe them vntill you haue neede: and whan occasion shall serue, dissolue one of these peeces in Rose water, the white of an Egge or womans Milke, and put it into your eye. This is most excellent to make cleane the eyes, sharpe the sight, and make it beutifull. *The beste learned of the Grekes and Latines vse this for sore iyes.*

Another for the same. Take Ceruse washed in Rose water. viii. sundrie times in seuerall waters. ʒ.i. whit gum, Sarcocol of Persia ℈.ii. Impli, Traganth. ana. ℈.i. Opium. ℈. iiii. all lightly beaten or grounde on a stone, put therbnto a little of the Mulsege or thicke decoction of Fenigrece, and so fashion them and make them drie, & kepe them cleane, you may put some of this into your waters for the eyes.

Sicknes.

How make you a Liniment to put away paine in the Pleuricie?

Health.

The Oyle of Camomill, the fatte of a Capon, ana. ʒ.i. of fresh Butter newly made. ʒ.iii. and a littell peece of new waxe, so make your Liniment to anoynt the stomacke. *A Liniment for pleuracie.*

Sicknes.

How make you a Frontale or a Forhedcloth to quench heate in the head, in the time of a Feauer, and to cause sleape.

Health.

After the minde of *Galen* prepare a double cloth of Linnen. iii. fingers broade, and in length from one eare to the other eare, put into this clothe as foloweth. Take Red Roses or their leaues, *A frontaile for hed ache.*

G.iii. Lettice

The booke of Compoundes.

Lettice leaues, Poppie leaues or the seedes, and twiste it, and make this frontall warme betwene twoo broade plattes or platters, with Rose water and Uinegar, and then binde it to the forehedde. An other for the same. Take water Lillies, Uioletes, Mellilot, Lettice flowers white Poppie heddes, ana. ℈.q. bruse all together, & put it into your clothe. If the hedde be colde, and haue no warmenesse, then make your frontale thus. Take Sage, Rosemary, Camomill, Betonie, Brioni, Mellilote, Bazel, Sauor, or soche like herbes broused, and putte into your clothe: And in hotte paines of the hedde, poure water of Roses and Uinegar together, vpon a hotte Tile stone, and receiue the vapor or smoke into your mouthe. In causes hot poure *Aqua vite*, & Sage water vpon a burnyng Tile or stone, & receiue the smoke. Comonly *Galen* in. xii. of his *Therapeuticis*, did anointe sicke folkes heddes with *Oxyrhodinum*, whyche is made of oile of Roses. ʒ.i. and Uinegar. ʒ.ii. mingled and shaken in a Uial of glasse, and colde, anointe the forehedde therewith.

For scape.

Uapour to smell vpon.

Sicknes.
How prepare you a Gargarizme or washyng gurgle, for the mouthe and throte.

Health.

A gargarizm to gurgull in the mouthe and throate.

You shall doe thus. Take the stilled waters of Roses, Plantan, Uinegar, Honie, Lettice, Straburie, Nightshade, water Lillie, and of Burnet, ana. ʒ.i. Diamoron. ʒ. vi. the iuce of Raspes, of Barberies, ana. ʒ. vi.ß. syruppe of Poppie, ʒ.ß. of Straburies. ʒ.iii. of Uinegar. ʒ.ß. mingle theim well, and this is a gargarizme, to skower the throte in all hotte diseases, and in the time of *Anginæ*. And here followeth an other for the same. Take Planten, Burnet, Straburie leaues, Knotgrasse, ana. ℈.i. Sorrell, Sage, ana ℈.i. redde Roses, ℈.ß. long Peper, Pellitorie, ana. ʒ.ß. ℈.ii. boiled in a pottell of water, till the halfe or more, then straine it, and putte to it Honie of Roses. ʒ.i.ß. Orimell, Scillitici. ʒ.i. mingle them together, & than it is perfitly made. An other very good, which haue doen much good, as Doctor *Leonarde Fuchius* reporteth. Take *Hyera Picra simplici*. ʒ.ß. Orimell, Scillitici. ʒ.ii. the stilled waters of Hysoppe, Betonie, and Orgain. ʒ.i.ß. mingle them, and make your gargarizme. Mustarde, Uinegar, Peper and Honie mingled together, doe make a good readie gargarizme. Prouided that you minister your gargarizmes warme, to drawe humours: But when you stoppe them, vse colde thynges, taken colde in your mouthe, as Uinegar, fountaine water. &c.

A gargarizm must be giuē warme to draw humours from the head.

Sicknes.
How make you Nasalia, or to stoppe blood in the Nose?

Health.

Nasalia.

When the bloode doe aboundauntly flowe out of the Nose, it is good to open the Liuer vaine in the right arme, to take the aboundance awaie, and sometyme small stringes or vaines wil breake,

The booke of Compoundes. Fol.xl.

breake, in soche cases moderate diate and colde thynges, is good to bee vsed, and this pouder to be put into the nose. Take the kates or wolly knottes, growyng vpon Sallowes, commonly called Palmes, beyng drie, Bole Armonie fine, that will cleaue to the tongue, and Dragons blood, ana. ʒ.i. beaten into pouder, and finely sifted, and the fine heere of a Hares bellie. ʒ.i.ß. cutte or minced moste shorte like pouder, put these together, and stuffe theim into the bloodie nostrell, or els dissolue them with the white of an egge, and so drawe thē into the nose: Often tymes the hedde is stopped, and the stomacke so disquieted, that starnutacions or nesynges will helpe. And also the saied starnutaciōs will helpe women to quicke deliueraunce, in the time of their trauel. Then doe thus. Take Margarū, Nigella, Cloues, white Peper, Ginger, ana. Ɔ.ii. Castor, Condisi, ana. Ɔ.i. make them in fine pouder, and putte them into the nose. Or thus. Take Nutmegges, Ireos rootes ana. ʒ.i. *Elleborus Albus*, called nesyng pouder roote. Ɔ.i. white Peper, Pellitorie. ʒ.ß. Calamus. ʒ.i. Ɔ.i. beate them in pouder, and kepe it to vse, as a mornynges and in child birthes. &c.

To stop blod in the nose.

The profite of nesyng.

Sicknes.

Reumes, weaknes of sight, dulnes of hearyng, slownes of speache, ouer moche slepe, somtime trouble me with foulenes in my mouthe, what helpe then to clense, or drawe forthe fleume.

Health.

Make a pretie linen bagge of fine clothe, put therein Mustard seede, Hysoppe, Ginger, Peper, Pelletorie, Stauesagre, Mastike, Organ, ana. ʒ.i.ß. beaten together, put part of this into this bagge, or els into your mouthe, without the bagge, or els tempered with the iuce of Beates and Honie, and so make your mansill or bityng thyng. It will drawe fleume, clense the iyes, comforte memorie, and quenche the salte fleume, that make the face high coloured, vse it a mornynges often times.

Apophlegmatismi, to putte in the mouth to draw forth filthe.

Sicknes.

How make you Pessis to molifie, to vnbinde, and to restraine, to be put into the secrit place of the brin of women?

Health.

Truly the makyng of them which doe molifie be thus made. Take Oesypi, whiche is an oyle sodden out of the woll that is clipped or shorne from the neckes or flankes of shepe, Hartes tallow or ye marth called Mary, Goose greace, Capons or Hens greace ana. ʒ.i.ß. flax or lint seede, fenigrece in pouders, ana. ʒ.ii. Melilot ʒ.i. Masticke. ʒ.i.ß. the yolkes of Egges, Oyle of Roses, and the Oyle of Flowerdeluce, ana. ʒ.i.ß. freshe Butter. ʒ.iii. put to a peece of waxe melt them together, and prepare woll rowled together in the forme of a finger or such like, dippe it in this liquor, whan it is stiffe let it be vsed.

Oesypi is an foule Oile made of woll but very good for Pessaris and other medicens.

A mollifyng Pessary.

G.iiii.

The booke of Compoundes.

How to vse a Suppositor. vsed, I meane into the secret place of Conseption, retainynge it in the place. iiii. or. v. howers with a threade in the ende therof, it may be made with a Sponge.   To prouoke termes menstrual. Take Mugwort Sutherne wood, Dyttan, Calamus odoratus, ana. ʒ. ii. the seede of Nigella. ʒ. i. ß. Bay beries. ʒ. ß. drie Rue. ʒ. i. Sauen. Ɔ. ii. Myrrhe Styrax liquid, añ. ʒ. i. ß. Sagapine, Ladani, ana. ʒ. i. beaten in a morter with Hony, and rowle it in the Pessary, and applie it accordyngly.

Sometime imoderate flux or termes passeth so much and so painfull, that in suche cases, Pessaris restrictiue be very holsome as example. **Pessaris to restraine.** Take the pouder of Hartes horne, Olybanum, ana. ʒ. ii. Dragōs bloud, Balaustia, añ. ʒ. i. ß. Damaske Roses. ʒ. ii. *Acaciæ*, or iuce of sower Ploummes dried, Hypocistidis, Mastike, ana. ʒ. i. Bole armeny. Ɔ. ii. Bistorta, Comfory, ana. ʒ. i. ß. bruse and stampe them well in a morter put in the iuce of Planten, and Oile of Roses, as will suffice to rowle in your woll and make your Pessari.

Sicknes

Against foule stinke of a corrupt ayre, a filthy house, and coldnesse of the braine. What smoke, fume, or sauour is then good.

Health.

How to receiue fume or vapor. Not only for a colde braine, but also against rawe humours, and vomityng of bloud. &c. If the pacient haue a few coales betwene the legges, stouppyng downeward, with clothes caste loose aboute the naked body, as a mantel gowne &c. receuing ye smoke at the mouth, through some Trunke or hollow thyng. Take the wod of Aloes. Ɔ. ii. Galia muschata. ʒ. i. Sage, Margarum, Rosemary, Maces, Bay leaues, añ. ʒ. i. stamped in a morter into fine pouder, put in fine Muske ℈. viii. and cast parte of this or al this, by littel and littell on the cooles, or thus as foloweth.

Take fine Frankinsence, Cinamon, Cloues, Maces, the rinde of a Pome Citron, añ. ʒ. ß. the wood of Aloes, Myrrhe, Mastike, Trochis of Gallia, Muskata. ʒ. ii.. beate all in a morter, and put some Styrax liquide, and your morter partly warme, beate altogether & make your sweet fume, puttyng in if you will Muske, Amber grece. ana. ℈. iiii.

Here is a good one. Take Ladani. ʒ. i. Frankinsence, Mastike, ana ʒ. i. Styrax, Calamita. ʒ. ii. Cloues, Cinamon, Nutmegges, ana. ʒ. i. wood of Aloes, Myrrhe. ʒ. ß. dead cooles of Salow, Syprus, Fur, or Geniper. ʒ. ii. beat them all in a morter somewhat warme, put in a little Uenis Turpentine, and cleane Rosewater, and worke al together with your pestill, and make your parfume, and this shall suffice, **Perfumes for ye mother.** but when women doe sodenly faule sicke with swellynge of the Matrix called the mother, then it is perilous to vse sweet parfumes, but then vse to parfume with Galbanum, Castor, Fethers, the paryng of Horshoues. &c.

Sicknes

The booke of Compoundes. Fol.xlj.

How make you Sacculum or Scutum, the childe or twilte for the breast.

Health.

They be verie comfortable for the breast and stomacke, to stoppe vomittes, and be good for the Hart, splene, and Belly, and thus it is made. Take flowers of Rosemary, Lauender, Camamell, Betonie, Roses, ana. ℈.ß. or Sage, Margarum, Mellilote, Mintes, ana. ℈.ß. or leaues of Sene. ʒ.ii.ß. Stichadus. ʒ.iii. Cloues, Nutmegges, ana. ℈.ii. and Maces. ℈.iii. stamped in a morter and twilted in a silke or fine linnen clothe, made in the forme of a shielde or a square Trencher. Another. Take flowers of Buglosse, Roses, Balme. ʒ.iii Cloues, Maces, wood of Aloes, Cardamon. ℈.ii. Saffrō. ℈.i. Galinga Spiknarde, the bone of a Hartes hart, an. ℈.i.ß. Muske, Amber grece ana. ℈.x. beate in a morter, and with soft Cotton twilted and applied to the breast, you may put in warme herbes as Sage, Wormewood, Mintes, Horhounde, Sothernwod, &c. put in a Twilt or Stomicher with the pouders of Calamus, Cloues and Comen, twilted and made verie warme with wine or Aqua vite betweene twoo platters, and so applied to a weake feble stomacke, and thus I ende of Saccutum or Twyltes.

Scuta.

This is an Emplaster, if oyle be put in.

Sicknes.

How is a Cerat made?

Health.

They be made of war, Oyle and pouders in a Twilt, in forme of a show soole, or an Oxe tongue, and is thus made. Take Cinamon, Cloues, ana. ʒ.i. Galingal Maces, ana. ʒ.ß. sweet Calamus. ʒ.i.ß. wood of Aloes, Gallia Moschata, ana. ℈.i. Flowers of Pomgranets, Mastike, Ladani, ana. ʒ.i. oyles of Mastike Roses, Mintes, an. ʒ.i. with war. ʒ. Turpentine, beat your drie thinges in pouder and put your waxe to them, and so melte them, and so kepe your Cerot. You may make the same in Leather or Sylke. You may for the Splene put in Melilot, Line seede, Fenegreke, Caper barkes, Calamus, Nutmegges, wax, Turpentine, according to arte, puttyng in Oyle.

A Cerot, and how to make it.

Sicknes.

How make you Insessus?

Insessus.

Health

For lacke of a Bathe, these are good for the belly and raynes. Take filipendula, Sarifrage, Mallowes, Holihoke, water Cresses, ana. ℥.i. the seedes of Flax, Smalage, Fenigrik seeth all together in sufficient water to the thirde parte and so vse it for the stone. Another. Take Mugworte, Sage, Betony,
Cala-

The booke of Compoundes.

Calamint, Orgaine, Peniroyall, Camamill, Mellilot, saint Johns grasse Sothernwood, ana. ℈.ß. the rootes of Yreos and Smalage, an ʒ.i. seeth your rootes soft and your herbes, this is good for the Matrix, Belly, for Collicke, swellyng winde, Timpany, colde. &c. Another against a blouddy flire. Take Planten, Knotgrasse, the rindes of Pomegranets, Shepardes purse, Horsetaile like a water sprinkle, the flowers of Pomgranets, ana. ʒ. iiii. seeth all in raine water, Uineger or Redwine to the thirde parte and applie it to the lower partes of the belly.

A goodlie remedy for the flixe.

Sicknes.

How make you Fomentum.

Health.

Fomentes moiste & drie.

Ther be twoo Fomentes one moyst and the other drie as Hipocrate saieth lib.ii. victu. acut, and now of a moyst one. Take malowes the flowers or toppes of Dyll, Camamill, Mellilot, ana. ℈.ß. the seedes of Line and Fenegrice. ana. ʒ.ß. sodden in. li.ii. of Fountaine water to the halfe, and so you may drawe it through a searse or a strainer, and with a spōge warme, you maie washe the belly, or any other greued place.

Sicknes.

How make you Dropax to clense the head, and pull of scaules, and filthy Glewe that children are infected withall.

Health.

Dropax will doo many thynges to the bodye, it may be made to humect and to drie, to clense, to coole & warme, but to your question to make a Dropax for an vncleane head, called the scaule or glewe, or els crust. Take Pix or Pitche, waxe, Colophoni, ana. ʒ. iii. Bytumen. ʒ.ß. Brimstone. ʒ.iii. Peper, Pellitorie, ana. ʒ. ii. Stauesagre. ʒ.i.ß. Euphorbii, Ellebori the white, ana. ʒ.ß. beat your dried thinges into pouder, and melt them together, spreade this vpon a Lether warme laied on the fowle head, beyng first shauen for. xxiiii. howers and so quickly rente of, and thus I make an ende of these kindes of Compoundes. And when I haue more quietnesse, with conuenient leyser I will say some thynge of Compounded waters: But it shall make no greate matter if I giue place to them, whome no man can mende, that haue written most plentifully, learnedly and compendiously, of the natures of Precious waters, bothe Simple and Compounde: yet shal I remember some good waters shortly, because time and place so moueth me in that case.

A Dropax for a skalde hedde.

where the harte is vnquiet, prosperous labour doe not goe forwarde.

Sicknes

The boke of Compoundes. Fol.xlij.

Sicknes.

Mine iyes beginne to bee dimme, my sight faileth me: I would learne to make a water, to kepe them from vtter blindnes. For when the sight is decaied and gone, the ioyes of this worlde is paste, and nothyng is left, but miserie and heauinesse of minde, and cõtinuall musyng.

Health.

A Merueilous water to conserue the sight, I shall teache thee, whiche I haue proued my self, to haue helped many one: and the greate learned manne in waters, called *Euonimus*, haue written it, whiche in distilaciõs was equal to any, that euer practised the same, and it is thus made. Take the leaues of Rewe, Minte, redde Roses, Sage, Maidenheere (other leaue out Minte, and Sage, and for theim putte red Fenel, Veruine, Euphrage called Iyebright, Betonie, Honie Succle of the Mountaine, and Endiue) of euery one. vi. handfulles, lette them be put into white wine, for the space of. xxiiii. howers, then let them be distilled in a Limbike: the water that shall first runne out, is compared vnto Siluer, the seconde vnto Golde, the third vnto Balme, and this must be close kept in a glasse: it is a water for all the diseases of the iyes, that bee curable, out of *Aegidius*, and *Lullius*, it is described. Emongest the waters, composed for diuers inward diseases by *wolstadius*. *A goodlie water for sore iyes.* *Three riche waters, Siluer, Golde, and Balme.*

In other water for the iyes, aboute the beginning of Maie, gather Selandine, Veruen, Rewe, Fenell, beate them seuerally, and take. ʒ. iii. of the iuce of euery one of theim, then mixe theim, put to a little of the grene braunches of Euphrage, called Iyebright, or Roses. ʒ. iii. of Sugar Candie. ʒ. iiii. of the beste Tucia, and as moche of Dragons blood, when all these are beaten, thou shalt mixte them together, and distille theim in a Limbicke of glasse, the liquere that runneth forthe, thou shalt let it stande twoo or three daies in a receiuer, and then vse it: it is of greate vertue, for the iyes that bee darcke, dimme, redde, or haue the webbe in the iye. The water of the Wine, together with Honie sublimated by the fire, cureth the blindnesse of the iyes specially. The Monkes in *Mesuen*, that is the water of the Wine (saied thei) whiche in euery Spring tyme, when the Vines are cutte, for certaine daies, this water without any distillacion pressed forthe, putteth awaie prickynges, and heate of the iyes, and clarifieth the sight, commyng by a hotte cause, if a man put it in bothe corners of the iye, one droppe of this water, it sharpeneth the sight, and cureth any disease of the iyes, within. v. daies, saieth *Euonimus.* &c. Rede after in the trimming waters, emongeste them that be ordeined to Diyng of the heere. Here is also a water for the iyes in Sommer, to preserue the sight, descrbed by *Ioannes Mainardus*, in his Epistelles, vi. iiii. three partes of Roses, the herbes of Fenell, and Rewe, of either one parte, and let them be well mixt together, and after three daies, let a water bee distilled, other in onely vapor of sethyng water, or in the Sonne, or in *Balneo Mariæ*, as thei call it, *A water for the webbe.*

so

The booke of Compoundes.

The maner of destillyng the water for iyes.

so that a handfull of the foresaied herbes, bee put into the receiuyng vessell, that the droppes maie fall vpon them, and the mouth of the receiuer, and the nose of the vpper vessell, must bee diligently ioyned together, and closed, that the vapours maie not gette out, but kept very close from aire.

And hereafter foloweth an other water, of an excellente vertue. Fill a still full of the leaues of Agrimonie, Veruen, Euphrage, Fenell, Rewe, redde Mintes, and Louage, cutte theim, sprincke vpon them a little white and clere wine, and destill theim in a claie stillitorie, this liquore represseth the swellyng of the iye liddes, of a colde cause, it drieth vp the blere iyednesse, it stoppeth the flowyng of teares, it cleareth the sight, it breaketh the blemishes, spottes, cornes, or pearles, if thou wilte haue it stronger to breake spottes or pearles, put vnto it *Gallirrium*, and Chickens weede, with redde flowers. You maie gette a water out of Fenell, also for thesame causes, for a liquore gathered out of the rootes and leaues of Fenell, sodde in water, with a Basen laied vpon the water, while it yet seeth, and kept in a glasse, and one droppe put in to the corner of the iye euery daie, mornyng and euenyng, for the foresaied causes, and this is proued. To breake the spotte or pearle, mixte with the foresaird waters, Mirrhe, and Aloes a pounde, and putte a droppe of the liquore strained, in either corner of the iye, early and late.

Goodlie waters for the iyes, whiche excelleth in vertue.

The water of white thorne and willowe for rednesse of iyes, comyng of heate. Water of Euphrage called Iyebright, for swellyng in the iyes, comyng of cold. Euphrage or Ophthalmica so named, because it is a herbe for iyes Gordonius water for iyes. Gordonius water for a Fistula.

A water distilled of the flowers of white Thorne, and Willowe, putteth awaie prickynges, heates, or rednes of the iyes, it stoppeth teares comyng of a hot cause, and breaketh the spottes, or pearles of thesame cause. A water of the leaues (flowers) of Euphrage, stoppeth teares, comyng of a colde cause, and maketh sleder the iye liddes, that swell of thesame cause, and restoreth thesame sight, that hath any impedimēt *Euonimus* doe saie, that Euphrage doe not heate, but is temperate, or els doeth coole moderatly in the first degree, and drieth in the seconde.

An excellent water for the debilite of the sight, described by *Gordonus*, take Selandine, Fenell, Rewe, water of the Mountaine Euphrage, Veruen, redde Rose with their buddes, ana .li. ß. Cloues, long Peper, ana. ʒ. ii. when thei are brused together, destill them in a Limbicke of Glasse, with a slowe fire, and put of it euery daie in the iyes.

An other of thesame mannes, for a Fistula, which he is certain wil heale, twoo pounde of good white wine, destilled in thesame vessell, that *Aqua vitæ* is destilled in: the waters of Rosemary and Sage, ana. li. b. Sugar. li. ii. when thei are destilled, put again to theim. ʒ. i. of Sage, and asmoche of Rosemarie, when thei are steped together eight daies, thou shalte straine it and vse it. A cancar in what parte of the body so euer it be, the herbe called Cancar, whiche is also called Doues foote, the flowers of Quinces, the flowers of Cerifolium, the flowers or leaues of the Breer, called Idea, whiche is like a swete white Rose, and a fewe white Roses, Honie, and white wine, and the Alume, whiche is called Alume Glasse, let all these be destilled together.

Andreas Fornerius water for a Cancer.

A good water destilled of a Molwarpe, for all kinde of Goutes, or dropsies

Dropses, *noli me tangere*, Scalles of the hedde, Saucie face, and the wolfe. If you will haue a water without destillyng, quickely to washe your legges or feete, to make your saied water to smell well. Set a vessell of runnyng or conduite water on the fire, seeth it well, and putte into it the flowers of Lauendula, or Lauender, and moche rather of that, whiche is comonly called Spike, bothe grene, and drie Baies, Basell, Sage, Fenell. &c. and so washe at night: put cleane runnyng or Conduite water, and white wine into a vessel wel stopped, and set it in the Sonne, putting in Lauēder, Spike, and Cloues, that thei maie make swete the said water and wine with their smell, but yet if the Lauender be grene and moiste, it will tourne the wine almoste into Uinegar whiche if it be drie, it doe not so, the liquoure shall bee made the more smellyng: If the flowers be dried in the Sonne, in a Glasse closed, and afterwarde white wine to be put into it, if so be it, a manne desire to haue a swete water forthwith, by and by, and let hym put a droppe of oile of Spike, vnto a good deale of pure welle or Conduite water, and chafe it together, in a glasse with a narrowe mouth, although thei be made without destillacion, the same notwithstandyng, beyng right destilled in the Sonne, specially if certain other thinges be mixt with them, as Muske, Imbre, Ciuet, Caphura, or meaner thynges, as Stirax, and Stacte, Mirrhe, or any other spices, chiefly Cloues, or els thynges of lesse estimacion, as Roses, the barkes, flowers, or leaues of Oringes, Limons, Baie leaues, common sweete herbes, Rosemarie, Margerum, Basill. &c. thei shalbe made moche the sweter. But if you will haue a very pleasant water, take. ʒ.ß. of good Muske beaten, in twoo poundes of Rose water, put in the belly of a Glasse stille, and destille it, by little & little, then put it in a Glasse well stopt, with Amber grice. ʒ.i. it is a water merueilous swete, and conuenient for fine persones, that their clothes maie be sprinkeled therwith: put. ʒ.ß. of good Saffron, in. li.ii. of Rose water (for the space of one daie) and destille it, this water is holsome to bee mixte with medicenes: also for smelle, and garnishing, put. ʒ.ß. of Cloues beaten, in a pounde and a halfe of Rose water. xxiiii. howers, and destille it, destille Camphere. ʒ.i. with a pounde of Rose water, and vse it in medicenes, for noble persones. After the same maner is Rose water, made with Saunders, and other spices (swete smellyng) what so euer a man will, some destille all this in puer water, in stede of Rose water, three leaued herbe, an herbe very swete of sauour, whiche thei destille for perfumes, and to make diuers other pretie swete sauours. The Monkes of *Mesuen*, make a water of swete sauour, where with the hedde, harte, and stomacke are reuiued.

℞. Fower handfull of the flowers of Lauendula, Roses white, and redde, of either twoo handfull, Rosemarie, Cloues, newe and freshe Ciperus, of euery one a handfull, Minte, Sage, Tyme, Baileaues, or Peneriall, of euery one halfe a handfull. ʒ. iiii. of Cloues, Galingall, Nucis Moschi, Calamus Aromaticus, Ginger, Cinamon, of Flowerdelice, of euery one. ʒ.ß. sixe poundes of white Wine (asmoche as shall suffice)

how to make swete water without stillyng, good for to wasshe the feete, or for Barbars.

A pleasaunte swete water.

The Monkes water for correction of the flesh, better then holie water, and more costly.

The booke of Compoundes.

suffise) when thei are brade and beaten in a Morter, let them bee put into a Glasse, well closed, for the space of eight daies, afterwarde vse them, as occasion shall serue: it is excellent to washe the handes, if you mixte a little of it, with a greate deale of pure water. A man maie vse it also destilled, and put in. ℈.i. of Muske, *Epiphanius Empericus*, writeth an other of thesame mannes, delectable, with a marueilous swetenes of sauour: Ciuet, Muske, of either. ʒ.i. let it be tied in a fine linen cloth, & let it be set to soke in.li.ii. of Rose water, a fewe daies in the Sonne.

An other of thesame *Epiphanius*, a very swete sauour, Basille, Minte, Marierum, Flowerdelice, Hysop, Sauerie, Sage, *Melissa*, called Balme, Lauender, Rosemarie, of euery one halfe a handfull, Cloues, Cinamō Nutmegges, the Pome Citron, of yellowe coullere, three or fower. let them be beaten, and set three daies in Rose water, then let them be destilled with a slowe fire: when the destillacion is finished, put to. ℈.i. of Muske, and set it in the Sonne: you maie adde Amber grice. ℈.ß.

An other of thesame *Epiphanius*, of moste exellente sauoure. ℞. Three poundes of Rose water, Cloues, Cinamon, Saunders, ana. ʒ.vi. twoo handfull of the flowers of Lauender. ʒ.vi. of *Assa dulcis*, Malmesey, *Aqua vitæ*, ʒ.ii. lette it stande a moneth to stille in the Sonne, well closed in a Glasse, or vpon the toppe of a Furneis: then destille it in *Balneo Mariæ* and at. ʒ.i.ß. of Muske, to the destillacion, then let it stande tenne daies in the Sonne, or aboue the Furnes, and so vse it. It is a marueilous pleasaunte in sauour, a water of a wounderous swetenes, for the perfumyng the shetes of a bedde, whereby the whole place, shall haue a moste pleasaunt sente: put into a little viall of Glasse. xviii. or twētie graines of Muske, and Ciuet, and a little of Ambergrice, after filled full of Rose water, sette it ouer the fire, and when it is hotte, take it awaie, then let it stande to coole, well closed, after you haue doen, let it stand twoo daies, you maie vse it frō thense foreward, it is as good as though it wer destilled: then thou wilt perfume thy napkins, or other linen, put it in a vessell with a wide mouthe, and sprede the clothes vpon it boiling, and that thei maie drinke vp the vapor and breth of it.

An other maner of sweete water, is called the water of the castyng glasse, into some little vessell of Siluer, a little Rose water made with Muske, and a little Ciuet, and Cloues, Agalā, Styrax calamita, whē thei are all punde against a fire, mixe theim, and perfume any clothes with the vapour or smoke thereof, it is a marueilous swete sauoure, whiche if thou wilte kepe close the vessell diligently, and when thou thinkest good, put more Rose water vnto it, that it maie be renewed.

An other. Thou shalt put into fower poundes of Rose water, *Assa dulcis*, somewhat grose beaten, Styrax, and Cloues, Camphere, Agalam, of euery sorte. ʒ.i. Muske, Ciuet, of either of them. ʒ.xx. putte these together in a glasse, shutte with a Parchement, prickte through with tenne or twelue smalle holles, and let the vessell boile fower howers in a kettell, full of cleane water, as though it were in *Balneo Mariæ*, after when it is colde, strain it through a fine linen clothe, and kepe it

Sweete water for linnen.

Agalam, or Agalugin, is the woode of Aloes.

iii

The booke of Compoundes.   Fol.xliiij.

in a glasse, in the whiche graines. xii. of Muske shalbe put, whiche beyng moisted, and steped with water, thou shalte stoppe the glasse, and sette it in the Sonne. viii. daies, so shalt thou haue a wonderfull well smellyng water, a sweete water, and a secrete, whereof one parte mixte with ten partes of pure water, maketh the whole moste swete, graines. xx. or there about of Muske, as the smell thereof pleaseth the more, or lesse, Nutmegges, Cloues, Galingall, Spicnarde, Graines of Paradice, Mace, Cinamon, of euery an. ʒ.i. all these beaten in a morter, let theim be put into a Glasse, fitte to destille in, with Rose water li.i.ß. powred vnto it, let it stand so, for the space of fower or fiue daies afterwarde put to it thrise asmoche of Rose water, and destille al this in a Limbicke, set in a kettell full of water sethyng, as in a *Balneo Mariæ*, thou shalt kepe the water gathered together, diligently stopped for the same purpose aforesaied, that the former serueth for.

An other excellent water, twoo pounde of the water, of the flowers of Citri, one pounde of the water of redde Roses, of Mirtes. li.ß. of Muske Roses a good quātitie, and likewise of the flowers, of Cloues, ana. ʒ.ß. of *Assa dulcis* ʒ.iii. well beaten an. ʒ.i. of Stirax Calamita, and redde Stirax, ana. ʒ.ß. all these stamped, and mixte with water, thou shalt distille them in a glasen Limbecke, the hedde and the receiuer diligently closed with claie, with a soft fire, or in a *Balneo Mariæ*, or in a kettell of sethyng water: a water of moste swete sauour, with the whiche oile is stilled also, the laste water beyng mixte, with a hundred tymes asmoche of pure water, doeth sauour with the swetenes thereof, so is this folowyng of greater vertue, health, and swetenes.

    There bé. ii. kindes of this Assa, one is called Assa fœtida, or Diuel's dungue, ye other is called Assa dulcis, whiche commeth from Syria, and is also named Syrenaicus liquor, or the iuce of Laserpitium.

Take a pounde of Mirrhe chosen, pure, newe and fatte, beaten into small peces, halfe a pound of the iuce of Roses, when thei are mingled together in a Limbicke, let them be distilled in asshes: where first thou shalt seperate the water, with a slowe fire: then make the fire bigger, and seperate the Oile: and at laste deuide the water from the Oile. It maketh the face bright, it closeth woundes effectually, as well old as newe, the oile is moste precious, and doeth thesame thynges that the water doeth, but moche soner, as for example: it doeth that in an hower that the water is about in. xxiiii. ʒ.i. of this water distilled, mixt with a pottell of pure water, maketh them all notable well smellyng, but ana. ʒ.i. of the oile, if it bee put to eight gallons of pure water, it doeth thesame.

    A water incomperable, for the singuler goodnesse, of the moste excellent vertue thereof.

A goodlie Rose water made with Muske, whiche is required, and vsed also in other composicions, put. ℈. xii. or more of Muske, and. ℈. xvii. of Amber grice.

Sicknes.

THese waters be very pleasaunte and profitable, but waters to make a man to slepe were comfortable, I praie you saie somewhat of them.

    Of slepyng waters.

Health.

The booke of Compoundes.

To cause rest and slepe.

If you will cause one to slepe, then doe thus as foloweth Take. ʒ. ii. of Henebane. ʒ. i. of the rootes of Mandragora. ʒ. vi. of Popie, Lettice, Orpin, Housleke, ana. ʒ. ii. the water Lillie one handfull, when thei are beaten, let theim bee put in twoo pounde of water of Popie, with ʒ. i. ß. of the sede of Darnell, for the space of twoo daies, and let them be stilled, and this is perfite.

An other causyng slepe. Take the seede of Darnell. li. i. of the seede of Henebane. li. ii. of the seedes of Purselen. ʒ. iii. of the seede, or roote of Mandrag, as moche of Alkakengi, when thei are beaten, powre to theim. li. i. of the iuce of Beanes, as moche of the rootes, or leaues of Henebane. li. ß. of the iuce of the leaues of blacke Popie, minister. ʒ. i. of this water, when it is distilled, it is vehement, and of great vertue.

A goodlie water for the stone, and helpeth the palsie and falling sickenesse.

A water for the stone, made by *Aegidius*, bicause it breaketh the stone, ℞. the sede of Pimpernell, Parsely, Smalage, Cokopryke, mustardsede, Bures, Mastiches, of euery one like moche, when thei are well beaten let theim bee mixte with the blood of a he Goate, and a little Vinegar poured to it, let theim stande a fewe daies, in a vessell well closed, and then at the laste, let theim bee well stilled, it is good for theim that bee troubled with the stone, what maner of stone so euer it bee, red, white sharpe, or plain, if so be it the stone be confirmed, and gathered to some straight, let the pacient drinke of this water euery daie, for so shal it be broken, and brought into sande, if so be scabed heddes be washed ones a daie with this water, thei shall bee made hole, and newe heere shall spring, and the scabbes shall be cured within nine daies (otherwise any kinde of scabbes washt therwith, is made holle within three or fower daies) if it be dronke fastyng, it maketh good blood, and good couler (more then any other medicen) marueilously it maketh strong the sinewes, and taketh awaie the fallyng sicknes, if it be dronke twise a daie, otherwise is added, it healeth cleane the Pallie, if it be not dedde and radicated in the members. Thus saieth *Aegidius*, and *Lullus*, with other learned Clarkes. Also. ℞. *Cauda equina*, Plantaine, redde Roses, the graine of Alkakengi, the rootes of holy Oke, shauen or scraped Liquoris, of euery one. ʒ. i. Iuniper, Sebesten, of either of theim. ʒ. vi. Bolearmoniake. ʒ. ß. Cummen seede, the greate cold seedes clensed, of euery one. ʒ. iiii. the seedes of white Popie. ʒ. vi. ʒ. ß. of Quinces, or the thinnest of Goates milke, li. vi. let them stand twoo daies in the infusion, and after let theim be distilled, giue the sicke paciente to drinke. ʒ. iiii. warme, so long as the disease continueth *Epiphanius Empericus*.

An other water cōposed of *Aegidius*, it is cōmended of *Lullus*, of waters, ℞. Rewe, Satirion with the handes, and Satirion with the stones, Agrimonie, Chelidoni, Sugar, and the stone called Calaminaris, all of one waight, and beat it in a morter, it must be distilled with a slow fire: this water excelleth in vertues, no disease of the iyes is so dull or dimme, or greate, but it wil banishe awaie, and giue place to this medicen: beyng dronke, it driueth awaie all poisone, or taken with meates,

The booke of Compoundes. Fol.xlv.

tes, for so it auoideth the poisone by vomites, it cureth the Dropsie, it purgeth the stomacke from al euill humours, it quencheth sainct Anthonies fire in one daie, if flaxe dipte in it, be laied vpon the sore: it is good also against the fire of a blacke Melācholy, and white apostume without the fire, but if it appere redde without, it shall in no wise be conuenient, to laie on a plaster. It also healeth the canker, if Aloes be mixte with it, and a little Towe or flaxe dipte in it, and laied like a plaster vpon it, twise a daie: this is a precious medicen, & neuer faile. *Sacra ignis.*

Sicknes.

These be excellēt waters. Be there any good waters against the fallyng sicknesse, and resolucion of the senewes and feuers. I praie you tell me them.

Health.

Here after I will shewe thee goodly waters, for the same purpose, as folowe. Take Hisope, Peneriall, Cloues, Cikory, ana. ʒ.i. let thē be beaten in a morter, and distilled in Sage water. li.vi. afterward take the stone *Tutiæ*, Persely, Rue, Setwall, Aloes, and the stone called Callaminatis, ana. ʒ.i. and Ualarion. ʒ. vi. when thei are beaten in a Morter, seeth theim in the foresaied water, till the thirde parte be consumed, and the liquore strained with a clothe, thou shalte kepe it in a glasse, diligently closed nine daies, afterward let it beé giuen in drinke, euery daie in the Mornyng before daie (by the space of tenne daies) to the sicke paciente fastyng, it is profitable againste the fallyng sicknes: If he that taketh it, continue fastyng after it sixe howers. And truely it is a moste effectuall remedie, it healeth all resolucions of the senewes, and the members are strengthened thereby, if it be dronke with Castorium, it is good againste all goutes, whiche hath not taken roote yet in the members, if it be dronk nine daies together fastyng, it putteth awaie all maner of agues, what matter so euer it come of, if it be dronke nine daies, euery mornyng earely. This water is also most profitable to wash woūdes, in which the sinewes are cut. *A goodly water for feuers generall.*

An other of *Aegidius*, the nineth in nomber, otherwise thei call it double, the seede of Smalage, the seede of white Popie, Ginger, Sugar, Cloues, ana equall waight, beaten in a Morter, put to it water (that is distilled of Persely) and distille it: this is the chifest remeady for the cough, and breast pained, if a man drinke it colde in the mornyng fastyng, and in the euenyng as hote as he can: If it be dronke hote with Castorio, it is good against the disease called Apoplexia, it healeth also the members sicke of the Pallsie, if so be the Pallsie bee not dedde in the members, it bringeth slepe and reste easely, it cherisheth all the members, it driueth awaie euill humours, and strengtheneth the hed and the braine. *Another water of Aegidius.* *Water agaiṅt the Pallsey, & to helpe the braine.*

An other emongest *Aegidius* waters, Gladiolus, Hisope, Sauin, Sothernewood, or the seede of Sothernewood, leauyng out Sauine, of

H.iii. euery

The booke of Compoundes.

A water to be vsed with discrescion.

euery one like quantite, beate them together, and let them stand a certaine daies, then distille it. This water is of greate strength, it withstandeth all Agues, bothe hote and colde: it prouoketh womennes termes, if it bee dronke thrise, but it is hurtfull to women with childe, it stancheth the bloodie flixe, and other flixes: It killeth wormes, beyng dronke fastyng. It cureth all the grief, which with Beuers stones healeth the Palsie (if it be dronke daily very hote) within three daies, the same descripcion is found in the boke of *Lullus* of waters moste excellēt.

Therbe some that vse this water to purge.

Here after foloweth a very good water. Take a Weather, that is al white, and fatte fedde in a good pasture, and well likyng, cut his throt receiue his blood, and stirre it while it is freshe and new, a good tyme, with a sticke of redde Juneper, and euer in the stirryng, cast awaie the lumpes, that is gathered of the blood, then cast in the shauings of the same Juniper, and the beries of Juniper that be red, to the nomber of xxv. and to this put a little Agrimony, Rue, Valarian, Scabious and Veronica, commonly so called, Pimpernell, Cicory, Peneriall, ana, if so be it, the measures of the blood excede three quarters, then put into it. ʒ. iii. Triacle of Jene, but if it be lesse : accordyng to the porcion of the blood, thou shalt make lesse the measure of the Triacle. Thei must all bee prepared ready at hande, that thei maie bee put into the blood, while it is yet warme : when thei are all mixte, drawe out a stilled liquore, whiche thou shalt kepe diligently in a glasse, and sette it in the Sunne eight daies, for it will endure twentie yeres, it is knowen by experience, that this liquore is excellent, and good againste the Pestilence, the impostumes of the hedde, the sides, or ribbes, or againste the diseases of the liuer, and lightes, the inflacion of the Splene, corrupte blood, agues, swellynges, tremblynges of the hart, the dropsie, vnnaturall heates, ill humours: and chiefly against poisone, and the Pestilent Ague. The sicke paciente that is taken, with any of the foresaied diseases, shall drinke a sponefull, or fower or fiue, and procure hymself to sweate, and shall be healed within his sicke bodie.

Distill this bloud, & kepe it close.

An excellent liquor agaist the pestilens and many other diseases.

Sicknes.

what are composed waters, I would gladly learne them.

Health.

Thei are to bee called composed waters, that are distilled of medicens composed, and stieped in wine, *Aqua vitæ*, or other liquore: certain composicions of spices and verbes, to restore the strength of the harte, and the spirites, are mixt with waters of Capons, dreste by distillacions, accordingly: also with burnyng waters, or called *Quinteƒƒence* of wine, against the Pestilēce, and poisones, as we declared before, but also hote medicens *Electuariis*, chiefly in the whiche *Dacridium*, and other vehement thynges hurtfull to the stomacke, are receiued, mixte with the liquores, specially with burnyng water rectified, or with wine (sometyme also with Milke and wine, or with waie: also in hotte natures and

The boke of Compoundes.   Fol.xlvj.

and diseases, it should doe well) and sometyme let stande in fusion, or sokyng, thei are artificially distilled, that thei maie be giuen to drinke to them that are weake or feable, or as thei call it deintie, or haue their stomackes abhorryng, againste other medicens, whiche *Lullus* also praiseth greatly, and certain practicioners, of antiquitie haue vsed it with praise, and commendacion.   *what composed waters be*

Sicknes.

I would learne to make Quintessence of *Antimonio*, if it would please you to shewe me.

Health.

Quintessence, of *Antimonio*, is thus made, incorporate, and mingle the pouder of *Antimoni*, moste finely beaten, with most sharpe white vinegar distilled, and let it stade vntill the vinegar be tourned, into a very redde culler, then pour this vinegar out, and kepe it. And in a clene vessell, put other distilled vinegar, vpon the *Antimonium*, and set it ouer a little fire, till the vinegar be coloured, this shall you chaunge so oft, till the vinegar will be coulered no more, and so moche of the vinegar as is coulered, thou shalt distille it in a Limbicke in asshes: first the vinegar it self will run out, after this, thou shalt se a matter issue forthe of sondrie coullers, and this is that *quintessence*, whiche is called of the Philosophers, the Philosophers Leade, and of some called virgines Milke (it differeth notwithstandyng from it) it is almoste like blessed oile in couler: putte this in a Pellican, to bee circulated by the space of fourtie daies, it drieth vp woundes, and it is profitable for all woundes, in stede of Balme, for it cureth all the saied woundes easely, and quickly: it is maruellous good for all impostumes, and *Quintessence* is extracted, and drawen out of white Leade, after the same maner, as out of *Antimonio*, powring distilled vinegar vpō it, that the vinegar be ouer it fower fingers depe, afterward let it be digested in a dūghit, as it is vsed in *Quintessence*, of herbes and flowers, then let it be destilled and first ye shall se the vinegar it self ascende vp, after that a liquore like to oile, and also this is called oile of Leade, or *Quintessence* of Leade, and it hath in it a certaine sweetenesse, like as the oile of *Antimoni*: it is good against all burnynges with fire, and hote water, as also against iches, as ryngwormes, and Chollerike bladders, but a man must note that the white Leade ought first to bee washed often, with water of Roses, driuyng it through a linen clothe, vntill none of the pouder of the white Leade remain in it, then when it is dried, reserue it to your vses. So doeth *Bulcasus*, and *Ioan* of sainct *Amandus*, vpō the *Antidotarie* of *Io. Mesue*, will to bee dooen: If the drawyng foorthe of *quintessence*, out of diuers metalles, as Golde, Siluer, Leade, Tynne, Vitrioll, or Coporas, Iron Coper, Brimstone, redde Orpement, yelowe Ocker, *Antimonio*, and *Marchasita* Leaden, who so listeth, let hym rede in *Lullus*, in his booke of *Quintessence*, the spirite of *Quintessence*, or Vittrioll, is commended of certain men

Antimonium is called Stibium, or a stō bright and shinyng foūd among siluer, this ston dō clense the eyes.

Philosophers lead.

A water that drieth vp woūdes and healeth them.

Quintessence is drawne out of many meatels.

H.iiii.   against

The booke of Compoundes.

againste the fallyng sicknesse, and Apoplexia, or the beginnyng of the sences. The spirite of Golde, against the diseases of the Liuer, the spirite of Birall, against the stone of the raines and blader.

Sicknes.

How make you *Aqua vitæ, after maister Raimundus Lullus*: whiche was a man moste excellent in waters.

Health.

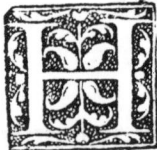

Raymonde Lullus, florished, anno 1322. he was a Spaynard

His water for the stone.

HE in his daies, did make the water of life, called *Aqua vitæ* of incomperable goodnesse. Mary he vsed to stille his waters, bothe simple and compounded: many tymes to make theim more heauenly or pure. But to the matter, of makyng this *Aqua vitæ*.

Take an herbe called wilde Mirte, like Butchars Brome, *Asparagus*, called Sperage, Rapes, Persellie, the Sea Thistle, called *Eryngium* Maiden heere, Grumill, called *Grana Solis*, Cichorie, Endiue, and wilde Carrites, Fenill rootes, ana of like quantie, cutte or braied grosly, and stille theim with your wine, vpon a soft fire. This water will breake the stone, and make moche brine.

Another precious water.

Here foloweth an other. Take Nutmegges, the roote called Doronike, which the Apoticaries haue, Setwall, Galingall, Mastike, long Peper, the barke of Pome Citron, or Mellon, Sage, Bazell, Margerum, Dil, Spicknarde, wod of Aloes, Cubebe, Cardamon called graines of Paradice, Lauender, Peniroyall, Mintes, sweete Calamus, Germander, Enulacampana, Rosemary, Stichados, Squinans of eche like quantitie, Saffron. ʒ. i. and the bone of a Hartes hart grated cut and stamped: but beate your spices grosly in a morter. Put in Ambergrice, Mulke, ana. ʒ. ſs. distill this in a common simple *Aqua vitæ*, made with strong ale, or Sacke leyes, and Aniseedes: not in a common still, but in a Serpentine, to tell the vertue of this water, againste colde, wind, fleume, dropsie, and heauinesse of minde, coming of melancholi. I can not declare, the excellent vertue therof, the tyme wer to long.

Sicknes.

How make you a water, that will kill the Cancre, and heale the place, whereas the saied Cancre haue been.

Health.

Sir Thomas Eliot. Sir Phillip Paris.

MAny good menne and women within this realme, haue diuers and sondrie medicens for the Cancre, and dooe helpe their neighbours, that bee in perill and daunger, whiche be not onely poore and nedie, hauyng no money to spend in Chirurgi. But some doe dwel where no Chirurgians be nere at hand, in soch cases as I haue saied, many good Gentlemen and Ladies, haue doen no small pleasure, to poore people: as that excellente knight, and worthie learned man, sir Thomas Eliot, whose workes be immortall. Sir Philippe Parris of Cambridge

The booke of Compoundes. Fol.xlvij.

shire, whose cures deserueth praise. Sir William Gaiscogne of Yorke shire, that helped many sore iyen: And the Ladie Tailor of Huntyngdon shire, and the ladie Dorrel of Kent, had many precious medicens, to comforte the sight, and to heale woundes withall, and were well seen in herbes. *(Sir William Gaiscoigne.)*

The common wealth hath greate wante of them, and of their medicens: whiche if thei had come into my handes, thei should not haue been written on the backside of my booke. Emong al other there was a knight, a manne of greate worshippe, a Godly hurtlesse gentleman, whiche is departed this life: his name was sir Anthony Heuenyngham. This gentleman learned a water, to kille a Cancre, of his owne mother, whiche he vsed all his life, to the greate helpe of many men, women, and children: he had also a salue, for sundrie grene woundes. But bicause I haue not the coppie therof, I will make report, but onely of that water, whiche I am assured he vsed, and it is not moche vnlike a water for the Cancre, whiche *Andreas Furnerius* the Frenchman, did make of a greate vertue, and thus it foloweth. *(Sir Anthonie Heueningham of Henyngham in Suffolke his medicene against the Cancre.)*

Take Doues foote, an herbe so named, Arcangell, Iue with the beries, young redde Brier, toppes and leaues, white Roses, their leaues and buddes, redde Sage, Selandine, and Woodbinde, of eche like quātitie, cutte or chopped, and put into pure cleane white wine, and clarified Hony. Then breake into it Alum glasse, and put in a little of the pouder of Aloes, Hypatici, & destill these together softly, in a limbecke of glasse, or pure Tinne, if not, then in a Limbecke, wherein *Aqua vitæ* is made. Kepe this water close, it will not onely kille the Cancre, if it be daily wasshed therwith: but also twoo droppes daily put into the iye, will sharpe the sight, and breake the pearle and spottes, specially if it be dropped in, with a little Fenell water, and close the iye after.

Sicknes.

Any men, women, and children, now a daies, be greuously bered with a shamefull disease, called the Frenche Pockes, paines in their iointes, no reste, palenesse of culler, fallyng of here baldnes of hedde and berde, lamenes of limmes, skabbes, filthe. &c. in soche cases what is to bee doen, I praie you tell me gentle Health, for this sicknesse waxeth common, but yet it would faine bee called, but onely a Feuer.

Health.

Any men haue written moche of this Pore, after sondry sortes, and diuers waies, & haue killed not a fewe with lōg diattes, but I will speake that, whiche I do knowe, proued and seen, to haue helped very many. Yet would I not, that any should fishe for this disease, or be to bolde when he is bitten, to thinke hereby to be helped: but rather eschue the cause of this infirmitie, and filthy, rotten, burning of harlottes. &c. As to flie from the Pestilence, or from a wilde fire, for *(A treatice of the pore.)*

what

The booke of Compoundes.

A treatise of the Poxe.

what is more to bee abhorred, then a pockie, filthie, stinkyng carcas. But if through blinde ignoraunce, sodain chaunce. &c. any haue gotten it: then doe thus to be deliuered from it.

Thre notable thynges to be obserued in this Guacũ drinke, and ye diate in the time of sicnes

First ye shall, prouide that the sicke bodie, muste haue a close chamber out of all grose ayre, and clene warme garmentes, bothe for the bodie and legges, and at risyng, and goyng to bedde, a fyre of Charcoles, for wodde is not holsom for smokyng, also they must not be troubled with any thyng to bryng them out of patience, for that corrupteth the bloud, whiche must be new altered: also the sicke body must eate but littell meate, and that kinde of meate as shall hereafter be prescribed, and at suche time as shalbe apointed, and let the sicke body vse plaiyng of some instrumentes, or here some plaiyng, or tell merie tales, and haue no company of women, for that is a moste daũgerous poison for the health of any persone in that case.

Although the pore be moste vncleane, yet to heale the same, requireth clenlines as moche as medicene.

Secondly, ye muste prepare twoo Brasse pottes, or els of Iron, one beyng .iiii. gallons, the other .vi. gallons, one for strong drinke, the other for smal drinke, also ye must haue close couers to them of brasse or Iron, ye must also prepare good earthen vessels with close couers to kepe your drinke in of bothe sortes by them selues. Also ye must haue a strainer of a Sears clothe, to straine your drinke after it is decockte: instrumentes to take out dead fleshe, and to searche a sore, and firing to clese any sore being depe with the same drinke. Also ye must haue a wodden bessell to bathe the sicke body in, at such times as here after shalbe apoynted. Also ye must prepare cleane clothes, to drie the sicke body after a sweate, beyng warmed well first, other instrumentes ye shall neede none, but only your wod raped small, or turned, and the barke of the wod pouned in a morter, and the drugges also small, and your water whiche ye shall decocke, the same must be of a cundite, or runnyng brooke, verie cleane without any kinde of filthe. Chalke water is good.

Howe to proue good Guacum.

Thirdly for your strong drinke, ye must take your potte of .iiii. gallons, & set him one a soft fyre of cooles, with .iiii. gallons of the fayre runyng water, then put into the same one pounde and a half of your wodde small raped or turned, at the Turners, but when you do bye your wodde, se it be not olde, and lacke moyster, the triall is best, take a littell coale burnyng and lay it on the blocke, before it be raped, and if it be good it will boyle vp on euery side of the coale, like Myrre, thẽ put therto. ʒ. i. or a littell more of the barke of the same wodde, made in small pouder, then take a quarter of a pounde of comen seedes hole into the same, and one halfe quarter of an ounce of Radyre, and Rubarbe, and then stoppe your pot faste, and laie paste aboute the couer, and so faste, that no ayre come out, then seth it on a soft fire, but euer

Softe fire maketh swet Malte, and ye like doe make good Guacũ drinke.

to kepe it boilyng, and let it boyle at the leaste .viii. houers, then set it by, and vnstoppe it not vntill it bee colde, then take your Sears, and strain it into a fayre yearthen potte, and couer it cloase: the sicke body muste drinke of this but one draught leuke warme in the mornyng,

and

The booke of Compoundes. Fol.xliij.

and one other at night.

Fourthly you must take your potte of .vi. gallons, and put in it .vi. gallons of runnyng water, and one pounde of the wodde raped, and a quarter of cummen seedes, and decocke it in al kinde of thing, euen as the other, beinge close stopped, and when it is colde straine it into an earthen vessell, or vessels: and that must the partie drinke at meale, & at all other times whē he list to drinke, and spare not but drawe it by. <small>Fourth rule.</small>

Fiftly the sicke body must be kept very warme, and not rise out of bed before .viii. of the clocke, and then eate a dosen or twenty Raisons of the sonne, and no breade, and about a leauen of the clocke, let the sicke body eate a littell meate as may suffice nature, and what meate, it shalbe hereafter shewed, then let the sicke body walke some whiles, in his chamber, or reade some booke, or play on instrumentes to kepe him from sleaping, then at .vi. of the clocke, a dosen of Raisons of the sonne, and nothing els but his draught of stronge drinke warmed at vi. a clocke in the morning, and at euening at eight. <small>Fifth rule. Note, also that Filtrum is good to clense the Guiacu water with.</small>

Sixtly, geue to the pacient to eate these meates folowing, Cheken Pertrige, Fesante, Henne, Capon, Rabbette, Conie, Veale, Mutton, and none other, nor any salt, nor leauened bread, nor Rie bread, & very seldom rosted, but boiled in water, and no broth, nor porrage, nor any kinde of sauce, if the sicke body haue roste, let it bee but euery thirde meale, and no kinde of Fishe, Milke, or fruites, Raysons excepted. <small>Sixt rule.</small>

Seuenthly, once in .iii. daies, for the first .ix. daies in the mornynge let the sicke body drinke a good draught of ẏ stronge drinke somthing warme, and then lay very many clothes on him, till he sweat, for the space of twoo houres, then ease some of the cloathes, and haue warmed linnen cloathes, and rubbe all the bodie drie or he rise, if he haue any sores that be depe, wash the sore with the strong drinke, and with a sypring, and depe a littell cloath in the stronge drinke, and lay it to the sore, whether it be sores or knobbes. <small>Seuēth rule</small>

Eightly, after .ix. or .x. daies be past, once in three daies let the sicke bodie be bathed on this sort. Set fayre running water on the fyre, & put therto a great deale of grounde Iuie leaues, and redde Sage, and Fenell also, and by a good fyre when the sicke bodie is goyng to bedde, put the water and herbes, into a vessell of wodde, and let the sicke bodie stande vpright in it, by the fyre, and take vp the herbes and rubbe the body of the sicke paciente downewardes, and then drie him with warme cloathes, vse this .iii. weakes, & by the grace of God the sicke body shalbe made whole, what soeuer they be, then if ẏ partie be very weake after .ix. or .x. of the first daies, then let them eate euery daie at .iiii. of the clocke at after noone, a new laied Egge poched in faire water, & as much new bread as will suffice nature, & a litle cleane wine, rede furder in the place of *Guiacum* for ẏ Pox, wheras is shewed greater secretes. And for this diat few men are to be cōpared in worthinesse & knowledge to Thomas Gladfeild a cunning Chirurgian of London. <small>Eight rule, Thomas Glanfeild.</small>

Sicknes.

H.i. Now

The Table of Compoundes.

Now I praie you maister Health make a brief rehersal of the Compoundes, and shortly their names, and to what sicknes they be aplied vnto.
Health.

That I shall gladly, & first I will begin as foloweth: wherfore thei doo serue, praiynge thee to be contented to reade them, and marke them diligently: and also of the common seedes, colde & hot, of ointments. &c.

Vreæ alexandria.
Mythridatum
Sirupus de Bizantijs.
Trochisci diarhodon
Pilles of Agarike. &c.

¶ **Against Tercian Agues.**

Aureæ Alexandrina
Oxysaccharo simplex.
Sirupus de acetosæ simplicis.
Sirup of tarte Pomgranites.
Syrupus de Bazantijs

¶ **Against Quarten Agues.**

Antidotum asincritum
Diasene.
Mythridatum andromachi.
Oxysaccharo
Vnguentum aragon

¶ **Against hot burning agues.**
Sirup of Violets.
Diaprunes **not laxatiue.**
Decoctio communis
Electuarium catholicum
Mel violatum
Oxysaccharo.
Sirupus de limonibus
Trochisci de camphora
Vnguentum populeon

Against agues coming of diuers humours.
Diaphænicon
Pilulæ Agregatiue
Pilles of Reubarbe.
Trochisci diarhodonis

¶ **Against long agues of colde.**

Diacurcuma
Diacoralium magistrale
Pilles of Reubarbe.
Sirupus de eupatorio
Trochisci de Rubarbaro
Trochisci de absinthio

¶ **The foure great hot seedes.**

Aniseede,
Fenell seede,
Cummen seede, & Carowaies.

¶ **The foure hotte and lesser seedes.**
Amij, Amonium, **Smalage,**
Yelow Carrets.

¶ **The foure great colde seedes.**
Gourdes, Cucumers,
Melons.
Citrons.

¶ **The foure colde and lesser seedes.**
Endiue, Chycory,
Lettice,
Purseline.

The foure hot ointments.
Vnguentum Martiaton, altheæ.
Aragon, et agrippe
Vnguentum Altheæ

The foure colde ointments.
Vnguentum album,
Populeum, Resumtiuum
Citrinum.

The fiue common opening rootes.
Smallage, Fenell,

Persely, Sperage.
Buchers Broume.
Kneholme.

¶ **The fiue waters whiche do comfort the hart.**
Endiue, Succorie,
Scabiose, Langdebefe.
Balme.

¶ **The viij. solutiue herbes.**
Mallowes, Mercurie,
Parietarie, Violets.
Colewortes, Holioke,
Acanthus. **Beetes,**

¶ **Against Lienteria.**
Aurea Alexandrina.
Theriaca Galeni
Trochisci diacorallion
Trochisci diambre
Trochisci de terra sigillata

¶ **Against biting of venimous beastes.**
Mythridatum.
Theriaca Galeni
Oleum de Scorpione

¶ **Against euill liking of the body.**
Diacurcuma
Diatragacantha frigida
Diacomeron.
Diasatirion.
Sirupus de eupatorio
Oleum Sesaminum
Trochisci de Rheubarbaro.

¶ **To aswage paine in any outwarde parte of the body coming of ache.**
Emplastrum oxycroceum.
Oile of Dill.
Oile of Juniper. &c.

Against

The Table of Compoundes.

Against inward diseases.
Antidotum asincritum
Aurea alexandrina
Mythridauum.

Against burning and scalding.
Electuarium palme.
Oile of Mirtes.
Vnguentum rosatum.
Oyle of Egges.
Oile of water Liliies.

Against broses.
Electuarium palme
Vnguentum aureum.
Vnguentum potabile.

Against paine in the spitting.
Emplastrum coroneum
Loboch de Pino.

Against belching of raw humors.
Diagalanga
Diatrion Pipereon.
Diatragacantha calida.
Loboch sanum
Oximel scilliticum
Sirup of Calamintes.

Against paine in the backe.
Pilule fœtide maioris
Oleum de Cheiri
Olium Scorpionis.
Diacassia

To drawe forth broken bones.
Emplastrum oxicrocium
Emplastrum contra rupturas. &c.

To purge the bladder of grauell.
Antidotum sincritum
Benedicta lax.
Diacurcuma.
Oximel diureticum

To aswage paine in the bladder.
Emplastrum de granis lauri.
Mythridatum Galeni.
Electuarij Ducis

Sirup of Iuiubes.
Trochisci de Alchachengi.
Oile of swete Almondes.
Oleum Cheiri

Against erulceracions in the bladder
Oximel scilliticum
Trochisci de Alchachengi

Against the colicke.
Antidotum asincritum.
Aurea alexandrina
Diaphœnicon
Trochisci de Rosis
Oile of Camamill. &c.

Medicenes to be vsed after lōg and hot agues.
Diarhodon abbatis
Rosata nouella

Against the colde and shaking in agues.
Mythridatum Galeni
Syrup of sticados.
Trochisci de eupatorio
Oile of Dill.
Oile of Sothernwood.

To cause an appetite.
Antidotum asincritum
Aromaticum rosatum
Miua simplex.
Conserue of Quinces.
Sirupus de absinthio
Electuarium confortatium Sto.

To comfort a cold brain
Electuarium de gemmis
Aromaticum rosatum
Conserue of Gladian.
Theriaca galeni
Oile of Maces

To comfort a moist braine.
Conserue of Rosemarie.
Diambre
Diaprassion
Diatragacantha calida
Electuarium indi maioris
Pilule alephanginæ

To aswage paine of the brest.
Decoctio pectorale
Loboch de squilla.
Oleum de cheiri
Vnguentum marciaton
Sirupus de Hyssopo. &c.

Against streghtnes of the brest.
Confectio dulcis de moscho
Conserue of Maidēheere
Diatragacantha calida.
Theriaca Galeni
Vnguentum Martiaton.

Against diseases of the brest.
Diacomeron
Diatragacantha frigida
Sirup of Horehounde.
Sirup of Maidenheere.
Galeus cerott for the stomack.

To cause bouldnesse.
Triphera magna.
Electuarium de gemmis.

Against gnawing in the belly.
Antidotum asincritum
Mythridatum

To kepe the boofe stronge.
Pilulæ lucis maiores
Rosata nouella
Sirupus ex infusione rosarum
Theriaca Galeni
Diasatirion.

Against spitting of bloud.
Mythridatum Galeni
Antidotum Asincritum
Electuarium inde Maioris
Emplastrum de granis Lauri
Pilu'e aureæ
Pilulæ Fætida maiores
Pilulæ sine quibus esse nolo
Theriaca Galleni

P.ij. Against

The Table of Compoundes.

¶ Against old coughes of humours.
Mythridatum
Pilles of Agarike.
Pilulæ Bechi.
Loboch de Pino.
Loboch sanum
Sirup of Horehounde.
Syrup of Mirtes.
Sirup of Hysope

Against a drie cough.
Julep of Violettes.
Sirup of Liquoris.
Sirup of Violettes.
Sirup of Popie comp.
Syrup of Jujubes.

¶ Againste the cough of the lunges.
Antidotum asincritum.
Diatragacantha frigida

¶ Against coughes, whiche come of superfluous humours in the stomack.
Aurea Alexandrina
Diamargaritum calidum
Diacomeron
Diacalamintha
Diaireos
Diapapaueris
Decoctio pectorale
Loboch sanum
Loboch de pulmone Vulpis
Sirup of Calamintes

¶ Against the Crampe.
Mythridatum
Theriaca Galeni
Sirup of Sticados
Oile of Flowerdeluce,
Vnguentum martianum magnum
Vnguentum Arogon

Against conuulcions.
Mythridatum andromachi
Theriaca Galeni
Vnguentum Arogon
Vnguentum Martianum.

¶ Against the consumpcion.
Aster.
Aurea Alexandrina
Diamargaritum calidum
Diacomeron.
Dierhodon abbatis.
Diatragacantha frigida
Mythridatum
Triasandali.
Loboch de pulmone Vulpis

¶ Against the canker, in any part of the bodie.
Confectio hamech.

¶ Against all aches, and diseases of colde.
Oile of Baie.
Oile of Spike.
Oile of Coste.
Oile of Camomill.
Oile of Flowerdelice.
Oile of Roses.
Oile of Masticke.
Oile of Lilles
Vnguentum Martianum magnum.
Vnguentuum Aragon
Vnguentum de althea

¶ Againste cliftes aboute the fundamente, or other places.
Oile of Mirtes.
Pomatum.

¶ To deliuer women of dedde children.
Theriaca Galeni. &c.

¶ To cause good colour.
Antidotum asincritum.
Electuarium de gemmis.
Oleum de Costo
Trochisci Diarhodon
Hiera picra Galeni

¶ To purge cholet.
Antidotum asincritum
Aromaticum rosatum
Conditum Cotoneorum
Confectio Hamech

Diacurcuma
Conserue of Langdebefe
Conserue of Borage.
Conserue of Maidenheere
Conserue of Succorie.
Conserue of Sorell.
Oxysaccaro simplex.
Electuarium de roses
Electuarium de psillio.
Pilulæ sine quibus esse nolo
Pilulæ de octo rebus

¶ For colde complexions.
Diatragacantha frigida
Sirup of Endiue.
Trochisci de Rabarbaro
Siripus de acetositate citri
Sirupus de succo acetosæ
Sirupus comp. de Fumiterre
Sirupus acetosus comp.

¶ To make good digestion.
Antidotum Asincritum
Aromaticum rosatum
Condicum cotoneorum.
Diacuminum
Diamber
Diacalaminthæ
Diatrion pipereon
Miua simplex
Pilulæ ante cibum
Oile of Mintes.

Against the dropsie.
Diacomeron
Diacurcuma
Emplastrum coronem,
Emplastrum de granis Lauri
Pilulæ de Euphorbio
Theriaca galeni
Trochisci de Eupatorio.
Trochisci de Rhabarbaro
Sirupus de eupatorio
Vnguentum Agrippæ

To cleare the iye sight.
Diaprasium
Pilulæ Cochiæ rasis
Colyrium album rasis

Hiera

The Table of Compoundes.

Hiera picra Galeni
Pilulæ sine quibus
Pilulæ de aureæ
Pilulæ de octo generibus mirabolanorū

Against pain in the iyes.
Antidotum asincritum.
Mythridatum androm.

Against all maner of exulceracions.
Oile of Violettes.
Emplastrum de Cerusa
Theriaca Galeni
Trochisci de alchachengi

Against deafnes and paines of the eares.
Mythridatum andromachi
Oile of sweet Almondes.
Pilulæ sine quibus esse noli

Against the faulyng euill.
Antidotum asincritum
Aurea Alexandrina
Confectio dulcis de moschu
Syrup of sticados.
Theriaca Galeni
Vnguentum Marceatum

To purge fleume.
Antidotum asincritum
Diacartami
Confectio hamech.
Diatrion pipereon
Conserue of Rosemarie.
Conserue of Gladian.
Conserue of Enulacāpa.
Mel rosatum
Pilulæ alephagine
Pilulæ fœtide maiores
Pilles of Euphorbe.
Pilulæ de Sarcocolla

To purge salt fleume.
Sirupus comp. de Fumiterre

To make a beautifull and a faire face.
Oleum de tartaro
Pomatum.

Against flures of the bodie.
Antidotum asincritum
Diacordion
Mythridatum andromachi
Mycleta
Miua simplex
Oile of Roses.
Sirupus de rosis siccis
Sirupus de agresta
Sirupus de Acetositate
Sirup of Mintes

☞ Against the flure of meate vndigested.
Mythridatum
Mycleta
Oile of Mirtes.
Sirup of Calamintes.
Trochisci Diacorallion

Against the bloodie flixe.
Diacodium Mesuæ
Mythridatum
Mycleta
Trochisci diacorallion

To prouoke the menstruall termes.
Mythridatum
Sirupus de absinthio
Trifera sarasanica
Trochisci de mirrha

To stoppe the menstruall termes.
Pilulæ de Bdellio
Trochisci de terra Sigillata

To stoppe the flure, after a strong purgacion.
Electuarium conformatium sto.

Against palenesse of the face.
Hiera picra Galeni

To cause newe flesh.
Vnguentum Apostolicum

To consume dedde flesh.
Vnguentum Apostolicum
Vnguentum Ægiptiacum

Against old fistulaies.
Vnguentum Apostolicum
Vnguentum Ægiptiacum

Against the Goute of heate.
Electuarium de rosis
Pilulæ Arthriticæ
Oile of Wormewood.
Olium Lumbricorum
Oleum de Cheririnum

Against the Goute of colde.
Benedicta laxat'ua
Electuarium inde Maiorū
Mythridatum
Antidotum Asincritum
Pilulæ Fœtida maioris
Oile of Baie
Oile of Spike.
Oile of Flowerdelice.
Oile of Mastike.
Oile of Euphorbe.
Vnguentum Marciaton
Vnguentuum Aragon

Against the Goute in the feete onely.
Æntidotum Asincritum
Benedicta laxa
Mythridatum
Pilulæ de quinque generibus myroba.
Pilulæ Fœtida maiores
Oleum Vulpinum
Vnguentum marciaton

Against gaulynges.
Emplastrum de Cerusa
Oile of Mirtes.

For Glisters.
Diacasia fistula pro Clist.
Hiera picra Galeni

To comfort the harte.
Diacorallium magistrale
Electuarium de gemmis
Sirupus de acetosa
Theriaca Galeni
Trochisci de gallia moschata
Aromaticum rosatum

H.iij.   Aroma-

The Table of Compoundes.

Aromaticum gariophillatum
Conserue of Roses.
Diambre
Diamargaritum calidum.
Diarhodon abbatis.

To engender heate in the inwarde partes.
Aromaticum gariophillatum.
Diacuminum
Diambre
Emplastrum stomachicum
Oyle of Rue.

Against trembling of the harte.
Confectio de musco dulcis
Electurrium de gemnis
Conserue of Borage.
Conserue of Langdebief.

Against heate of the harte.
Iulep of Roses.
Iulep of Violets.
Sirup of Violets.
Sirup comp. of Endiue.
Sirupus de infusione rosarū viridium.
Sirupus de succo acetosæ.

Against horsenesse.
Decoctio pectoralis,
Lohoc sanum.
Oleum senaminum.
Syrup of Iuiubes.
Theriaca Galeni.

Against the Hickup.
Antidotum asincritum
Syrup of Mirrhe.

Against falling of the heere.
Oyle of Baye.
Oyle of Coste.

Against ache in the hyppe.
Aurea Alexandrinæ
Pilule fetidus maiores,
Pilule de quinq̃ generibus mira.
Oyle de Baies.

Oleum vulpinum.
Vnguentum marteaton.
Vnguentum aragonum

Against al maner of hardenesse.
Mythridatum.
Oile of sweet Almondes.
Oyle of Bay.
Oyle of Wintes.
Oile of Holioke.
Oleum Sesaninum
Oyle of Flowerdelice.
Oyle of Mastike.
Emplastrum diachilon album
Emplastrum diachilon magnum
Emplastrum de mucelagenibus
Emplastrum de melilote.
Emplastrum oxycroceum
Vnguentum apostolicum
Vnguentum Martiaton

To purge the head.
Pilulæ aureæ
Pilule Cochie

Against olde hedache.
Antidatum asincritum
Pilule Cochie Rasis
Pilule agregatiue

Against hedache of heate.
Electuarium de Rosis.
Oyle of Roses.
Oile of water Lillies.
Oile of Poppie.
Vnguentum rosatum.

Against hedache of colde.
Mythridatum.
Aurea alexandrina.
Oyle of Dill.
Oyle of Spike.
Oyle of Flowerdelice.
Oleum de euphorbio
Vngentum Martiatou

Against the Hemerodes.
Mycleta
Pilule de Bdellio

To kepe the head from basenesse.
Oyle of Coste.

Against vermen and scurfe of the head.
Oyle of Bay.
Oyle of Lilles

Against the yellow Iaunders.
Antidotum asincritum
Diarhodon abbatis
Electuarium de ribis
Syrupus de Bizantinj.
Theriaca galeni
Trochisti de Camphora
Trochisci de rubarbaro
Trochisci de eupatorio
Triasandali

Against Ilica passio.
Antidotum asincritum
Theriaca galeni
Mythridatum Andromachj
Hiera picra
Pilule sine quibus
Vnguentum martiaton.

Against inflamacions
Antidotum asincritum
Cerotum stomachicum

Against hot impostumes either in the stomack or liuer.
Cærotus pro stomacho

Against inwarde impostumes.
Trochisci de reubarbaro
Trochisci de eupatorio
Olium violarum

Against hot impostumes in the throate.
Diamoron potio

To ripe impostumes.
Emplastrum diachilon magnum
Emplastrum diachilon paruum
Emplastrum diachilon album
Oyle of Flowerdelice.

Oyle

The Table of Compoundes.

Oyle of Masticke.

Against insensibilitie.
Mythridatum
Theriaca galeni. &c.

Against inflamacions of choler.
Conserue of Uiolets.
Vnguentum rosatum.

Against paine of the Liuer.
Antidotum asincritum
Diacurcuma
Pilulæ aggregatiue
Pilule de euphorbio
Trochisci de rubarbaro
Sirup of Cetrac.

Against heate of the Liuer.
Julep of Roses.
Julep of Uiolets.
Electuarium catholicum
Mel violateum
Sirup of Uiolets.
Sirup comp. of Endiue.
Triasandali
Trochisci de champhori
Trochisci de spodio
Vnguentum rosatum

Against coldnesse of the Liuer.
Theriaca galeni
Diagalanga
Diarhodon abbatis
Trochisci de gallia moschata
Trochisci de absinthio.
Trochisci de eupatorio
Emplastrum stomachicum
Oyle of Euphorbio.
Sirupus de eupatorio
Sirupus de absinthio

Against hardnesse of the Liuer.
Emplastrum diachilon album
Pilule de euphorbio

To make a man laxatiue.
Antidotum asincritum
Hiera picra galeni
Conserue of Uiolets.
Diacassia fistula pro enematibus

Against daunger of life.
Antidotum asincritum
Diacomeron

Against heate of the Lunges.
Diatragantha frigida
Diarodon abbatis
Triasandali
Sirup of Uiolets.
Sirup of Endiue.
Sirup of comp. Endiue.
sirupus de infusione rosarū viridarum

Against coldenesse of the lunges.
Confectio dulcis de musco
Conserue of Maidenhere
Theriaca galeui
Trochisci de absinthio

Against drinesse of the lunges.
Oyle of sweet Almondes.
Sirup of Liquoris.

Against the Lepzie.
Confectio bamache
Theriaca galeni
Trochisci theriaci
Pilule fetide maiores.

Against the Mesels.
Theria galeni

Against madnesse.
Aurea Alexandrina
Diasene

Against the Mother.
Antidotum asincritum

To asswage paine of the Matrice.
Emplastrum de granis lauri
Oile of sweet Almondes.
Trifera

Against colde diseases.
Antidotum asincritum
Diambre.
Electuarium de gemmis
Oyle of Lilles.
Emplastrum pro matrice
Emplastrum Ceroneum
Oile of Flouerdeluce.
Oyle of Wormewood.

To cause Myrth.
Diambre
Diamargaritum calidum
Diacameron
Diasene
Electuarium de gemmis
Conserue of Borage.
Sirup of Langdebief.

To purge Melancholy.
Antidotum asincritum
Alipta muschata
Confectio dulcis de musco
Diasene
Mithridatum
Sirupus de epithimo
Conserue of Roses.
Conserue of Maideheere
Conserue of Succorie.
Conserue of Langdebief.
Conserue of Rosemarie.
Conserue of Borage.
Pilule fine quibus
Pilule de lapide lazuli
Pilule aggregatiue
Pilule lucis maioris
Trochisci de absinthio
Trochisci de eupatorio.

Against all diseases about the Medrife.
Mithridatum
Theriaca galeni.
Pilulæ Cochiæ Rasis
Oyle of Spike.
Oyle of Euphorbe.

Against sores in the mouthe.
Diamo.

The Table of Compoundes.

Diamoron potio
Mythridatum Cleo

Against bledyng at the nose.

Trochisci de terra sigillata
Trochisci de Carabæ

¶ Against stenche at the nose.

Oile of Flowerdelice.

Against wrythyng of the necke, on the one side.

Confectio dulcis de moscho
Sirup of Sticados

Against obstructions.

Oile of bitter Almondes
Oile of Coste.
Oile of Dill.
Oile of Camomill.
Oile of Flowerdelice.
Oile of Wormewoode.
Oleum de Cheiri
Sirupus de radicibus
Sirup of Bizantes
Sirup comp. of Endiue.
Sirup of Maidenhere
Sirup of Ceterac
Trochisci de Rabarbaro
Trochisci de Absinthio
Trochisci de Eupatorio.

To cause good odour and sauour.

Electuarium de gemnis.
Oile of Coste.

To comfort the principall partes.

Aromaticum rosatum
Aromaticum gariophillatum
Electuarium confortatum stomacum
Diamber
Diamargaritum calidum
Miua simplex
Sirup comp. of Femita.
Sirup of Buglosse.
Electuarium indum maius
Conserue of Roses.

Sirup of Calamintes
Oile of Coste.
Oile of Masticke.
Oile of Quinces

Against the dzinesse of the principall partes.

Oile of swete Almondes.

To mollifie the principall partes.

Conserue of Roses.

Against the Paulsie.

Antidoium asincritum.
Confectio dulcis de moscho
Mythridatum
Pilulæ de Euphorbio
Sirup of Sticados

Against the Pleurasie.

Diatragacantha frigida
Sirup of Violettes.
Julep of Violettes.
Lohoc of Squilla.
Conserue of Maidenheere
Oyle of Violettes.
Sirup of Liquoris.
Sirup of Hysope
Sirup of Endiue.
Syrup of Jujubes.
Vnguentum de althea

To purge the winde pipe of grosse humours.

Diaphasium
Theriaca galeni
Loche de Squilla
Loboch sanum
Sirup of Liquoris.
Sirupus acetosus compo.

¶ Against the pestilence or poison.

Theriaca Galleni
Mythridatum
Puluis contra pestem
Siripus de acetositate citri
Sirupus exacitosa
Sirupus de infusione

Rosarum viridium
Oile of Scorpions

Against Pimples or wheales.

Oile of Mirtes.

¶ Parfumes.

Confectio dulcis de musco. &c.

¶ Against reumes.

Antidotum asincritum
Aurea Alexandrina
Mythridatum
Diaprasium
Sirup of Sticados.
Sirup simp. of Popie.
Oile of Rue.

¶ To purge the Raines of grauell.

Antidotum asincritum.
Benedicta laxa.
Oximel diureticum
Sirupus acetosus comp.
Sirup of Maidenheere.
Sirup of Cetrac.

¶ Against pain in the Raines.

Aures Alexandrina
Mythridatum
Diacomeron
Diacurcuma
Electuarium inde maiores
Oleum vulpium
Oleum Cheiri
Emplastrum de granis Lauri

¶ Against ringwormes.

Confectio Hamech
Oleum de Tartara

¶ To comfort the stomacke.

Theriaca Galeni
Diacoralium magistrale
Diamargaritum calidum
Diaprasium
Diagalanga
Aromaticum rosatum
Aromaticum garyophillatum
Trochisci de gallia muschata

Trochisci

The Table of Compoundes.

Trochisci de alchachengi
Mythridatum
Mitua simplex
Electuarium confortatum stomacum
Electuarium de gemmis
Electuarium inde Maioris
Emplastrum stomachium
Sirup of Mirtes
Sirup of Sticados
Sirup of Wormwood
Sirup of Langdebefe.
Sirup of Quinces.
Sirup of drie Roses
Conserue of Langdebefe
Conserue of Enulacāpa.
Conditum Cotoneorum.
Oile of Coste.

¶ To purge the stomacke of grose humours.

Hierapicra Galeni
Pilulæ Fætida maioris
Pilulæ de Sarcocolla
Pilulæ lucis maiores
Pilulæ Stomachiæ.
Pilulæ de agarico
Oximel simplex.
Oximel Scyliticum
Emplastrum coronem
Theriaca Galeni
Sirup of Hysope.
Sirup of Horehounde.
Sirup of Maidenheere.
Sirupus acetosus compo.
Sirupus de limonibus

¶ Againste heate and burning of the stomacke.

Trochisci de Spodio
Trochisci de Camphroa
Diarhodon Abbatis
Triasandali.
Sirupus de succu acetosæ.
Iulep of Roses.
Vnguentum rosatum.

¶ Against coldnes of the stomacke.

Sirup of Mintes.

Sirup of Calamintes.
Oile of Wormewood.
Vnguentum de Althea.

¶ Against hardnesse of the stomacke.

Pilulæ de Euphorbio.
Emplastrum Diachilon album.

¶ Againste paine of the stomacke.

Emplastrum de grranis Lauri.
Emplastrum ceronem.
Pilulæ Fætida maiores
Pilulæ Agregatiue
Trifera.

¶ Against diseases of the Splen.

Antidotum asincritum
Diacurcuma.
Electuarium catholicum.
Pilulæ de quinque generibus myroba.
Sirup of Calamint.
Sirupus acetosus comp.
Oleum de euphorbio

¶ Against hardnesse of the Splene.

Trochisci de Absinthio
Trochisci de eupatorio
Emplastrum meliloti
Emplastrum diachilon album
Emplastrum coronem
Vnguentum marciaton

¶ Against sighyng.

Antidotum Asincritum
Diamargaritum Calidum.

¶ To cause the spittle to auoide.

Antidotum asincritum
Sirup of Pineaples.
Loboch de Squilla.

¶ To restore the speache.

Deaireos

¶ To breake the stone.

Aurea Alexandrina
Theriaca Galleni
Mythridatum
Oleum de Scorpione.

¶ Against the strangurion.

Aurea Alexandrina.

¶ Againste sounyng and fainting of the harte.

Diamargaritum calidum.
Diasene cum Manna.
Aurea Alexandrina
Sirup of Langdebefe.
Conserue of Langdebefe
Conserue of Borage.

¶ To prouoke sweate.

Oile of Dill, and other hotte oiles.

¶ To prohibite ouermoche sweating.

Rosata nouella.
Oile of Quinces
Oile of Mirtes.

To cause a man to slepe.

Diapapauer
Sirup of Popie.
Oile of flowers of Popie
Oile of Dill.
Oile of Nenuphar.

☞ For children, whiche can not slepe, or doe speake in their slepe.

Trifera.

Against strangurion.

Diamoron potio. &c.
Venise Terebentine

Against the scabbes.

Confectio Hamech
Oile of Baie
Vnguentum pro pueris scabiosis.
Vnguentum contra scabiem.

To purge the instrumentes of the sences.

Pilulæ Alephagine.
Pilulæ agregatiue.
Pilulæ lucis maioris.
Therica Galeni

Against the squincie.

Mythridatum

gainst the stifnesse of the inward members

Mythridatum

The Table of Compoundes.

Mythridatum audromachi
Conserue of Rosemary.
To mollifie and ripe all swellinges
Diachilon paruum
Emplastrum de granis lauri
Emplastrum Diachilon album.
Oile of Flowerdelice.
Vnguentum Apostolicum
Vnguentum Agrippæ

To increase seede.
Oile of sweet Almondes
Oleum Sesaminum

Against the slepe or forgetfull diseases.
Oleum de euphorbio

Against depe diseases in the sinewes.
Sirup of Sticados.
Oile of Quinces
Oile of Mastike.
Vnguentum agrippæ

Against colde diseases of the sinewes.
Oile of Euphorbe.
Olium Lumbricorum
Oleum de cherua.
Pilles of Euphorbe.

Against shoting of humours.
Emplastrum palmeum

Against great and colde sores.
Tela gualterii
Emplastrum de cerusa
Emplastrum de minio
Vnguentum Ægiptiacum

To drie vp sores and biles.
Emplastrum de Siccatiuum rubeum
Vnguentum Apostolorum. &c.

To quenche the thrist
Trochisci de camphora
Trochisci de Spodio

Rosata nouella.
Sirupus infusione rosarum viridium
Sirup of Quinces.
Sirup of white Popie.
Siripus de acetositate citri
Mel violatum
Julep of Roses.
Conserue of Violets.

Against the falling sicknesse.
Antidotum asincritum
Aurea Alexandrina
Confectio de moscho
Electuarium de rosis
Electuarium de psillio.

Against the touth ache.
Antidotum Asincritum
Aurea Alexandrina.
Mythridatum
Diaprassium
Pilulæ de Hiera simplici

Against roughnes of the tongue.
Diatragacantha frigida
Diamoron potio.
Sirup of Violettes.
Julep of Violettes.
Oleum sesaminum
Oile of sweet Almondes
Oile of Violettes. &c.

Against shortnesse of winde.
Antidotum asincritum
Mythridatum
Confectio dulcis de moscho
Alipta muschata
Diaireos.
Diacomeron
Sirup of Calamintes.
Theriaca Galeni
Pilles of Agarike.
Sirup of Horehounde.
Sirup of Hysope.
Sirupus de pino
Loboch de Squilla.

Loboch de papauere. &c.
To breake winde
Antidotum asincritum.
Aromaticum gariophillatum
Pilulæ aureæ
Diagalanga
Diacurcuma
Electuarium indum maius
Sirupus de eupatorio
Oile of sweet Almondes.
To stop vomiting.
Antidotum asincritum.
Aromaticum gariophillatum
Miua simplex
Rosata nouella
Sirup of Mintes.
Syrup of Quinces.
Oile of Mintes.

To cure the disposicion to vomitinge, whiche is whan a man would vomit & can not.
Aromaticum gariophillatum
Miua simplex
Rosata nouella
Sirup of Mintes

To prouoke vrine.
Antidotum asincritum
Aurea Alexandrina
Diacurcuma.
Diacassia cum Manna.
Diasatirion
Oximel diureticum
Vnguentum agrippe

¶ **To prouoke venus.**
Diasatirion, &c.

¶ **To heale woundes**
Balsamum artificiale
Emplastrum palmeum
Vnguentum apostolorum.

¶ **To scower and clense woundes.**
Tela Gualterij
Vnguentum Apostolicon Auicenæ.
Vnguentum basilium
Vnguentum Ægipsiacum.

Against

The names of the Compoundes.

¶ Againſt wormes in the belly.
Puluis contra Lumbricos
Sirup of Lemmons.
Oile of Wormewood.
Hyera picra Galeni
Mythridatum &c.

Vnguentum contra Lumbricos.

¶ And thus I haue ended the notes of the *Compoundes,* **with Common ſeedes. &c.**

Sickenes.
What be the names of the Compoundes, and in what leaues may I finde them, I pray you tell me.

Health.
Fyrſt I will begin at the letter *A. &c.*

A.

Alyptæ Moschata.	*Folio.j.*	**Conſerue of Maidenhere**	**Fol.ib.**
Aſincritum, a goodly *Antidotari,* of ſinguler vertue.	*ibidē.*	**Conſerue of Gladen.**	**Fol. ibi.**
Aromaticum Roſatum.	*ibidem*	**Conſerue of Enulacampana.** *Folio.*	*ibidem.*
Aureæ Alexandrina	*Fol.ij.*	**Conſerue of Succorie.**	**Fol.v.**
Aromaticum gariophillatum.	*Fol.ibid.*	**Conſerue of Sorrel.**	**Fol. ibid.**
Acatiæ	*Fol.iij.*	**Conſerue of** *Diagalanga*	**Fol. ibi.**
Aurilj	*Fol. ibidem*	*Collyra & ſief.*	*Fol. xxxviij.*
Aquæ odoriſera	*Fol. ibidem*	*Cerotte,* **how to make it.**	**Fol. xli.**
Apophlegmatiſmi, **to draw fleame from the hedde.**	**Fol. xl.**	**D**	

B
Benedicta laxati.	*Fol. ibidem*	*Diaſiminum nicolai.*	*Fol.ibid.*
Balſamum artiſicial.	*Fol.ibid.*	*Diambra meſuæ.*	*Fol. ibidem*
		Diamargariton Calidum.	*ibidem.*

C
Confectio dulcis.	*Fol. ibidem*	*Diamargariton frigidum*	*Folio.vj.*
Confectio Hamech.	*Fol. ibidem.*	*Diathamaron* **of Dates.**	*Fol. ibidem*
Cerotum ſtomachale	*Fol. iiij.*	*Diarhodon Abbatis*	*Fol. ibidem*
Confection for the iyes.	**Fol. ibid.**	*Diacalamintha.*	*Fol. ibidem*
Conſerue of Bugloſſe.	**Fol. ibid.**	*Diatrion pipereon.*	*Fol. ibidem*
Conſerue of Roſemary.	**Fol. ibi.**	*Diaireos Salomonis*	*Fol. ibidem*
Conſerue of Borage, and Bugloſſe.	**Fol. ibid.**	*Diatragacantha Frigida.*	*Fol.vj.*
		Diameron	*Fol. ibidem*
Conſerue of Roſes.	**Fol. ibidem**	*Diacodium*	*Fol. ibidem*
Conſerue of Violets.	**Fol. ib.**	*Diaphraſſium*	*Fol. ibid.*
		Diapapauer.	*Fol. ibidem*
		Diacurcuma	*Fol. ibid.*
		Diaſatirion	*Fol. viij.*

Diapru-

The names of the Compoundes.

Diaprunes	Fol. ibidem	Fomentum	Fol. xlj.
Diaphænicon	Fol. ibidem	**G**	
Diacarthama	Fol. ibidem	**Clifters.**	**Fol. xxbiii.**
Diacorallium magistrate.	Fol. ibidem	**Gargarisme.**	**Fol. xxxix.**
Diacassia fistula	Fol. ibidem	**H**	
Diasæne	Fol. ix.	Hyera picra galeni	Fol. ibidem
Decoctio pectorale.	Fol. ibidem	**I**	
Decoctio comunis	Fol. ibidem	**Julep of Uiolets.**	**Fol. ibi.**
Dropax.	Fol. xlj.	**Julep of Roses.**	**Fol. ibidem**
E		**Insessus, bsed for a stoue.**	**Fol. xli.**
Electuarium Catholicum.	Fol. ibid.	**L**	
Electuarium Rosatum	Fol. ibid.	Loch de Pino	Fol. ibidem
Electuarium de Spillio	Fol. ibid.	Loch de Squilla	Fol. xiiij.
Electuarium inde maioris	Fol. x.	Loch sanum	Fol. ibidem
Electuarium stomachi	Fol. ibi.	Loch de Caulibus	Fol. ibidem
Electuarium de gemmis	Fol. ibid.	Loch de pulmone vulpis	Fol. ibidē
Emplastrum Diachilon album.	Fol. ibid	Lyniment,	Fol. xxxix
Emplastrum diachilon magnū.	Fol. ibid.	**M**	
Emplastrum de mucilaginibus.	Fol. xj.	Mythridatum manardj	Fol. ibid.
Emplastrum pro stomacho.	Fol. ibid.	Mythridatum **very noble against**	
Emplastrum de granis lauri.	Fol. ibidem.	**poyson.**	**Fol. xxxix.**
Emplastrum meliloti.	Fol. ibid.	Mycleta	Fol. xv.
Emplastrum Coronem	Fol. ibid.	Miua simplex aromatica.	Fol. ibidem
Emplastrum oxicroceum	Fol. ibidem.	Mel Rosarum	Fol. ibidem
Emplastrum de Ianua	Fol. xj.	Mel violarum	Fol. ibid.
Emplastrum contra rupturas.	Fol. ibi.	Mel Anthosatum	Fol. ibidem
Emplastrum de gratia dej.	Fol. ibidem	Manus Christi	Fol. ibidem
Emplastrum pro dolore matrice.	Fol. ibi.	**N**	
Emplastrum diuinum.	Fol. ibidem	Nasalia **for the nose.**	**Fol. xxxix.**
Emplastrum de minio,	Fol. ibidē.	**O**	
Emplastrum de serusæ	Fol. ibidē	Oximel simplex	Fol. ibidem
Emplastrum Palmeum	Fol. xij	Oximel diureticum	Fol. ibidem
Emplastrum triapharmacum	Fol. ibidē	Oximel Squilliticum	Fol. ibidem
Epithema,	fol. xxxviij	Oxiosaccharum simplic.	Fol. ibidem
Emplastrum desiccatiuum rubrū.	fol. ib.	Oxiosaccharum compositum.	Fol. ibid.
F		**Oile of sweet Almondes.**	**Fol. ibi.**
Frontall for the head.	**Fol. xxxix.**	**Oile of bitter Almondes.**	**Fol. ibi.**

Oile

The names of the Compoundes.

Oile of Baie.	**Fol. ibidem**	Pilulæ Cochiæ	ibidem
Oile of Sesamynum.	**Folio. ibidem**	Pilulæ de octo rebus	ibidem
Oile of Spike.	**Fol. xvii.**	Pilulæ de Mirabolanis	ibidem
Oile of Coste.	**Fol. ibidem**	Pilulæ Elephanginæ	ibidem
Oile of Rue.	**Fol. ibidem**	Pilulæ Aggregatiue	ibidem
Oyle of Dill.	**Fol. ibidem**	**Pilles of Rubarbe.**	**ibidem**
Oile of Camomill.	**Fol. ibidem**	Pilulæ de sarcocolla	Fol. xxiij.
Oile of Mirtes.	**Fol. ibid.**	Pilnlæ fetide maiores	ibidem
Oile of Flowerdelice.	**Fol. ibid.**	Pilulæ de Euphorbio	ibidem
Oile of Roses.	**Fol. xviii.**	Pilulæ lucis maiores	ibidem
Oile of Violettes.	**Fol. ibid.**	Pilulæ lucis minores	ibidem
Oile of Quinces.	**Fol. ibid.**	Pilulæ de lapide Lazule	ibidem
Oile of Masticke.	**Fol. ibid.**	Pilulæ de Bdellio	ibidem
Oleum Castorej.	Fol. ibidem	Pilulæ de Hermod.ctylis	Fol. xuiiij.
Oleum de Euphorbio	Fol. ibidem	Pilulæ Arthiticæ	ibidem
Oleum vulpinum	fol. xix	Pilulæ stomachicæ	ibidem
Oleum de Tartaro	fol. ibidem	Pilulæ ante cibum	ibid.
Oleum Scorpionum	fol. ibidem	**Pilles of Agarike or Agarici.**	**ibi.**
Oile of garden Lilies.	**Fol. ibid.**	**Pilles of Fumiterre.**	**ibidem.**
Oleum de papauere	fol. ibidem	Pilulæ Comunis	ibiaem
Oleum nimphæatum album.	fol. ibidem	Pilulæ de Asseieret	ibidem
Oleum Menthæ	fol. ibidem	Pilulæ Bichiæ,	ibidem
Oile of Wormewoode.	**Fol. xx.**	Pilulæ imperiales,	ibidem
Oleum Lumbrecorum	fol. ibidem	Pilulæ de Hiera picra	Fol. xxv.
Oleum de Violaceum album.		Pomatum	Fol. xxvj.
or Hartes ease	**Fol.**	Pessis,	Fol. xl.
P		**Pox, how to hele them, with. viii.**	
Pomander.	**Fol. xx.**	**thinges considered.**	**Fol. xlvii.**
Pouder of Violets.	**Fol. xxi.**	**and. xlviii.**	
Puluis contra pestem	ibidem	**R**	
Puluis de bolo armenio,	ibidem	Rosata nouella,	ibidem.
Puluis contra Lumbricos	ibidem	**S**	
Puluis Bezeardicus	ibidem	Syrupus de Acetositatis citri	ibidem
Penidias	ibidem	Syrupus de Acetosæ. Simpl.	ibidem
Pignolatum	Fol. xxij.	Syrup de Agresta labrusca, **or vnripe**	
Pilulæ sine quibus esse nolo,	ibidem	**Grapes.**	**ibidem**
Pilulæ Auriæ	ibidem.	**Sirup Calamintes or of** Calamiata.	

I.i.   Syrup

The names of the Compoundes.

Syrup de Menta.	ibidem.	Sirup de Limonibus.	Fol.xxxj.
Sirupus de Absinthio.	ibidem	Sirup de Cetrach	ibidem
Syrup of Fumitarie	**Fol.xxvii.**	**Sirup of Buglosse.**	**ibidem.**
Syrupus de Fumoterre simplex	ibid.	**Sirup of the same**	**ibidem.**
Sirup of Liquoris.	**ibidem**	Sapo Moschatus	ibidem
Sirup of Hysope.	**ibidem**	**Suger Roset**	**Fol.xxxviii.**
Sirupus de Marubio.	ibid.	Sacculum or scutum	Fol.xli.
Sirup de Epithymo	ibidem	T	
Sirupus de Eupatorio	Fol.xxviij	Theriaca galenj.	ibidem.
Sirup of Sticados.	**ibidem**	Trifera sarasenica	ibidem
Sirupus de Violes, or **Violets**.	ibidem	Trochisci Diarhodon abbatis.	fol.xxxii.
Sirup de Papauere simp. or **Popie**.	ibi.	Trochisci de Violetes	ibidem
Sirupus de Papauere compositum,	ibidē	Trochisci de Squilla	ibidem
Sirup of Myrtes comp.	**ibidem**	Trochisci Theriaci	ibidem
Syrup of Myrtes simp.	**Fol.xxix**	Trochisci diacorallion.	ibidem
Syrup of Acetosus simplex	ibidem	Trochisci de Camphere	fol.xxxiij.
Sirupus Acetosus compositus	ibid.	Trochisci de Alchachenge	ibidem
Sirupus de succo Endiuæ or **Endiue**		Trochisci de Myrrha	ibidem
simplex.	ibidem	Trochisci de Moscho	ibidem
Sirup of Endiue compositus.	**ibidem**	Trochisci de Rubarbaro	ibidem
Sirup of Suckery or Cichori.	**ib.**	Trochisci de Spodio	ibidem
Sirup of Quinces	**ibidem**	Trochisci de Absinthio.	ibidem.
Sirup of Nenuphar, **or water Lilles.**		Trochisci de Eupatorio.	ibidem
	ibidem.	Trochisci de terra sigillata.	fol.xxxiiij
Sirup of Barberies	**Fol.xxx**	Trochisci de Ambra.	ibidem
Sirup of tarte Pomgarnets.	**ibi.**	Tela Galterij.	ibidem
Sirupus de Bizantiis	ibidem	V	
Sirupus de infusione Rosarum viridium		Vnguentum Apostolicum	ibidē.
or **greene Roses.**	**ibidem**	Vnguentum Rosarum.	ibidem.
Sirupus de Rosis succis, or **Dried Roses.**	**ibi.**	Vnguentum basilicum maius.	ibidem
Sirupus de succo Rosarum	ibidem	Vnguentum Aureum.	ibidem
Sirupus de Iuiube.	ibidem	Vnguentum basilicum minus.	ibidem
Sirup of Maidenhere comp.	**ibi.**	Vnguentum populeon	fol.xxxv.
Sirup of Maydenheere simp.	**ibi.**	Vnguentum martiaton.	ibidem
Sirup of the same	**ibidem.**	Vnguentum Arogon.	ibidem
Sirup of Mugworte	**ibidem**	Vnguentum Dialtheæ.	ibidem
			Vnguentum

The names of the Compoundes

Vnguentum Agrippæ.   Fol. xxxvj.
Vnguentum Diapompholigos ibidem
Vnguentum de Enulacampana ibidem
Vnguentum contra scabiem ibidem
Vnguentum pro pueris scabiosis ibidem
Vnguentum desiccatiuum Rubrum. ibi.
Vnguentum contra lumbricos ibidem
Vnguentum Resumptiuum   ibidem
Vnguentum Album   ibidem
Vnguentum Matritum   Fol. xxxvij.
Vnguentum Ægyptiacum   ibidem.
Vnguentum Citrinum.   ibidem.
Vnguentum Neapolitanum   ibidem
Another Vnguentum. &c.   ibidem
Vnguentum Galeni   ibidem
Vnguentum pro Combustione ignis, to heale white fire.   ibid.

Vapors and Parfume.   Fol. xxxix.

W

Water for sore iyen.   Fol. xlii.
Water for the webbe.   ibidem
Water of Furnerius for Cankers.   Folio. xlii.
Water most sweet.   Fol. xliii.
Water to make sleape.   Fol. xliiii.
Water for the Palsie   Fol. xlv.
Waters composed.   ibidem
Water of the Quintessence. Folio. xlvi.
Water of life, called Aqua vitæ. ibidē.
Water to kill the Canker, by syr Anthony Heuenigham knight, Folio. xlvii.

And thus endeth the names of Compoundes.

¶ The ende of the Booke of Compoundes, and here after foloweth the booke of the vse of certain Compoundes.

J. ii.

The names of the Compoundes

Sicknes.

NOw you haue ended your Table, with the names of compoundes. There are certain wordes, very harde for me to vnderstand as when you doe name *Apophlegmatismus, Dropax, Linement. &c.* I knowe not what thei doe meane, by their proper names, I praie you tell me the significacions.

Health.

When you come to *Apophlegmatismus*, it is a singuler good medicen to purge flegme by vomite, or els to drawe from the hedde, euill and grosse humours, and is vsed somtime, as I haue rehersed in the proper place of *Apophlegmatismus*, before spoken.

And by mixture vnderstande, what sondrie *Confections* and *Electuariis*, bee mingled together, to be taken in the mornyng, or els three howers before repaste of meate and drinke, to purge choller. &c.

Confectura, is a medicene mingled of simples, or some meate digested: as *cibus confectus*, meat digested. There are sondrie cōfectiōs, as *Confectio Hamech. & c*

Electuarium is commonly knowen, made moiste with Honie, Suger, and pouders for to clense humours, beyng taken in the mornyng, in Bolo, that is in the same masse, rolled with Suger, or els in Potione, or drunke with waters, accordyng to the complexion: as to the chollericke least, and moste to the Melancholie persone, by the reason of his yearthly nature. And of *Electuarijs* be diuers, and of sundrie inuencions, as *Rasis* made one for an Heathē king, whose name was *Almonsor*. To this kyng he writeth moche, concernyng bodily health, and to put awaie pensifenes, heauines, and Melancholie, he made *Electuarium Læticans Rasis*.

Electuarium de succo Rosarum of Roses, *Electuarium frigidum Cophonis* of one called Cophe. Reade of this man, and many mo, in the worke of *Mesue*.

Electuarium gemmarum of precious stones. &c. with many mo worthie Electuaries, profitable for mankinde: some warmyng, and some coolyng. &c.

Tragia, are sondrie pleasaunt pouders, mingled together, whiche are caste vpon delicate meates, or put in wine against cold in the stomack or Collicke, wholsome for the Melancholie, or Flegmaticke bodie, whiche is colde or windie.

Conserue is knowen, as of Prunes, Barberies. &c. and will cōserue and kepe the strained fruites, wherein the spices with Suger, and sometyme swete waters are sodden together, to make it bothe to laste in it self, and pleasure moche the receiuer, whiche shall eate thereof, Mornyng and Euenyng. Also young fruites, as Nuttes, Peares. &c. and flowers maie bee conserued, preserued, and condited in Syrupes. Kepyng their forme and goodnes, with moche vertue.

Trifera saracenica against fransie, Melancholie, and coldnes. &c. was inuented of the Saracens, to be dronke in wine.

Esdra was made by Eldras the holie man, when the people of Israel were in captiuitie, the great miserie and affliccion of mynde: this was the bodily remedie for all the paines of the hedde, commyng of cold.

Auria Alexandria was made in Alexander, and for the singuler vertue against

and the Apoticaries rules.

gainste colde reumes, and to comfort the brain: like as golde excelleth all other mettalles in riches, so doe this all other in vertue.

Loboch is a pleasaunt thyng, as *Loboch Sanum, Loboch de Pino. &c.* This *Loboch* is to licke or melte vnder the tongue, against paines in the throate, and lunges, and are good to helpe the cough.

Syruppe of Liquorice, Horehounde. &c. are made Simple, or Compounde, to be taken a mornyng and euenyng, some be hotte, and some bee colde.

Rob is a certaine thing made harde, and put into medicines: there is *Dia Rob*, very wholsom for the liuer, and put in medicins for the mouth as in gargarisme.

Decoction is a drinke moste wholsome to clense the bodie, or to restrain or els maie bee put in Clisters, either to purge, or stoppe, accordyng to the nature of the sicknesse. When ye will purge, take openyng seedes, leaues, barkes, rootes. &c. with Suger, and seeth theim, then straine them through a cleane wollen clothe, adde to Suger: and let the paciente drinke a Mornynges, twoo or three daies. And when you stoppe, decocte Planten, Shepherdes purse, gumme Arabike. &c. straine it and drinke mornyng and euenyng. Note also, that Syruppes and decoctions be best newe, specially the decoction, whiche wil not last lōg.

Iulep is not sodden so thicke as Syrup, but is clere made with sonderie good waters and clene Suger, and are wholsome for the liuer, as of the waters of Chicorie, Endiue, or Sirupes and waters together.

Infusion, is when the Apothicarie doe for twelue or xxiiii. howers, put purgyng medicenes in water, as *Rhabarbe, Agarike, Succo rosarum. &c.* and then straine them forthe to drinke, and purge in the mornyng.

Trochist are many, as of Cappers, Wormwoode, *Rhabarbe. &c.* and are drie like small table men, vsed in medicenes, beaten into pouder, and maie be long kepte.

Sufuf is a goodly *Aromatike* pouder, made of spices, as *Galanga. &c.*

Sief is made for sore iyen, white and hard, in the forme of a little Suger lofe, but skant an ynche long, whiche must be steeped in Rose water, and womannes milke, to be applied to the iyen, to helpe them.

Collyrium is made of *Sief*, when it is soft, or dissolued for sore iyen.

Pilles are of sundrie kindes and natures, of greate strengthe and vertue, to expulse euill matter, and maie bee taken at euenyng, morning, and *Ante Cibum*: according to their natures, as I haue written. But old Pilles are daungerous, newe are good, howbeit, perilous for very fat bodies. There are also Pilles restraining, or stopping, as for flixes.

Subsimentum is sondrie pouders for womē, cast vpō coles, whose smoke doe subtilly passe into the bodie, or matrixe, and sometyme for menne.

Nasalia is a wholsome thyng, to be put into the nose, to comforte the braine: and stoppe the bledyng at the nose.

Frontaria is good to reconcile slepe, to bee applied to the forehedde, the length twelue inches.

Masticatorium, to champe vpon, to drawe forthe flegme from the hedde,

and

and to clense the teeth.

Gargarismus, is to gargle in the mouthe, not to swallowe it doune, to clense the mouthe, throte, and teeth, put in warme to.

Clister is ministered bee neathe, and are of sonderie kindes: relaxyng, bindyng, and restoryng, and muste bee ministered, neither to colde, for wind, nor to hot, for excoriacion or skalding. But temperate to clense and worke his proper effecte. Clisters are good for the stone, and when one can take no Purgacion by the mouthe, Clisters are moste beste.

Athanasia is no named, because it is so excellent in goodnesse, againste the immoderate fluxe menstruall in women, it is called a medicen immortall: of whiche I shall speake of more, in a perticuler booke by it self, God willyng.

Epithima, are used inwardly for the liuer, and also fine wolle, or rawe silke twilted, and steped in waters and pouders, accordyngly. Scarlet in Graine, is wholsome for the same purpose.

Liniment is made to anointe, or make softe, hauyng no waxe there.

Pessis is made to be applied, into the secret place of a woman, to helpe the euilles of the matrixe.

Sacculum is a bagge or twilte, wherein spice cordiall, with wholsome herbes are put in, and made warme with wine, vineger, or swete water, and so applied to the stomackes of sicke folkes.

Cerot is made of Waxe, Spice, and Oile, spread vpon leather, and applied to the breste. &c. as *Cerotum Galenj pro stomacho*.

Insessus is sweete herbes sodden in sweete water and wine, in whiche the pacient must sit at euen.

Suppositor, is to put vnder in at the fundamente, for to relaxe the bellies of weake bodies.

Fomentum is to washe the sore bodie with herbes, whiche muste bee moche sodden, and applied to the sore place. &c.

Dropax is good for skalde heddes, to clense them: and for women that would haue high forheddes, againste nature. For a *Dropax* will pull of the heere.

Emplastrum is commonly knowen, and is groslie made of herbes, Spices. &c. and warme to be applied to the sore, or pained place of the body

Frication, is rubbyng or chafyng of the bodie, with warme clothes in the mornyng.

Dentifricj, is to make thinges to cleanse the teethe, and make theim white: as with dried Mallowe rootes. &c.

With many more pretie and apte notes of medicins, but these shall suffice for mannes healthe: whiche the preparers of medicenes, muste wisely make and obserue, these. xxi. notes followyng.

Firste

and the Apoticaries rules.

i. Muste first serue God, forsee the ende, bee clenly, pitie the poore.
ii. Must not be suborned for money, to hurte mankinde.
iii. His place of dwelling, & shop, to be clenly to please the sences withal
iiii. His garden must be at hand, with plentie of herbes, sedes, & rootes.
v. To sowe, set, plant, gather, preserue and kepe them in due tyme.
vi. To reade *Dioscorides*, to knowe the natures of plantes and herbes. &c.
vii. To inuente medicenes, to chose by colour, tast, odour, figure. &c.
viii. To haue his morters, stilles, pottes, filters, glasses, boxes cleane and swete. &c.
ix. To haue Charcoles at hande, to make decoctions, syrupes. &c.
x. To kepe his cleane wares close, and cast awaie the baggage.
xi. To haue twoo places in his Shoppe, one moste cleane for the Phisicke, and a baser place, for Chyrurgi stuffe.
apothecary
xii. That he neither increase, nor diminishe the Phisicians bille, and kepe it for his owne discharge.
xiii. That he neither buie, nor sell rotten drugges.
xiiii. That he peruse often his wares, that thei corrupt not.
xv. That he put not in *quid pro quo*, without aduisement.
xvi. That he maie open well a veine, for to helpe the pleurisie.
xvii. That he medle onely in his vocacion.
xviii. That he delite to rede *Nicolaus Myrepsi, Valerius Cordus, Iohannes Placaton ỹ Lubik. &c.*
xix. That he doe remember his office, is onely to be the Phisiciãs Coke.
xx. That he vse true measure and waight.
xxi. To remember his ende, and the iudgement of God: and thus I doe commende hym to God, if he be not coueitous, or craftie sekyng his owne lucre, before other mennes health, succour, and cõfort.

Sickenes.

I Assure you, if the Apothicarie, dooe Godly obserue these plaine rules, he can not dooe amisse: but shall please almightie God, profite the common wealthe in his callyng. Finally, quiete his conscience, and liue well. I praie you shewe vnto me, a little of the waightes and measures, and so make an ende of this parte, whiche is of medicenes.

Health.

If I should speake moche of waight and measure, that I could not well dooe, without I should alight the learned man *Georgius Agricola, de mensuris & ponderibus*, whiche maketh the destinction of all the measures of this worlde, of euery age and people. Whiche I dooe wishe that you doe often tymes reade, and for this present tyme, lette this suffice for waight, as followe, for this little booke, that is passed before.

The waight of { I pounde. ℔.
In vnce. ℥.
I Dragme. ʒ.
I scruple. ℈.
I graine. G.

The waight of { of ech part, ana
I quarter. q.
Halfe. ß.
I handfull, M.
I. iiii. Note

The names of the Compoundes.

Note also, that the Apoticaries, doe deuide a pounde thus.

li.　　ʒ.xii.　|ʒ.i.　ʒ.viii.　|ʒ.　Ə.iii.　|Ə.i.　Ꝑ.xx.

Another note for waightes and measurs.
Furder, there is a measure called *Pugillum*, or a little handfull, noted thus. P.

And euer measure your herbes by the handfull. M. your flowers by the. P.

Your rootes and seedes by waight as. Ə.ʒ.ʒ. &c. But sometyme the rootes are vsed in nomber, as in decoction. &c.

The liquors and pouders, by waight, as the seedes.

Fruites are vsed in nomber, as Apples, Prunes Myrabolans. &c. not by waight, as.ʒ.ʒ.li.but.i.ii.iii.iiii.v. &c.

Also when you dooe come to decoction, or sethyng of your thynges: Consider that you firste haue pure cleane vesselles, as Iron or stone, auoide stinkyng Brasse, as moche as you maie, and prepare white mettalle, to make in your decoctions, with verie cleane water: then you haue your rootes cleane scraped and sooden. Why the rootes firste?

Why rootes are first sodden in decoctiō : and why flowers are last put in decoction.
Mary because thei be harder, then any other thing, in sethyng or decoction: therefore thei had nede of moche sethyng, to make theim tender, next after them, put in your seedes. And laste of all your flowers, or Sene leaues, for because thei bee tender, and will quickly passe awaie by smoke, vaupour, and aire: lette it seeth neither vpon a sharpe quicke fire, nor vpon a slowe, but vpon a meane, vnlesse it requireth moche haste. But after the seethyng, let it stande by, in some conuenient place: and then straine the same decoction, through a cleane white wollen, or Skarlet in grain clothe, and so reserue it to vse of medicen.

Howe to make Suppositours.
Suppositours muste be made of Honie, sodden to a thicknesse, and tempered with a sticke, and when it is almoste sodden, then put your Salt, and *Hiera picra simplex*, when your Honie is almoste thicke, or els the *Hiera* will lose his strength: then roule it with butter, in the forme of a spindle, smaller at one ende, then at the other in length, accordyng to the bodie, as a finger, twoo fingers in length.

Clisters.
Clisters you haue the makyng of theim before, but because trouble and time haue preuented me, I could not doe so moche in Clisters, &c. as by Goddes grace, I doe intende hereafter. Therefore I commende thee to *Nicholaus Myrepsi, V. Cordus I. Placatom*, and also to one of this tyme, of little fame, because he haue written but a little boke, but yet this worke is excellent good for a Pothicarie, his name is *Petrus Gorius Bitriscensi*. Note also, that you muste haue your Clister pipe, and bladders in store, to minister the Clisters, neither very hotte nor cold, for feare of winde, or skaldyng in the guttes. Also I haue said before, your Clisters must be first of decoctiō with your rootes, then sedes, last Sene, then strained, and so your oiles, and *Hiera picra. &c.* with a little recoction, and so giuen a pinte. &c. Euen so there be Clisters, restrainyng and stoppyng. &c.

Syrupes, simple, and compounde.
Sirupes some be simple, that is made of one thing, puttyng thereunto Suger, or Hony: and this sirup is made of the iuice of herbes, or fruites, as Borage. &c. Either the iuce is stamped and strained, and clarified,

and the Apoticaries rules.

rified, or els the herbe is sodden in water, vntill the water bee consumed to the third parte, then strain it, and put the decoction again into the kettell or panne, and recocte it again, puttyng in the Suger, compounded with sondrie Sirupes, as grosserie, as spices and seedes, are decocted and sodden together.

Juleps must be sodden but lightly, made thinne and cleare, and is made of Violettes, Roses, or Sirupes and waters together.

Infusion must stand all the night togither, as Agarike, Rhubarbe Sene. &c. and stilled water, and in the mornyng strongly pressed forth into a cleane vessell, to the vse of potion, to purge.

A stone of Marble must be prepared, to caste Manus Christi, or Losenges: whiche Losenges muste bee made of Suger, put into the pan with Rose or sweete water, sodden to a thicknesse, and when it is so thicke, that a droppe thereof will be cleare, like Venice Terebintyne, then putte in you Cordiall pouders, or Dias, stiryng it with a sticke, caste it abroade vpon your stone. Note also, that your stone bee either anointed, with oile of Almondes, or els sifted ouer with the pouder of Sinamon, whereby you maie take vp your Table, to make your Losenges. The names and quantities of them, are before rehearsed in the Compoundes.

Electuarij muste bee sodden thicke, and kepte close, as *Electuarij de succo Rosarum. &c.* and ʒ.i. of any Electuarie, is sufficient to be taken at ones in the mornyng, with distilled waters accordingly.

Pilles ʒ.i. made in fiue or seuen pilles, is sufficient to purge the bodie withall. Pouders, Sirupes, and waters must bee alwaies prepared for Pilles, and to make them newe, beaten in a cleane morter togither, and kepte close.

For moiste or liquid thinges shortly to be saied.

Amphora is. xlviii. *Sextarijs*, and this *Sextarius* dooe containe a pinte and a halfe, whiche is vnces. xxiiii. that is. ℔.ii. Romain waight.

The measure of liquors, & their names.

Vrna is halfe of *Amphora*, whiche. xxiiii. *Sextaries*, here in England is two gallons and a halfe. And thus I doe ende of these medicenes aforsaid and what faultes be escaped, amendes shall be made, God willing.

Hec sunt vsitata Medicamina quæ in officinis Medicamentarijs vbique fere prostant, reliqua ad præscriptum Medicorum parentur, quod non difficile est in comunibus exercitato.

Valeto.

Gulihelmus Bullenus.

Ianuarij, anno salutis.
1562.

¶ *Hereafter foloweth the booke of the vse of Sickmen, and wholsome medicen.*

The booke of the vse of sicke men, and medicens.

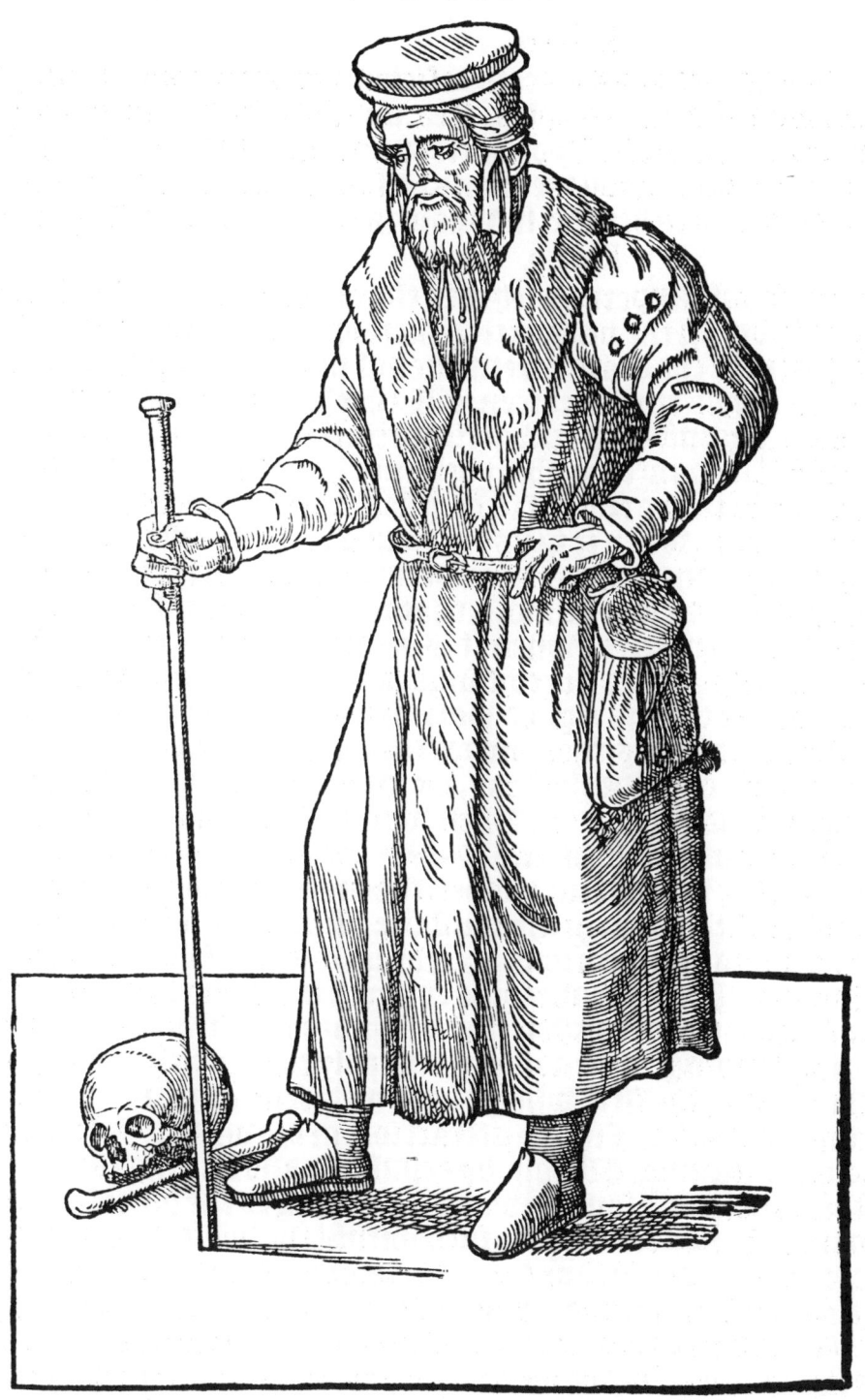

Surfeite, age, and sickenes, are enemies all to health,
Medicenes to mende the bodie, excelleth worldly wealth:
Phisicke shall florishe, and in daunger will giue cure,
Till death vnknit the liuely knot, no lenger we indure.

The booke of the vse of sicke men and medicines.

Sickenes.

Although medicens, as composicions, be well made in all pointes, wanting no Simples. Yea, and also the Simples are good and newe, and the Apoticarie cunning: yet it often times happeneth that the same good medicens do hinder me more, then my long paintull dolorous sickenesse: in whom is then the faulte? I praie you.

Health.

The fruite of rashe ministracion of medicenes.

It should appere, neither in the medicen, nor in the Apoticarie, but in the vndescrite giuer, or rashe Phisicion, whiche men, be the death oftentimes of many, that put their trust in thē, as euill medicen is. I therfore shall shew thee, what is to be doen, against such euil accidentes, if thei doe chaunce, how to remoue thē. And how thou shalt behaue thy self wisely, in receiuing pocions. &c. For in the time of sickenesse, sometime wee loose, or make the belly laxatiue, when it is stopped, euen so we do restraine, stop and binde the belly, when it doeth imoderatly run with laxis. Sometime we do mortifie or kil euil humors, that rebelleth against nature. And also we restore to nature, when it is decaied thinges restoratiue, as Cordials, Dias, & Sirups accordinge, with Kitchin phisicke: whiche

A good kitchin is a good Apoticaries shoppe.

Kitchin I assure thee, is a good Poticaries shop. When we make euacuacion with laxatiues, then vse we *Seamone*, Rubarbe, *Cassiasistula*. &c. But whē we restrain or binde the body, we giue *Acacia* and *Opium*, in restoring, repatring, or binding nature. Then we minister in meates & drinkes, and other conuenient medicens, *Diarhodon, Triasandali, Diamargariton, &c.* And there is an other kinde of cure, when the matter is not mature or ripe crude and couched fast whiche must bee displeased with decoctions, warme syruppes and medicens according, whiche I shall declare hereafter. But here I will speake some thing of medicens solutiue, or laxatiue: and then next of constrictiue, or binding. Thirdly, of the maner of restoring, helping, or mending. Fouerthly to digest, chaunge & alter

Fower thinges cōsidered attractiō, dissoluyng. &c.

Now concerning the first, whiche be of medicens solutiue: we vse thē three maner of waies. First by attraction or drawyng. Secondly by dissolucion or wasting. Thirdly, by expulsing and driuing forth. Then we do this diuers and sondrie waies, according to the diuersitie of the place where the matter is contained within the bodie. Then we loose & relax, with *Benedicta laxatiue* or *Catarico imperale*, or suche like *electuariis*. We make attraction with Aloes, and certain of the Opiattes &c. We doe expell with *Scylla*, washen in the waters of *Tamarindes*, and suche like: and as the matter is, so doe we worke, and prepare pocions, accordyng to the diuersitie of the place, where the euill humour or matter lieth hidden, whiche we intende to dispatche, by Gods grace, without whose furderaunce, nothing cometh to good lucke, and all our labour is in vaine, although we watche, rise, studie, labour &c. Therfore let the minister of the medicen diligently foresee, the veritie of the matter, so that he may minister one or twoo pocions of medicens, accordyng to the

The boke of Compoundes.   Fol. xlix.

the propertie and place. As for example, if the matter bee in the stomacke, liuer, or places nere the same, one pocion shall suffice to euacuate and expulse the same: but if the euill matter dooe lye in places distant, and farre from the stomacke, as it happeneth to them that haue the goute, whose grief is in the feete. We giue more medicens, to dissolue, remoue, and open the matter, whiche is so farre of the stomack: then we giue the iuce of Polipodie, and Agarike, and the pilles called *de Serapino*, or pilles *de Lapide Armenio descriptione Mesue*, and soche like. Then secondly, we vse to giue medicens whiche haue vertue, to alter, to draw attracte the losed humours to the stomacke, and so to dissolue theim with *Benedicta, Hieralogodion*, and *Hiera picra.&c.* For bitter thinges do penitrate and pearse soner to the extreme partes, and doe purge more, then doe any other medicens. Thirdly, we giue an expulsiue, and expell the humours, that be gathered and alredie in the stomacke with *Psilium.&c.*

Propertie & place, must be obserued.

The vertue of bitter medicens bee greate.

Sicknes.
But I praie you, how doe you vse these medicens?

Health.

IN maner folowyng. Medicens to expell, we giue one in the Mornyng, the second at Noone, the third at Night: The cause maie so require, the one at euening, an other at midnight, the thirde in the mornyng. Take hede also, that the humours bee not to moche dissolued, in the seconde ministracion: but after the firste pocion, the paciente maie slepe, bicause the pocion is more weaker, when it is ones drunke, then when it is taken twoo tymes, for beeyng dronke twise, then it is double in strength. Some men maie not awaie with many medicens: well, to soche we giue but onely a digestiue, and an expulsiue. And to them that are not able to receiue twoo, we giue them but one, but that one in effecte, must be as good as the thre: whiche muste dissolue, attracte, and expelle, whiche waie of purgacion is not hurtefull. For Phisicions seldome tymes doe giue twoo, or three pocions, but it is the greater ouersight: for if one pocion will purge, how moch more will twoo or three, for one strong pocion, haue not that vertue, and efficacie, that three mennes pocions haue: although one stronge pocion, and vehemente medicen, doe quickly purge the nether partes of the stomacke, euen so it maie bee so quicke, that it will penetrate to the extreme partes, as the hedde, handes, and feete. Also the vertue of the medicen, if it bee weake in operacion, it doeth banishe awaie, thorowe the passage of the vnapt partes, whereby that it cannot obtain to the extreme members. And also, when wee dooe intende, to purge the extreme partes, then we doe giue twoo preparatiues: to the intent that the thirde, maie haue the freer waie, and more effectuall passage. If we must nedes giue but one, then let it bee doen by little and little, and oftentymes, so that the matter maie bee purged, faire, and softly, and not rashely, nor sodainly, as it chaunceth in many places, where

A pocion must bee geuen at three sondrie tymes, to remoue and expulse matter from the stomacke. A Caueat, to beware.

Mens natures must be obserued, a little medicen will worke moche of some men, and a stronge medicen, will skant worke, on some other manner.

I.i.   the

The booke of Compoundes.

Requiem eternam, with a spade

the pacient doeth receiue soche medicenes, that he goeth fourtie, or three score tymes to the stoole. Soche medicenes ones dooe cause the pacient, to haue sunge for theim: *Requiem eternam, dona eis domine,* whiche is, O Lorde, giue theim euerlastyng reste, for suer we be, through soche medicenes, in this worlde, thei shall neuer haue rest, nor health. For these swifte, strong purgacions, doe weaken the bodie, drieth vp the blood, consumeth nature, bryngeth conuulcion, or palsie, and finallie retaineth euill humours, and letteth the good humour out. Therefore *Hippocrates* saieth, after sodain euacuacion, or replexion, to hotte, or to colde, be deceiptfull, and vtterly aduersaries to nature.

Sicknes.

I Had thought to haue made no more to do, but whē my bely had been costiue, or bounde, to haue taken any thing, that had been laxatiue, but now I perceiue by so doyng, I should haue dooen my self more hurte then good: for by soche actions and doinges, I am brought into this case, but from hence forthe, I will take better hede, and God aforne. For so helpe me God and hollidame, gossope Health,

Like as heat consumeth, euē so do Phisike money.

I gotte soche a sicknesse in Flaunders, that by the space of twoo yeres, consumed my money emong the Phisicions, that in the ende, thei had all my riches and gaine: and I nothyng but sicknesse and paine, then likewise men, thei counsailed me, to go home into my natiue countrie where saied thei, the aire should be my chief Phisicion. Euen so I did, but my sicknesse is so veterate and olde, that the aire was vnsufficient to bee my helpe: yet the countrey is very pleasaunte, ye knowe it verie well, it is Suffolke, whereas very fewe Phisicians dooe inhabite, of myne acquaintance, but onely an old imperike, called Jhon Preston,

Jhon Preston, called Jhon of Stoneham.

some take him to be a greate clarke, but I thinke he is learned beyond the marke. For of all men in that countrey, he is greatly sought vnto: for he plaieth our Ladie of Wallyngham, giuyng as moche healthe for a penie, as she did holinesse: yet custome hath cōmenced him, emongeste the common people, to be their doctour, I was this mannes pacient a greate tyme, but yet I neuer heard hym talke of *Hippocrates*, and *Gallen*, he troubles not his house with any of their bookes. What shall I saie, all the tyme that I was with hym, he vsed to minister his purgacions by chaunce medley, to his pacientes, happie man by his dole some spede well, but I doe remaine sicke still. And as I dooe perceiue by these three rules, that the fault was in abusing, misusyng, and not duely ministryng of his medicenes, how, and in what maner therfore should I receiue, or giue my friende medicene, without errour accordingly, I beseche thee gentle Health tell me.

Health.

whē purging medicenis giuen, first minister herbes & drinkes to prouoke vrin

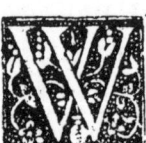
When you will giue any purgacion, or medicen, diate your pacient first, by the space of a daie or twoo, with meates or suppynges, to prouoke vrine: as the brothes of flesche and fische, boiled Onions with fatte Porke. Also giue the pacient two

The booke of Compoundes.   Fol.1.

or three tymes poched Egges, sauced with a little wine and Peper, or els herbes molifiyng or softening the bellie, as Irage, called Itriplex Mallos and Mercurie. &c. For whiche cause saieth *Hipocrates*, when any man will purge the bodie, he must first prepare, the matter to be flowyng, that when the purgacion doe come, it maie easely passe, and cary awaie all the euill humour, without grief or hurte. And this must be giuen to harde complexions, whiche will not easely giue place to purgacion, for in case the medicen lose not: it will rather inprison, shutte vp and close, bothe the humour and the purgacion, rather then purge accordingly. Upon whiche occasion saieth *Galen*, these Methodians, while as thei make light of medicenes preparatiue. Thei inclose the matter, and make no euacuation, therefore thei cause not onely the sicknesse of the lunges, but also of the iointes, as handes and feete.

Preparatiue must be firste giuen, & then purgacion.

Methodici, bee Phisicions that obserue certain rules by art.

Sicknes.

NOw sir, for that you are very sensible, and talke in good order, I praie you furthermore, if you be not wearie of my poore companie: shewe me how that I maie beste prepare medicen for me and others accordingly.

Health.

FOR as moche as I doe lacke many of my companions, whiche bee now a daies, all on thy side: intised bee idlenesse, surfette, and their companion glottonie, and now are thei all with thee, I knowe them well by sight, but I kepe very little companie with theim. For if I so did, I should lose my name, and be called no more Health. But miserable wretched Sicknesse, as feuer, Dropsie, palsie, blinde, lame, Frātike, Cōsumed, Rupture, Goutie, Pore. &c. Yet would God, would God, if thou and thei bee not paste cure: I wishe you all on my side againe. For I confesse, many of you haue moche wealthe, but all you lacke Health. But to want bothe, if age approche, I promes thee, it is the first hell, the greatest extreme miserie, and moste wretched enemie to mankinde, that can be inuented, how saiest thou, is it not so? Thou canst not denaie it. Well, yet it is a manifest signe of health to seke it. Cōtinue therin, & thou shalt find it: and for this thy honest demaund, how medicen should be prepared. You shall prepare theim in this maner, if you wil quicken your purgacion with Scamonie, quicken it. x. or. xv. daies, before it be giuen: so that thesaied Scamonie maie be incorporated with the spices. But note that the Scamonie be well rubbed betwene the handes, or chafed in a morter, with Oile of Roses, or Uiolettes, or Syruppe of Roses, well wrought betwene the handes, puttyng thereunto a little Masticke. For Masticke haue a propertie, that it will let, and not suffre Scamonie, to cliue to the softes of the stomacke, whiche oftentymes causeth a bloody flixe, and excoriacion of the guttes. But by this mixture, the malice of the medicen is excluded, and will dooe no harme: but if any chaunce happen in any soche

The causes of sicknesse.

How to prepare medicen

          I.ii.   case,

The booke of Compoundes.

Scamonie is perilous, except it be wel prepared, and doe kill many one.

case, it will bee sone helped. But there bee many blooddie villaines, whiche will giue medicenes immediatly, after thei haue put in Scamonie, before it be well incorporated with spices. For the longer it be incorporated: so moche it will purge the more effectually and gently. Now if you haue not this medicen prepared, and of necessitie it muste be giuen, or ministered in soche case: lette the Scamonie be rubbed or chafed, as is aforesaied, with oile and Syruppe of Roses, and a little cleane Masticke, and thus beyng quickened, it maie bee giuen after ii. or iii. daies: you must also rost the medicen, in this maner folowing

Take a graie Costarde, or a Quince, cut it a sunder ouerthwarte in the middes, pike out the Core, then put in the pouder of Scamonie, then putte it together againe: when this is doen, wrappe it close in a weat linen clothe, and couer it in the hotte emers of smale coales and asshes. When it is well rosted, then take it forthe, and mingle it with a medicine, and being thus prepared, it maie be giuen after two daies But take hede still, that it be not finely poudered, for feare of cleauing to the stomacke, through whiche maie come a blooddie flixe, and excoriacion of the guttes: but it must be beaten grossely, that it maie tary the longer, or more tyme in the stomacke. And why so? Mary, then it shall dissolue the lurkyng humers, whiche be hidden priuely, in the extreme partes, as hedde, handes, and goutie fete. But if you either wil

Lurking humours, howe to finde them and expulse theim.

receiue, or giue a pocion, then temper it with Rubarbe, Mirobalans, or Agarice: and let it stande a daie and a night, accordyng as the medicen shall require, wherewith the matter shalbe purged, at Mornyng, sometyme at Euen, as I shall declare hereafter. If a man bee stronge, lustie, and not weake, then he maie take the substaunce in the pocion. If he be feble, tender, or weake, then to straine it, and drinke the liquor onely: thus, or after this maner, is to prepare medicenes.

Sicknes.

How and in what maner, doe you giue solutiue medicens?

Health.

Medicenes solutiue, why thei are giue.

Solutiue medicens, bee sometyme giuen to the whole, and sometyme to the sicke. To the sicke, to expulse sickenesse: to the whole to preserue theim in healthe. Then when thou mindest to minister to thy self, or to any other, first consider the sicknesse, and the matter whereof it groweth, and the place infected. When these thynges be well noted, then as the matter shall require, euen so minister accordingly, as is saied before. But consider this, that the medicen must not bee offered, vntill soche tyme, as the matter or humour bee decocted, riped, and made softe, whereupon saieth *Hippocrates*, we must purge digested matter, but not moue crude, rawe matter. &c. The digestiõ of matter is knowen, by thicknesse of vrine, in case a thinne vrine passed before the saied thicke vrine by attenuacion, but if a thicke vrine, come before the thinne, then it is a feuer. Wherefore knowe first the distinction

The chief signe of digestion.

The booke of Compoundes. Fol.lj.

tion of the matter in this behalfe. Now if it be vndigested, vse incisiues, and thynges that prouoke vrine: then after you haue prouoked vrine with herbes accordingly, then maie you minister your medicen. But on the other side, when you will giue a medicene laxatiue, to the whole body. First, consider what humour doe abound, and thesame is that, whiche causeth the paine and sicknesse in the bodie: and therfore purge this cause, and then the effecte shall cease, by Gods grace. Now furthermore, if there be twoo humours, equall aboundyng together, extremely in superfluite, then there must be more Simples, put vnto the composicion, accordyng to the qualitie or quantitie of the humor, to purge thesame. As when choler and blood doe abounde, then purge with confectio Hamech. &c. For if twoo humours bee superfluous. And then if you giue to purge but one humour, then the bodie will be molested, sicke, and greued: and for this cause Hippocrates saieth, *Si qualia oportet purgari purgentur, confert & bene ferunt, si vero non: contrarium*: whiche is, if soche thynges bee purged, whiche ought to be purged, is good and auailable and menne bare it well, if not, then it is cleane contrary and euill.

It helpeth moche to nature, to prouoke vrine.

That humor whiche do abound, purge thesame.

The cause of sickenesse.

Hippocrates. Purge that, which should be purged, or els medle not

Sicknes.

What signe or manifest token, is then to be giuen, whereby a man should perceiue the humours by. I praie you saie on.

Health.

Partly thei maie bee knowen by certaine thynges, what humours to abounde, or ought to be purged or clensed, within the bodies of men or women. As example, if any man be leane, or wante his fleshe, yea, or whiteshe of complexion or fleshie, & haue salte spittle in his mouth, with bitternesse of taste in soche bodies, salte fleume do chiefly abounde, and nedeth purgacion: but thei whiche feele the moisture, or spettle sweete in their mouthes, and haue plentie of swellyng vaines appere in their faces. And also haue noisomnesse and abhorring in their stomack, with aptnesse to vomite, and vrine redde, thicke and oilei, this is a manifest signe, of the aboundance of swete fleume. Furder, if any manne doe feele tartnesse, or sowernesse in his mouthe, with quicke apetite, no thurst or desire to drinke in this case, doe tarte fleume greatly aboudeth, and doeth raine, when all the spettle semeth like Winegar. Some tyme the mouthe dooeth feele no taste, and is vnsauerie, feelyng nothing but like welle water: neither haue apetide or drinesse, desiring neither meate nor drinke: this is an vnsauerie fleum, and nedeth purgacion. Nature haue ofteetimes rebellyng, against her bitternesse in the mouth, but no saltnes, the brine thinne, yellowe or reddishe in colour, this doe declare that redde colour haue the victory. Greate strong bitter vomites, as bitter gaule in the mouthe, without vomites, and vrine yellowe or ruddishe, not very thin: these signes do declare, there doe raigne in the bodie, euill corrupted and infected couler. But if it be of lesse thinnesse, rednes, and bitternes: then it is coul-

Howe to knowe what humour doe abounde, by his propertees ken.

Of swete fleume.

Tart fleume

Signes manifeste declarpng what humours beareth the greateste rule, in the bodies of men and women, without whiche it is

J.iii. ler

The booke of Compoundes.

not possible to purge, accordyng to arte, but rather to kille.

ler, vitelline or like yolkes of Egges, that dooe abounde. Well, if the vrine be yellowe and thin, hauyng small residence in the bottome, and greate bitternesse in the mouthe, then Citrine couler, is a Lorde, and ruleth aboue nature, therefore this and the reste, ought to bee purged with medicenes, made accordyng to the arte, to putte these cruell enemies awaie, whiche els will putte the whole bodie, with all the members, in perill of desolucion and death. Marke when slothfulnes, dulnes, idlenes, wearinesse, and heauinesse be greater, then thei bee accustomed to be: the appetite increased, and thirst deminished, and all the members, as though thei had been wearie, after some painfull labor, whē these signes doe appere, then Melancholy must nedes be purged with spede: If the vaines be full, moste chiefly in the face. Also when as the pulses be verie full, with plentie of swete spettle in the mouth with swellyng, and the blushyng in the face, heauinesse, painfulnesse, and wearinesse in the shoulders, as it happeneth after labour, or bearyng some heauie burden: and the vrine thicke and redde, in these mē blood doe plentifull abounde, whiche maie be helped, by the openyng of the vaine *Mediana* or *Cephalicæ*, or appliyng of boryng glasses, with skarifiyng the place first, if either purgyng doe seme to long, or els the openyng of the vaine, is not dooen accordyngly. &c. *Electuarii* of *Succorosarum.* &c. be good to purge blood.

Signes to knowe when Melancholie doe approche, after whom commeth the quartaine.

Sicknes.

How then doe you purge fleume, whiche is one of the fower humours. I praie you tell me: For lacke of medicen, conuenient for the same: there be many, whiche be daily caste awaie, as it appereth by the rules of Phisike.

Health.

Purgers of fleume.

To speake of fleum simplie, it must be purged with these medicenes, as with *Benedicta laxatiue, Catarico imperiali:* decoction of Polipodie, Agaricke. &c. But salte fleume is purged with the holie bitter medicene, whiche the Grekes call *Hiera picra simplex, Theodoricon, Anacarde, Hyperisticon. &c.* Swete fleum must be purged with *Hyeralogodion* of *Memphis*: and the strongest *Hiera picra*, and soche like thinges. For purgyng swete fleume, as appereth in the compoundes of medicens.

Sicknes.

How doe you purge burnte redde Choller, whiche is hotte and drie?

Health.

The Manna of Calabria is the beste of the worlde, & falleth doune in the nighte, as dewe vpō flowers and leaues.

To purge soche choler, is with *Trisera Saracenica, Electuario frigido, Oxyphænieum*, with the decoction of Mirabolans, Cassiafistula, Tamarindes, violettes, and Manna of Calabria. Choler infected, must be purged with Anacardium, or *Agni cordis*, which groweth vpon a tree in India, whiche tree, giueth fire of it self, and vringeth

geth

The booke of Compoundes.

geth forthe fruite like vnto Lambes hartes, but very small, hauyng a bloodie iuce: of this Rasis maketh a good confection, for simple taken it is venemous. There is also an excellent *Antidotum*, in the .ccxvii. Cha. of *Nicolaus Mirepsi*, in his booke of *Antidotaris*, called *Theodoretos*, or Gods gifte, wherein Anacardus is brought in. &c. Whiche medicen doe helpe the hedde, lunges, stomacke, liuer, splene, goute. &c. And also purgeth choler, so doe with *Hiera picra simplex*, Rubarbe, Diaprunes, &c. But when melancholi, that colde, drie, wretched Saturnus humor crepeth in, with a lene, pale, or swartishe couler, whiche raineth vpon solitarie, carful musyng men: whiche humour at length, bredeth and bryngeth forthe a terrible childe, called the feuer quarten, whiche if he bee not corrected, and banished awaie, will be his fathers death. When he appereth correcte hym thus, as with the strongest Hieralogodion, with the decoction of Sene epithimum, Hamech. &c. But in case the humour bee compounded, then you muste also vse compounded medicen: for medicen simple, dooe rather hurte, then helpe in soche cases. And why so? Mary beyng simple, it purgeth but one humour, and suffer the other corrupted humours to remain: and what is the cause thinke you? Truly none other, but that it is to weake, and lacketh strength and force, whiche the compounded medicenes haue. As example. George Tomson of Kelshall in Suffolke, haue a feuer tercian (well) your good will is to helpe hym, and you giue hym a simple medicene: but what dooe your simple medicen profite him? Nothyng at all. For he whiche haue a tercian, must be purged of choler, and in soche a case, because fleume is mixed with choler: your simple maie rather putte foorthe fleume, whiche is moiste, and not moue choler, whiche is hotte and drie. Yea, the very cause and woorker of the rigour in this tercian, and so when nature haue moister drawen awaie from her, whiche should quenche the heate, then to conclude, choler shalbe come the more hotter, vehementer, and cruell to nature, through a simple medicen, foolishly giuē of a good intent.

When blood doe abounde, or breaketh forthe at the nose, commonly on the right nostrell, or spettyng of blood. &c. then deminishe it, as I haue saied by descrite openyng the vaine, with a fine lansette, and no flem with a bearde, like to a blood Iron, that Smithes doe lette their horse blood withall. For thei will sometyme cutte a vaine through bothe the sides, and cause a crampe. &c. Also in diminishyng of blood, let not the Chirurgian without counsaill, or auncient experiēce, take or open the said bain or baines. As example, Williā Downaby of Iken haue a greuous pain in his hed with ache, he cā take no rest. &c. there is no remedie, but to let him blood: the common Barbar doe take his lanset, and openeth a vaine, as the blind man shote the Crowe, he taketh the first that come to hande, or appereth greatest, perhaps a Sinewe, whiche maie chaunce let out the spirites of life, and kille hym, well, in case this Barbar, for the paines of the hedde, intende to open Basilica, whiche is *vena interna*, or *axillaris*, growyng through the arme

Theodoratos a diuine gift.

Melancholie the worst humor of nature he begette a sonne called the quarten.

Compoūded humour maie not be purged with simple medicene, for thei are to weake.

An example betwen a simple and a cōpounde medicene.

The fire will get the victorie, if the water bee not equall, or haue the masterie. Good intentes and good actes, be two thynges.

hole

The booke of Compoundes.

Ignoraunte Barbars, their fruites,

hole, and bryngeth bothe from the harte and liuer, whiche is his rootes, and through ignoraunce, dooe open a greate sinewe harde by it, whiche is like a vaine: in whiche sinewe the spirites of life doe swiftly run vp and doune, mixte with the blood of life. What haue he doen now? Mary slaine one. And what is their refuge in soche a case? The signe saie thei, was in that place: and he would be nedes letten blood. But in case if the Barbars cunnyng be better, and if he open Basilica without hurt, what doe this helpe the hed? Nothyng, or els very little at al. But if you will helpe M. Downabes hedde, open Cephalica, called *vena externa*, with a long cut, to let out grosse blood, and foule matter, and cut not depe, for feare of apostumacion: this vaine I saie, helpeth his hedde, to purge first with. Ʒ.i.ß. of the pilles of *Hiera simplex*, a daie before is better. Now if his paines bee in his breaste, or right side, ye or pleurasie, then open the vain called Mediana, the middle bain, whose parentes be Basilica, and Cephalica: this Mediana or Cardiaca must bee opened somwhat ouerthwarte, and so shall he blede well, to helpe

Obseruaciõs in bloode lettyng.

the greues aforesaied: but when the matrix, raines, bladder, or yarde, be troubled with grief, stoppyng or swellyng, & moche paines, then in a vessell of warme water, open *vena talii* the ancle vain, called Saphena, for this olde crepyng vulcans, or lame sicknesse, called Sciatica, with paines in the hucle bones. Can neuer be better helped, then to purge with Hiera, to anoint with oile for thesame: as appereth in the Compoundes, and to open the foresaied Sciatica vaine, whiche is one of the middle, & towarde the out side of the foote. And thus to open vaines in order, is the beste waie: and when tyme of blood lettyng, is not conueniente, then aplie boxis with skarissaction, euen as the place, humour, and tyme dooe require, and this shall suffice of purgyng humours, with blood lettyng.

Sicknes.

I Truste to obserue these your saiynges very well, deare frende Health. But how should I knowe, when medicenes haue takẽ their effecte, and wrought accordyngly, to the ende of their forse and vertue?

Health.

To knowe whẽ medicen haue wrouzt their effecte.

Thus you shall knowe, first, there is no man, but dooe take medicen, to putte awaie some grief: and when the grief is past, and the bodie quiet, and no pain in the stomacke, then the medicen haue wrought his good effect. Then you maie giue the brothe of Capon, Chicken, or Hen, sometyme Almonde milke, or cleane stewed brothe, drinke small wine, of colour yelowe and cleane, and vse moderacion in eatyng and drinkyng, vnlesse there folowe an ephemerall agewe. Now the next daie after purging the pacient maie go to the stophe, hothouse, or bathe: so that he go thither, takyng no colde, or doe no labour, by the space of three daies, and then to vse moderate exercise, and to feede vpon meate, that will ingẽder

der good humours. And thus to conclude, the bodie, or any that are sicke before time, shall now be conuerted into a newe nature, through the helpe of nature and medicen.

Sicknes

What els I praie you, is to be obserued in medicen?

Health.

Three thynges are to be noted, Tyme, Humour, and Region: where purgacion is to bee ministered. Firste, as touchyng Tyme, there bee twoo diuersities: the one is the tyme of the yere, and the other is the tyme of the daie & night, in whiche euery humour haue his being. For accordyng to the variacion, alteracion of the tyme of the yere, the maner of the purgacion must bee altered and chaunged. And *Hippocrates* saieth, we muste purge the vpper partes of the body in Sommer, and the nether or lower partes in Winter (for why?) The humours doe folowe the propertie of tyme. In Sommer purge with vomites, in Winter by the stoole, and not without a good consideracion of the tyme, age, and kinde of disease, and habite of the bodie. For thei, whiche haue straight throtes, maie not bee purged with, or by vomite, for feare the spirit and breath of life be stopped and strangled, & so through chokyng, the bodie be killed. Again purge not old men, by the reason of the coldnes of complexion. In Sommer purge aboue, earely in the mornyng. In Winter purge beneth, late at night. In the *Equinoctial* tyme, prepare at euen, and the next mornyng after your preparatiue, purge by Electuarii. &c. In extreme hot regions no purgacions: nor in extreme colde regions, none also. Neither in the daies, whiche be not temperate, as to hot with the Sonne, or to colde with frost. &c. nor in the *Caniculer* daies, except greate nede require.

Tyme, humour, region are chiefly to be considered

Purge vpward in Somer, & dounward in Winter.

Sicknes.

How must the daie and night be considered, in purgacions?

Health.

Whereas the tyme of the daie & night, be in length xxiiii. howers, whiche is called the artificiall daie, and artificiall night, whiche xxiiii. howers, maketh but one naturall daie, deuided into fower tymes sixe, for the fower complexions. For euery complexion haue his gouernement, and dominion sixe howers. First the blood beginneth at nine at night, and continue vntill three in the mornyng. And choler from three after midnight, vntill nine before noone. And so the other twoo humours: first melancholy and fleume, haue eche of them sixe howers, wherein thei doe raigne, and gouerne the bodie. Now if it be Sōmer, and then you be minded to purge choler by vomite, then you must giue thesaid vomite, a little before the hower of the daie. So that when it haue remained, and staied it self a while in the stomacke, it maie woorke in the howers of choler, to purge thesame. In the like appoincted

The daie natural, and the daie artificial

The fower complex, raignyng euery one sixe howers.

The booke of Compoundes.

appoincted howers, so purgyng melancholi dounward, in his hower and make euacuacion of it. If thou wilt purge fleume, let the pacient reste a Gods name, by the space of three or fower howers in the night, and then wake, and take his pocion, or medicene, a little before Midnight, and not slepe after it, vntil it be purged. Now if you will purge blood, in the mornyng open a vain, except verie old, or yong, or people consumed, or women with childe, with soche I dare not haue to doe. If you will purge humours, other waies then thus: that is obseruing the howers, yea, and the mansions, or course of the Moone, els thou shalt greatly erre, and doe more hurte then good.

The aged, & very younge, weake folke, and women with childe, maie not bee let blood.

Furdermore, consider the diuersitie of humours, if blood abounde, he must be letten forthe by the vain, as Cephalica, or Mediana. &c. If choler be to moche aboue nature, then purge by vomite: but if choler be mixed with blood, then let blood as I haue saied, vnles the matter be contained, in the neather partes of the bellie, then purge by glister or pocion. &c. If fleume or melancholi be beneath, purge dounwardes vnlesse it be aboute the mouthe, or entrance of the stomacke, or the vpper partes of the bodie: marke and wisely consider the tyme, in al these thynges, for that is the chifest poinct of all. For euery thing, saied the wiseman haue his proper tyme vnder heauen. &c. And regions by whiche here in this place, the humours be considered: also the places of purgyng, the vpper part, the neather part, the nostrelles, rofe of the mouthe, pores of sweatyng, and vaines of bleedyng. &c.

Matter in vaine must be put forthe by blood lettyng and in the bellie by glister, in the breaste by vomite.

Sicknes.

What saie you then of place, in whom the matter is contained?

Health.

Place where medicē shuld be ministered conuenientlie ioyned with tyme.

THE place in deede, as I haue saied, muste be considered in whiche a medicen shalbe giuen: whether it be to hot in Sommer, or to colde in Winter. If the daie be to hot, you maie caste Vinegar, Sallowe braunches, Violettes, water Lilles: and bee in a lowe vaulte, or from the Sonne. And temper the place, where you will purge, on the other parte if the place be to colde, make a fire of Charcoales, or a stoue, whiche is a fire secrete felte, but not seen. Close windowes from wind, in a pretie warme chamber, with good hole hanginges or selyng. The pacient to haue light warme clothes, and slippers cleane, and well lined: swete linnen, as sheetes, shurtes, and kerchiffes, a close chere, lined softly with a backe, hauyng a cleane rounde bason, or vessell within the same, to receiue the stooles or purged matter. And then to haue soft Cotten or clothe, to make clene natures priuie place, you knowe my meanyng. Forget no sweete perfumes by arte, for nature will plaie the stinkyng beaste, I tell you truely. Also in this place no noise, nor vtter Monkishe silēce, but be mindfull of some honest merie matter, or pleasant tale, or thinges that wil reioice ÿ spirites. &c. And this place must be thus vsed, in the time of purgacion: but still I saie,

beware

The booke of Compoundes. Fol.liiij.

beware that you take not colde, or rather colde take not you. For in soche a case, if he get the victory, then he will put you into a shete, and sende you to the God of *Qui Lazarum.* Colde doeth take, and is not taken.

Sicknes.

WEll good sir, after *Qui Lazarum: Credo videre bona domini, in terra viuentium:* And that dooe I beleue, euen to see the goodnesse of the Lorde God, in the lande of the liuyng, where I shall receiue all my bodie whole and sounde, in as goodlie a forme, as my father Adam was in, before his moste lamentable fall: by whom I am thus punished, with miserie, care, heauinesse, labour, ingratitude of myne owne fleshe, and frendes, sicknesse, paines, sorenesse, & daily daunger, to haue my blood spilte for myne owne gooddes, prisone, affliction of minde, and sometime the periured enemie doe preuaile, with fierie tongue of slaunder, with a thousand crosses, whiche make me to stoupe. And to despise the worlde, whiche is trapped with snares before myne eyes, in eche place and then I crepe, within my self, wheras I doe se in myne own breast and conscience, written the carefull woordes of Job, Chapiter. xiiij.
Homo natus mulieris paucorum dierum est, & repletur inquietudine. &c. Man saieth he, that is borne of a woman, liueth but fewe daies, and is ful of miserie: fewe daies, and yet spente in trouble. Truely there is none other purgyng place, or purgatorie but this: whiche Job haue poincted here with his finger. The very maner, condicion, place, and turment, whiche is onely miserie, deuided into twoo kindes, the one is the greuous affliction and miserie, whiche is seen with mortall iyne, as I haue saied before, as penurie, prison, sickenesse, &c. The seconde miserie is not seen, but felte, as the inwarde agonie, affliction of the spirites: no inward consolacion. Continuall thought, sometyme wishyng that death might conquere life. Broken hart, and vexed spirite, full of sondrie inwarde affections, and alteracions of minde, small rest or quietnes, sorowfull for the death of kinred, or frendes, being changed into bitter enemies, whiche is a greate plague. Or goodes loste, or actes doen insolently in tymes paste: and moste fearfull of thynges to come, as doyng hurte, or suffring harme by enemies, or turning with a sodain fal, from the fortunate happie whele, if it so chăce, of riches, health, worship, pleasure, the victory of thenemy, and pleasuring the frede & hartes rest, &c. Into the pit & darke lake of aduersitie, sodainly depriued of these vaine slippery thynges, and eftsones linked, fetred, and intangled, withall soche euils, as the hart, and spirites, do vtterly deteste, feare, and abhorre to thinke vpõ: besides ỹ slepyng passions of the night, with carefull troubles of the spirites, & dreames most dredfull, of strange shapes, fearfull sightes: and pitifull appering of the ded parentes, frendes, brethren, & old acquaintance. And somtime tharmed enemy, with frounyng face, gnashyng teth, bloodie handes, doe mercilesse approche to kill me, the slepyng naked manne, embrasyng my delighte: eftsones the flatterer

The hope of the life to cum

In Adã wee haue our fall.

Acab wil kill Naboth, for his vineyard

When one descēde into him self, he shal beholde fearfull thynges.

Mannes life is bothe short and miserable

In this life we haue our purgatorie, & that we feele and perceiue. Two sondrie kindes of miseries.

Sorowe for thinges paste and feare of thynges to come.

Prosperitie is very slipperie.

Horrible dremes in the night.

doe

The booke of Compoundes.

doe please the eare, and pleasaunt thynges approche. And the fleshe is sone moued, through wicked luste, and in the twinkelyng of the iye, from dreame to dreame, the spirites bee so variable: that the night to the carefull manne, is the very Image of helle, and specially to theim which feare not God: thus he punisheth theim, as Job saieth, in the night, to reforme thē: And by soche affliction of the night, in the time of slepe, whiche is brother to death. In whiche tyme the almightie do schoole mankind, rebuke hym, and suffer the wicked enemie to scurge hym, with strange visions, &c. Mankinde maie sone thereby, vndoubtedly beholde and perceiue the soule, whiche is liuely occupied, when as the grosse sences of the bodie be stopped, and in a maner dedde: neither seing, hearing, &c. Now whether it be dreame, elusion, vision, &c. As some doe saie, or the effectes, or workes of the fower complexions, as the cholorike man, to dreame of fire, fightyng, &c. The flegmatike, to dreame of water, &c. And so in the other twoo complexions, or as *Artemydorus* in his booke of dreames saieth, thei dooe presage, deuine, or shewe before, what thynges doe folowe, or come after, good or badde. All these thynges bee greate miseries, and greuous afflictions of the soule, whiche I moste humble desire God, to deliuer vs from: and comfort vs with his holy spirite, against all soche euill spirites, which do molest & vexe our spirites: whiche is a thousand tymes more greuous inwardly, then the outwarde miseries of the bodie: as pouertie, prisonment, and extreme age. &c. For looke how moche the soule, is purer then the bodie, euen so the ioies, and cares of thesame, be more plentifull. And this occasion haue moued me, beyng a sicke man, to wander from our former talke. And why? Onely because you spake of *Qui Lazarum*, whiche I haue heard song, in a lamentable tragidie, perhaps: but my song shalbe, *Beati mortui, qui in domino moriuntur.* Blessed be the dedde, which dieth in the Lorde: and happie are thei, whiche liueth in hym also: whiche is the chifest signe of their election, and endlesse estate, in that place wheras no ende shalbe of perfite felicitie, and life for euer: wher as neither enemie, sicknes, woundes, prison, or pouertie shall vexe the immortall bodies, whiche now be subiecte to all calamities: yea from the Kyng and Quene, whiche, of all be honoured, obaied, or flattered: vnto the poorest bondman, and his wife, with his wretched children, that be shamefully despised, contemned, and vtterly reiected. But because no manne shalbe perfectly happie before death, as the Philosopher saieth: yet thesame death shalbe swallowed vp in victorie, which victorie is Jesus Christ, the conquerer, beginnyng, and endyng of all thynges, to whom be praise for euer. *Amen.*

Yet because I am a man, of the creacion of God, scorged with many infirmities in this worlde: by, and through thesame God also, many goodly medicines be prepared to helpe me, to reliue and comforte me, vntill soche tyme, as it shall please GOD, to call me to the ende of my pilgrimage. Therefore good maister Health, beare with me, although I haue spoken in my greuous passion, to ease my mynde: and now by
your

of sicke men and medicens.   Fol.lv.

your paciencs, whereas you haue shewed me, immediatly before, in what place medicen should be giuen. Now I praie you, shew me what tyme, medicen should be ministred?   *Of the tyme of medicen.*

Health.

I am sorie for thy double affliction, bothe bodie & mynde, thou hast tolde a lamentable tale: well, I will saie thus moche to thee, many handes make light woorke. Bare these greues quietly, & haste many to helpe thee in this worlde. For there is nothyng vnder ye sunne, but vanitie & affliction of minde. Euery liuinge man hath trouble, this must nedes be wisely suffred, because it cannot be auoided: & wise men maie not dispaire in aduersitie, for comfort will come I warrant thee be neither to effeminate or childishe, whē trouble assault thee, for then thou art cleane gone. But arme thy self wisely w magnanimite, foresee thende, holde vp thy hed, and sinke not. Use this worlde like a Stadge, play thy parte thereon in thy vocation, for the time honestly, serue God reuerently, despise not ciuill policie. Profite the common wealth, kepe good companie, be not ingratefull to thy frende. Depart from thyne enemie, and yet beware of thy friendes. Speake gently, truste not them, that commonly vse swearyng, slaunder, drunkenesse, and be full of ielousie. Liue of thyne owne, though it be but poorely. Be not bonde, if thou maiest stande at libertie. Go not to Lawe with Lawers, for thei will hinder thee. And beware of a flatterer, he will betraie thee. Bee not variable in Religion, obseruyng tyme, and the maners of men: But obaiyng God, whiche doe not chaunge. There be three sondrie men, whiche haue doen thee neuer good: The winker in his tale, the laugher in his rage, and the Foxe coloured, whiche will not sticke for blood sheding, false witnesse, or periurie. Yet praie for thē and let go displeasure. Bee angrie and synne not. Let not the Sonne go doune on thy wrathe. Truste not to the worlde, yet beholde it, and thou shalt see marueilous thynges wrought therein. Thou shalte see moche wrong doen daily vnder the Sonne, and beholde the teares of soche as be oppressed, and there is no manne to comforte them, or that will deliuer or defende theim, from the violens of the oppressours, but onely God: Therefore, followe the counsaill of the wise man, there is nothyng better saieth he, for a man, then to bee ioyfull in his labour, for that is his porcion. And for as moche as mankinde, haue labour, trauell, heauinesse, sorowe, and disquietnesse all his life, and yet shall leaue al his labours to others, whiche neuer sawe them, is it not better then, for a man to eate and drinke, and his soule to be merie in his labour, and this is the gifte of God, saieth the wise man. And thus to conclude, if thou bee troubled in mynde, praie onely to God, and aske counsaill of the wise: if thou be sicke, seke the Philicion. Honour him because of necessitie, God hath created hym. For of the highest cometh medicen, and he shall receiue giftes of the kyng. The wisedome of the

Eccle. v.

A three strin ged whippe.

Eccle. iiii.

Eccle. iii.

What thynge is best for mā kynde.

R.i.   Philicion

The booke of the vse

Phisicion, bryngeth hym to greate worship: in the sight of the greate men of this worlde: he shalbe honourably taken. The lorde haue created medicen of the yearth, and he that is wise, wil not abhorre it. Was not the bitter water made sweete with a tree: that men might learne to knowe the vertue thereof. The Lorde haue giuen men wisedome, and vnderstandyng, that thei might bee honoured in his wonderous workes: with soche doeth he heale man, and taketh awaie the paines, of soche doe the Apoticarie make a confection, yet can not a man performe all his workes. For of the Lorde cometh prosperous wealth, ouer all the yearth. My sonne despise not this in thy sicknes, but praie vnto the lorde, and he shall make thee whole. Leaue of fro synne, and order thine handes a right. Clense thine harte fro all wickednes: this is the counsaill of Iesus the sonne of Syrach, in his holie booke. Capit. xxxviii. And now shall I shewe vnto thee, what time medicen shal be giuen. Then doe thus. Somtyme medicen is giuen to slepewarde, or before slepe: and sometyme before daie, in the mornyng, to the wakyng tyme. Firste, in the tyme of wakyng, then giue liquid or moiste medicenes, and also easie: and specially when we must purge light humours in the stomacke. For as a moiste liquide medicene, in potion is sone disolued: euen so she will spedily and quickly, doe her duetie, and worke her feate effectually in her place, wheras she haue power to conuert actiuely, and chaunge thynges into her nature. Euen so nature haue power, to chaunge meat and foode, into her own proper vertue. Therfore note this, that whē soche medicens be ministred: if y pacient should then slepe, at soche tyme, as the naturall heate beginneth to encrease. Then thesaid slepe letteth the vertue, and good operacion of thesame medicene: resoluyng the bodie into painfull sweate, and attracte and drawe humours out of order, makyng the paciente sicker. Item, in as moche as liquide and light humors, be sone dissolued: then it foloweth, that thesame humours doe eftsones, come to the place of expulsiō. Therfore to conclude, if thesaid pacient do slepe, at that presente, it might then chaunce that the medicene, would not conuerte, chaunge humour or cast it forthe: but rather resolue humours in the body, whiche would cause moste painfull perill, and noisome sickenes and disease, while as the putrified matter, remaine still in the bodie, not purged. But when as the pacient haue taken but a light supper, he maie take pilles, so that thesaid pilles be newe, and the pacient not very fatte: for fatte menne and women, haue small guttes, and pilles maie chaunce hurte theim. And when we purge harde matter, or humours in the extreme partes of the bodie, we minister pilles. But for as moche, as pilles bee harde of resolucion within the bodie, one maie slepe well vpon theim, before thei be resolued. For slepe bryngeth inward warmnes: and warmnes maketh resolucion, and furdereth the workyng of pilles, whiche muste take their effecte, in the extreme partes, as hedde, handes, and the feete. And thus I saie, pilles maie be giuen without hurte, when the pacient go to his naturall rest and slepe

Prouided

Exod. 15.
3. Regum. 4.

Eccle. 38.

Good counsel in the time of trouble.

Medicen do chaunge, and meat is chaūged.

Why purgacion worke not natutally

One maye slepe after Pilles, but yet beware of olde drye Pilles.

Prouided, that in the mornyng, when thei beginne to worke: then the saied pacient muste slepe no more at that tyme. And note, that pilles maie be confected, of all kindes of medicenes: and there be pilles giuē before meate, for them whiche haue euill digestion, called *Pilule ante cibum*.

Pilles maie be made of all kindes of medicenes.

Sicknes.

Somtyme it commeth to passe, that in a maner vnaduisedly, or sodainly, the Phisicion doe giue a purgacion or medicene, not consideryng the complexion of his pacient, therein doe he well or no? I praie you.

Health.

THE complexion would bee knowen, but when there is no oportunitie or leasure, to knowe the complexion: whether it be hote, cold, moiste, or drie. In this cause let vs vse a preuentyng medicen, or an *Antidotarj*: wherby we maie bothe prepare the waie, and also knowe whether the matter bee hard or softe. To remoue with thesame preuentyng medicen, either yea, or no: also in this case, let some thing be ministred before, whiche maie gently resolue the humours, as *Benedicta laxatiuæ, stomathicum Cartaticum imperialæ*. Or els lette vs giue to the paciente some gentle pilles, and decoction of Polipodie, Agarice, and Hermodactilis, tempered with white wine: puttyng therevnto purified and cleane Honie, and then giue it to the pacient, when it haue stande, vntill it commeth to a residence, doe thesame with Polipodie, Esula, sodden in wine, puttyng in a little Sinamon. For this dooe resolue, and vnbinde flegme, and purge it well, or els gather solutiue and losyng herbes: as is Mercurie, Beates, Mallowes. &c. seeth theim in fatte Porke, puttyng in a little Sene. And in case this lose the saied sicke pacient, if he marke the quantitie of the euacuacion, or thynges purged: so he maie be contented therwith. If he feele more grief in the bellie, or pain burnyng, or noisomnes: he maie then prepare a stronger, or one weaker, accordynge to his humour, age, or tyme of the yeare, or habite of the bodie. And in all medicens, beware of this, that nothing be taken in the fitte, rigour, terrour, or hower, when the pacient shall be vexed, tossed, or turmented with quotidian, tertian, or quartein. &c.

The obseruacion of complexions.

To giue medicene, in the fit of a feuer, is perilous.

Sicknes.

FVrthermore it cometh to passe, as is daily seen, that there be many feble stomackes, and fearfull iyes, that doe not onely abhorre to se medicens. Some for their blacknes to behold, as *Cassiafistula*, or bitternesse in taste, as *Hiera picra*, or fulsome to smell: as strong pilles, yea, it no lesse greueth them to beholde, or se the vessell, in whiche the pocion is kept in, then to drinke thesame pocion, or bitter medicen, contained within thesame. Soche be the weake, feble, nesse stomackes of many, God knoweth: for why, nature haue made theim no stronger. For the feble stomacke of a tender gentlewoman,

weake stomackes can not awaie & strong medicenes.

K.ii. maie

maie not be cōpared in forse, to the boisterous, rough, gredie, or strong stomacke of the Carter. The sight or smell of vile thinges, doe hym as small displeasure: as the swete odours, and pleasaunte aspectes, dooe hurte the dilicious sences of the tenderlynges, or carpet muses. I saie the barbarous vplandishe Jenkyng, with torne hose, and clouted bootes: foule shurte, and thredbare bonet, long lockes, and crompled handes, and grined, scuruie countenaunce. With gantlettes made of Sorrelles hide: armed with a pece of a Mottly mantell. Boldly chargyng a long whipstocke, with croppe and laniard, against Rudde, or blinde Baiarde: whiche traile, and drawe, the laden Carte, and bende their backes, with continuall burdens, rewarded with vnpleasaunt foode.

Cowe, shepe and Plough, be our nurses

This vnsemely grome or Carter, driuyng his Carte I saie, yet is he a childe, and a feeder of the common wealthe: with Cowe, Shepe, and Plowe, in the clottie field, following the Share and Culter. After the dreamyng steppes, of the deepe treadyng Oxe: whiche treadeth on the foote, of eche poore man in the countrey. These tillions, which vse no Speres, but Spades, and fight their cumbates, with flailes: in solatorie Barnes, emong the Sheues, fraiyng the Mise into the Chaffe.

The life of the plain people in the countrey.

When Snowe and Froste, maketh Cowe and Calfe, to tremble in couarte: and Swine to lurke in cotte, for feare of the Northren, sharpe, cuttyng winde. Long blacke nightes, and short colde rainyng daies: vncouered naked trees, shrouded with Snow, vnder who lurketh the hungrie birdes. At soche tyme as the plain people, do spend, consume, and bring to nothing their substance emong their labouryng hindes, Sōmers frutes: not without winters trauell God wot. If Saturne caste forthe, then from his high cold throne vpon them, his malicious euill infortunate influence: when he with Sithe in hande, and graie horie lockes, doe crepe into the sixt house of the heauen, or fallyng angle. From whence he poureth forthe, saieth *Haly*, emong men, greate infirmities, melancholie, fallyng euil, madnesse, leproses, quartens, and also euery sicknes that cometh of coldnesse, and drinesse. &c. And drineth the plain people, to their wittes ende, which lacketh prouidence, to forsee and prepare medicene, fitte for their defence. Of whom, God taketh the onely cure and charge: From an higher place, then where as olde Saturnus doe dwell. Vpon the simple sort of mortall menne, he careth for the straunger, fatherlesse and widdowe. And open his hande, and fill euery liuyng wight with plentiousnes: and is nere vnto them, that dooe call vpon hym faithfully, and there is none of his, that are fallen into any miserie, but he see their fall, whether it be pouertie, prisonmēt, exile, care, agonie, affliction, or vexaciō of mind. &c. Then with mercie and pitie, he putteth forthe the hande of his prouidence: and lift them vp, and help them in the daies of their caresulnes, makyng them pleasaunt. Giuyng theim reste and quiet slepes, while as the vngodly, doe remoue their neighbours lande markes. And rob them of their cattell: and by extorcion, kepe them from their own, and oppresse the widdowe and fatherles. Making them go naked, yet these people

Hali de iudicijs Astrorū pars octaua Capi. vij.

Psal. cxlvii.

Psal. Cxlv.

Job. xxiiii.

of sicke men and medicens. Fol.lvj.

people prospere for the tyme, although thei murder the simple. But at length the shadowe of death, shall come vpon theim: and thei shall goe into horrible darknesse. And thus haue I redde, in a lamentable booke of one, which had experience, of miseries infinite: Sicknes and sorowes, yea, this Job was onely sicknes: whose seruaunt I am, and what is the chief helpe, or to whom shall I the sicke, poore, feble man resort. Euen to him that my maister Job went vnto. Who was that I praie you? Was it the Chirurgen, Apoticarie, or Phisicion? &c. No, no. It was the almightie God, without whom euery artificer, bothe in Philosophie and Phisike, their woorkes taketh none effecte, nor any good successe, although thei dooe excell in knowlege, learnyng, iudgement, and practise. Therefore I doe saie deare frend Health, with the Prophete Dauid, in his Hymne or song. I doe lift vp myne iyes vnto the mountaines: from whens cometh helpe to me? My helpe cometh from the Lorde God, whiche made heauen and yearth: and here I doe gather, if I bee sore or sicke, weake or wounded, troubled or vexed. Although I liste vp myne iyes, vnto mountaines of this worlde, for the health of my bodie. Is to the best Chirurgians or Phisicions, whiche as I haue saied, doe excell in knowlege and practise. This is nothyng if my helpe cometh not out of heauen: from the fountain of Phisicke, euen so for the health and regiment of the soule, when it is sicke. The mountaines of sainctes, angels, and men, can not preuaile, except the very saluacion, attonement, healthe, praise, and quietnes: proceadeth onely from God, whiche is very *Salus*, that is health: or *Sospes*, the healthe giuer, and vpon hym I do onely depende, whiche dwelleth in heauen.

The ende of the wicked menne.

God the very Phisicion.

Psalme.

Health.

If he be on your side, who can be against you? Nothyng in heauen, yearth, or hell, to molest you: if you be vnder the shade of his winges, you are safe from all stormes. I dooe commende your Godly zele, and faithfull affection to almightie Godward: albeit you seme vnto me, to wander in this your communicacion, from the path or line, whiche was laied out straight, betwene you and me, whiche was the regiment and health, onely of the bodie. And you doe declare of the miserie of the common people, and of the calamities: and saie when thei fall sicke, thei lacke prouidence, and helpe emong them selues, but onely God. Mary I saie also, onely God. But how? That God doe alwaies sende health, without meane? No, for almightie God do woorke by miracle, and by meane: by miracle, as when he raisedt he dedde, clensed the lepre. &c. By meane, when with claie, he opened the iyes of the blinde: and with spattle, he caused the deafe to heare. Yea, and commaunded the Apostles, to cary Oile with theim, to heale the sicke. Why doe you then talke thus, leauyng out this woorde meane? Whiche is like vnto an hande, whiche worketh for euery thing, bothe without, and within the bodie. By whiche meane, the holy spirite of

Roma. viii.

God do work by miracle, & meanes.

K.iii. God

The booke of the vse

God is perceiued, as example. The Apostle. i. Corin. xii. Chapiter. The gifte of the spirite is giuen to euery man, to edifie withall. To one is giuen through the spirite, the vtteraunce of wisedome. To an other the vtteraunce of knowlege, by thesame spirite. To an other is giuen faithe, by thesame spirite. To an other the giftes of healyng, by the same spirite. &c. Lo, here you se healyng, is the gifte of Gods spirite, whiche is God the holy ghost. And although the gift of healyng, was plentifully shewed and powred in, and vpon the holy Apostles, which wrought bothe with miracles, and meanes. Yet it can not be denaied but diuers, whiche had no faith heauenly, or the gift of faith: yet thei had the gift of healyng. For thei be seuerall giftes of God.

The holie Ghoste.

Hippocrates. Galen, Auicen. &c. had not the gift of faith, and were Infideles, beleued not in God, nor in his soonne Christe: yet God bestowed vpon thē, excellent knowlege of natural thynges, as appereth by their learned bokes, whiche be candles, to giue light to Phisicions, to the worldes ende. For the incomperable learnyng and cunnyng, whiche bee written in theim. Thus God haue made the very Infideles, meanes to helpe the Christians, whiche you maie not denaie. Neither thinke the plaine people to be so ignoraunt, but when thei be sicke, thei can sende to the Phisicion, or Chirurgen for helpe: as well as thei will sende to the Mill, to haue their corne grounde. Or to the Shomaker for Shoes, to defende theim from goyng barefoote. What would you haue the Carters (as you terme them) so miserable, or without wit, or worse then the Dogge: whiche can licke his wound, and chose his bomityng grasse. That should appere by the fruites of poore menne, I meane their children. I praie you, be not mitours set vpon the heddes of Plowmennes soonnes: and doe not the children often tymes, of obscure, skant yomen, and very abiectes, possesse bothe riche houses and landes. Where somtyme their parentes, would gladly haue serued in the Kichen. &c. What is the cause? It should appere, vertue auaunceth and learnyng helpeth. Exclame not, neither bewaile these pooreones estates: for thei can see daie at a little hole, and liue as merie, the olde Prouerbe saieth, as white Bee in Hiue. I praie you pitie theim with measure, vnles your large lamentacion, should giue occasion, to nourishe idlenes. Nor that men yet should disdaine the poore. But who so stoppeth his eare at the crie of the poore: shall crie hymself, and not be hard of God. Nor also that poore people, should disdaine, murmour, or speake euil against theraltacion, or aduauncement of them, whō God haue plucked out of ỹ dust, to be his ministers in ỹ rule of this worlde. And as for thoppressours, be pacient: for thesame God that giue them preparatiues with warnynges, as plague will also giue thē a purgacion, and expulse them frō him, except thei doe repent. For gather thei neuer so moche, beware the third heire of an extorcioner: and often times he doe not enioie, his goodes hymself. For Salomon saieth: *Hereditas ad quam festinatur in principio, in nouissimo benedictio carebit:* The heritage that cometh to hastily at the first, shall not bee blessed at the ende. And in an other place.

Infideles haue singuler giftes of God

Poore men bee exalted through vertue.

Math. xxv.

Psalm. cxlvii

Prouer. xx.

of sicke men and medicens. Fol.lviij.

place, saieth he, whoso hurdeth vp riches, with the deceiptfulnesse of tongue: he is vaine, and a foole, and like vnto theim, that seeke their owne death, this is their ende. Therefore my brother, disquiet not thy mynde, contente thee in thyne estate: kepe thyne owne goodes, spende them to Gods glorie, desire none other mannes. And when thou doest see the wicked, in greate prosperitie, disdain them not: neither fret thy self, thou hast nothyng to doe with them. But to make accomptes for thyne own self: and be not forgetfull of the Prophetes wordes, whē he said: *Noli emulari in malingnantibus. &c.* saith he: fret not thy self, because of the vngodly. Neither be thou enuious, against the euill doers, for thei shal be cut doune like grasse: and be withered, euen as the grene herbe. Put thou thy trust in the Lorde, and by doyng good, that thou maie dwell in the lande: and verely thou shalt be fedde. Delight thou in God, and he shall giue thee thy hartes desire. Commit thy waie vnto the Lorde, and put thy trust in hym, and he shall bryng it to passe. &c. If thou art troubled in thy minde, resorte vnto his holy worde: and ministers for the soule. And wheras thou art sicke, and sore in bodie, despise not his ordinarie meanes, but honour the Phisicion, because of infirmitie: the almightie haue created hym, for that purpose. That through the vertue of Phisike, thy name shall bee chaunged, from Sicknesse into Health. I therefore will now cease, and giue place vnto the Deuines, and Moralle men: whiche with tongue and pen, can giue good counsaill, and heauenly Cordalles for the sicke, sore, afflicted spirite.

And now to the firste parte of your question, concernyng Phisike, whiche is the rase, wherein we begun to run. Let vs now come again into that plain pathe, holde on still, and then we shall the soner come to our waies ende. And then sit vs doune, and reste vs quietly a Gods name: for rest is an image of heauen, after labour. Your question was thus, of them, whiche doe abhorre the sight, or smellyng of medicene: beyng redy to vomite also, to behold the vessels, wherin medicen was giuen, to that question, you answered your self. The cause was, the stomacke doe abhorre those thynges: that offende the sences, as in seeyng, smellyng. &c. (But in deede our sens of smellyng, is worse then any other liuyng beastes. As *Aristotle* saith, in his booke of sences: *Odoratum peiorem habemus quam alia animalia.* Furder saieth he, man onely dooe smell, and doe delight in the odours of flowers, or swete thynges: Euen so do his nature abhorre stinkyng thynges. But specially thei, whiche be clene of nature, or by accidentes. And this is knowen by naturall Philosophie, and Phisike: and whereas the Philosopher doe leaue, there the Phisician doe begin. Although there be many secrete, hidden desires within nature, knowen onely to the same, and hidden from the Phisicion. As example: some women beyng with child, desire Tarre, yea, I haue seen them eate Sope, and hurte them not, with other vile thynges, that I will not name. Without nature had them, death would folowe: yet Phisike compt them deadly. These be the secret hidden thinges within nature.) But now to the question.

K.iiii. When

Sidenotes:
Sodain gotten substance remains not longe.
Let no man bee angerie with an other mannes follie
He whiche loueth God, shal haue hartes reste.
Ecclesias.
Aristo. in libro de Sens.
Nature haue many hidden desires, vnknowen to the Phisiciōs

The booke of the vse

When nature is so weake and feble, that it doe lothe and abhorre, to see or smell medicen. The beste remedie is thus: that you giue laxatiue Claret, made after this maner.

Medicenes for feble stomackes to purge gently

℞. Clene Clarit or whyte .li.x. of Polipodie, Honie, ana .li.ii. Igaricke .ʒ.ii. Sinamon, Cloues, Spicknard, Ginger, Galingall, ana .ʒ.i. of Peper .ʒ.iii. Firste make it thus: temper the clarified Honie with wine, and drawe it through a Colander. And stampe the Polipodie, and strongly strain it, and seeth it to the thirde parte, then beate your spice into pouder. And put them into a bagge, made of a pece of a sers or bulter: then put your tempered wine, Honie, and iuce of Polipodie together, put in your bagge with spice, & seeth all in a close vessell well tinned, and straine your bagge often tymes. And then receiue this drinke, and geue a draught to your weake, feble, stomacke, accordyng to your strength. And for Honie, you maie put in clene Suger, and to your spices, you maie put to Sene .ʒ.iii. And when you drinke of this you must drinke clene colde water, or running water after it. Now sir if you will restraine, or stop the bodie, when it is to moche laxatiue: or draweth nature to behemently. Then giue hote water to drinke, and this is bothe pleasaunte, and profitable to nature: though to many it semeth to be vnpleasaunt. Then take spices in pouders, accordyng to the propertie of the humour, or complexion, whiche ought to bee purged. Puttyng the water, and thesaid spices, with a little Sugar, into a close vessell of glasse: and seeth it in a vessell of water. Prouided, that thesaied vessell of glasse, be wrapped in Haie. Or els stande in a plaine stillitorie: makyng a good fire vnder thesame, and then you maie take it forthe, after it be well, and close sodden and strained. And either receiue it your self, or els giue it to others. But if it be bitter, so putte in more Sugar into thesame, to please your stomacke. The more spice you do take, the more vertue it hath, for the melācholie or flegmatike.

Item, also you maie doe thus, take a meane quantitie of *Elleborus albus*, chopped small with a cuttyng knife, seeth it with Barley, with clene water, into a thicknesse. Then feede an Hen eight daies, with thesame corne, and *Elleborus*, & at eight daies ende: Kill thesame Hen, and seeth it, and put in no Salt, but cromes of bread and Sugar, and drinke this broth. Put in *Manna* if you will, and eate the fleshe of thesame Hen, and it will purge thesame: without any molestacion, or hinderance to nature, I assure you, and that I haue proued. Euen so haue a greate nūber, proued *Elleborus albus*, to their greate hurte, and perill of death by bomityng, yea, almoste expiryng emong the Dogge Leches, and murderers. But beware of theim, and then thou shalte be called Health, and no more sicknes, by Gods grace.

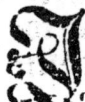
Elleborus albꝰ the poisone therof.

Sicknes.

IS there no consideracion to bee had, in the ages of men, or women: maie the medicen giuer, giue hande ouer hedde, to the tender childe, middle age, and olde men, all a like without hurte to them:

of sicke men and medicens.   Fol.xlix.

them: I would faine knowe, what to doe in this case. For in the countrey, the medicene that is giuen to a woman, of. xxiii. yere olde: is also giuen to a man of. xlvi. yere old.

Health.

YEs surely, diuersitie of age muste bee considered, in the ministracion of medicenes laxatiue. For purgyng or relaxyng medicens, bee giuen to sondrie sortes of ages: as to boies, springaldes, lustie yong men, and to the aged. Euen so to womenkinde, in their degree of ages: euery one of these, haue his, or their proper purgacion. As *Manna* of *Calabria* to yong thynges, and the same to olde folkes: or els some gentle solutiue medicen. And to women with child, no laxatiue medicene, vntill the. v. moneth be paste: and then but gentle ones, as *Cassia*, *Manna*, or the Syruppe of Roses, solutiue. Euen so she maie haue some Sene of Alexander, their leaues sodden closse in brothe of a Chicken or Mutton, within a couered yearthen, or Tinned potte. Also suppositours maie be giuen to these foresaid folkes, that be excepted in purgacions. And furdermore, with discrecion, the aged maie receiue a gentle glister: bicause the said aged bee greued, with corrupcion of the raines, blader, and guttes. For if children bee purged moche, because the humour is light: thei shalbe in daunger of their liues. And liuyng the said purgacions will make wretched, alter the complexion, and expulse the naturall moister, whervpon thei should increase and growe As we see yong children hauyng laxes, be wretched, leane, swelled bellies, crampe and conuulsion. &c. The aged also in soche, shall lose moisture of blood, and fall into melancholie drines, feblenes, lacke of slepe and consumpcion: through resoluing of a strong laxing medicen. But yet to them that be not in extremnes, either of age or sicknes: there be many gentle resolucions, or clensyng of humours, and maie be giuen without daunger. As Reubarbe infused in Cichory water, or the water of Milke, and Mirabolans. But by the waie of Parenthesis, lette euery minister of medicene feare, to giue any thyng that dooe, or will drie the bodie, or bodies to moche, of yong or olde menne: yea, or in the middle age, specially of chollorike men. As example, I did knowe one, beyng then a yong practisioner, seuen yeres paste, did minister a purgacion, wherein was Scamonie, vnto a right worshipfull and a famous knight, called sir Robert Wingfelde of Lethingham, which eftsones, gaue hym twentie stooles. &c. The cause was, as I doe suppose now, this Scamonie was not prepared accordyngly: and also the pacient chollorike, and then partly weake of nature, before the receipt of the saied noughtie purgacion. Therefore, looke diligently to all that I haue saied before: marke the tyme of the yere, the age, qualitie, and complexion of the paciente. The Region or dwellyng place, the goodnes, quantitie, and mixture of your medicene. &c. And then you shall doe no harme, nor plaie the ignoraunt murderer.

Men, women and children, muste take medicens, accordynge to their strégth and age.

Beware of dryng medicens in Somer, for chollorike persons

Now

The booke of the vse

A cauiat for Sommer.

Now again to our matter, neither purge yong children, nor old men in the heate of Sommer: and if you will nedes doe so, then you shalbe commenced Doctor of Phisike, wearyng William Sommers hudde, for your labour, whiche will bryng you to no small estimacion. So trimly to set the carte before the horse, and to plaie blind Baiard your self: therefore be warned, or you bee reproued, or ashamed. For in the heate of Sommer, resolucion of humours be quickly made with purgacion: after whiche insue euacuacion, to moche aboundantly, to the vtter hurte of nature. Yong lustie or sickly persones, maie bee purged at any tyme: so the saied purgyng, doe agree to the tyme, and the complexions. And thei maie take more of the purgacions, then the childrē or old people maie, because of their strength. But yet the Spring time is best, and the Dogges daies worst to purgacion: but sicknes cometh at all tymes, and muste at all tymes bee diligently watched for. As a these that will steale awaie, the moste precious thing called life, whiche is our beste iuell, through the benim of death. But yet death finisheth, and maketh an ende of euery matter, and of euery persone, good and badde. Before whose battell bee fought, we liue but vncertainly: although we flatter our owne selues. For happines is not common to euery liuyng creature: but life and death, be cōmon to euery liuing thing. As *Aristotle* saieth, in his booke of life and death. *Vita & mors sunt communia omnibus animalibus*. And life is but dwellyng of the soule, and bodie together for a tyme. And in the meane season, clouted and patched vp, with meate, drinke, clothe, slepe, &c. And when life is in perille, then helpe Phisike, Phisike, I praie you helpe: we be afraied to die Godlie, bicause we haue liued wickedly. I praie God this Caroll be not to cōmon, yea, or rather there be many doe so liue, that thei feare no punishment or hell, after this life, doe thei neuer so wickedly. Excludyng god cleane out of their hartes, or rather God refusyng them, for their wickednes. There is a Psalme, wherein Dauid lamenteth, the wretched estate of fooles, saiyng: *Dixit insipiens in corde suo non est deus*. The foolishe manne hath saied in harte, there is no God. Would God that there were fewe of them, oh Sicknes, Sicknes, although thou sekest Health. And parhaps maiest obtain it: yet thou shalt ones chaunge this life, and se an other worlde. And also God, for no manne can se hym parfitly before death, nor be saued: whiche in this life, beleueth not in hym.

Sicknes.

Your conclusion, although it did not belong, to your *Exordium*, is yet very godly: I praie God graunt vs to be his, and to forsake sinne. Whereby we shall so quiet our consciences, that when our arriuall shal bee, into the nexte land: we feare not our passage, or iourne from hens thither, for awaie we must. But in the meane tyme, the Image of death, is to all fleshe so fearfull, that menne would be glad to nourishe, helpe, and comfort life, bothe man and beast, doe vndoubtedly *of sicke men and medicens.* Fol.lx.

ly feare death. Nature haue taught one beast, to be in dred of an other, the shepe be afraied of the Wolfe: the Dere of the Dog. The small birdes of the Hauke. And if thei escape woūdes curable, there be medicēs: yea, nature haue taught diuers beastes, and foules, to help thē selues, moche more man should do the same. We therefore thanke God for his grace, ȳ he hath giuē vs reason: which other liuing beastes haue not, which do excel vs, almost in al other thinges, ioyned to their natures. As the Vnicorn to haue an horn, to withstand poison. The Lion void of dread. The Horse strong and swifte. The Shepe, whose caste coate, maketh vs apparell. The birdes to flie, whereas no man can clime the waie. The fishe to swim, where as no man dare folowe them. &c. But onely reasō I saie. What make vs els superiours to beastes? Nothing. Well, take that awaie, and then we be the moste vilest, and the worst: and can leaste helpe our selues, of any other liuing thinges vpon the yearth: as appereth by the foolishe, or madde people, or els yong babes. Thei be in shape and likenes as we be. And why are thei so miserable. Bicause reason is not there, whiche should gouerne them, and this is a lamentable case, deare Health: to se so goodly Images, lackyng their principall beautie and gouernemente called reason. Like Shippes without their helmes, subiecte to euery hurte and storme: excepte the prouidence of almightie God, their onely defence, watched them. Els should thei perishe sodainly, in the mouyng of an hande, as God doce knowe: And bicause God haue giuen reason, by whiche, artes are perceiued, and good thing from the bad, the sicke from the whole: and folishnes from wisedom. Els how eshouldest thou haue shewed me reasonably, the natures of medicenes, complexions, age, time, place, qualitie, and quantitie. &c. And therfore to the matter, in my last question I demaunded, of the age of men and women, to whom medicen should be ministred. I haue in that case recieued myne answere, for whiche I giue you hartie thankes, for your curtesie, and greate gentlenes: specially for your reuerent and godlie zeale, wherin you doe neither smel of the Papistes, which is the mother of al disobediēce to Princes, and the spring of errours. Nor of thē, whiche be of no Religion. But some doce saie, it is better to bee of one euill Religion, then of none at all. Now sir I praie you, after our diuersitie of ages, what doe you saie to the barietie of complexion, in giuyng purgyng medicen.

Health.

ALL is in vaine deare frende, if we doe forget the temperamente, or complexions of men, or women. You therefore doe very well, in callyng theim to remembraunce: for one complexion, can not bare so moche as an other in purgyng. No more then a little weake boie, or yong ladde, can beare as heauie a burden, as a greate lubber: whiche is sturdie and stronge to laboure. Wee therefore giue more of a purgyng medicen, to the flegmatike bodie, then to the chollorik, and

yet

Nature haue prepared that one creature dreadeth and feareth an other.

The booke of the vse

Purge fleum more thã choler and Melicholie more then fleume.

yet more to the melancholie, then to the flegmatike. Why so? Bicause melancholie is an harder humour, then the flegme is: and humiditie, or moisture, more aboundeth in the flegme, then in the melancholie. As example. Therefore when you will giue Scamonie, to any cholerike persone, giue hym a penie waight: to the flegmatike, twoo penie waight: but to the melancholie, giue three penie waight. For a chollorike man, must haue but little giuen hym. The cause is, the said choler is hotte and drie: and if he should take as moche Scamonie, as the melancholie, it would inflame hym, and rather consume the pure naturall humiditie, then purge the noisome filthie humour, whiche is the cause of the sicknes. For the slender man, maie bide worst a quicke

choler is sone drie, therfore purge but little: But the fleshie bodie hath moche moister, therfore purge more.

purgacion: as on the other parte, the more fleshie, I meane flesh, and not grosse fatnesse, soche maie abide a good strong euacuacion, or strõg medicen. By the reason thei haue the more moisture and mumiditie, then the saied chollerike haue.

Of the quantitie of matter to be purged.

Furthermore, as concernyng matter to bee purged, sometyme it is moche: and at other tymes, it is scars, or of quantie. Therefore the medicen must be giuen accordyng: somtyme moche, and somtyme little, small matter is dispatched with small medicen. Except it be wrapped compacted, and thrust togither: and then a preparatiue must be giuen, and after purged. But whereas moche matter is, there it doe require

Moche humour must be purged by little and little, and not attõs

a greater medicen, notwithstandyng, it ought not to be euacuated all at ones, but by little, and little, and by tymes. If it bee in the extreme partes of the bodie, as hedde, handes, and feete, be the extreme partes. And in this case, we haue that noble famous prince of Phisicions, for a witnes: how this matter should bee handled, in the beste maner, saiyng.

Hippocra.

Nam secundum multum est repente euacuare: siue replere fallax est: & omnino inimicum nature. (that is) to make a large or a quicke euacuacion, or purgyng: Replexion or fillyng, is a deceiptfull thyng: and an vtter enemie to nature. Therfore, beware of extremite in all thinges, & vse the meane and best waie, a Gods name, what els haue you to saie?

Sicknes.

I Haue almoste forgotten, how to receiue moiste, or harde medicens: it would please me very moche, and not displease you a little yet again, to put me in remembraunce. For Sicknes God knoweth, is forgetfull. *Ferendum est imbecilitatẽ hominis.* The weakenes or feblenes of man, is to be borne withall. Good sir, should thei be giuen hote or colde. What saie you to the matter?

Health.

Colde medicenes to the whole, but warme to the weake must be geuen.

T O the healthfull, liquide or moiste medicenes, be giuen cold: and to the sicke persons, it is giuen warme, bicause the vertue of the medicene shall in theim lose, deuide, and expulse matter, whan the saied medicene standeth, in the stomacke or guttes: whiche in the whole bodies, the potion or medicen, wil take

his

of sicke men and medicens. Fol.lxj.

his effect in good part, and this must be doen at mornyng. The harde medicine, as I haue saied, at euenyng moste, as pilles: lo enges after midnight. Pouders at noone in brothe: clarified posset ale at euening And why be pilles giuen at night? Bicause a man maie slepe well after them. What doe slepe then preuaile? Bicause slepe maketh the body warme within, and pilles be very hard: and therefore thei must be resolued with warmnes. To what maner of men? To them, which haue the riche mennes sicknes. What is that? Forsoth the goute, which many gentlemen bee turmented withall: as example. Sir Richard Fulmerston knight, Barthram Anderson esquire. &c. For the goute is sore a fraied to dwell emong poore menne: for thei kepe him so hardly, and punishe him with cold, and labour. &c. But the bitterest pilles of all inward medicenes, dooe fardest pearce to the handes and feete, to purge and heale them. And in the feete the goute is placed: therfore pilles be good for the feete. Who can denaie it, whiche I haue spoken?

The Goute loueth riche men, but is a fraied of poor folkes.

Sicknes.

After purgacions, often times it happeneth, that the pacient falleth into a feuer, called *Ephemera febris*, or a light ague: whiche maie doe more hurte to nature, if it bee not helped quicly. What is the cause I praie you tell me?

Health.

Truly, there do often tymes chaunce, soche euill accidentces after purgacions, through sondrie causes. Is sometyme by to moche euacuacion, clensyng, or purgyng, whereupon the Spirites cause vnnaturall heate, and thereof insueth an vnnaturall flamyng or heate called on *Ephemeral*, and likewise it chaunseth by ouermuche eatyng or drinkyng as wine. &c. and also by cold or by attraccion of ouer many humers to the stomacke, or the lacke of the quantitee of medicen, which haue no vertue or strength to be purged, but remaineth stil in the stomacke, and therby do continue putrified, hurting the bodie & maketh a feuer, if this do chaunce, then put the pacient into a bathe, if he bee able. And let there be made a good fire, or hote house, for this patient, and anoynt him before and behind with *Vnguentum dialthes*, or els with *Vnguentum Martiaton*, and bring him close with clothes, from the balne or bathe to his bedde, and kepe hym from sleape eight howers: and so shall he bee dispatched cleane, and made whole, beyng purged againe, to clense the inward partes, as the stomacke. &c. But if the pacient be to weake to come to the bathe: refreshe him in his bed, with wholsom suppinges. Kepe hym warme, in a swete chamber, and then giue hym an easie laxatiue, of drawen *Cassiafistula*. ʒ.i. with water of Burage. ʒ.iii or els with swete *Calabria Manna*. ʒ.ß. And often it chanceth, that men are drie after purgyng, then giue theim small Ale clene brued, or Ptisane or els clene colde water, wherein Gumme Arabicke, and Dragantum be sodden. And to gargarisme these thynges in his mouth and throte:

Of ouermoch purgyng the bodie. the remedy to helpe the same.

and

The booke of the vse

To coole the mouthe. and to put Prune stones in cold water, and chafe them with the tong vp and doune in his mouthe, and so renue theim still. And kepe the mouth, teeth, and tongue clene with washing, clensing, and scraping: and this shall comfort the sicke man, whiche els shalbe corrupted, defiled, and so anoied, that it shalbe as painfull to himself: as hugly and noisome to the beholders of the saied sicke man or pacient.

Sicknes.

Well, then I doe perceiue, that this should suffice to help theim, whiche be not well purged before: and also to coole theim, in their greate thrist and drines.

Health.

No not so: it is not sufficient to quenche. For, first you must vnderstande, the occasion of this thrist: firste of hote chollor not purged, of whiche I speake not. But when the bodie is well purged of drie, yea, or of moiste humours, then lackyng moistnes, it must nedes folowe, drines will eftsones ensue. Then we giue water, wherein the fower cold sedes, gum Arabike, gum Dragagantum, and crumes of bread haue been sodden: drawen through a strainer, this is giuen blood warme. Now sir, there is a drines, as I haue saied: whiche when it cometh, declareth the body is well purged, as some menne suppose. But therein I take, that thei doe mistake the wordes of **Hippocrates.** *Hippocrates. Quicunq; in pharmacijs purgantur: non siciunt, non quiescunt: donec sitiunt, non enim semper bonam purgationem significat:* that is: Who so euer be purged, and thrist not, and the pacient take no reste, vntill thei doe thirst: this doe not alwaie signifie, the purgyng to be good. Take this for an example. One **Example.** called Beumaine, haue a pletorike bodie, that is a body full, or replenished with grosse humours, aboundauntly compacte together: this grosse body must be purged, well he taketh a purgacion by Electuarii, it woorketh vpon Beuman. Now if he feele hymself very drie, with a great thrist, desiryng to drinke, after fiue, sixe or seuen stooles: what is this, a signe good or badde? No it is an euill signe, and is proued thus: cholorike or drie humours be attract, and drawen vp into the stomack and therefore thei are not expulsed. Whereof there riseth a hote and a **Howe to knowe whether Choller be purged, or no.** drie fleume, smoke, or vapour, into the throte, and Spirituall partes: causyng the thirst aforesaid. What remedie for this grosse bodie, then I praie you? None other, but with spede to giue him an other laxatiue medicen, to purge the saied choller, and drie matter, and then the thirst will sone, or quickly cease. And so in the ende, he shalbe better purged of the grosnes of humours, perhappes then clensed from the corrupcion of euill condicions. For a bodily medicen can smally preuaile, or take any effecte, in the regiment of the mynde or soule. Also, if soche a grosse bodie as I haue named, whiche is called *Pectorike*: doe waxe drie or thristie, after. xii. xvi. yea or. xx. stooles: then is not hotte Choller alone, in the stomacke, but in all the members of the bodie. Purge hym still with gentle Electuaries, by little and little: vntill he felety moister

of sicke men and medicens.   Fol. lxij.

ster in his throte, and moche. And to conclude, whosoeuer beyng grosse, and is very drie, before his purgacion, and is sicke of the feuer quotidian or tercian: thesame must be purged, in thesame maner, as I haue said before. But the leane cholorike man, is sone purged, and when he is drie: take his remedie, as is aforesaid, a Gods name. It happeneth also oftentymes, that the pacient can not awaie with cold water: yea and vnknowen to the Philicion. The saied pacient doe drinke wine, to his greate daunger, hurte, and perill: for thereof followeth hotte inflamacion, and turment with paines in the bellie. If this doe happen, then with spede prouoke a vomit: with drinkyng warme water, and Sallet oile, thrustyng a fether into the throte, or a finger as farre as it maie go, and so to vomite. This helpeth, but dooe it spedely my good frende, for sondrie causes, to auoide soche daunger, as els would followe. *what harme wine dooeth in a feuer, or after purging*

Sicknes.

ONe question I will aske you, bicause, cause moueth me so to do. I haue taken oftentimes purgacions: And as the Philicion haue saied: thei were excellent good, well compounded, newe, the quantitie, place, and tyme conuenient, to receiue them. But to conclude, thei would not worke accordingly. What is to be saied therein, I praie you tell me?

Health.

DOe cause, cause you to moue this question to me? I will shewe you three sondrie causes: whiche letteth the medicen to make euacuacion, or workyng. The firste cause maie be, by the reason the purgacion is to weakly made: els the dose or quantitie is to little, which remaineth to the hurt of the body vnpurged. The second cause maie be that the bodie is to moche cold, & subiect to melancholie, as me thinke yours is. The thirde cause is, the resolucion or wastyng of humours, dooe extinguishe, or quenche the vertue of the laxatiue medicen: as it happeneth somtime in the flegmatike bodies. In whom, when soeuer the fleume beginneth to dissolue, eftsones and by and by: it quencheth euen as waxe will sometyme and quenche a burnyng charcole, when it is melted vpon it. And bicause grosse humours are resolued, and can not bee expulsed: then there dooe followe an importable dolour, and a mightie turment about the stomacke, and intrailes. And in the ende, soche solucion: or none other but a manifeste signe, or perille of death to followe. *Certain causes, whiche letteth medicen to worke. Example of waxe and fire. Signes of death, thorowe purging the body*

Sicknes.

MAry, this is a poinct next the worste, and an extreme case: it is hye tyme for a manne to bee wise, and diligent to his pacient, now, or els neuer. God helpe, what remedie?

Health.

L.ii.   The

The booke of the vse

When the paciēt is in peril the remedy to helpe hym.

THE beste remedie is this, when soche perill approcheth, with the strength of mennes handes: take vp the paciente warmely with clothes, folded aboute hym, not harde, boisterous, or comberous about thesaied pacient. But diligēt quicke, easie, and trim: and bryng into a hotte Stophe, or Bathe. Or hauyng none soche, then prepare a verie good fire, as thei terme it, made of Charcoale, if you maie: and then anointe his backe bone, with the oiles of Chamemill, Capers, and Roses. And then anoint the bellie, breast, and sides with thesame: then put a warme tile stone, in a double linnen clothe, and applie it very warme to the belly. Wherefore is this doen? To the ende that the naturall heate maie be made strong: and also that therby, the medicen maie be excited, stirred or moued to expulse, and doe his feate. Now if this moueth hym not to go to the stoole, then giue hym a molifiyng glister, made with Mallowes, Mercurie, Polipodii, Agarike, braied and soddē in water strained, and mingle the decoction with oile of Olife: and putte in a little *Hiera picra simplex* therevnto. But if *Euphorbium* be in medicenes, as in a glister it will excoriat the skin of the guttes, and cause a bloodie fluxe to run forth: it is also helped this waie, as to drinke oile, and warme water, or els the fatte brothe of Porke a ladlefull, wherin .xii. of Asarabaca leaues, the iuce of thē bee strained, and drinke this, it will prouoke vomites, rather to helpe, then hinder the body. If the pacient fele no dolour aboundantly in the guttes: then purge not moche, vnlesse moche purgyng, wherin Scamoni is, doe cleue to the stomacke. But if soche thynges chaunce, giue the paciente to drinke, water of Mirrhe. It is often tymes seen, that when medicen beginneth to worke, within the body, in the waie of purging. Then nature is so weake, that it cannot take his effect, as it should doe accordingly: and by the meanes thereof thesaid medicen remaineth, chokyng the stomack, and neither cometh vpward, neither dounward. What is then the best remedie to be vsed? None other, but folowe *Hippocrates*, whiche saieth: *Elleborum mouit corpus. &c.* Elleborus moueth the bodie. Therefore, let the bodie be moued therewith, in drinke halfe a dragme, whiche is corrected in a Radishe roote: and so bomite will followe, but walke still in the close house, and take no winde. And so the medicene shalbe disperced, and banishe through vomites and sweate, in vehemente mouyng of the bodie. Now if he can not walke, let hym sit, but slepe not: and then after three howers, giue hym *Oxicatarticum imperiale, saccarum violatum. &c.*

A glister to molifie the belie in the time of daunger.

A good note to be obserued when nature is weake.

In Elleborus you shall knowe howe to correct the same, folio. 19 *Simplici*. He meaneth Elleborus albus. ʒ. ß.

Sicknes.

Extremes be perilous thinges.

LIke as some men, in theim medicen will skant worke: in other men, medicen doe so moche worke, that it will not cease, vntill it haue (almoste, yea, or altogether) slain the bodie. What helpe for them then?

Health.

There

of sicke men and medicens.   Fol.lxiij.

There be twoo waies, death or life. If the bodie be dedde, there is no remedie, no medicene, no counsaill, nor comfort, to call it againe. But pacience, and farewell, well, we shall all followe in the ende of our liues: when we haue run our race. Therefore, burie hym that is dedde, let hym reste in peace, and cease from sorowe. But vnto the liuyng that is in hope of cure, if his medecine bee to violente, cruell, and daungerous: Causynge flixes, consider the faute is in the Phisicion, whiche hath giuen to sharpe a purgacion, or in the vnwise paciente, whiche will not kepe the house with a cloase stoole, but sitteth in the winde abrode in the ayre, yarde, or garden. &c. Or els in the vndiscrecion of the Ipothicarie puttyng in to much Skamony, or this may be the cause: the aptnes of humers prepared to expulsion as it chaunceth often to children that haue repletion with hot humers. And after purgacion excoriation or scaldyng of the guttes do follow, which is no small daunger to nature. Therfore to withstand this we stoppe the flixe with Planten water, or water wherin Planten, Bursa pastoris, & Comphorie is sodden, with Bolearmony, gum Irabicke and sower plummes &c. or we minister Almonde milke with Rice. &c. or Glisters stoppyng as appereth in the compounded medicens, here before: also comfort the pacient with a Diacodio, syrup of Myrttels, or of Quinces with warme anointyng the pacients belly & his backe against the warme fier with cleane clarified Hony. Now you shall perceiue a blooddy flixe by the greate paine in the belly, and porynge foorth blood and scraping like leather. Well do as I haue sayd before, and applie a plaster of Barly bread crommed into strong Vineger and apply it to the belly: and giue him to drinke the foresayde Syruppes or Planten water, wherin the flowers of Pomgranets or Mulberies haue ben sodden in &c. And giue him Diacodion, euery night to bedwarde and in the night also. Mary there is a perilous grief in y̆ bellie called Tenasmus, hauynge a will or despre to go to the stoole, and yet cannot voyde or purge any thyng at all, this cometh of the acuite or sharpnes of the medicen or els of the ouer sight of the pacient: let the pacient therfore, sit ouer a Porzmate or decoction of Pomegranettes flowers, barkes, or rindes of Pomegranets, knotgrasse, Roses, Coriander, Peache leaues, Planten, Oke leaues, or the water wherein Mulberies haue ben sodden, *Acacia*, and *Hipoquistes*, and Quinces, beaten together and sodden, and the pacient to sit warme and close therin, and to drinke Diacodion, put in a litle pouder of Saffron, to cōfort the hart.

Death is the ende of life.

The causes why medicen worke vnmoderately.

A plaster for the flixe.

Tenasmus what it is, and how to helpe it.

Sicknes.

You saie this is a good remeadie for the flixe. It often tymes chaunceth, that a man after suche turmentes in the belly cānot be without muche noisomnes in the stomacke: and whā the stomacke is anoied, how is it helped, or w̄ what medicē

Health.

                              L.iij.   Like

The booke of the vse

The yearth is mother of euery liuyng thyng.

LIke as the earth is the mother and nourishe of euery liuyng thyng, and feedeth al creatures good and badde: so is the stomacke the storehouse or kitchen, which do nourishe bothe the members and euery parte of the body, noble and ingnoble: as the harte whiche is the kynge within the body, and to all the subiect members in order, the place from whens thei all be fed is onely the stomack, whiche must be kept cleane, as a pure vessell, and must not be offended, greued or anoyed, but nourished, fortified and pleased: now if it haue lost apitite through lothsomnesse, anoynt the same with Oyle of Maces or of wormewoode, and applie Galen his proper plaster to the stomacke, and drinke the tarte Sirup of Pomgranets, or with sower Grapes with grose Pepper therin, and giue the pacient in his sauce the iuce of Mintes, and of Parcelie, put in Ginger and Suger: whan he hath eaten his meate, giue the saied pacient sirup of Roses and Diarodon, and this shall helpe his stomacke with moderat drinking. And keping the body from sweating heate, and quaking colde, vse temperance only for the meane diate is best of all. And who so dooe vse it, shall neuer falle into the snares of surfites or sicknes.

How to quitken the stomacke.

Extreme heat and cold be euill.

Sicknes.

THe chief thynge that I had thought to haue demaunded, and the very marke, that I woulde haue thee to shote at, is to tell me some thinge of dietinge my selfe with meate and drynke, in Health and Sicknes.

Health.

A consideracion in eating and drinking to be had, and of the variete of meates.

THere is to be considered, in eatynge, and drinkyng, the time of hunger, and custome the place, of eatynge, and drinkyng, whether it be colde or hotte. Also the time of the yeare, whether it be winter or sommer: also the age or complexion of the eater, and whether he be whole, or sicke: Also the thinges which be eaten, whether thei be fyshe, or flesh, fruites or herbes. Note also the complexions, and tempramentes, of the said meates, hotte, or colde, drie, or moyste, and most chiefly marke the quantite, and so foorth. And like as Lampes do consume the Oyle, whiche is put vnto them, for the preseruacion of the light, although it cannot continue for euer: So is the natural heate, whiche is within vs, preserued by humidite and moistenes of bloud and flegme, whose chief engender, be good meates & drinkes. As *Auicen* saith, *de ethica*, When naturall heate is quenched in the body, then of necessitee, the soul must depart from the body. For the workman can not worke, when his instrumentes is gone: so the spirites of life can haue no exercise in the bodie, when there is no naturall heate to worke vpon. Without meate saith *Galen*, it is not possible for a man to liue, either whole, or sicke: and thus to conclude, no vitall thyng liueth without refeccion and sustenance. Whether it bee animall, reasonable as man,

A cause why the soule departeth from the body.

of sicke men and medicens. Fol.lxiiij.

or animall, as brute beastes, without reason, as Tree, Gum, mettall, stone, herbe, or any vitall thyng insensible. All these thynges be nourished, with the influence, or substaunce of the fower elementes.

Sicknes.

Truly thou knowest well my complexion, & disorder of my diate what remedy for me, that haue liued without order of diate?

Health.

I knowe it well, thou art flegmatike: and therefore it is long, or thy meate be digested. When thou doest eate fishe and fleshe together, it dooeth corrupt in thy stomacke, and stincke: euen so doeth harde Chese, and cold fruites. And olde poudered meates, and rawe herbes, ingender euill humours: so that diuersitie of quantitie, and quātitie of diuers meates, doeth bryng moche paine to the stomacke, and doeth engender many diseases. As thou maiest rede in the first booke of *Galen: Iuuamentis membrorum. cap.iiij.* And the prince hymself saith, in *iii.pri.doc.ii. cap.vii.* saiyng nothing is more hurtful, then diuers meates, to be ioined together. For while as the last is receaued, the first beginneth to digest. And when the table is garnished with diuers meates some rosted, some fried, and baked, some warme, some colde, some fyshe, some fleshe with soundrie fruites and sallettes of diuers herbes, to please thine eye. Remember with thy self that the syght of them all, is better then the fedyng of them all. Consider with thy self, thou art a man and no beast, therfore be temperate in thy fedyng, and remēber the wise wordes of Salomon: be not gredie in euery eatyng, and be not hastie vpon all meates. For excease of meates, bringeth sicknesses, and glotony, cometh at the laste, in to an vnmesurable heate. Through a surfet haue many one perished, but he that dieteth him self tēperate y, prolongeth his life. Therfore grose fyshe, Lambes flesh, and the inwardes of beastes, rawe herbes, Pigges braines, and all slimie meates, be euell for thee: but late suppers bee worste of all, specially if they bee longe, for thei cause painfull nightes to folow. But *Galen* saith in his booke *Dieuschymia*, the meates whiche be without all blame, be those whiche be betwene subtile, and grose. Good bread of cleane wheate, fleshe of Capones or Hennes, Fesantes, and Partriches, Pingions, and Turtell Doues, Blacke birdes, and small fielde birdes, rosted Veale, and Mutton: These dooe engender good blood, saieth *Galen.* Note also that any other meate, that thou doest eate at supper, although it seme repugnaunt to a flegmatike stomacke, if thou slepe well after it, and fele no pain, thou maiest vse it, as a meate necessary. And when thou canst not slepe wel, if the defaulte, came through meate: marke that meate or drinke, although it seme pleasaunt, refuse it as an enemie. And where as thou hast vsed euill diete, as accustome in abusyng time, quantite, and qualitie, by little and little: bring thy self into good order, and to time, both for thy breakfastes, diner, and supper. Prouided alwaies, to eate good

L.iiij. thynges.

To eate both fish & flesh together hurteth the flegmatike.

Galen.

Hipocrates.

To fede of diuers sortes of meates corrupteth the body.

Eccle.37.

Good diet prolongeth life.

What kindes of meats doth cause good bloud.

A good rule to be obserued

The booke of the vse

thynges: but not many thinges. For like as repletion, or a boundance of meate, is an enemie vnto the body and soule, and bringeth sudden death: euen so is emptinesse, a shortner of time, a weaker of the braine a hinderer of memorie, an increaser of winde, choler and melancholy. And oftentimes to many, bringeth sudden death also, excepte nature haue some thinge to worke vpon, as I did tell thee before: vse some light thinges, at brekefast of perfet disgestion. Within .iiii. houres after thou receaue thy dinner, obseruing the good order of diet, drinking Wine or Beare oftentimes, and litle at once, eschuyng great draughtes of drinke, whiche be vsed amonge beastes, and mingle thy meate with myrthe, which is euer the best dishe at the boarde, and be thankfull to God. And so leaue with an appetite passyng the time wysely betweene dinner, and supper, with exercise, labour, studdie, or pastime, vnto thende of .vi. houres, and then begin thy supper: prouided that if it be shorter then thy dinner, eatyng thy meate by litle and litle: for greedie eatyng is hurtefull to nature, as *Galen* saith in his Dietarie. Note also, that thou must eate more meate in winter, then in Somer, because thy naturall heate is closed within thy bodie in Winter, but vniuersally spred in sommer. Also cholerike men may as lightly disiest Beefe, Baken, Venison. &c. with asmuch speede, and littell hurte, as the flegmatike man may eate, Rabet, Chicken, and Partrige. &c. But the Melancholie man, throughe the coldenesse of the stomacke, hath not the strengthe in the stomacke, as he hath promteness in wil to eate thinges warme, & moist be good for him. The sanguine man, is not so swift in his disgestion, as the hotte cholerike man is. But not withstanding, he hath good disgestion, through the humidite, and warmenes of bloud, and coueteth to eate sweet thinges, which greatly augmente the bloud: Therfore sharpe sauces, made with Vineger Onions, and Barberies be holsome, Purslene, Sorrel, smalle fisshes that feedeth vpon the stones, in fayre runnyng waters, Cucumbers, and pure Frenche wine, partely delayed with water, bee good for the Sanguine men: to kepe them from much encrease of flesshe.

Sidenotes: what hurte cometh of an emptie stomacke when ye go to bed. An order of dieting. Galen. die. Cholerike. The melancholie. The sanguin.

Sicknes.

Thou hast shewed vnto me a very discreate, and holsome order, of diet perticulerly to my self, and partly to other complexions but what rule or pretie gouernement, is there for sicke folkes, that be sodenly vexed or other waies?

Health.

They that be sodenly vexed with sharpe sicknesses, must haue thinne diets, with water gruell, thinne Mutten, or Chickens, Potage without any fatte or thicknes, Violet leaues, Endiue leaues, and suche like colyng herbes, and let their drinke be made of Tizantes. Thus doo to them, that haue hot sharpe sicknesses, occasioned of choler. And also colde syrups of Endiue, Violets, Sugar, water and Vineger, sodden together be verie holsome.

Sidenote: An order for the dietyng of suche as bee sicke of sharp feuers.

But

of sicke men and medicens. Fol. lxv.

But if sicknesses be longe of continuance, their diet must bee the thicker, and their meates made the stronger, specially if their diseases be colde, with the fleshe of Cockes, Capons, temperat wine, stewde brothes, with holsome herbes, as Buglose, Burrage, Basel, Parsely, and Fenell rootes, with some Maces, Dates, Damaske prunes, Raysons of the Sunne, and suche like. Siruppes of Isope, and Citron: prouided that they neither take meate, nor medicen, immediatly before, or soone after their fittes. Posset ale with clarified herbes accepted, whiche they may take for their comforte, accordyng to the estate, of their disease. Suche as bee sicke, must haue meate contrarie to their complexion. For they that be colde, must haue hot meate, and medecines. And they that be drie, must haue moiste thinges. But they that be hot must haue cold thinges, for the hardēt heate of the fier, is quenched with the moistenes of the water, and so the quantitee of one element ouercometh the qualite of an other. And in dede, Phisicke saith, the bodies that be hot, must be fedde with thinges like thē selues, as thei that be moiste fed: with moist thinges to preserue their moistnes: they that be hote with hot thinges to preserue their heate, & suche like. But when they doe exceede in heate, colde, moist or drie: then let the qualites of moistnes, be tempred with drienes, and the coldnes, with warmenes. For like as man deliteth in thinges of like, as the cholerike man, cholericke thinges: euen so do beastes, and fruites, as the *Coloquintida*, which is bitter, deliteth in bitter ground. Hote spices delight to grow in hot ground, and euery fruite, and herbe, doth delight in the thing, that is like it self: beware of distemperance, surfets, or replecion, rere suppers and dronkenesse, make thy bellie no shambles or kichen.

Shorte sickenesse, thinne brothe: longe sicknes thick brothe.

Of Syrupes and drinkes.

As the complexion is, so mā requireth his foode, in the tyme of health, thynges like to his nature, but in sicknesse the contrary.

Sicknes.

But if a man feleth greate grief after meates, or drinkes, what waie is there then, for to helpe hym?

Health.

Se walkyng vp and donne, and perhaps, that will digest, as *Auicen* saieth: And *Rasis* saieth, to walke an hundred paces after meate, is wholsome. For it comforteth digestion, prouoketh vrine, and giueth one power, and strengthe of stomacke, to eate his supper. But the counsaile of *Galen* muste here be obserued, whiche saieth: there is no meate, but it will corrupt, or stincke, if the bodie bee caste into a sodaine heate, by stronge trauell sone after meate, whiche corrupcion of digestion, is the mother of all diseases, and the beginner of all infirmities, as *Auicen* reporteth. And if you see, this will not helpe to digest, your ingorged full stomack, then prouoke your self to slepe: liyng vpon your right side, leanyng toward your breast and bellie, laiyng your warme hande vpon you breaste, as *Auerois* saieth: The power of digestion is made strong, when a man sleapeth. For naturall heate, that is drawen inwardly with warmenesse, or heate, hath power to digest: but if sleape ease you not, prouoke vomite,

Auicē the .iij. doctrine, the vij. chapiter. Moderate walke after meate, profiteth.

Galen in. vj. de accidenti & morbo. Capitu i.

Auicen in. 13 Theo. iij. trac. iij. Capit,

The booke of the vse

Auicen in se-
cundo doc. ca-
pitu. 6.

mite, or caste it out: and this is the counsaill of many learned menne. For it is no maruell, although many meates corrupt one man, which be of sondrie workinges in the stomack, liuer, and vaines, for the qualities do hinder nature, almoche as the superfluous quantities. And take hede these signes, & euill tokens, be not found in you. The paines of all your mēbers, with idlenesse, and wearinesse to go, or moue your body: Sodain greate blushinges, or rednesse in your face, vaines swelled and puffed vp, redde vrine, and grosse skinne, extended or stretched out, with fulnesse, like a blowen bladder, and pulses ful, smal desire to meate, ill reste, & grief in slepe: semyng in the slepe, to beare some intollerable burden, or dreamyng to bee speachlesse: these bee the euill and daungerous tokens of replecion. And of this I giue you warnyng, for it hath slain as many by aboundance: as hunger hath killed through scarcitie. Therfore forget not vomites, wherof I doe intende to speake shortly hereafter: how to vomite by medicene accordyngly.

Daungerous
tokens.

Sicknes.

Of aire.

I Haue heard thee saie, that wholsome aire, is a greate comforte to mannes nature: but corrupt aire, doeth moche harme. I shal require you therefore, to tell me of the good, and the badde aire, that I maie learne to vse the good, and refuse the badde.

Health.

Phisicions
ought to haue
a perfect kno-
ledge of the
nature of pla-
ces, and aire.

GALEN *in lib. de Sectis* saith: A wise Phisiciō ought to knowe the natures of menne: of waters, of aire, of regions, and dwellynges, generally. Particulerly, to thy self beyng a naturall Englisheman, of birthe and educacion. This lande is verie temperate, how bee it, our dwellynges in this lande bee variable, as Fennes, Marrishe, Woodes, Heathes, Valleys, plaines, and rockie places, and neare the Sea side. But the saide *Galen*, geueth counsell in his Regement of health, saiyng a good ayre, whiche is pure and holsome, is that, which is not troubled in standyng water pooles. Therfore Marrish groundes, and places wher Hempe, and Flaxe is rotten, and dead carions be cast, or multitudes of people dwellyng together, or houses inuironed with standyng waters, where into priues, or sinkes, haue issues, or wallowyng of swine, or carrion vnburied, or foule houses, or suche like places be daungerous, corrupt the bloud, whiche is worse then corrupcions of meate. For *Hippocrates* saieth, that all places of concauites, as Sellers, Voltes, holes of Mineralles, where mettales be digged, or houses, or walles, ioyned together, wheras the sunne with reflexion beateth in with soden heate, whose absence bringeth colde. These ayres are distempered, but plesaunt cleare ayres, sweet gardens, goodly hilles, in daies temperate, when one may se far of: these be good. There be certain starres called also infortunates, in their exaltacion, whose influence bringeth corruption to creatures, rot, and pestilence, to men and beastes, poysonyng waters, and killyng of fisshe, blastynge of fruite

Note which
is the moste
holsome ayre,
to dwell in.

What ayres
corrupteth y
bloud.

Corrupt ay-
res bringeth
sondrie disea-
ses.

in

of sicke men and medicens. Fol.lxvj.

in trees, and Corne in the fieldes, infectyng men with diuers diseases Feuers, Paulsies, Dropsies, Fransies, Fallynge sickenes, and Leprosies. Against the saied influences, all christian men must pray to God to be their defence, for thei be gods instrumentes, to punish the earth. Example, we haue of mortall pestilence, horible Feuers, and Sweatyng sicknesse, and of late a generall Feuer, that this lande is often plaged with all. Then make a tier in euery Chimnay within thy house, and perfume, sweet perfumes, to purge this foule ayre. And now in conclusion to answer thy question, for the health of dwellyng *Auicen* saieth, to dwell vpon Hilles is colde, and in balleys, comprised with hilles, is hotte. Upon a Hilles side, against the Northe, is colde and drie. Towarde the Weste, grose, moiste, very subtill towardes the East, and cleare and warme, towardes the Southe. And *Rasis* saith: in his first booke *Afforie*. A man dwelling neare the Sea side, or great waters, can not liue long, nor can not be without weaknesse of members or blindenesse, but the best buildyng of an house is vpon a drie ground and a hill towardes the west side, and southe weste doores, and windowes open towardes the East, and Northeast, hauyng near vnto the said house, sweet springes of runnyng waters: from stonie or chalkie grounde, which is bothe pleasant and profitable to the house, for *Hypocrates* saieth in his booke of ayre, and water, the second chapter: cities and townes, placed toward the Easte, be more surer, then the townes builded towardes the Northe, for temperate ayre, or winde, and sickenesses be lesse. And in the saied boke *Hippocrates* greatly comēdeth plesant riuers, runnyng towardes the risyng of the Sunne, the dwellers in such places (sayth he) be fayre & well fauoured, smothe skinned, cleare and sharpe voyces, and this shall suffice, what and where, good and pleasaunt dwellynge is. Note also, that thou must obserue ayre, as thou doest meate: colde sickenesses, warme ayre, drie sickenesses, moyste ayre. And so in the contraries to them that be sicke, and they that be whole, ayre of like qualite, is most holsome. They that haue longe sicknesses, change of ayres is a great help, both in Feuers, Dropsies, Faulyng sicknes, and Rumes. Rede *Hippocrates* in his booke of aire.

Feruente prayer vnto God doeth mitigate his wrathe.

Sweet ayre to be made in the time of sicknes, with perfumes.

What situacion is beste for a house.

Plesant people, their aire.

Ayres are to be obserued in sickenesses as in health.

Sicknes.

I Haue founde very much disquietnesse in my body, when my seruauntes and labouryng familie, haue felt ease, and yet wee are partakers of one ayre, and my foode is fine, and theirs grosse.

Health.

The cause why thy laboryng seruanntes, in the field at Plough Pastures, or Wood, haue suche good health, is exercise & labor, and disquietnes cometh partely of idlenes, and lacke of trauell whiche moderately vsed, is a thing moste sufferain to nature. Rede of exercise in the booke of houshold, written by Erenophon: wherein he sheweth, that princes would labour, plante, &c.

Moderate exercise is a sufferaine thing.

Sicknes

I pray thee tell me some thing of exercise.

Health.

Health.

Fulgen, in lib. 2

THE well learned man *Fulgentius* saith: that exercise is a file, and chafer of the heate naturall, whiche chaseth awaie slepe and consumeth superfluous humours, wastyng the natural vertues. Redemyng of time, enemie vnto Idelnesse, due vnto yong men, ioye vnto olde men, and to saie the truthe, he whiche doeth abstaine from exercise, shall lacke the ioyes of health, and quietnesse, bothe of body and mynde. And *Galen* saith, in his Regement of Health, if we will kepe parfecte Health, we must begin with labours, and moderate trauell, and then to our meate and drinke, and so forthe to our slepe: and this is the cause why Faukeners, Shouters, Hunters, runners, Tenisplaiers, Plowmen, and Gardeners, and lifters of waightes. &c. Haue so good digestion and strength of bodie. Who be stronger armed menne then Smithes. Why so? Because of the exercise of their armes: stronger bodied then Carpenters, whiche lifte greate blockes, and Masons, whiche beareth greate stones, not onely in their youth, but suche men will take maruelous trauailes in age, whiche to Idell people, semeth very painfull, but vnto theim selues that trauell, no pain, but pleasure, because of custome. These people can digeste grose meates, eatyng them with muche pleasure, and slepyng soundly after them vpon harde beddes: where as the idell multitudes in Cities, and in noble mennes houses, greatnumbres for lacke of exercise, doe lothe meates of light digestion, and daintie dishes, Mary in deede thei may be very profitable to Phisicions. But if trauell be one of the beste preseruers of health, then is idelnesse the destroier of life, as *Auerois* saieth: and *Hippocrates* saieth: euery contrary is remoued, and helped by his contrarie, as Health helpeth Sicknes, exercise putteth awaie idelnes. &c. But euery light mouyng or soft walkyng, maie not bee called an exercise as *Galen* saieth: therfore Tennis, Daunsyng, Running, Wrastlyng, Ridyng vpon greate horses, ordeyned, aswell for the state of mennes healthe, as for plesure, whereas it is now conuerted in many places, rather to the hurte of many, then the profite of fewe. Exercise doeth occupie euery parte of the bodie, quicken the spirites, purge the excrementes bothe by the raines, and guttes, therefore it must be vsed before meate. For if strong exercise be vsed immediatly after meate, it coueieth corrupcion to eche parte of the body, because that meate is not digested. But when thou seest thy water after meate, appereth somewhat citrine, or yellowe: then maiest thou begin exercise, for digestion is then well, but sicke folkes, leane persones, yonge children, women with child, maie not muche trauell, to conclude. The exercise of Dice, Cardes, sityng, drinking, footbaule, and castyng of the stone, with lustes imoderatly vsed, and suche like, maie bee called an exercise of fooles, rather then of wisemen. I might haue spoken moche of exercise of hande laboure: and of the noble profession, or worthie estate of a true soldiour, but this shall suffice.

what profit cometh by exercise.

Use maketh labour easie.

Apho.

Idelnes the mother of all mischief.

Exercise before meate.

Little trauell for the sicke.

A signe of digestion.

of sicke men and medicenes. Fol.lxvj.

Sickenes.

There are many idle people in citees, and in noble houses, dooe thinke the chief felicitie onely, to bee from bedde to bellie, and then from bellie or borde, to bedde again: none other liues thei wil vse, then Cardes, Dice, or pratlyng title tatle excepted. Spendyng their tymes in slepyng, eatyng, and laughyng: and somewhat els to small effecte. Now for asmoche, as thei neither can, or will trauaile, what saie you to the matter?

The practise of idle people.

Health.

Mry this kinde of life, would quickly make of a noble, or worshipfull persone, a deformed monstrous man: with a life short and painfull: and eftsones chaunge a yoman into the miserable estate of a begger. For idlenesse and plentie of victualles, is fitte for soche citezeins, as wer in Sodoma and Gomorha, which perished in their lust, idlenesse and fatnesse. And although perhaps, there be a greate nomber, whiche saieth in their hartes, *Non est deus*: and looke for no life to come. Yet because thei haue the shapes of men, not forsyng for the immortalitie of the soule (for whiche dampnacion is due) yet lette theim not appere, worse then brute beastes, in this poincte. Or the Heathen infidell, whiche Heathen are bothe comely, cleane, worldly wise, valiaunte, nette and fine: and also haue goodlie (although not godlie) prouided to preserue bodily health. For it is reason, thei should so doe seyng thei are carelesse for the soule: but the idle Christian, careth litle for bothe, the bellie excepted. Well fare the Heathen, in this honest manlie poinct to preserue nature.

Idlenes bringeth mischief to the bodie & soule, and pouertie. Gene. xix.

The Heathen are better than many Christians.

The fatte Oxe, or vglie brauned Bore, although thei can not come out, from their frankes or staules, lackyng libertie: yet nature haue taught theim, a trim wholsome exercise, called fricacion, or rubbyng of theim selues: chafyng forthe by the poores euill humour, wherein thei dooe finde pleasure and healthe. There is no kinde of beaste, that might bee longe without filthie itche, sores, or skabbes, without thei vse fricacion, comyng. &c. Fricacion is one of the euacuacions, yea, or clensynges of mankinde, as all the learned affirmeth: that mankinde should rise in the mornyng, and haue his apparell warme, stretchyng foorthe his handes and legges. Preparyng the bodie to the stoole, and then begin with a fine Combe, to kembe the heere vp and doun: then with a course warme clothe, to chafe or rubbe the hedde, necke, breast, armeholes, bellie, thighes. &c. and this is good to open the pores. Further, if any haue the Crampe, or is full of Melancholi, or heauinesse of mynde: or els fallen into a sodain colde, through watchyng in a colde house, or field. Or els haue a moiste reume. &c. What is better then fricacion, or chafyng with warme clothes. This is the verie beste wate, but it must be doen a morninges, before meates: but at night it is not good. For then it openeth the pores of the bodie, and is an enemie to

An example of brute beastes.

Of fricacion, the vertue thereof.

when to vse rubbyng or fricacion, and wherefore.

M.i. slepe,

The booke of the vse

<small>Three thynges to be obserued in Fricacion.</small>

slepe and quiet reste, and letteth forthe naturall vertue, whiche should nourishe slepe. Now, as concernyng the diuersitie of fricacion, or rubbyng, note three thynges: The firste is, harde fricacion doeth open the pores, let forthe the smoke, and binde the bodie. Soft fricacion doeth molefie, and relaxe the bodie, as it is writen. *Dura frixione ligaturi molle vere soluitur.* But the .iii. whiche neither is soft, nor hard, but meane, doeth neither deminishe, nor increaseth, but indiffretly warmeth. Neither is the spirites or smoke of the naturall heate, therby letten forthe by the pores of the skin:

<small>It is not good to bee trimmed of the Barbour at night, but in the mornyng.</small>

And all men that vseth to bee trimmed, washed, or rubbed at the Barbours at euening, doe erre from the regiment of health, but in the mornyng, it is verie good and comfortable, and augmenteth naturall heate, and strength, expulsyng slogishnes and slepe. So that the bodie lifteth some waightie thing from the grounde: or els drawe a Bowe, accordyng to his strength. Furdermore vnderstande, that all drie and whole bodies, maie vse fricacion, with warme and moiste oiles: And all moiste and colde bodies, to vse the contrary. There is also

<small>Gestacion the profite therof</small>

ioyned to fricacion, twoo other exercises: the one is called Gestacion, that is to be carted of an other thyng, without any trauaill of the bodie it self: and as easie rockyng in a cradell, to be carsed vp and doun in a chaire, either in faire weather, to be rowed vp and doune, in a tilted Boat or Barge, & this is verie good for weake people, which haue had long agues. &c.

<small>Equitacion is very wholsome.</small>

The second part of this exercise, is Equitacion, which maie bee moderatly vsed of sicke menne and women: that bee weake through Feuers, or timpanie. And that must be vsed, vpon a soft easie goyng horse, in a plaine pleasaunt fielde, in the cleare aire, vpon the faire daies. These exercises doe not onely reconcile slepe, but augment and make strong the naturall vertues. And thus I ende of Fricacion, Equitacion, and Egestion: of this you maie read *lib. iiij. capi. vi. Aetius. Cornelius Celsus lib. iiij. capi. xix.* Whiche writeth profitable, and plentifully of the same no lesse pleasaunt then good, to mannes nature: sodaine exercise after meate, maketh the blood foule: corrupteth digestion, letteth forth na‑

<small>when to trauell, or plaie.</small>

turall heate, maketh the stomacke colde, bryngeth skabbes: as *Hyppocrates* affirmeth. *Si impurgatus laborauerit, vlcera erumpent,* therefore in the mornyng, and twoo howers after meate, exercise is beste.

Sicknes.

This is well, I assure you. But yet I haue seen, strong vomites haue chaunsed to menne, after their meates. Exercise or Fricacion. &c. what is the cause thereof?

Health.

<small>The cause of vomite, and when it helpeth, & when it hurteth.</small>

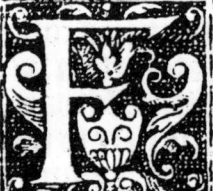Irste, weake stomackes in sicke people, or women with childe, thei will quickely vomite, as we see by custome: also Replerio through meates, or strong drinkes, bryng vomites. Notwithstandyng, vomite is a goodly euacuacion, for those persones, whiche be molested and greued in their breastes or stomackes: or them, which be vexed

with

with fleume, or choller, with soche like foule humours, whiche grieue the stomacke. And specially to people, whiche haue shorte neckes, greate breastes, and wide mouthes: For all these maie easely vomette without hurte. Also thei, whiche haue narrowe breaste, and longe small neckes, maie not well vomet, without hurte, or perill of deaffenesse, and strangling: howbeit *Hyppocrates*, the Prince of Phisicions saith who so hath a vomet, without coaction or medicene, it healeth them, whiche haue had a long flixe or laxe. The same *Hyppocrates* saieth, who so euer vomiteth blacke choller vpwarde, without a medicen giuen, it is a token of death. Vomits be also perilous, to them that be in consumpcion, or weake of nature. The beste time of vomites is in Sommer, as *Hyppocrates* affirmeth. *iiij. Aphoris. Æstate quidem superioris magis ventr. Hyeme autem inferiores medicamentis purgare conuenit.* It is more conueniente, for to purge the bodie douneward in Winter, but vpward in Sommer: specially in haruest tyme. Howbeit, *Cornelius Celsus* affirmeth, that to vomet in Winter, is better then Sommer: by the reason the stomacke is full of crude, rawe fleume. *Galen lib. primo de ratione victus,* counsaileth to vomette twoo tymes in the monethe is good, that is to saie, euery .xv. daies. But note this, that you vomet twoo daies together, for that whiche is lefte the firste daie, shalbe clensed by vomet the second. But in some vomites, vaines are broken through great straining of the body: and like as to procure a vomet, we doe minister *Oximell, Squillitiej,* warme water and Honie, and sometyme oile, or the leaues of Azarabaccha. &c. Euen so we minister when an euill accidence commeth, of ouermoche vomette, to the sicke bodie Minte water, with the pouder of Mumie, Sage, Mirobolans, Chepoli, the pouder of Mastike. And giue to drinke *Diacodion*, small wine with tosted breade: and thus I dooe ende with vomittes, whiche are good before meate, but better after the same two howers: as affirmeth diuers men, of greate experience.

What persones maie best vomette.

Who maie worst vomet.

Vomet helpeth the flixe.

When to vomette.

How to prouoke vomet, and how to staie it.

Sickne.

After strong vomettes, there chaunceth often tymes the hickop, or yeskyng, what helpe for that?

Health.

That is verie perilous, I assure you: for after strong purgacions or vomettes, saieth *Hyppocrates*. If either conuulcion, or the hickoppe, called yeskyng doe come, it is perilous, and moche to bee feared. Furder saieth he in his *Aphorism. Conuultio a veratro lethalis est.* A conuulcion saieth he, after one haue drunke *Elleborus albus*, is deadly, by the reason that the strength of this venemous herbe: doe draw from the senewes moistnes, and contract them with a sodain emptines, and drines that scant help maie be had, but rather dedly perill to folowe, or euen as if thei were aged, paste nature, and redie prepared to the place of silence, or the graue. Yet notwithstãdyng do thus, and refuse not this meane, whiche haue greate vertue. ℞. Meale of fenigreke, of fleeworte, of

An hickop after a vomette is perilous.

To helpe the hickoppe.

M.ij. cleane

cleane Barlie, ana ℥. iiii. and the oiles of violettes, water Lillies, and red Roses, ana ℥. i. ß. Honie. ℥. i. mingle all, and temper theim in a morter then seeth Mallowes, and Violettes together, ana ℳ. i. put theim into a morter, beate theim well, and make twoo emplasters: appliyng vnder the breastes and arme holes, metyng towardes the raines of the backe. And giue the pacient Goates milke, or womans milke with Suger: and wasshe his hedde with warme wine, wherein is sodden Roses, Violets, Mallowes, Barlie, and fiue finger. And then warme anoint the hedde with the oiles, of Roses, water Lillies, and Hennes greace, and then make a bathe for the pacient to sitte in. Of Violettes Roses, Henbane, Mallowes, Poppie, Lettice, and water Lillies: and thus I doe ende of the yeskyng, whiche is an euil accidence, folowyng vomet of twoo extremes, that is of replecion and emptinesse: a meane is left therefore in euery thyng. For extremes you see, are hurtfull, bothe in matters politike, and Phisicke. &c.

A goodly waie to helpe hickoppe, comyng after vomette.

A meane is beste.

Sicknes.

There is euacuacion, called *Sternutacion*, or nesyng: what doe that profite?

Health.

Of nesyng, the profite thereof.

HYPPOCRATES, of neesyng saieth thus, *Sternutamentum fit ex capite, Cerebro calfacto, aut humectata capitis parte inani: Aer enim nitus contentus extra erumpit, sonat autem quoniam per angustiam exit: Aphor. 52.* That is, neesyng that cometh from the hed, is made either of brain, whiche is hotte, or els the emptie or voide place of the hedde, beyng verie moiste. For the aire contained therein, breaketh forthe, through a small narrowe waie: and so cometh the sounde or noise forthe. This is wholsome, that the strength of nature forseth forthe winde, specially ones or twise in the mornyng, puttyng awaie belchyng: but more is not good, and who so can not neese, it is a signe of weakenesse, sickenesse, coldnesse, and age. And to neese after meate, is not wholsome, but when a woman labour with childe, or haue the mother, then neesyng is wholsome and healthfull: and will sone helpe them, but somtyme through strong neesyng, bledyng dooe quickely ensue, by the breakyng of some vaine. Then applie the *Nasalia* and *frontarij*, as I haue written before, in the ende of the Compoundes.

Neesyng doe helpe women in their trauel

Sicknes.

Then what saie you of bledyng, what profite or perill is in it?

Health.

When it is good to blede.

I Haue spoken thereof sufficientlie before: therefore, I saie remember, that to bee letten blood, in the Spryng tyme, is the beste season, as *Galen* affirmeth, *in libro de Flobothomia*, and through the same, these euilles are helped. Replecion, Pleuricie, hotte Tercians, Frenses, Pestilence. stoppyng of the termes. &c. Al the orgaines of the sences, are cleansed thereby. And finally, the bodie is

of sicke men and medicenes. Fol.lxviij.

of a weake bodie, made strong to them, whiche are in lustie yeres. But prouide, that neither people in consumpcion, old folkes, women with child, or yong children, be letten blood. And no man letten blood, after that good blood appereth in bleeding, for feare of Crampe, Palsey, or dropsie. Nor none to slepe, after thei are letten blood. 8. howers. Rede Galen vt supra, and Rasis lib. 4. ad Almanso. There are a newe kind of instrumentes to let blood withall, which bring the blood letter, somtime to the gallowes, because he strik to depe. These instrumēts ar called, the ruffins tucke, and long foining raper: weapons more malicious, then manly. *who muste not bleede.*

Tucke and Raper.

Sicknes.
Will boxyng doe any pleasure?
Health.

Ye forsothe, verie moche: As example, if you haue any causie loughte, or loitryng lubber within your house, that is either to busy of his hand, or tongue: and can do nothing, but plaie one of the partes, of the 24. orders of knaues. There is no pretier medicen for this, nor soner prepared, then boxyng is: iii. or. iiii. tymes well set on, a span long on bothe the chekes. And although perhaps, this will not alter his lubberly condiciōs, yet I assure you, it wil for a time, chaūge his knauishe complexiō, and helpe him of the grene sicknes: and euery man maie practise this, as occasion shall serue hym in his familie, to reforme them. *Boxyng is good for a lubber.*

But for the Boxing, whereof *Galen* speaketh, calling it Boxing, Cuppyng, with *Cucurbitula. &c.* Saieth he, Boxyng dooe helpe swellyng, and let forthe winde, stoppe the termes immoderate, and the bloodie flixe, helpeth apetite: And when a woman doe swoune, it is good to reuiue the spirites againe. There are twoo kindes of the bentosas, or Boringes, the gentilest is without scarifficacion: the other is to drawe forth water, and asswage harde swellyng, and cleanseth Melancholi, specially in weake bodies. And it will remoue humour, from place to place as from the hed to the necke, from the necke to the shoulders. &c. And what stoppeth the termes soner, as *Hyppocrates Apho. Si muliere menstrua sistere vos lueris, Cucurbitulam quam maximam, sub mammis defige.* If thou wilt stoppe the termes of a woman, then put a greate bentos vnder, or vpon her breastes, for the vaine, whiche is in the matrixe, come from the breastes. *Boxyng doe drawe forthe euil humor. &c.*

Boxyng doe stop the termes, when thei do aboūd

Sicknes.
Doe sweatyng profite any thyng at all, to mankinde?
Health.

Sweatyng is no lesse pleasaunt to nature, then profitable to a common wealth: and somtyme sweatyng is vnprofitable. As example. If any Artificer, or Husbande man, haue any seruaunt, that is so diligent, that he can sweat at his labor, and not at his meate, this is a good sweate: But if his man, doe eate vntill he sweate, and labour without heate, this fellowe, if you giue *Of sweates profitable, & vnprofitable, to a common wealthe.*

M.iii. hym

The booke of the vse

him not an expulsiue, out at your haule dore, vndoubtedly he will els shortly bomette you, into the backhouse diche, with a threde bare cap. Therefore, take hede to soche sweaters, and idle eaters, except you bee *Abunde Diues*, and yet let all men, bothe poore and riche: remember what almightie God saied vnto Adam. *Manducabis herbam agri, in sudore vultus tui vesceris pane, donec reuerteris in humum.* Thou shalte eate the herbe of the fielde, in the sweate of thy face, thou shalte eate breade, vntill thou bee retourned backe againe, into the yearth or grounde. And in an other place it is written: thei which will not labour, shall not eate. And also there is a promise of God, by the mouthe of the holy Prophet: whiche affirmeth saiyng *Nam labore manuum tuarum edes, beatus eris, & optime habebis* : that is. For of thy labour of thy handes, thou shalt eate, thou shalte be blessed, and haue the beste thinges: as prosperitie, and the fruictes of the yearth. &c. Lo, here you see, here is no hunger, beggyng, idlenes, loitryng, pickyng, slauerie, disyng, horyng, theuyng, prisonyng for thesame, or Tiburnyng, appoincted to labourers, but to loiterers. Here you haue the promise of God for thesame: that thei whiche wil honestly labour and sweate, shall bee in good health to eate. As we daily see the honest labouryng husbande men, and their familie do trauell, toile and sweat: thei haue therfore Gods blessyng, good health, and long life. For if the husbande man and carter did not sweate, eche other daie, the Curtier and Citezein would crie well awaie. Now sir, to Phisicall sweate, whereof I will shortly conclude, whiche are twoo kindes: the first of them is naturall, as when men do voluntarily sweate, without force of medicene: as hotte drinke, or hotte house, or stoue, this will easely open the pores, and disolue grosse humours, clense the blood, comforte the spirites, put awaie colde, consume crude humour, amende the senewes, put awaie ache or numnes, feuers, dropsie, and the pestilence: Sweate helpeth all these. And if one bee sicke in his sweate, he ought not to slepe: and this is a token, that he shall dooe well in sweatyng, if he sweate in all places, and by little and little, fele the paines aswage then it is a signe, that health will followe. But if he sweate, in one or twoo places onely, and finde more grief, it is an euill token.

The artificiall sweate, is made in stoues, bathes, or bladders, with hot water, hot stones, put in clothes, and applied to the bodie liyng in bedde. Or els with moiste bathe of herbes, or parfumes with Masticke, Stirax oile, &c. Whiche haue vertue to clense skabbes, iche, pox. I saie the pore, as by experiens we se, there is no better remedy, then sweatyng, and the drinkyng of Guiacum, vsyng it in due tyme and order. Prouided alwaies, to sweate at euenyng is better, then in the mornyng: as Phisicke affirmeth, and reason proueth. For when the bodie haue nourishement within, the spirites shall not be vtterly drawen forthe, to the extreme partes, through the outwarde heate. Furder, lette leane drie folkes, or feble persones, vse lettle to sweate: for it will hurte them moche, but fatte folkes maie sweate well, it helpe thē moche, howbeeit, sweate is not good for the iyes. Because it drieth to moche

of sicke men and medicenes.   Fol.lxix.

moche, leane bodies ought to bee anointed with oile, after thei haue sweate. Sweate is euer good in sharpe agewes, in the daies of the Crises, or iudgemente of sicknes, saieth Hyppocrates in his *Prænostico*, but the contrary. *Sudores optimi sunt, in omnibus acutis morbis, qui in diebus iudicatorijs. &c.* Rede here after, in the signes of death, of sweatyng. what sweate is good.

Sicknes.

What saie you of abstinence, or fastyng, is it verie profitable for the bodie?

Health.

Yea truely, and also for the soule: as it is written by the Prophete. *In ieiunio humiliaui animam meam:* In fastyng, saith he, haue I humbled and brought lowe my soule. Fastyng is a singuler instrument, to correct the fleshe, and make it obediente, and seruaunte to the spirite: if it be ioyned with faithe, otherwaies it is vaine, concernyng perfite religion. But neuerthelesse, profitable in Phisicke, is abstinence for the bodie. For take this for example: If one haue taken a surfete, with replecion or fulnesse, or els dronkennes, nothing is better, to bring the bodie into good quiete order, then abstinence, whiche will consume matter superfluous and hurtfull. But yet not of it self, but by a certaine waie or meane: for it is not quickly restored, whiche with longe abstinence haue been wasted. Fastyng is not vtterly to refuse meate, but to eate that, whiche preserueth life onely: Oh that moderacion wer vsed in a comon wealth, then should not the riche die in glotonie, and aboundaunce, nor the poore perishe for lacke of bread. Extremes are euill, to moche fastyng, or to moche hunger. *Galen* affirmeth, people whiche haue narrowe vaines, thei haue but little blood, and soche maie not suffre long hunger, but shall faule into sicknes. But thei, whiche haue greate vaines, haue plentie of blood: and maie fast without hurte. So maie all soche, as haue moche rawe crude matter, whiche is helped through fastyng: Abstinence is hurtfull, to Chollerike and Melancholike persones. Or them, whiche are sicke and weake, or to yong children: so euery one must be considered in order accordingly.

The greate goodnesse of fastyng, bothe for the soule, and the body.

The rich vse glotonie, and poore, penury

Cholorike people, muste not fast moch.

Sicknes.

When I haue been werie and sore vexed, bothe in mind, and bodie, nothyng haue dooen me so moche pleasure, as slepe haue doen, and reste in the night tyme: what saie you to slepe.

Health.

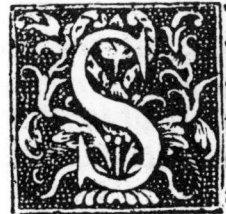

Slepe is brother vnto death, sauyng the one doe not walke again, and thother doe recouer the sences: and of necessitie, all creatures that waketh, or watcheth, must slepe and reste. For the holie Prophet saieth, in the boke of Psalmes, or Hymnes to almightie God. *Ego iacui & dormiui atque euigilaui quoniam dominus me suffulcit.* I laied me doun (saith

The vertue or benefite of slepe, or reste. Psal. iii.

M.iiii.   he

The booke of the vse

No manne or beast, can liue without rest.
he) and slepte, and also waked againe: for the Lorde did onely comfort me. Truely that God, that made vs also, made our accions and doynges: as labour, reste, eatyng, drinkyng, slepyng, and wakyng, without whiche wee can not liue. *Aristotle* saieth, all liuyng thynges haue slepe, as swimmyng, fliyng, and goyng creatures. Furder he saieth, slepe is like the fallyng euill, by the reason all the sences are depriued: for slepe is the ligament of sences, and wakyng doe vnbinde them, and slepe is giuen to eche liuyng creature, for their health. And furder, *Aristotle* she-

Arist. de som.
weth the cause of slepe, saiyng: *Somnus causatur ex vapore cibi, qui vadit ad cerebrum. &c.* Slepe is caused of the smoke, or vapour of the meate, goyng into the braine: and cometh backe againe colde, and maketh slepe. Therefore men after meales, are sone giuen to slepe, as we doe see by experience: and without slepe, wise men should be chaunged, into ideotte fooles. Note this, that all slepes doe not make thin, dissolue, or warme alwayes, but that soche slepes, that followe either labour, greate excersice or hunger. And furder, when manne is slepyng, the naturall heate is

How the stomacke muste be prepared toward slepe.
drawen inward, whiche when the saied slepe, findeth no nourishment or thyng to feede vpon: then like a Lion, it doeth forthwith consume, and waste the beste humour, or one of the radical vertues. And in conclusion, to drie vp the blood, and make the bodie leane: therefore, let al leane folkes, or theim, whiche haue been aboundauntly purged, or els letten blood, beware of very moche slepe, slepe after sweate, labour, as running, tenis, moche daunsyng, which doe open al the pores, and let

When slepe is perilous.
forthe all the euill vapours, betwene the skin and the fleshe. Whiche slepe doe reuoke, retract, and drawe backe again, through the inward heate, wasting the same moister, & if one haue flegmon in his guttes, that is to saie, a postumacion of Choller and blood. Nothyng is more perilous then slepe, by the reason that the burning & heat encreaseth, whiche wil augment the dolour: euen so in our Englishe sweate, and the Pestilente slepe, is to bee forborne, and also before blood lettyng, and after, duryng twelue howers, or els the poison will approche to the hart. Or whē the first of an Ague do begin, or in drinkyng any benime. &c. For in soche case, it will make either rigour, or horrour, leauyng the outwarde partes cold, drawyng through vnnaturall heate, the benime to the nutrimentall partes, or els to the partes vitall: and so this waie slepe is not well, but rather hurteth. Euen so it hurteth the drunkardes, bench wislers, that will quasse, vntill thei are starcke staring madde, like Marche Hares: Fleming like Scinkars, brainlesse like infernall Furies. Drinkyng, braulyng, tossyng of the pitchar, staryng, pissyng, and sauyng your reuerence, beastly spuyng vntill midnight: these fellowes abuse the tyme of slepe, and in soche case if thei should slepe, perhaps apoplexia, and sodaine death would followe, as

Drunkardes what thei do.
Hyppocrates affirmeth. *Aphoris. vij. Si ebrieus quispiam repente obmutuerit conuulsus moritur, nisi febre, corripiatur, aut vbi ad horam peruenerit qua crapulæ soluuntur vocem recuperet.* That is (if a drunkarde dooe sodainly lose his speache, and become dombe: he shall die of a conuulcion, excepte he bee taken of an Agewe, or els receiue againe

of sicke men and medicenes. Fol.lxx.

gaine his speache, at the same hower, when the surfite is digested. He herein speaketh reasonable: for drunkennes flieth into the brain, and so distill into the senewes, whiche bryngeth conuulcion, and after conuulcion insueth death, through the crude, colde moistnesse. Except the heate of a Feuer doe concocte, and waste it. &c. Therefore, let men take hede of dronkēnes to bedward, for feare of sodain death: although the Flemishe nacion, vse this horrible custome, in their vnnaturall watching all the night. But remember his wordes, whiche haue made vs all, and knowe what diatte is beste for vs, euen Jesus Christ hymself, saiyng: *Cauete autem vobis, nequando grauetur corda vestra, crapula, & ebrieate. &c.* And a wise manne saith: *Omne nimium naturæ inimicum*, all extremities are enemies to nature. So is to moche labour, meate, slepe, watche, or to little is euill also: a meane therefore is good, and the beste of all. And a dewe tyme, place, maner, and order of slepe. The night is the best time: the daie is euill, to slepe in the fielde is perilous. But vpon, or in the bedde, liyng firste vpon the right side, vntill you make water: then vpon the lefte side is good. But to lye vpon the backe, with a gaping mouth, is daungerous: and many thereby, are made starke ded in their slepe: through apoplexia, and obstruccion of the senewes, of the places vitalle, animall, and nutrimentalle. And all soche as feele intolorable paines in their breastes in the night, whiche growne, and can not drawe their breathe: the verie cause is, liyng or slepyng on their backe. And not through the Mare, or night spirit, as thei terme it: after the iudgemēt of supersticious Hypocrites, Infidelles, with charmes, coniurynges, and relickes hāgyng about the necke, to fraie the Mare, thou foole I should saie. Let soche people, bothe kepe good diate, cleane lodging, lye in order, as I haue saied, and specially commende, bothe their slepyng and wakyng, to Jesus Christ, that thei maie liue honestlie, goe to bed merily, slepe quietlie, and rise earely. To serue GOD deuoutly, and doe their businesse in their vocacion diligently: to helpe them selues, and their neighbours charitably, and not to be carfull, for any dream in the night. But wisely consider this, if thei dooe dreame of fire, to take it for no euill presage of strief. &c. But rather that fire doe signifie, yellowe hotte Choller doe abounde, and would be purged by good pocions, Diasene, or the Siruppe of Rhabarbe. And to beware of a tercian Ague. And when thei dreame of cloudes, darcknes, or to lye in darcke dungions. &c. Remember it is Melancholi, that vexe the bodie and spirites in the slepe: and would bee purged with Hamech, Pilles *de lapi de Lazule &c.* If dreames be of cold, Snowe, Ise, water, then fleume would be diminished tō pociōs accordyng, & Pilles *de Agarico, &c.* Some in the night, seme in their slepes, as though a great blocke were, pressyng doune their legges: this is the resoluciō of the senewes, or the aboundaunce, whiche would be letten forth, by the Median vain. And to vse bathing to bedward in warme water, with swete herbes: and to drie their legges, and so goe warme to bed. And thus I ende of slepyng and wakyng, whiche saieth *Hyppocrates Aphor. Vehemens vigilia tum cibi tum potionis cruditatem*

The cause why a drunkard doe dye sodainly.

Luke.xxii.

Of good and badde slepe.

Fooles be afraied of the Mare i their slepe.

How to auoide euill dreames.

What dreamies dor signifie.

Hyppocrates vpon slepes.

The booke of the vse

Moch watch causeth rawe humours in the stomacke.

ditatem efficit. That is, vehement watchyng doe bryng crudetie, and rawnes, bothe to meate and drinke in the stomacke: Moderate watche is good for studientes, to make theim learned, for aprentises, to giue the knowlege in their facultie: to the man of warre, or watchman, to preuente the enemie. To the fatte bodie, to diminishe grosenes: But watching at Dice, Cardes, &c. Make many watch men in lanes endes, for the purse: soche watches I say make many miserable wretches, whose rewardes we see daily, to be daungerous and shamefull in the ende.

To whom watche is good.

Sicknes.

Thaffliccios of the mind is harde to bee helped.

There is one thing, whiche haue troubled me verie long, it is a sicknes, that hetherunto I could find no Phisicion so cunnyng, wise, or learned, that euer was able to helpe the same. Neither did I euer se, or tast of that medicen, that had vertue to releue me in that poincte. Furdermore, the chaunge of aire, were it neuer so swete or pleasant, with the sightes of faire fieldes, gardeins, hilles, woddes, and valleis, couered with all coloured kindes, of swete smellyng, and plantes, herbes, or flowers, did neuer helpe this sickenesse. The daiely beholdyng of iewelles of stone, golde, riche apparell, faire buildynges: yea, manly feates of armes, with triumphaunte sightes, did me neuer a pinsworthe of pleasure. But when the tyme was paste, my sicknes double assaulted me again.

Pleasure is noysom to the disquiet hart.

The .ix. heauenly ladies can smally comfort some careful hart, when it is in care.

The Sacred heauenlie *Musæis* or *Heliconiades*, the daughters of Jupiter, whom I haue knowen: those .ix. celestial damosels, whiche did washe theim in the well, with siluer streme, where as the swift flyng horse called *Pegasus* pearced with hard houe, the frosen hard diamonde flint, as Poetes affirme. These ix. ladies, called the *Nimphes*, haue infinite vertues, to please the eare withal in Musicke yet haue not pleased me: as example. The first called *Culliopen* haue a voice moste heauenly in pleasure, to moue thaffeccios withall. The .ii. named *Clio*, a matron of grace to all damosels, for womanly behauior: yet with a glorious comly gesture, mouing her beholders, inwardly to sigh, or breake their slepes in the night. Soche grace she haue, to wound the hartes of lustie youth, and make the aged dispaire, whiche are past hope, to renue their age again. The iii. is the amorous ladie *Erato*, with her sweete songes of louers delite: whose tunes are of soche heauenlie vertue, equall to the Angell: whiche haue soche force, that it will banishe all louers weping lokes, yea, care, and louyng spight, and make eche amorous subiecte, or prisoner free to them selues, without mistruste. Castyng from theim, their cold willowe crounes of mournyng: and foorthwith, this tune will cause to renue them selues, in that victorious diadem of warme Laurell, against all cold passions. And giue them their delites, through this her swete pitifull song. The fowerth will caste a swete water, on the face of euery slothefull louer, and quickly wake theim, out of their flatteryng or fearfull dreames: and shewe them gladnesse, and all pleasant grene thinges, to forgette their follie, or pleasaunte purgatorie, her name

The Sacred gifte, that the ix. heauenlie Museis haue and can giue to others, to comfort them in trouble.

of sicke men and medicenes.   Fol.lxxij.

name is *Thalia.* Then followeth dame *Melpominen* with her songes, seperatyng of *Mars* from *Venus*, Prophesiyng of warre, and fearfull Tragadies, she is the. v. The sixte named *Terpsichren* pacifiyng warre, and noise of bloodie Trumpet, reconsiling all again, with heauenly Harpe, and Musical instrumētes of cordes by her: vnder the swete arbour, sitteth her sister *Euterpen*, with instrumentes of winde, agreyng with her sister, in true Musicall concord or vnitie, she is the seuenth. The eight is *Polyhymniā*, with a memorie passyng al creatures : this *Museis* driueth Musicke into nombers, by whose knowlege, the velositie or swiftnesse of the soule is perceiued. The. ir. and laste is *Vraniam*, whiche through the sacred song, moueth eche liuyng man, to be heauenly mynded, religious, and giue them selues to a blessed life. Her songes be lamentable, pitifull, drawyng the hartes frō yearthly vanities: desiryng a change into a happier lande, aboue the bright shinyng starres. These *Museis* I saie deare Health, haue helped me before these daies: but now can not at all for all their pleasaunt pipyng. For their delites to me, be rather lothsome, and vexe my mynde: sauyng the laste *Musa*, called *Vraniam*, moueth me, for els none. For thei are but plain vanitie.

<small>The names of the nyne Muses, with their giftes.</small>

Health.

What sicknes is this, that neither Phisicke, nor all these delites, can giue cure vnto: it is a merueilous disease, bee like it should appere, that it is no sicknesse of the bodie, but rather the passions or perturbacions of the mynde.

Sicknes.

YOu haue spoken the truthe, it is euen so: but I take it to bee no newe sickenesse, emong foolishe men. For the wisest man hymself, complainyng thereof, saiyng: *Ecclesiastes Cap.i.Prospexj enim omnia opera quæ sunt facta,& ecce omnia sunt inanitas,& animi molestia.&c.* Truely I did behold all thynges, that are wrought vnder the Sunne: and beholde, thei are all but vanitie, and vexacion of the minde. &c. And so this afflicciō of the mind, is the greatest grief: that I haue with my perturbaciōs. But in a maner, I do not vnderstand, eche of their causes, thei are so variable, painlfull, and endlesse. For my delite and pleasure is gone, and brought in bondage to them through long trouble.

<small>All the wōrkes vnder the Sonne, are nothyng but vanitie, and affliccion to the mynde.</small>

Health.

THei are called perturbacions of the minde, after *M. Cicero*: but *Galen* terme theim *Pathemata vel affectus animi*, that is the affeccions, or sodayn mocions of the minde, chaunged or altered thorowe some cause. From the right waie of reason into some passion, and these mocions of the spirites, must be as well considered, and diligently obserued of the Phisicion, in the tyme of sickenesse, as moche as any other common knowen sicknesse. For these perturbacions, or painfull affeccions of the spirites, do chaunge the estate of the bodie, marueilously and sodainly. As we within fewe daies past, haue seen

<small>The perturbacion, or sodaine mocion of the minde must be well obserued.</small>

The booke of the vse

Of the sodain alteracion of the minde, frō ioye to care.

seen a persone beautifull, well fauoured, pleasaunt, &c. but now wee skante knowe hym: Iesus saie we, how this man is altered, and clene chaunged, within these fiue daies, as though it had neuer been he. &c. This is our talke, of the sodain alteracions of our acquaintances: we therefore, muste resort vnto certain reasons, in soche cases. As example.

Of feare what it is.

Feare is after some euill tidynges, or doubte of mischief, as losse, prisonment, or death, will quickly insue. Then these thinges wil folowe, The spirites & blood are all drawen inward: and then al the outward mēbers are pale and colde, with tremblyng, & faintnesse of speache. By the reason that all the vertues, bothe animall and naturall, are made feble, and sodainly weake: through whiche, often times it haue been seen, that sodaine feare, haue brought sodaine death: as example.

Examples of sodain feare.

When Ely the high Priest, ouer the people of God, in the day of the greate battaill, when the Philistines preuailed against Israel: as he satte vpon a stoole, lookyng towardes the waie, his harte feared hym, for the arke of God, in the meane tyme, there ran a manne hastly into hym, with a lamentable looke, in mournyng clothes. Declaring vnto hym, first how that Israel was fledde and slaine. Secondly, that his twoo sonnes, Ophni and Phinehes were slain. Thirdly, that the vncircumcised had taken the Arke of GOD, at whiche tidyng, soche sodain feare came to his hart, that forthwith he fell doune backward and brake his necke. And this same euill tidynges, slue with sodaine care, his doughter in lawe, the wife of Phinthes, saiyng in her death, the glory is gone from Israel. This was Elies plague, for sufferyng his children, to liue wickedly. For where as God is not feared, at lēgth God will sodainly feare them. Feare I doe saie, is a marueilous monster, an infernall Image, and a terrible bision to the soule: for feare is not for thinges paste, but onely for thinges to come, and to take thynges in the worste part. Was not Iesus Christ our God and sauiour afraied, what tyme as he sette before his iyes, the paines and sharpnes of death.

Goddes vengeaunce. Regum. i.

Euill parentes, and euill children.

Feare is like a monster of helle.

Dolore afficitur anima mea vsq; ad mortem. My soule said he, is made heauie euen vnto the death: yea, his feare was soche, that for agony, his droppes of sweate, was like vnto blood. This was a greate feare, euen in Christ: but yet it made hym not giue ouer, forseyng the sealyng of our eleccion by his death. But the feare, whiche taketh mortall men, make them cowardly oft tymes. Through it Peter did sweare, he was none of Christes cōpanie: & that he knewe hym not at all. Feare made Dauid to counterfette, and go like a madde manne, for to auoide Saule, whiche persecuted hym. Feare made Athanasius, the Bishop of Alexandria: to hide hymself, sixe yeres in a Caue, from the crueltie of the Arrians. It causeth the Christians to flee, in the tyme of persecucion: And sometyme the Christian through it, is forced to plaie the Idolater. As example. When the tyrant Diocletianus Themperour, in his cruell murderyng of the Christians: did commaunde euery one to bee slaine, that would not honour, and offer to his Idols. Marcellus the Bishop, as Eusebius affirmeth, in a greate feare, did Sacrifice to the Deuelles.

Feare in Christe.

Feare in S. Peter.

Feare in Dauid.

Athanasius feare.

Feare of the Christians. Fear maketh men offer to Idolles.

Example of Marcellus.

of sicke men and medicenes.

Diuell: Lo here doe feare trie religion. Sometyme feare will crepe so far into the consciece, that it letteth in dispaire. As example of Judas whiche is a good president to all traitours: and many tyrauntes thorowe it, haue slaine them selues, fear ofte tymes, is verie intolerable. For there is no touche stone, can better declare, the diuersitie of mettalles, then feare will bewraie the worthie, or vnworthie manhode of menne. As example. There was a lustie blood, or a pleasaunte braue young roister at *Athenes*, whose name was *Aristogiton*, as the Historiographer affirmeth: whiche commonly would talke and bragge, of what good seruice, that he could do to *Mars*. All his talke was of warre, how to deuise weapons of inuacion, to destroie the enemie: to train forthe men, to giue the vnsette, with all lustie courage. And vpon a time, the *Athenians* prepared a mightie strong armie, againste their enemies, and emog al others, thei had this *Aristogiton* in no smal price: supposyng him to be in deede, as he was in woorde. Callyng hym foorth to a charge, whiche when he harde, an acte to bee doen in deede: Oh God, how his hart was in his hose, for feare he trembled, and quaked, like an Aspen leafe, as though he had begon, the fitte of a tercian ague. He could not tell what shift to make, or whether to go to hide hymself: but at legth dame shame, wispered hym in the eare. And badde hym wrappe one of his legges with roulers and cloutes, as though he wer lame: so he did and with pale face, and staffe in hande, he came haltyng and crepyng foorthe, like a shepishe loute, lamentyng his case, that soche euill had chaunsed him. But his hart was with the all said he, yet durst he not trauell, vntill his legge was whole: But when the people did see him daunse so liuely, like a lubber in a nette, Lorde how thei laughed this Carpette Squire to skorne. I praie God, the like feare be not founde, emong a greate nomber of our people, that can roiste, crake, braule, sweare, and bragge, in the tyme of peace: quarellyng with quiete people, and lifte vp lookes, frounyng like Tegers. And when the Quenes maiestie shal haue nede, to withstand thenemie, or suppresse the rebel: that then thei become not like vnto *Aristogiton*, with sore legges, Agues, broken armes, tremblyng, lamentable lokes, as bolde as Geese, or Lions of Coteswolde Heath. Sendyng their water to the Phisicion, to cloke their knauerie, for lacke of manhode, or els with *Vnguentum aurum*, cã anointe their Capitaines hande, to blotte theim out of their muster booke, whiche is a good medicene. For feare in soche case, there is not the like receipte, in all Bucklersburie, I assure you: many mo thynges could I speake of feare, but my matter is of Phisicke. But this Cordiall shall suffice, for a coward.

Now followeth anger, whiche doe increase, inflame, and set their bodies vpon a fire, with a sodain burnyng heate: Cleane contrarie to feare. For feare drawes the heate and blood inwardly, with feble pulse: but anger dooe caste it to the outwarde partes, with swifte pulse, as *Galen* affirmeth, *lib. ij. de tuenda sanitate*. Counsailyng euery one, that will preserue naturall healthe, thei muste vse soche exercise, as maie keepe warme-

Marginalia:
- Feare bryngeth desperacion, example of Judas.
- To proue a coward by example of a Greke which was a greate bragger.
- A shifte for freshe water souldiours.
- What the passio of anger is

The booke of the vse

Gal.de.Sans tuen. warmenes, temperatly, neither to moche cold, nor heate aboundyng. And although exercise, commonly bryngeth warmnesse, yet to the idle bodies, when thei haue no naturall heate, then their bodies are made warme, of an other thyng, as oile, bathyng in warme water, or goyng into the stoue. &c. But soche heates are artificiall, to moue the heate naturall, but thei are all without, and not moued of the principall inward heate. But anger or perturbacion, is moued of naturall heate, it nedeth no meane to helpe it: as we fele by our selues in colde weather, let our enemie sodainly appere before vs, or if we heare our selues shamefully rebuked. We nede no fire, to kindle the flame of our cholour, forthwith we are in the house toppe, the holiest of vs all. For heate aboue nature, will quickly inclose the harte, and with swiftnes go further, sekyng vengeaunce. Unto this euill be Cholozicke menne moste bent, whiche must vse often, to correcte Choler: or els to obserue an order, whiche a worthie Philosopher, taught a hastie Prince, that he should, before he did any thing, moued by quicke and sodain affection. First, saie ouer the Alphabet, or the nomber of letters: this Heathē rule, against anger or rashenes, will not hurt the Christians. It declareth great pride and anger, to be sodainly moued. As example. At euery light wind, weake trees will moue, and tremble with their braunches, from ground to the toppe of the same: whiche with great storme and wind, will skant moue the great strong tree. Prouidence and pacience, maketh men strong, and get the victorie of themselues: and able to withstande anger, whiche is a common passion of cruell beastes, tirauntes, and fooles. It should seme by *Domitius Nero*, that he was an angrie wretch, to murder his mother, to poyson his scholemaister and finally to sticke hymself. In his maners at the borde, he was sone inflamed with anger: that vpon a tyme, hearyng but the Frenche nacion named. Foorthwith he brake twoo moste costly drinkyng vessels, of an incomperable value, thei wer so riche and beautifull: he cast doune al the maete frō the borde, fallyng out with all the discombentes, without any other cause (a verie temperate man, I assure you). When *Ecelinus* the tyraunte, in battaill had receiued a wounde, forthwith he caste his weapon awaie: and roared like a madde beaste, and in his cruell anger, rent his skin from his owne fleshe, whiche, when his enemies espied, thei so laughed, that in a great rage and anger, he slue himself, (a verie meke persone). Oh what a victorie had he vpon his enemies, thus to handle hym self.

A wrathfull part of Alexander, in killing of Clit. *Alexander* the Greate, sittyng in a drunken bankette, vnsemely for a Prince, beyng admonished reuerently, of a noble wise man called *Clitus* his owne nourishes soonne: to liue like a Prince in vertue, reioysyng therin, more then in victorie. &c. But the ingratfull Prince at his banket, with his owne handes, strake him through the body, lettyng forth the sprites of life frō good *Clitus*, that would not flatter a prince. For an opē rebell is not so hurtful, as a secret flatterer to a prince, for thei are like Cancers, most hurtfull to thē. What anger had Cain against Abel

and

Of heate artificiall, and naurall.

Of cholorick heate.

A lesson againste anger.

Examples of wrathe in Nero.

A wrathfull wretche in battaile.

of sicke men and medicenes. Fol.lxxiiij.

and Herod, in killyng the hurtlesse children, that neuer offended hym.

The Popes, whiche are so charitable (as you knowe to the liuyng Christians) that thei will sende them, in burnte Sacrifice to heauen: emong theim haue torne one an other with violence, out of their graues, rendyng out of their pontificall apparell, cutting of their fingers And buriyng them emong the common harlottes, yea, drawen forthe againe and hedded: a fitte Sepulture for soche sainctes. Rede *Planten* in the liues of Steuen the sirt, *Sergius* and *Formosus*. *The Popes Lawe.*

Bubalam an excellent Painter, did so liuely set forthe, the monstruous Image of a deformed Poete, called *Hypponax*, whereat the beholders had greate pastime, and laughed. But in the meane tyme, the Poet wrote soche nippyng sharpe tantyng verses, against this Painter: that in a sodaine rage, he ran into his house, and hanged hymself. And to conclude, Saul was in soche a rage, that he destroied the Sacred high Prieste, and the Leuites, with the people in the citee of Nob: for receiuyng of Dauid, the elected of God. And this shall suffice to warne you from the passion of anger, by these examples. *Hypponax the Poet made soche sharpe verses agaist a Painter, which caused hym to hange hymself in his rage. Saul killed hymself.*

Then there is an other perturbacion of minde, called Sorowe or care, whiche is the greateste passion of the spirites: because it is some folkes turment. Again in an other, it make shorte worke. For care doe wound and smite the hart, with a depe stroke, & draweth it togither as a purse: suffring nothing to be caried thether, to cofort the same again. And so the generacion of the spirites are letted, and the vitall partes, by little and little, doe wither and waste awaie, and in this poinct, sorowe doe differ from feare: sorowe receiue his mischief at length, and feare at ones. But in colour pale, in pulse feble, in countinaunce heuie in stomacke weake, thei are like: but yet care is for thinges past. As example. Some for loue haue slain them selues, as *Cleopatra*, a Quene of Egipt: after she had spent her pleasaunt yeres in loue, mingled with lust, when her husbande. M. Anthonie was dead, she fell into soche sorowe and care, that in thend, she caused her self to be inclosed in a tombe, suffring two serpentes, to sucke at her breastes, vntill she had finished her miserable life with lamentacion, for all her riches and pompes, could not heale her sorowfull sickenes: but death onely was her refuge, so greate was her care. But *Iosephus* handle her death otherwaies. *The cause of sorowe and care, whiche bee meruaylous plagus. The differece betwene sorowe & care. Cleopatras death.*

Into what lamentable case, fell Quene Dido of Carthage, whiche was the doughter of Belus the kyng of Tire, whiche carefully finished her life in fire, for the losse & loue of Eneas, as the Poet feinethe. Leander a worthie young man, whiche was so rauished, for the loue of a faire maiden, called Erus, whiche dwelled in an Ilande in the sea Helle sponte: and this Leander in a toune called Abidus, the sea passyng betwene theim bothe, whiche water and salte streame could not quenche his loue, that he bare vnto Erus, his affeccion was so greate that euery night he would swim ouer this flood, vnto his deare Erus vnto a place called Sestos, where as she dwelt, supposyng his pain to be heauenly pleasure. He vsed this so longe, that in the ende Neptune *Didos death. The storie of Leander, whiche died for loue of Erus*

N.ii. frouned,

The booke of the vse

The death of Leander and Erus for loue.

frouned, and commaunded Aeolus to raise vp storme and tempeste, against Leander, in whiche he carefully finished his life. In the mornyng Erus looked ouer the walles, beholdyng the dedde bodie, tossed emong the rockes: therewith she was sodainly wounded, by sorowe and care, and with a petifull crie, caste her self from an high Toure, into the sea, whereas she finished her life, for the loue of Leander.

A noble woman wept to death, for the death of her husbande.

The wife vnto Duke Protesilaus, did continually weepe, for the death of her husbād, vntill she died. Soche loue of late in this realme, haue been inclosed in the harte, of some worthie ladie, that for the absence of her liuyng housbande, haue ended her life with care, that after the nomber of many Salte teares: Salte water was her laste drinke, and death her refuge. This affeccion called Loue, bryngeth more sorowe with it, then either prisonmente, pouertie, or sicknes: as we maie read, and se by experience, into what seruitude and bondage, it bryngeth people. And dooeth degenerate many, in a maner out of kinde, makyng them more effeminate then women: chaungyng Mars into Uenus. It altereth complexions, maners, and condicions, and maketh of free men, slaues, of wise men, fooles, of riche men beggers: it bryngeth many sicknesses, yea, incurable, through longe sorowe and care. Sometyme it doeth depriue the wittes, and sences reasonable, and maketh men more madder then dogges: crueller then Wolfes, shamlesse as Apes, rentyng their clothes, wakyng in their beddes, fastyng at their bordes, as wise as Geese, yea, and finally. What a great nomber dooe kill them selues, by stranglyng, stickyng, and drounyng: when thei can not obtaine their purpose, and incurable sute. Thus thei bee rewarded, that falleth into soche dolour and care, in this foolishe affeccion of minde, called Loue. And if thei might obtaine their purpose, in their foolishe fishyng in the flood of fantasie: what should thei then get, perhaps nothing, but a serpent, whiche would alwaies styng theim, or els a weate Ele by the taile, whiche would quickly deceiue theim.

Loue is a cōquerour.

Loue maketh beastly foles.

The fruites of Loue,

Ielousie is cosē germain to Frensie, marke the frutes thereof

The helle of Ielousie.

There is an other affeccion of the minde, verie perilous, daungerous, and incurable, whiche is cosin germain vnto fransie, whiche is called Ielousie: or a gredie foolishe affeccion of the minde, neuer quieted, but euer tourmentyng it self, burnyng in a continuall fire. This inwarde spirituall vengeaunce, dooeth make domesticalle debate, betwene man and wife: and tourne their house of libertie, into a miserable prisone. Double bondage to eche other, with quarelyng in presence, mistrustyng in absence: fearing them of their owne house, doubtyng the straunger, yea, and men often tymes, mistrustyng their own children, not to be of their owne generacion, when thei haue no argumente to the contrary, but deuilishe gelousie. Ielousie often tymes breaketh chastitie, emongest them that doe professe Godly Matrimonie: and causeth the one parte to desire libertie, to be out of the fire, of that louyng gelous Purgatorie. For some there be that doe saie, there is no more tormente in helle, emong the infernall furies, then there

is

of sicke men and medicenes. Fol.lxxv.

is here in this worlde, emongeste Jelous women, whiche neuer had good opinion of their housbandes: and some men also of their wiues, although thei wer locked vp in a closset, thei hauyng the keie, and sealyng the doore, yet thei thinke thei are begiled. Yea, some be so friendly, that thei be Jelous of other mennes wiues: and some women folowyng that example, doe the like to other womens husbandes. Here is marueilous kindenesse, thus to crucifie them selues, in the fire of follie: but the effect thereof, worketh mischief to them selues, and others. As it is written of one Phanus, whiche loued his wife with soch Jelousie, that he would neuer suffer her, to go out of doores: he also prouided, that none came in at his gates, or dores, but a great noies was made through crackyng and tinglyng of belles, whiche hanged at the at whiche sounde with all spede, he would run to see who came in. He so longe vsed this order of watchyng at the gate, that in the meane tyme, his deuoute wife, gaue hym a Barnardes blowe, lettyng in her companion, when it was darcke, by a broken place in the roffe of the house. Whiche, when it was perceiued, by the next neighbours: Lorde how thei commended Phanus, for so diligente and wittie kepyng of his gates. Here you doe see, that Jelousie bryngeth adulterie, yea, and sometyme it causeth murder: as Helena after the death of Menelaus, fledde for succour vnto Poliso, wife to Clipolemus the kyng of Rhoedes, soonne vnto Hercules, whiche burnt with soche Jelousie towardes her husbande, that she commaunded her, to be hanged vpon a tree.

Procris, daiely burnyng with Jelousie of her husbande Cephalus, whiche was taken in loue, with an other woman, did daiely pursue him, from place to place, through fieldes and wooddes. &c. And vpon a tyme, when Cephalus went foorthe, with his darte in his hande, into the forest, to seke his praie: his Jelous wife pursued hym, and closely shrouded her self in couerte, emong the Brackes, to beholde what her husbande did. But as she moued her self, the couert did shake, wherein she was hidden: her housbande perceiuyng that, supposyng that she had been a wilde beaste, foorthwith caste his darte, and vnwares slue his Jelous wife. Well ridde of an euill sore: O how craftily she did begile hym.

O what Jelousie was betwene Intiopa, and Licus her husband, the king of Egipt: and what a cruel murder came therof. I nede not to fetche no more examples from old, of the forgotten worlde, & time past for this euill is to common, as we doe see by daiely experience: and a merueilous plague, bothe priuate and publike, the effectes therof is nothing but miserable, veracion, dolour, care, agonie, and dispaire. And this is to cōclude, there is no remedie, but pacience perforce: for the old prouerbe is, that Heresie, Frāsie, and Jelousie, be so bred by the bone, that thei will neuer out of the fleshe, therefore vse no Phisicke for it.

There is also an other euill, ioyned to condicions of wicked mēne, whiche is none of the passions of the minde: nor yet an infirmitie of nature, but rather to be nombred emong the synnes mortalle, whiche is an euill moste intollerable, and moste odious of all vnto good nature: which is called Ingratitude, churlishnes, or vnkindnes. I count it not onely ingratitude, to be vnthankfull to theim, of whō we haue receiued benefites, but also to do harme to them, by whom we be preferred. As example. There was no greater dignitie, next vnto Christ, then to bee one of his Apostelles, as Judas was. Also none could bee more trusted then he, whiche kept the purse as he did. Christ gaue him power to doe miracles, equally with the twelue. He suffred hym to sit at his borde, and fedde with hym in his owne dishe: there could bee no greater kindnesse then this, a mortall manne, to sit with Gods onelie soonne. But this villaine, vngraciously and ingratefully, respectyng none of these benefites: but like a traiterous chorle, sought his maisters blood, betraiyng him to the shamfull death of the crosse. This ingratitude of Judas, is a goodly president, vnto all traitours againste Princes: by whom thei haue receiued benefites, and many seruauntes, whiche haue been brought vp, from rascalle and beggers states, through their maisters, haue been preferred, into the calling of estimacion, wealth, and worship. Whiche afterwarde haue sucked the blood of them, whiche gaue them first their sucke, and nourishment in their aduersitie. O what a monster, and a difformed infernall Serpente is this ingratitude, it is the mother of treason bredde in hell: enemie to liberalitie and gentelnesse, and is of the right line of wrathe and enuie, sprong of a deuelishe petigree, worse then wilde beastes. Whiche, when thei are made tame, and receiue any benefite of their kepers, thei will not rent and teare theim: but phaune vpon theim, waggyng their tailes, and run about and leape for ioy. As by example, we maie see of Horses, Dogges, Beares and Apes, whiche will reioyce in the sight of their maisters: and many tymes, put their life in venture for theim. Although I might bryng foorthe, many notable examples to proue this, it neede not, it is so manifest: The scriptures of God crieth out against it, the Lawe of nature doeth vtterly reiect it. There is no man worthie to be called a gentleman, although he can auaunce him self of a petigree infinite, and boaste neuer so moche of his birthe, and is a gentelman borne in deede. If he bee infected with ingratitude, he is degenerated from his right kinde: and is become a counterfeit gentleman, and a naturall churle, of the right line of Naball the carle, whiche abused the gentlenesse of Dauid, whose wrath was quenched through the beautie, lamentacion, and liberalitie of Abigael his wife Who can forget, or remember without teares, the traiterous ingratitude of Theseus, the sonne of Ageus the kyng of Athenes, which was a lustie, beautifull, and valiaunt knight: wantyng no gifte nor grace, that nature might doe vnto hym. He excelled all men in his daies, in manly actes, sauyng Hercules: he slue a terrible cruell Bull in Attica in his young yeres. And when he was, xxiiii. yeres olde, by lot and destinie, of the people of Athenes, he was appoincted and condempned, to be caste vnto a horrible monster, in the Labyrinthe of Crete: whiche

monster

Ingratitude or vnkindnes called churlishnes.

Luke. xxii. Math. xxvi. The treason of Judas, that moste ingratefull vilain, his example to all churles.

Gratitude of dumb beastes

Bothe God and Nature doe abhor ingratfulnesse.

To knowe a very gentelmanne.

The shamful ingratitude of Theseus, the soonne of Ageus the kyng of Athenes.

of sicke men and medicenes. Fol.lxxvj.

monster had deuoured many thousandes before, his foode was onelie the fleshe of mankinde, he cried and rored out for his praie. This giltlesse knight, was inclosed in a dungeon harde vp, voide of all comfort, bewailyng his fatall destinie: thus to be cut of, in his youthfull daies beyng a kynges soonne. Now voide of all frendship, helplesse, hauyng no succour, criyng out againste the Goddes: Cursyng the date of his birthe, that he receiuyng his life, within the bodie of his mother, beyng a noble Quene. Should eftsones now bee buried, within the infernall bowelles, of this horrible monster: voide of all mercie, dedly to beholde, with venemous teeth, and flamyng iyen, pouryng forth poison at his mouthe, with moste noisome aire and stincke, in his infernall kenell. Thus death approched nere vnto Theseus, whiche greued hym nothyng so moche: as to remember the pleasaunt life, whiche he somtime had, accōpaniyng the amorous ladies, whiche wer full of al courtly curtasie. And the worthy knightes, emong whō he alwaies achiued euer the victorie: yea, his Musick was turned into mournyng, and his libertie that somtime he had, in the swete woodes and feldes. Is now chaunged into a little darck dungeon, for there is no greater aduersitie, then in miserie, to remember prosperitie. But lady fortune smiled vpon Theseus, & opened the eare of kyng *Minus* doughter, called the ladie Iriadne, and her sister Phedra: which so pitied Theseus, that with all spede, priuilie sent for the Porter of the dungeon, not far distaunt from the Labyrinthe, whom with faire wordes, thei intreated to open the prison doore, and so entred in, beholding this lamentable knight: whiche moste humbly kneled doun vnto Iriadne, cōmendyng himself, to be her graces bonde & thrall, during his life. To this ende yf it would please her honor, to inuēt some spedie waie, to deliuer him from this dedly monster. Iriadne then cast her pitifull iyes, vpon this lamentable Theseus, beyng secretly wounded, with the worthines of his person, pitiyng his miserable estate, saiyng it was more fitter that she should serue him as a wife, then he hers as a thrall being a kinges sonne. And thei concluded of the enterprise, how to kill the Monster: & afterward, she, her suster, and the Porter, al to be imbarked in a barge for Theseus sake, to flie her fathers lande, for feare of death. With all spede she prepared balles of waxe and heere, that Theseus might caste into the mōsters mouth, to kepe him occupied, vntil with sharpe weapon Theseus, might kil his griesly course, or bryng his monstrous carkes to the groūd, whiche came to passe withall spede accordingly, within the secret caue, or Labyrinth: frō whens Theseus came, by ẏ gidyng of a Clue of threde deliuered hym, by the hande of the Ladie Iriadne, whiche came secretly forthe frō the caue, and these .iiii. with all spede passed awaie in the night tyme, to a countrey called Enupie, whereas thei wer richely embarked, hauyng winde and weather toward their iourney, vntill at length thei came vnto an Ilande, in the middeste of the raging seas, whereas no man did inhabite, but wilde beastes onely. There he arriued with his wife and suster, the Porter, and Mari-

The Monster of the Labyrinthe.

The greate greife and lamentacion of Theseus whē he was in prison.

The noble pitifull Lady Iriadne, did comforte the miserable Theseus and set hym at libertie.

Iriadne fled awaie for Theseus sake forsakyng her fathers land.

N.iiii. ners

ners, whiche after their longe trauell vpon the sea: were sodainly begiled with swete slepes vpon the land. After the whiche awaked Theseus, and secretly commaunded his Mariners, to waie their Anckers,
and spred their sailes, without the sound of whistell, or other noise for
feare of wakyng Ariadne, whom he lefte slepyng soundly, emong the
swete flowers, which a little before he had embraced, with foldyng armes. And secretly taking Phedra by the hand, traitorously he toke his
leaue with silence, aborde thei wente, and awaie thei sailed. At length
Ariadne awaked, puttyng her hande a side, felyng the couche all cold,
where Theseus laie: vp she starte with a tremblyng harte, lamentable
looke, and dedly crie, running to the rockes of the sea. When the shippe
was almoste out of sight, she did holde vp her handes to the heauens,
and cried out, bewailyng her miserable estate, thus to bee lefte alone,
without any cause, forsakyng her owne fathers lande, for the loue of
Theseus, whiche had forsaken her for her suster. Then called she to remembraunce, how he was by her deliuered, from a Monstrous beast:
and he had left her, in a solitarie Ilande, imprisoned within the Sea,
to liue emong the wilde beastes, moste ingratefully forsakyng her.
Then Ariadne rente from her, her womanly apparell, making a weffe
thereof vpon the ende of a pole, standyng vpon the toppe of a Rocke,
criyng out: Returne, returne, Theseus again, my deare Theseus, take
pitie vpon me, whiche moste loueth thee. And when she was paste all
hope, she kneled doune, and did kisse his foote steppes: cursing her slepe
liyng her doune in the bedde, where Theseus laie, bewailyng her fa-
talle destinie. That he should preferre the beautie of her suster, before
her vertues: and finally, forgettyng her benefites. This lamentable
storie she did write, in barkes of trees: but some doe affirme, her tongue
was cutte foorthe, and how she wrought her miserie in a clothe, and
thus finished her wofull life.

    Ouid doeth tell this lamentable storie at large, describyng the vise
of Ingratitude, whiche emongest all other euils, is moste intollerable
and the greatest grief to them, that be of good natures. And nothyng
soner doeth wound the hart, as whē the child shal shewe Ingratitude
to the father: the wife to her husband, the friend tourne to an enemie.
These be soche griefes, that it passeth my poore pen to describe: what
paines it bringeth to the harte, of a gentle mynded man. Thus doce I
ende of Ingratitude, or churlishenesse, whiche haue ended many.

    There is a passion of the minde, called a sodaine Ioye, whiche is of
soche force, that the harte casteth from her, the vitall blood: that often
tymes it cometh to passe, that for lacke of stregth, and liuely power in
the hart, that the bodie is killed, before the harte doe call backe again
the warme Spirites, or blood of life, as wee maie reade by example.

    There was a noble matrone of Rome, whiche, when a false messen-
ger tolde her, that her sonne was slain in battell: she paste the tyme of
mournyng, accordyng vnto nature. But vpon a daie, her sonne yet beyng a liue, came vnto her, whose presence moued her spirites, to soche

sodain

Marginalia:
- The craftie treaso of false Theseus.
- The death of Ariadne.
- Ingratitude haue killed many a man.
- Of sodain ioy
- Example of sodain ioye.

of sicke men and medicenes. Fol.lxxvj.

sodain Joie, that in his armes she fell doune ded, and neuer reuiued again. *Valerius Maximus Capite de morte non vulgo,* saith of a noble consull of the Romaines, called *M. Iuuentius Thalna,* as he was in a Temple doyng worship, and offring to his goddes, in the Ile called *Corsica*: letters were sent him from the whole Senate, whiche brake vp and reade theim. And was smitten with soche sodain ioye, passyng all measure: that or he had finished the readyng, he fell doune dedde, in the presence of all the people, before the Sacrifice in the Temple. *(Iuuentius the Cousull died sodainlie for ioye.)*

Who can forget the noble olde learned *Diagoras Rhodius,* when in his presence, his three valiaunt soonnes, preuailed in the victorie of worthie knighthode, aboue al other men. And were crouned with the garlandes of honour, with the praise of all the multitude, at the hille *Olympus*: These noble young men came, and caste their crounes with flowers vpon their fathers hedde: whiche for sodaine ioye, gaue vp the soule, and died in their armes. This was a swete pleasaunt death, of noble Diagoras. Reade this storie, *Cicero lib.i, Quæsti Tuscul,* whiche saieth, Diagoras had but twoo sonnes. But *A. Gellius* saieth he had three sonnes. *(Diagoras Rhodius did expire ỹ breth of life, for sodain ioye. A pleasaunt death.)*

Some doe dye with extreme laughyng, as did the Poete Philemon saieth (*Valerius Maximus*) when he satte at Dinner, an Asse came stalkyng to the table: and with his swete face, stretched foorthe his necke, waggyng his eares. The Poete beholdyng his aunciente countenaunce, and his sadde comelie grace: began to smile at this loutishe beaste, or foolishe Asse. But when the Asse, licked a figge from the table, he did eate it so manerly, writhyng, and mouyng with his lippes: where at the Poete so conceited, was smitten into an incessable laughyng, vntill death did ende his pastyme. Againe there bee, whiche are smitten with soche inwarde ioye, that thei haue sodainly died for ioye. When thei haue doen a mischief, in bloodshedyng, vengeaunce, or cruell murder, as many Tirauntes haue. Example of the Tirauntes *Sophocles,* and *Dionisius,* as affirmeth *Plinius secundus lib. vij. cap. liij.* In which chapiter, you maie reade of many sodain deathes, moste fearfull to be heard. Thus many for gladnes, of the destruccion of their enemie, haue quickly died: a iuste rewarde, to ridde the worlde of Tyrauntes, whiche haue died in so hellishe, an enuious infernall zeale, reioysyng in takyng vengeaunce. *(Philemon the Poet died laughyng at an Asse. Some do reioise so moche in vengeaunce that thei haue died for gladnesse.)*

Also there is an other passion, verie fearfull to mankinde. As when lustie wealthie people haue spente, spoiled, and prodigally consumed their gooddes: then loke thei behinde them, and call to remembraunce their pleasaunt daies, their honor, riches, and greate possessions. And when their olde friendes, forsake theim, when wealthe doe flie theim: and miserie imbrace theim, then eftsones for lacke of magnanimitie, despaire dooe imbrace theim. As by example. It did to *M. Otho,* a noble young man, whiche prodigallie consumed, emong the lustie gentlemen and Ladies of the Romaines, an infinite substaunce: and when he had run beyonde his race, he thought there was no waie, to be his relief, but to kille his maister the Emperour Galba, and through his riches, to paie his debtes. But when he missed his purpose of riches, *(Some dooe kill them selues whẽ thei haue spoyled their goodde, and falle into debte: or els become murderers and traitours.)*

although

The booke of the vse

although he was Emperour. He became like vnto a noble Shippe, whose Mariners had caste out all the ballis, ouerwhelmed the barke of their sauegard, emong the fearfull streames, and rough rockes: In soche case was Otho, to redeme honour and libertie, sought to kille his Maister Galba the Emperour, whiche he so died, and was Emperour for fewe daies. But to conclude, in fine for lacke of wealthe, to furnishe his pompe and grace, to guyde hymself in meane: with sharpe Dagger, he pearsed his carefull harte, and lette foorthe the spirites of life. Looke further of *Sueton* in his life. This manne lacked the worthie magnanimitie, of some worthie kynges: that when thei were expulsed, and banished from their landes, and honours. As Deonisius the tyraunte was, beyng a kyng, whiche for his greate crueltie, and shedyng of the giltles blood, was deposed from his croune and honour: and banished like a vagabonde, from his landes and people. What, did he crie out? wepe, or dispaire like a beast, and hange himself? No forsoth, not at all. What then? Mary with a lustie manly courage he defied the spight of Furtune: and forthe he went to Athens, where as he became a poore schoole maister, teachyng young children, goodly letters, bothe in the Greke an Latine, and liued quietly. Read Tullie of hym. Suadocopus the kyng of Bohem, when his lande and citees were subdued, through Arnophus the Emperour: he killed not hymself, but did chaunge his princely apparell, and put on the habete of an Hermite, and accompanied with twoo solitarie men. Went into a wildernesse, whereas he continued still, vntill his death: quietly seruyng God, imbrasyng the crosse of pouertie, as a pleasure, to bee ridde from a wicked worlde.

Valerius, of whom Eutropius writeth, being a noble Emperour, makyng warre against Mesopotamia: he was ouercome by Sopores the kyng of Perse, and euery tyme the said Sopores, did take his horse Valerius did lie doune prostrate, and was his foote stoole, all his life: yet would he not kill hymself for care. As many miserable men haue dooen, when thei haue spent their tyme, moste prodigally consumyng their landes, treasure and richesse: with dishonour in abhominacion, wastyng their wealthe baingloriously, foolishely, and moste beastly, emongeste a greate nomber of Parisites, Baudes, Curtisaines, and knaues, and common hores. In fine, whē thei haue gotten the hatred of good people, which moste do abhorre wickednes, then thei run vnto their owne conscience, whiche moste doeth feare them. Then for lacke of grace and magnanimitie, thei flie into the dungion of desperacion: ledde thether, through feare and shame, not foreseyng their presente paine, and endlesse tormentes in the life to come. Forthwith in a mase thei droune, hange, sticke, poisone, burne, and breake their owne neckes, as did Nero the Emperour: whiche slue hymself, with his owne knife, when he was .xxxii. yere old. Reade *Pontanus de stellis lib. xxxv.* ¶ Eutropius of his death.

Did not *Sardanapalus*, the last Emperor of the *Assirians*, which was more effeminate

The death of Otho for care

The wisedō of Deonise the tiraunt in aduersitie.

The kyng of Bohem what he did in the tyme of pouertie.

Valerius the Emperours miserie, to Sopar the Persian king

The ende of men in desperacion.

The ende of Sardanapalus.

of sicke men and medicenes.   Fol.lxxviij.

effeminate, then a woman, and more Lecherous, then a beast, with al his pompe, willingly burne hymself in fire. Of his death read *Sabellicus*. Deoclesian, the persecutour of Christes churche, did poison himself. Judas the traitour hanged hymself. Brutus, whiche was one of theim, that gaue Cesar the .xxiiii. dedly woundes, whereof he died in the Senate, when as he was slain by treason: In the ende the saied Brutus killed hymself in despaire, with his owne sweard, and his wife Porcue hearyng therof, strangled her self with eatyng of coales. Reade thereof in *Plutarcus*. Some do kill them selues for shame, as *Lucretius* did, whiche was violated by *Tarquine* the proude, the laste king of the Romaines. Other some, rather then thei would make their bodies vnchast, & begile their husbades: haue slain thē selues, as did *Saphronia*, a noble womā of Rome, to be rid from the temptacion, of *Decius* a Prince of the Romaines. But fewe women now a daies, will take the matter so vnkindly, or putte them selues in soche daunger, I warrant you. Of this woman reade in *Eusebius*. Other many haue had soche torment of conscience, or els the weakenes of the spirites, haue drouned them selues: as did Sergeant Hailes of Kent, whiche was a well learned gentleman, in the Lawes of this realme. And finally, was ouerthrowen in the battaile of Antichrist. Many examples of Desperacion, I could bryng in, of the moste fearfull deathes of men and women: aswell in this our age, as frō old. But these shall suffice for our exāples, what euilles doe come, through these passions of the minde, and perturbacions of the spirites, whiche bringeth men to despaire, & then to death, and finally to dampnacion.

For thei whiche kille thē selues, doe lose their hope in God, because that thei synne, against their owne soules, and dye in murder: for it is writtē, Thou shalt not kill. And God doeth abhorre the blood thurstie and no man ought for to dye, but by the iudgement of the lawe of Nature: that is, when he can no longer liue. Beyng preuented by sicknes, age, or els valiantly to dye, in the defence of his countrey: the gates of heauen be not shut against soche, no nor against them, whiche be hanged, and suffer condempnacion for their offences, by the lawes of men if thei doe die in the Christen faith, and not like to desperate ruffians. But who so killeth hymself, there is no hope left, but the gates of hell shall receiue him: because he lacketh faithe, in the tyme of trouble, and pacience in aduersitie. As Saul did, whiche slue hymself. But Ezekias, when he heard tell he should dye, and the daie of death appointed hym: he despaired not, but humbly made his praiers vnto GOD, whiche prolonged his daies. And seyng that God hath putte the soule within the bodie, of reason it is he, that must let it forthe againe. For what seruaunte is he, that dare take foorthe his maisters treasures, from his cheste: without thei haue his keye, or other his lawfull warraunte. What souldiour dare be so bolde, to goe out of raie, before the capitain commaunde him. And who dare kill hymself, before it please almightie God to take hym: none but thei, whiche will refuse to dye honestly which in their liues, haue neither been faithful, nor fruitfull

pacient,

paciente, nor pitifull. Or hath been subiect, to any singuler heauenly bertue. Job in all his troubles, when his goodes and cattell were destroied: and his owne naturall children slaine, his bodie sore deformed yea, and for agonie, did curse the daie of his natiuitie. And finally, his greateste plague was, the ingratitude and malice of his owne wife, whiche moste wickedly gaue hym counsaill to curse GOD, despaire, and die: For all this he killed not hymself, but paciently reserued his plagues, saiyng: The Lorde hath giuen me, and he hath taken awaie, his will bee doen. And in the ende, you maie reade, what consolacion he receiued at the handes of almightie God: and vnto this marke, let all Christian menne flie. Like as in Adam we be all dedde, so in Christ we dooe all liue. Furdermore, we haue no plagues that fall vpon vs, what trouble so euer it be, either of the bodie, or the soule: but Adame was the cause, whose children we be, whose plagues we suffer. Is miserie of mynde, bondage, sickenesse, pouertie. &c. Euen so on the other side, there is no consolacion for quietnesse of minde, pacience, ioye, or long sufferyng, or any other giftes of nature, or grace. And finally, life euerlastyng, but all doe spring through Christe: whiche is the beginnyng, the ende, and the reward of all good thynges. And for as moche as we be all inbraced with miseries, and infinite afflicciōs, and daily cares mouing vs, to be wearie of this worlde: And that we haue no dwellyng place of continuaunce, here in yearth. Let vs humbly obeie the commaundementes of God, whiche is for our owne profites, that is to saie: to hope, trust, and looke for helpe at his hande, as the womā of Canane did. Whiche came to Christe, in the tyme of her trouble, hopyng in hym: neither killyng her self, neither her doughter. The fruites of her faithe and hope, was quietnesse of conscience, and health of bodie. And why so? Because she came to Christ, in the time of her trouble, not onely by her, but by al the holy scriptures: we be taught to go to Christ, in the tyme of trouble. For there is a promise made, call vpō me in the daie of trouble, and I will heare thee, help, and deliuer thee. Also there is an other promise of God, saiyng: If we dye with Christ, we shall liue with hym. If we bee paciente, we shall also raigne with hym for euer: now this we see to dye with Christ, is not to dispaire, or to be more vnpacient then wilde beastes, whiche in moste of their rages, will not kill them selues. Now to conclude, for all infirmities of the bodie, let vs seke the comfort of Gods meanes, whiche is the Phisicion, and for the griefes of minde: imbrace the heauenly Phisicke, contained in Gods woorde, whiche is the principall regimente. And furder, for a meane betwene theim bothe; that eche of vs doe walke in soche callyng in this life: that wee maie bee necessarie members, one vnto an other, in the common wealthe, to profite eche other, and hurt no bodie. To trauell for the fruites of the yearth, or any other riches, gotten by honeste policie, and after to spende theim accordyngly. By prouidyng for our selues, against the tyme of aduersitie: To obeie rulers, and pitie the poore, to doe as we would be doen vnto. To despise

of sicke men and medicenes. Fol.lxxix.

a wicked life, and feare no kinde of trouble, that it shall please God to laie vpon vs: that is the somme of Christen religion, of a honeste life, and of a happie ende.

Sickenes.

These perturbacions of the minde, are wounderous fearfull, God deliuer vs all, from soche infernall plagues from hence forthe. Now I thanke you, that you haue shewed me them, euen as I haue felt thē. Furder by good examples, you haue well perswaded me: and finally, with good consolacion, you haue healed my woundes of carefull miserie. But when all our Phisicall remedies will not helpe, good maister Health: I praie you, seyng that death is the ende of our mortalle rase, and finisher of life. Teache me the signes and tokens, of that moste monstrous fearfull death, and how I might knowe theim. Whereby I might not vainly truste in this life: whiche is but lent for a tyme.

Health.

After the daie, followeth the night, and after life, approcheth moste fearfull death: the ende of all thynges, and these haue their tokens & signes before theim. As when the daie passeth awaie, it is manifest to euery creature: the Sonne withdraweth his excellente light, drawyng home his beames from vs. Hidyng hymself, or through his swifte course in his circle. The darke vnmoueable yearth doe take from our iyes, the benefites of his brightnesse: and eftesones it is called no more daie, but night, and the time of silence or darkenes. Euen so, when the spirites of life, haue worne their vesselles, or instrumentes: or when the grosse humour of Melancholi, or yearthly complexiō, with extreme colde. Haue conuinced, quenched, and with force haue ouercome the warme moistenes, and vitall liuely welle spryng of the blood, the fountaine of life. Then the bodie and soule, waxe wearie of eche other, or whē thei faule to deuisiō, or begin to be at debate, within them selues, then thei neuer sease, vntill thei do come to vtter desolucion. For thynges with theim selues, beyng at debate, shall quicklie be desolued, whether it be a publike wealth, or a priuate bodie. And al for the waute of vnitie. As example. When there is good agremente, that is perfite temperamente, in the fower complexions: then the bodie, standeth in good case. But when one humor doe greatly abounde his thre felowes, gettyng the victorie, then for lacke of vnitie, or agrement emong them selues: the whole bodie is in daunger to giue place to one, and yelde to death. As example. If choler get the preheminēce, then he will putte his three felowes to the walles: he bryngeth in against hymself, and them also. Iaunders, Tercians, redde Lepre, Frēsie, hedache, Pleuricie. &c. When flegme getteth the rule, then Dropsie with a swelled bealie face and legges. &c. Doe giue the onsette against nature. Euen so in the colde Melancholi, Consumpcion, quar-

O.i. ten. &c.

The cause of the night.

Whatmischief doe chaunce to the whole bodie, for wāt of vnitie.

The booke of the vse

ten. &c. when it beareth the rule. All these haue their proper tokens and signes, goyng before them: and their effectes are death, when thei doe extremely rule, vnlesse thei through the wisedome of the learned, be helped. But if thei doe meanly abounde, it is not moche a misse: as if choler doe somwhat excede in drinesse and heate, then the coldnesse and moister of flegme, will pacifie her, & bryng her againe to her good estate. If Melancholi, through coldnesse and drinesse, dooe harme the bloode with his warmnesse and moistnesse: will reduce and call her backe from killyng the bodie, and thus one neighbour, will naturally helpe an other. And when thei will not accorde, or gree in vnitie, then purgacions. &c. are prepered to helpe the weaker: and expulse the vsurper, within the common wealthe of the bodie, whiche is the mansion of the soule, or spirites of life, after the Philosopher. And as for the moste principall humour, or blood in Sanguine persones, when it beginneth to corrupt, or the bodie at poinct of daunger: these signes will come together.

(marginal note: when the complexciōs dooe wante vnitie then the body can not longe cōtinue a liue)

Signes of sicknesse of blood.
- Slownesse.
- Idlenesse
- Dulnesse.
- Yaunyng or gapyng.
- Stretchyng forthe the armes and legges.
- No delight or pleasure.
- Swete spattle mingled with bitternesse.
- Moche heauie slepe, with dreames of redde colour, or bearyng burdens greate and heui.
- Perturbacion of the sences.
- Redde grosse vrine stinkyng.
- Little appetite or none to meate.
- Redde face with moche sweate.
- Of these signes cometh stinking Feuers, Pestilence, Squinaunce, bloodie flixe. &c.

Signes of the sickenes of choler.
- Yellowe colour in the skin.
- Bitternesse in the mouthe.
- Prickyng in the mouthe, of the stomacke.
- Heate aboue nature.
- Lothsomnesse to meate.
- Lamentacion, or greate grief of mynde.
- Drinesse, couetyng drinkes of sondrie kindes.
- Womettes of yellowe and grene.
- Small or no slepe, but fearfull fierie dreames of strief. &c.
- Yellowe vrine little residēce, & moche yelowe fome.
- Of these signes cometh Iaundes, Tercians, Pleuricies, madnes, Collickes. &c.

Pale

of sicke men and medicenes. Fol.lxxx.

The signes of sickenesses of Melancholi.
{
- Pale colour in the face.
- Sowernesse in the mouthe.
- Belchyng of winde.
- Little slepe, yet horrible and infernall dreames
- Moche thought, pensifnesse and care.
- A desperate minde.
- Woxe leaner then before, in the bodie.
- Straightnesse in the stomacke.
- Eluishnesse of countenaunce, & taunting in wordes
- Coldnesse, startyng, and fearfull.
- White thin vrine.
- Of these cometh Quarten, Morphewe, Lepri, Cancer, madnesse, hardnesse of the Splene. &c.
}

The signes of the sickenesse of Flegme.
{
- Sluggishnes, and dulnesse of memorie.
- Forgetfulnesse.
- Moche spittyng.
- Moche slepe.
- Paines in the hedde, specially in the hinder parte.
- Swellyng in the face and chekes.
- Euill digestion.
- White dropsie like in colour.
- Pacience with doltishnes, lacking liuely quicknes.
- Dreming of going naked, drouning, or of snowe. &c
- Of these cometh Quotidians, Dropsies, Pallsie, fallyng sickenesse, &c.
}

And to helpe all these, there are singuler good medicenes: bothe in the Simples, & chiefly in the compoundes. But yet brother Sicknesse, note *Hyppocrates*, the well & chief Tree, from whence the good order of Phisicke first did spring, whiche is a generall texte. Upon whose woordes *C. Galen. &c.* doe coment, and write at large, their great workes. He wrote one smal worke also called the *Aphorismes*, wherein is greate knowlege. But to our purpose. For this place of signes dedly, marke what he saieth in some of those *Apho. and Præno.*

Whosoeuer beyng an healthfull bodie, is sodain pained, and quickly after, haue loste his voice, and starteth with all: he shall dye with in seuen daies, next followyng after. It is not onely through the inflamacion of the spirites: but also by the vniuersall matter, drawen into the braine, from the stomake. &c. *Quicunque sani dolore capitis repēte. &c Apho. Hyppo.*

If one be a mased, and fall into idle talke: of the pricke into the hed, it is dedly. *Ex capitis ictu. &c. Aphori. vi.*

A conuulcion, shrinkyng, or crampe in the senewes, after a purgacion, is veric perilous, or dedly.

A conuulcion, after the takyng of *Elleborus* is dedly. *Conuulsio a veratro letha lis est Aphor*

A conuulcion after a wounde, is dedly.

D.ii. Who

The booke of the vse

Who so is dredfull or beaule in a franſie, the ſigne is dedly.

Conſiderare vero conuenit etiam oculoriū præno. Hypp. Capi. 4.

It behoueth the Phiſicion, to conſider the iyes of his pacient, whē he ſlepeth: if there appere any white thyng, betwene the iye liddes. If he haue had no laxe, nor receiued any pocion to purge before: it is a ſigne verie terrible, and preſent death.

To be deafe in a lōg feuer, if the body be weake: it is a tokē of death.

It is an euill ſigne, whē one haue a crampe, in bledyng at his noſe, or els ſwouneth withall.

A ſtoppyng in the throte, or ſuffocacion fallyng to one, which haue a feuer, and a ſwellyng in the throte, is a perilous deadly token.

Who ſo in Agewe, can neither tourne his necke, nor ſwallowe his owne ſpattle, death is at hande.

Si ebrius quiſpiam repente obmutuerit. Aphor. pars. j. vij.

If a drunkarde doe ſodainly loſe his ſpeache, he ſhall ſodainly dye of a crampe, or conuulſion: vnleſſe he fall into an Agew, or els receiue power to ſpeake again, when he haue digeſted the ſurfette.

Thei whiche be ſwelled in the backe, before thei come to age of. xiii yers: if it chaunſe of the ſhortneſſe of breath, or els a very ſtrong cough ſhall ſone dye.

A volentarie laxe, comyng after a pleuricie, or the ſickeneſſe of lunges, is a dedly token.

Who ſo in the emptie place in the ſtomacke, haue foule rotten matter, or els the dropſie: if thei be either ſo cutte, or burned, whereby all the water runneth forthe, ſurely it is preſent death.

Who ſo haue his ſpattle ſtinke, when it is burnte vpon the coales, and alſo if his heare doe eaſely fall from his hed, it is a ſigne of death.

A laxe or greate cough, with ſpittyng filthie matter, is dedly.

Who ſo often tymes are weakened, and loſe their ſtrength, without ſome manifeſte cauſe, ſhall haue ſodain death.

Mulieri grauidæ ſi mumma. &c. Apho. pars. 3. x.

When a womans breaſt dooe deminiſhe, beyng with childe: it ſignifieth the childe is dedde.

To be diſcontent in the tyme of ſickeneſſe, when thynges are giuen in medicen, is an euill token, for the contrary is good.

Inquibus morbo mente &c Apho. pars. 31

In euery ſickneſſe, if Melancholy, or blacke choler, be either purged vpward, or dounward, without medicen, it is bothe perilous, & dedly.

Who ſo euer bee Splenetike, and haue a bloodie flixe, if it long continue: then thei fall to the dropſie, or els their foode ſhall pas through their guttes, not digeſted: this is a dedly ſigne.

Quibus hepar aqua plenum Apho. pars. iij. vij.

Who ſo euer haue their liuer repleted, or filled full with water: and if the ſame water breake dounward to the bellie, it is preſent death.

Quibus in febribus mors bus regius & Apho pars. 5. xxxv.

Who ſo in hot feuers, bee taken with the yellowe Jaunders, in the ſeuēth. ix. xi. or the. xiii. date, it is good: ſo that his right ſide waxe not harde: but if theſe daies want, and the ſide waxe hard, it is dedly.

A wounde in the braine, harte, diaphragm, or midriffe, ſmale guttes, ſtomacke, and liuer, is euer death.

If the yelowe Jaunders cometh before the. vii. date, it is perilous.

In laxes, blacke ſtooles are euill: except purgacions cauſeth it.

To

of sicke men and medicines. Fol.lxxxj.

To haue any Melancholi stoole, in the beginnyng of any sicknesse: it is a signe dedly.

So is a bloodie flixe, beginnyng with a Melancholi sicknes, little peces of fleshe, apperyng in a bloodie flixe, present death.

If a woman with childe be sodainly taken, with any greuous sicknesse, present death.

It is perilous for a woman with childe, to haue a greate laxe. *mulierē vtero gerentem. & Apho pars.3.*

A woman with child, if she be letten blood, it kill her childe: the nerer the birthe, the greater perill.

A woman hauyng crampe or conuulcion, in the temperate tyme of her termes, is perilous.

He whiche haue an ague, beyng taken with conuulcion, is in danger: who so haue conuulcion before his feuer, is in no soche perill.

Feuers, whiche doe not giue ouer the third daie, are perilous. *Of Feuers.*

In a long ague we, if the outwarde members are very colde: and the inward partes hotte and drie, death at hande.

In a long feuer, when the lippes, nose, or mouth, be drawen a wrie or disgrased: so that the pacient can neither se or heare, and is in weakenesse, death at hande.

If any hauyng an ague we, sweate in these daies, it is good, if not, it is perilous. ii. v. vii. ix. xi. xiiii. xvii. xxi. xxvii. xxxiiii. *Of Sweate.*

Who so haue the pestilence, and bledeth not, before twelue howers, or slepeth eight howers after bledyng, death at hande.

Colde sweate with a sharpe Feuer, signifie death.

If the face of a sicke manne, be changed from the healthfull estate, with a sharpe nose, hollowe iyen, writhen temples, colde eares: contracted in the extreme partes, like a leafe when it dye, harde skinne in the forehed, and drie, pale fased, little or no slepe. Bityng or trembling of the lippes. &c. These are signes of death, saieth *Hyppocra.in libro primo præ no.capit.ij.* beginnyng at *Considerare porro hoc modo conuenit in morbis acutis &c.* *The signes of death by the face.*

If the pacient can not abide the light of Sunne, fire, or candle, but flie the same, or wepe inuoluntarily, without cause: or make one iye appere lesser then the other, or goggle with theim, lookyng moche a squinte. Except the iyes were so in health, or els haue the whites turned into bloodie redde: or haue darcke or blacke small baines in them, with vnstablenesse, and concaue holownes. Or open in the slepe, with the nether lippe hangyng doune, and the vpper lippe drawen vp. &c. Surely death is at hande *Hyppoc.prono.* *The signes of death by the iyen.*

Feele also the pacient, when he lieth in his bedde, his armes, sides, necke, breaste, and legges, whither the partes be pained, or flexable or haue loste their strength, and are stiffe, if he lye vpward: except it were his olde custome, and shrinke to the beddes feete, with castyng abrode the handes and feete: slepyng with a wide open mouthe, and couet to lye naked, death, death, and the graue at hande. *Hyppocra prono.* *The signes of death by lying in the bed*

If the pacient lye in his sickenesse, vpon his bellie, excepte custome moue it, and so doe slepe: it signifie a greate sickenesse in the breaste, or

O.iii. bellie.

bellie. Or els to be madde, and lose his wittes, through the malignitie of the spirites: and to sitte vpon their buttockes, in their sickenesse, of a sharpe sicknes, it signifieth the perill of death, or greate inflamacion in the lunges. As *Hyppocrates* saith in the *Præ. Capi. vij. at in ventrem decumbere. &c.*

Signes of death by the tethe.
To gnashe or grinde the teeth in feuers, is either a greate veracion of the minde, or madnesse at hande, or els death: For it is an affeccion of the senewes. Notwithstandyng young childzen, tormented with wormes, are not in this peril alwaies, when thei doe gnashe the teth.

Signes dedly by woundes.
In a stroke of a depe wounde, when conuulcion followeth: and no matter, or corrupcion come to the wounde sone after, if the bodie bee pale and swarte in colour, and drie with weakenes of digestion, death approcheth. And this affirmeth *Hyppocra. de signis ex vlcere Cap. viij.*

Signes dedly by the handes.
Who so in a sharpe Feuer, sicknesse of the lunges, frensie, or paines of the hedde: doe writhe the hande to his nose or face, as though he would kill Flees or Flies, or knitte a knotte, or brushe his clothes. Or els pulle vp Rushes, this is a presente signe of death, saieth *Hyppocra. lib. primo. præ Capi. ix. de gestaculo manuum.*

Signes dedly by the breath.
Shortnesse of breath, and of little forse, doe signifie greate dolour: inflamacion and madnesse, cometh of greate breathyng, like a Bulle, or a wilde beast. Cold breath, with the coldnes of the nose and mouth, death draweth nere, with fare well vain world, with fleshe, and blood Rede *Hyppocrates præ. vbi inquit spiritus densus dolorem significat. &c.*

Signes dedly by sweate.
Sweates are beste in sharpe Feuers, in the daies of their decrees, or iudgementes: but the contrary are perilous. As when sweate is cold, specially in a sharpe feuer, death approche: for colde sweate, cometh from grosse matter, without the spirites of liuely warmnes. But if it bee but a meane leuke warme sweate, called a fainte sweate: then it doe signifie a long sicknesse.

Signes dedly by swellig.
If the breast be swelled with throbbyng, beatyng, or trouble in the breast, or the vpper parte of the same: and therewith vnstable, fearfull iyen, vtter madnesse, or death dooe approche. But bledyng at the nose will helpe it, specially in young persones: but hardnesse in those partes, dolour, and swellyng, is death.

Signes dedly by spattle.
Spattle when one spittes, beyng white, light, and swetishe, not variable in colour, and also very easie drawne forthe, is good: but if it be sweatie filthe with matter, or blacke and stinkyng, with yelownes, grenesse, or blacknes. &c. Filthe is called *pus a putredine,* and perill of death. And that whiche is good, is of the benefite of the blood: and goodnesse of digestion, and the goodnesse of flegme and blood.

It is perilous, not to neese, in the tyme of sicknesse: but to neese vehemently, is perilous also.

Water, as dropsie betwene the skinne and the fleshe, commyng of a sharpe feuer, is euer perilous and euill in this case: when the nailes appere darke and pale, and the priuie members and stones doe swelle, it is a greate token of death. Reade of this, *Hyppocrates in libro secundo præno. De aqua inter cutem.*

of sicke men and medicenes.

Who so doe wake long, and can not slepe, either a greate sicknesse do approche, or els madnesse, throughout inflamacion. Who so breake his slepe of his commō custome, and fall into moche wakyng in the night, this is an euill signe, and goeth before a perilous euill. *Somnus atque vigilia. &c. Apho Hyppo.*

In all sickenesses hardnesse of the beallie, or costiffenes, vile stinke, blacke stooles, or bloodie fluxes, are verie perilous, but breakyng of windie dounward, at the stoole is good.

To vomette white flegme, not very grosse or yellowe, is good: but muddie darcke, or blacke, it is perilous. But to vomet sondrie colours of eche sorte, it is moste perilous, and dedly.

To be vnnaturall drie, with a feuer, hedache, shortnesse of breathe, moche swete spattle, high coloured, greate vaines, prickyng in the side it is the signes of the perilous Pleuricie, and death, excepte digestion and blood lettyng. Of blood lettyng, I haue spoken in place: and thus I doe ende, because tyme is so passed, or els I would haue spoken more of the Crises, or Iudgement, and of pulse and vrine, with a regiment, against the sweate, and the fearfull plague called Pestilence: whiche I praie GOD deliuer vs from. I praie thee take all my talke in good parte: and thus I commende thee, to the liuyng God, that haue made bothe heauen and yearth, to helpe and preserue thee, with his healthfull medicenes, and good defence againste all sickenesse, sornesse, and woundes. Contained within my little Bulwarke. *The signes of a pleuricie*

Sicknes.

I Moste hartely thanke thee, gentle Health, GOD bryng it so to passe: and graunt vs after this life, a blessed estate euerlastyng, where as is no miserie and wretchednesse. But happinesse, and perpetuall blessednesse, with Christ our God. Amen.

*The ende of the Dialogue, betwene Health
and Sicknes. By William Bulleyn.
Marcij. Anno salutis. 1562.*

*Though our giftes be neuer so small,
Yet let vs giue thankes to God for all:
And who of talentes, haue greate store,
Their accomptes to God shalbe the more.*
w.B.

The index of the booke

A.

A Good Kichen, is a good Apothicaries shop. Fol. xlix.
A pocion muste bee giuen at three sonderie tymes, to remoue and expulse matter from the stomacke Idem.
A caueat to beware. Idem.
An example betwene a Simple and a compounde medicen. lii.
Acab did kill Naboth for his vineyarde liiii.
A cauiat for Sommer lix.
A Clister to molefie the bellie, in the tyme of daunger lxii.
A good note to be obserued, when nature is weake Idem.
A plaster for the flixe lxiii.
A consideraciō in eating and drinking to be had, and of the varietie of meates Idem.
A cause why the soule departeth from the bodie Idem.
A good rule to be obserued lxiiii.
An order for the dietyng of soch as be sicke of sharpe feuers Idem.
As the cōplexion is, so man requireth his fode in ye time of health thynges like to his nature, but in sicknes the contrary lxv.
Aires are to bee obserued in sickenesses, as in health. lxvi.
A signe of digestion Idem.
An example of brute beastes. lxvii
An hickop after a bomitte in perilous Idem.
A goodly waie to helpe the hickop after a bomette Idem.
An expulse for an idle loute. lxviii
A good reward for diligēt labor. id
All the workes vnder the Sonne, are nothyng but vanitie, and affliccion to the mynde. Idem.
Athanasius feare
A shift for fresh water souldiors. 73
A lesson against anger Idem.
A wrathfull wretch in battail. idē
A wrathfull part of Alexander, in killyng of Clitus. Idem.
A noble woman wepte to death, for the death of her husband idē
Ariadne fledde awaie for Theseus sake, forsakyng her father land. Folio lxxvi
A pleasaunt death lxxvii
Adam began our plagues. lxxviii.

B.

Beware of dryīng medicens in sōmer for cholericke persons. xlix.
Boxing is good for a lubber. lxviii
Boxing doeth drawe foorthe euill humour. Idem.
Boxyng dooe stoppe the termes, when thei doe abounde Idem
Bothe God and Nature abhorre ingratfulnes lxxb.

C.

Compounded humour may not be purged with simple medicene, for thei are to weake Fol. lii.
Cowe, Shepe, and Plowe bee our nurses lvi.
Colde doeth take, & is not takē. 58.
Choler is sone drie, therfore purge but little, but the fleshely bodie hath moche moisture, therfore purge more. lx.
Colde medicenes to the whole, but warme to the sicke must bee giuen Idem.
Certain causes, which letteth medicen to worke lxii
Corrupte aires, bringeth sonderie diseases lxv.
Cholericke persones must not fast moche lxix.
Christ giueth all comfort. lxxviii.
Cleopatras death lxxiiii.

D.

Dreames do admonishe menne, to feare God Fol. liii.

Death

of Sicknes and Health.

Death is the ende of life. Fol. lxiii.
Drunkardes what thei doe   lxix.
Didos death   lxxiiii
Diagoras Rhodius did expire the breath of life, for sodain ioy. 77.
Deoclesian slue hymself.   lxxviii.

E.

Elleborus albus, the poison therof xlviii.
Example of waxe and fire.   lxii.
Extremes be perilous thinges. idē
Extreme heate & cold be euil lxiii.
Exercise before meate   lxvi.
Equitacion is verie wholsom idē.
Examples of sodain feare   lxxii.
Euill parentes, & euill childrē. idē.
Example of Marcellus.   Idem.
Examples of wrath in Nero. lxxiii
Example of sodain ioie.   lxxvi.
Example of Saul, whiche died in desperacion.   lxxviii.
Example against desperacion. idē.

F.

Fower thinges considered, attraccion, dissoluyng   Fol. xlviii.
Feruente praier vnto God, dooeth mittigate his wrath.   lxvi.
Feare is like a monster of hel. lxxii
Feare in Christ.   Idem.
Feare in sainct Peter   Idem.
Feare of the Christians   Idem.
Feare maketh men offer to Idolles   Idem.
Fooles bee afraied of the Mare in their slepe   lxx.
Feare bringeth desperacion. example of Judas   lxxiii.

G.

Good coūsaile in the tyme of trouble.   lb.
God the very Philicion   lxvii.
God dooe woorke by miracle, and meanes.   lxiiii.
Gods vengeaunce.   lxxii.
Good intentes, and good actes bee twoo thinges   lxii.

Gratitude of dombe beastes. lxxv.

H.

How to prepare medicen   Fol. l.
How to knowe what humour doe abound by his proper token.   li.
He whiche loueth God, shall haue hartes reste   lxiii.
How to knowe, whether Choller be purged or no   lxi.
How to quicken the stomacke lxiii
How to prouoke vomet, and how to staie it   lxviii.
How the stomacke muste be prepared toward slepe.   lxix.
How to auoide euill dreames. lxx.
Hyppocrates vpon slepes   Idem.
How a gelous foole begiled hymself   lxxv.

I.

Jhon Preston, called Jhō of stoneham.   Fol. xlix.
It helpeth moche to Nature, to prouoke vrine   li.
Ignoraunt Barbours, their fruites   lii.
In Adam, we haue our fall. liiii.
Infidelles haue singuler giftes of God.   lvii.
In *Elleborus* you shall knowe how to correct thesame.   lxii.
Idlenes the mother of mischif. 66.
Idlenesse bringeth mischief to the bodie & soule, and pouertie lxvii
It is not good to bee trimmed of the Barbour at night, but in the mornyng   Idem.
In this life we haue our purgatorie, and that we feele and perceiue   liiii.
Jelousie is cosin germain to frensie: marke the fruites therof. 74.
Jelousie causeth adulterie.   lxxv.
Ingratitude or vnkindenes called churlishenes   Idem.
Ingratitude haue killed many a man

manne lxxbi.
Iuuencius the Consul, died sodainly for ioye. lxxbii.

K.

Kynges and Quenes be subiect to the miseries of this worlde, and haue no perfite felicitie, before their mortalle ende, and beginnyng of immortall life. liiii.

L.

Like as heate cōsumeth snow, euē so doeth Phisicke money. Fol. xlix
Lurkyng humours how to finde them, and expulse them l.
Let no man be angrie, with an other mannes follie lviii
Little trauell for the sicke lxvi.
Loue is a conquerour lxxiiii.
Loue maketh beastly fooles. idem
Lucretius lxxbiii.

M.

Mēs natures must be obserued, a little medicen wil worke moche of sum mē, ẽ a strōg medicen wil scāt worke on some other mē 49.
Methodici be Phisiciās, that obserue certain rules by art l.
Medicenes solutiue, why thei are giuen Idem.
Melancholi the worste humour of Nature, begat a sonne called the quarten lii.
Matter in the vaines, must be let out by blood lettyng, and in the bealli byglister, in ẽ brest by vomet. liii.
Mannes life is both short and miserable lriii.
Midicene doe chaunge, and meate is chaunged lb.
Medicenes for feble stomackes, to purge gentelly lviii.
Men, women, and children, muste take medicenes, accordyng to their strength and age. lix.
Moche humor must bee purged by little & little, and not at ones lx.
Moche watche causeth rawe humours in the stomacke.
Moderate walke after meate profiteth lrb.
Moderate exercise is a suffraine thyng. lrbi.
Men doe dreme, accordyng to their temperament or complexion 54.

N.

Nature hath many hidden desires vnknowen to the Phisiciō.lviii
Nature hath prepared, ẽ one creature dredeth & fereth an other lx
Note, whiche is the most wholesome aire to dwell in lrb.
Nesyng doe helpe women in their trauell lrbii.
No man or beast, can liue without slepe. Fol.lrix.

O.

Of swete fleume. Fol. li.
Obseruacions in blood letting. lii
Of the tyme of medicene lb.
One maie slepe after pilles, but yet beware of old pilles. Idem.
Of the quantitie of matter to bee purged lx.
Of ouermoche purgyng the bodie, the remedie to help the same lxi.
Of Sirupes and drinckes lrb.
Of fricacion the vertue therof. 67.
Of nesing, the profit therof. lrbiii.
Of sweates profitable and vnprofitable to a common welth. idē
Of twoo kinde of sweates, naturall, and artificiall Idem
Of good and badde slepe lrx.
Of the sodaine alteracion of the mynde, from ioye to care. lrxii.
Of feare, what it is Idem.
Of heate artificiall, & natural. 73.
Of cholorike heate Idem
Of sodain ioye lrxbi.

P.

Propertie

of Sicknes and Health.

Propertie & place must be obserued   xlix.
Preparatiue must be firste giuen, and then purgacion.   Fol. l.
Purge that whiche should be purged, or els medell not   li.
Purgers of flegme   Idem.
Purge vpwarde in Sommer, and dounward in Winter.   liii.
Place where medicene should bee ministred, conueniently ioyned with tyme   Idem.
Prosperitie is verie slippery.   liiii.
Pilles maie be made of all kind of medicenes.   lvi.
Poore menne bee exalted through vertue   lvii.
Purge flegme more then choller, & melācholi more then flegme.   lx.
Phisiciōs ought to haue a perfect knowlege of the nature of places and aire   lxv.
Pleasaunt people thei are   lxvi.
Pore is clensed by sweate   lxviii.
Pleasure is noisome to the disquiet harte.   lxxi.
Procris did seke her owne death, through ielousie   lxxv.

S.
Scamonie is perilous, except it be well prepared, & do kil many.   l.
Signes manifest, declaryng what humors beareth y greatest rule in the bodies of men & women, without whiche it is not possible to purge accordyng to arte, but rather to kill.   li.
Signes to knowe whē melancholi approche, after whom cometh the quarten   Idem.
Sorow is for things past, & fear is for thynges to come   liiii.
Sodain gotten substance remain not long   lviii.
Signes of death, through purging of the bodie   lxii.

Short sicknesse, thin brothe, long sicknes thicke brothe   lxv.
Swete aire to bee made in y tyme of sicknes with perfumes.   lxvi.
Signes of death by the teth.   lxxxi.
Signes dedly by woundes.   Idem.
Signes dedly by the handes.   Idē.
Signes dedly by the breath.   idem.
Signes dedly by sweate.   Idem.
Signes dedly by swelling.   Idem.
Signes dedly by spattle.   Idem.

T.
The fruite of rashe ministracion of medicenes   Fol. xlix.
The vertue of bitter medicens bee greate   Idem.
The cause of sicknesses   l.
The chief signe of digestion.   Idem
That humour whiche doe abound purge thesame   li.
The Manna of Calabria is y best in the world, & falleth in the night as dewe vpō flowers & leues.   idē
The fire wil get the victorie, if the water be not equal, or haue the maisterie   lii.
To knowe when medicene haue wrought their effect   Idem
The humour region, are chieflie to be considered   liii.
The daie natural, and the daie artificiall.   Idem.
The fower complexions raigning euery one sixe howers.   Idem.
The aged, the very young weake folke, and women with childe, maie not be let blood   Idem.
The hope of the life to come.   liiii.
The soule neuer slepeth   Idem
The troubles of the minde be greater then y crosses of the body.   idē
The obseruacion of complexiōs   56
To giue medicene in the fit of a feuer, is perilous.   Idem.
The life of the plain people in the countrey   Idem.

is

The ende of wicked men. Fol.lvij.
The goute loueth riche men, but is afraied of poore folkes. lxi.
To coole the mouthe. Idem.
The causes why medicēs worke immo. lxiij
Tenasmus what it is, & how to uelpe it. id̄
The erth is mother of euery liuīg thing. id.
To feede of diuers sortes of meates, corrupteth the bodie. lxiiij.
To eate bothe fishe and fleshe together, hurteth the flegmaticke bodie. Idem.
The Melancholie. Idem.
The Sanguine. Idem.
The practise of idle people. lxvij.
The Heathē ar better, thā many chrīstiās. i.
Thre thinges to be obserued in fricaciōs. id.
The cause of vomete, and when it helpeth and when it hurteth. Idem.
To helpe the hickop Idem.
Lucke, and Raper. lxvij.
The Carter do daily helpe the Curtier. id̄
The greate goodnesse of fastyng, bothe for the soule and bodie lxix.
The rich vse glotony, & ȳ poore penurie. idē
The vertue or benefite of slepe or rest. idem
The cause why a drūkard du die sodaily. 70
To whom watche is good Idem.
The afflicciōs of the minde, is harde to be helped. Idem.
The ix. heauenly Muses, can smally cōforte some carefull hart, when it is in care. idē
The sacred gifte that the nine heauenlie Muses haue, and cāh giue to others whē thei be in trouble. Idem.
The names of the nine Muses, with their giftes. lxxj.
The perturbacion or sodaine mocion of the minde, must be well obserued. Idem.
The telousie of Antiopa. lxxv.
The treason of Judas, that moste ingratefull villain, his exāple to all churles. idē.
To knowe a very gentleman. Idem.
The shamfull ingratitude of Theseus, the sonne of Ageus, the kyng of Athenes. idē
The Monster of the Labyrinthe lxxvi.
The greate grief and lamentacion of Theseus, when he was in prison. Idem.
The noble pitifull ladie Ariadne, did comforte the miserable Theseus, & set hym at libertie. Fol.lxxvi.
The craftie treason of false Theseus. idem.
The death of Ariadne. Idem.
The death of Otho for care. lxxvij.
The wisedome of Deonise the tyraunte, in aduersitie. Idem.
The kyng of Bohem, what he did in the tyme of pouertie. Idem.
The ende of men in desperacion. Idem.
The ende of Sardanapalus. Idem.
The death of Judas. lxxvij.
The death of Brutus. Idem.
To dye in desperacion, is to renounce saluacion. Idem.
The pacience of Job. Idem.
The best regiment of life. Idem.
The cause of the night. lxxix.
The signes of death by the face. lxxxj.
The signes of death by the iyen. Idem.
The signes of death by lyīg in the bed. idē
The signes of a pleuricie. lxxxij.

V.

Vse make the labour easse. lxvi.
Uomet helpeth the fire. lxvij.

W.

Whē purging medicens ar giuen, first minister herbes & drink to prouoke vrīn. xlix
When one descende vnto hymself, he shall beholde fearfull thynges. liij.
Wicked spirites, to molest our spirites. idē
What thing is best for mankinde. lv.
Why purgacion worke not naturally. idē.
Weake stomackes, can not awaie with strong medicenes. lvi.
What harme winde doeth in a feuer, or after purgyng. lxij.
When the pacient is in perill, the remedie to helpe hym. Idem.
What kindes of meates doe cause good bloed lxiij.
What hurt cometh of an emptie stomacke, when ye go to bedde. Idem.
What aires corrupteth the blood. lxv.
What situacion is beste for a house lxvi.
What profite cometh by excercise. Idem.
When to vse rubbyng, or fricacion, and wherefore. lxvij.
When to trauaile or plaie. Idem.
What persones maie beste vomet. Idem.
Who maie worst vomet. Idem.
When to vomet. Idem.
When it is good to blede. Idem.
Who must not blede. Idem.
Who ought to sweate, and who not. Idem
When sweate is not good. lxix.
When slepe is perilous. Idem.
What dreames doe signifie. lxx.
What spirite gelousie is. lxxv.
Who must help vs in ȳ time of trouble. 78.
What mischief doe chaunce to the whole bodie, for want of vnitie. lxxix.

FINIS.